# Orthopedic Taping, Wrapping, Bracing, & Padding

**4th**


**Joel W Beam** EdD, LAT, ATC

Professor and Chair
Department of Clinical & Applied Movement Sciences
Brooks College of Health
University of North Florida


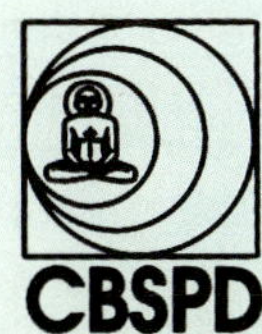

CBSPD


**CBS Publishers & Distributors** Pvt Ltd

New Delhi • Bengaluru • Chennai • Kochi • Kolkata • Lucknow • Mumbai
Hyderabad • Jharkhand • Nagpur • Patna • Pune • Uttarakhand

Original American edition published by:

FA Davis Company, 1915 Arch Street, Philadelphia, PA 19103, USA



Last digit indicates print number: 10 9 8 7 6 5 4 3 2 1

As new scientific information becomes available through basic and clinical research, recommended treatments and drug therapies undergo changes. The author(s) and publisher have done everything possible to make this book accurate, up to date, and in accord with accepted standards at the time of publication. The author(s), editors, and publisher are not responsible for errors or omissions or for consequences from application of the book, and make no warranty, expressed or implied, in regard to the contents of the book. Any practice described in this book should be applied by the reader in accordance with professional standards of care used in regard to the unique circumstances that may apply in each situation. The reader is advised always to check product information (package inserts) for changes and new information regarding dose and contraindications before administering any drug. Caution is especially urged when using new or infrequently ordered drugs.

**Library of Congress Cataloging-in-Publication Data**"

Names: Beam, Joel W, 1963–author.

"Title: Orthopedic taping, wrapping, bracing & padding/Joel W. Beam.

Other titles: Orthopedic taping, wrapping, bracing, and padding

Description: Fourth edition. | Philadelphia, PA : FA Davis Company, [2021] | Includes bibliographical references and index."

Identifiers: LCCN 2020034788 (print) | LCCN 2020034789 (ebook) |

ISBN 9781719640671 (paperback) | ISBN 9781719640688 (ebook)

Subjects: MESH: Athletic Injuries—therapy | Athletic Injuries—prevention

DDC 617.1/027–dc23

LC record available at https://lccn.loc.gov/2020034788

LC ebook record available at https://lccn.loc.gov/2020034789



**This edition is authorized for sale only in India.**

Published in India by CBS Publishers and Distributors Pvt Ltd under arrangement with FA Davis Company

**ISBN:** 978-93-48385-00-0

**CBS Edition: 2025**

Published by **Satish Kumar Jain** and produced by **Varun Jain** for

## CBS Publishers & Distributors Pvt Ltd

4819/XI Prahlad Street, 24 Ansari Road, Daryaganj, New Delhi 110 002, India

Ph: 011-23289259, 23266838          Website: www.cbspd.com          e-mail: delhi@cbspd.com

*Corporate Office:* 204 FIE, Industrial Area, Patparganj, Delhi 110 092, India

Ph: 011-49344934          Fax: 011-49344935

e-mail: publishing@cbspd.com; publicity@cbspd.com

*Branches*

- Bengaluru: Seema House 2975, 17th Cross, KR Road, Banasankari 2nd Stage, Bengaluru 560 070, Karnataka, India
  Ph: +91-80-26771678/79          Fax: +91-80-26771680          e-mail: bangalore@cbspd.com
- Chennai: No.18/8B, Subbarayan Street, Shenoy Nagar, Chennai 600 030, Tamil Nadu, India
  Ph: +91-44-42032115, 26681266          e-mail: chennai@cbspd.com
- Kochi: 42/1325, 1326, Power House Road, Opposite KSEB, Power House, Ernakulum 682018, Kochi, Kerala, India
  Ph: +91-484-4059061–67          Fax: +91-484-4059065          e-mail: kochi@cbspd.com
- Kolkata: 147, Hind Ceramics Compound, 1st Floor, Nilgunj Road, Belghoria, Kolkata 700056, West Bengal, India
  Ph: +91-33-25330055/56          e-mail: kolkata@cbspd.com
- Lucknow: Basement, Khushuma Complex, 7 Meerabai Marg (behind Jawahar Bhawan), Lucknow 226001, UP, India
  Ph: +91-522-4000032          e-mail: tiwari.lucknow@cbspd.com
- Mumbai: PWD Shed, Gala No. 25/26, Ramchandra Bhatt Marg, Next JJ Hospital Gate No. 2, Opp. Union Bank of India, Noorbaug, Mumbai 400009, Maharashtra, India
  Ph: +91-22-66661880/89          e-mail: mumbai@cbspd.com

*Representatives*

- Hyderabad   0-9885175004
- Jharkhand   0-9811541605
- Nagpur   0-8692091830
- Patna   0-9334159340
- Pune   0-9664372571
- Uttarakhand   0-9716462459

*Printed at* Nutech Print Services, Faridabad, Haryana, India

# Dedication

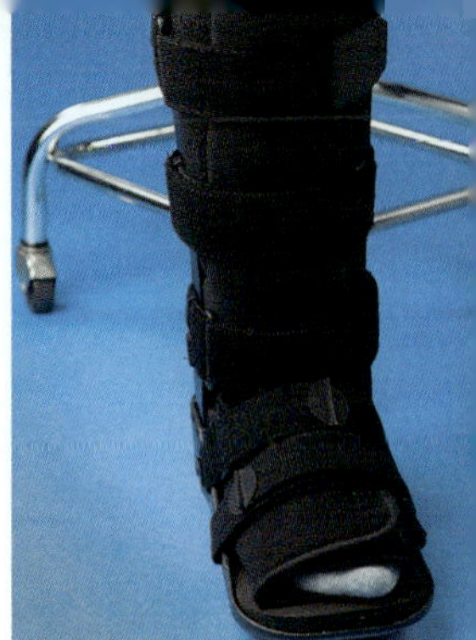

*To family, colleagues, and students—I thank you.*

# Acknowledgments

*There are many people whom I wish to thank for their time and willingness to assist in this fourth edition. At F.A. Davis, Quincy McDonald and Julie Chase provided assistance for the revisions. The photographs were made possible through the expertise of Jason Torres. His dedication to his craft will benefit each athletic training student and professional who uses the text. The student models, Michelle Charko, Marshay Greenlee, Dan James, Kara Janokowski, Courtney Schnorr, Jim Sommers, Daniel Buckley, and Jerry Buckley demonstrated patience and adaptability to create a successful photo shoot. Bernadette Buckley, PhD, LAT, ATC, provided her instructional expertise to guide the development of the instructor materials and contributed to the revisions of each chapter. Cassie Ettel conducted the literature searches for the revisions of the evidence summaries. Michelle Boling, PhD, LAT, ATC, assisted with several areas of the text and provided another viewpoint. During the writing of this book, many health care professionals served as chapter reviewers. I would like to thank each of them for their time and expertise. Their suggestions helped to strengthen the text.*

*A project such as this is not possible without the assistance of numerous manufacturers and others associated with taping, wrapping, bracing, and padding products. I want to thank the following manufacturers and people.*

Johnson & Johnson

3M

BSN Medical

Active Ankle

Sports Health

Henry Schein

Breg

DJO

Med Spec

Ultra Ankle

Douglas Protective Equipment

Pro-Gear

Hartmann

Andover Healthcare

Kinesio Taping Association International

Kinesio University

University of North Florida

Jacksonville University

Jacksonville Orthopaedic Institute

Episcopal High School

Hausmann Industries

Dr. Richard Salko

Western Michigan University

Stone Ridge School of the Sacred Heart

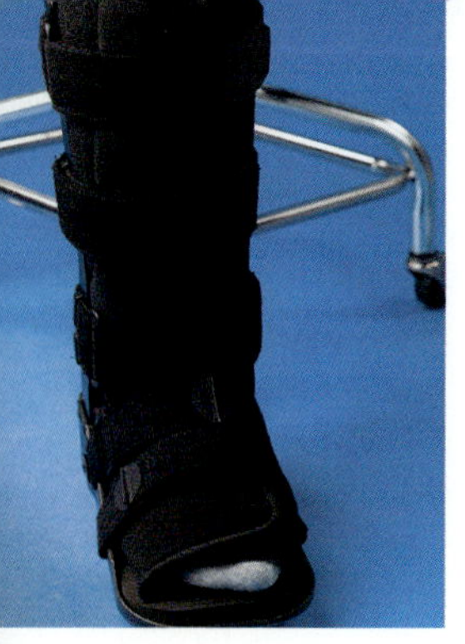

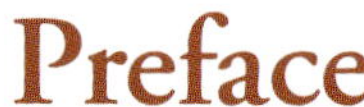

# Preface

The fourth edition of *Orthopedic Taping, Wrapping, Bracing, & Padding* continues the comprehensive presentation of taping, wrapping, bracing, and padding techniques. As the educational content of programs and profession of athletic training continue to evolve, updates and revisions were made throughout the text to provide the reader, instructor, and clinician a framework for clinical decision-making in the prevention, treatment, and rehabilitation of injuries and conditions. New clinically relevant research from the literature focusing on taping, wrapping, bracing, and padding techniques was incorporated into evidence summary boxes to provide the best available evidence for technique efficacy. New brace designs and steps of application replaced old techniques to reflect current clinical practice. Revisions to NCAA and NFHS mandatory protective equipment and standards and testing procedures highlight changes made among agencies and organizations to enhance protection for wearers from injury. Updated web references and further reading sections provide additional resources for the reader, instructor, and clinician.

The overall goal of *Orthopedic Taping, Wrapping, Bracing, & Padding* is to facilitate learning of the knowledge, skills, and clinical abilities required to effectively tape, wrap, brace, and pad patients. The book is intended for professional athletic training students, practicing athletic trainers, and other health care professionals responsible for technique application. Among students, the text is designed to first be used in the didactic setting, then taken to the clinical setting for practice and skill development. The all-inclusive, step-by-step technique focus of the text requires that students possess a general knowledge of anatomy, biomechanics, injury evaluation, treatment, and rehabilitation. This general knowledge can be obtained through either prerequisite or concurrent courses in an Athletic Training program. Several steps in the process of evidence-based practice require research knowledge and skills; as such, students may require guidance from instructors and preceptors at times. The material in the text covers the Board of Certification's Practice Analysis and the Commission on Accreditation of Athletic Training Education Curricular Content Standards related to taping, wrapping, bracing, and padding. Among practicing athletic trainers and other health care professionals, the text can serve as a practical resource guide for evidence-based practice.

While much of the fourth edition remains the same as the third, key revisions, updates, and additions have been made to support the overall goal of the text. Chapter 1 introduces tapes, wraps, braces, and pads and includes types, objectives, and recommendations for application. A discussion on evidence-based medicine and evidence-based practice presents an overview and example of the five step process for implementation of tapes, wraps, braces, and pads into clinical practice. Chapter 2 provides information on current and long-range needs and structural considerations of the application area. Chapter 3 includes the foot and toes; Chapter 4, the ankle; Chapter 5, the lower leg; Chapter 6, the knee; Chapter 7, the thigh, hip, and pelvis; Chapter 8, the shoulder and upper arm; Chapter 9, the elbow and forearm; Chapter 10, the wrist; Chapter 11, the hand, fingers, and thumb; and Chapter 12, the thorax, abdomen, and spine. These chapters begin with a general review of injuries and conditions that are common to the body region(s). Next, the chapters present step-by-step taping, wrapping, bracing, and padding techniques used in the prevention, treatment, and rehabilitation of these injuries and conditions. Chapter 13 discusses liability issues, standards and testing, and construction and application of NCAA and NFHS mandatory and standard equipment and padding.

Revised and expanded pedagogical features are used throughout the text to enhance the material to assist the reader in developing the knowledge, skills, and clinical abilities to implement evidence-based medicine into practice.

## Injuries and Conditions

Chapters 3 through 12 contain a brief discussion of common injuries and conditions for the particular body region. This feature allows readers to further develop an understanding of the purpose of the technique for each injury and condition.

## Photographs and Line Drawings

Color photography in each chapter plays an integral role in the presentation and learning of the techniques. The photographs are arranged to provide the reader with visual representation of the specific instructions for each technique step. Color line drawings illustrate the basic anatomy of each body region to assist the reader in developing an understanding of the purpose and effect of each technique on bone and soft tissue. Pathophysiology line drawings and diagnostic imaging and injury photographs provide the reader with realistic and actual depictions of injuries and conditions to assist with transferring knowledge, skills, and abilities from the didactic setting to clinical practice.

## Key Words

Anatomical structures and positions, injuries and conditions, and important terms are boldfaced to assist readers in recognizing key words.

## Helpful Hints

Helpful hints, identified by the icon below, provide quick tips and other "tricks of the trade" to assist in technique application.

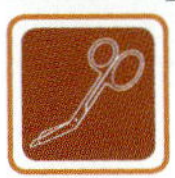

## Evidence Summary Boxes

Revised evidence summary boxes provide the available evidence from the literature on the efficacy of the techniques. The evidence can be integrated with student, instructor, and health care professional expertise and patient goals and values for the implementation of evidence-based practice.

## IF/THEN Boxes

IF/THEN boxes guide the student in choosing the most appropriate technique in a given situation.

## Details Boxes

Details boxes offer additional information on technique origin, construction, and application.

## Clinical Application Boxes

Clinical Application boxes are located throughout each chapter to allow the reader the opportunity to critically synthesize technique use and application. Answers to the questions are provided at FADavis.com. Instructors and preceptors can facilitate additional discussions with students to further expand the answers and incorporate evidence-based practice with actual clinical situations.

## Evidence-Based Practice

Evidence-based practice activities in each chapter present a clinical case within an actual injury prevention, treatment, and rehabilitation protocol to allow the reader the opportunity to select techniques using the five progressive steps of evidence-based practice. Instructors and preceptors can perform assessments of student performance with each step.

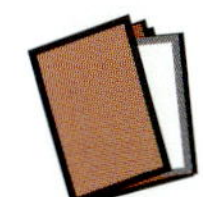

## Wrap-Up

The wrap-up summarizes the most important content of each chapter.

## Web References

Revised and updated web references provide resources for supplemental information on the prevention, treatment, and rehabilitation of injuries and conditions, online journals, surgical procedures, photographs, and other educational materials.

## Further Reading

Revised further reading provides additional information for in-depth examination of selected topics.

## References

Each chapter contains a list of cited references to give both the reader and instructor the opportunity to locate additional information and evidence.

## Glossary

Key words from each chapter are located at the end of the text.

## Index

The index allows for cross-referencing to locate specific techniques and information within the chapters.

## Kinesio® Taping Appendix

A Kinesio® Taping appendix presents an overview of the technique, physiological effects, strip types, general application instructions, and contraindications and precautions. Color photographs provide step-by-step instructions for seven Kinesio Taping techniques for upper and lower extremity injuries and conditions. An updated evidence summary provides the best available evidence from the literature on the effectiveness of the techniques.

## FADavis.com

Online resources are available to instructors and students at FADavis.com.

- FADavis.com resources, identified by the icon, are located throughout the chapters and contain additional taping, wrapping, bracing, and padding techniques with complete steps for application. A list of each chapter's techniques is located following the chapter Wrap-Up.
- Revised PowerPoint presentations are available for each chapter.

- A video containing 21 common taping, wrapping, bracing, and padding techniques is included. Individual techniques contained in the video are identified by the icon to the right throughout the chapters.
- The updated Instructor's Guide contains an image bank, revised test bank, class and clinical activities, syllabus, and lecture notes.
- Revised student review questions are available for each chapter.

I wrote this text to provide athletic training students and health care professionals multiple taping, wrapping, bracing, and padding techniques and alternatives. The best available research evidence, skill and experience levels of health care professionals, patient goals, values, injuries, and conditions, material availability, and facility budgets and sizes require a diverse set of strategies for the implementation of evidence-based medicine in the prevention, treatment, and rehabilitation of patients. I hope that after athletic training students and health care professionals have had the opportunity to read the text, both groups will develop the necessary knowledge, skills, and clinical abilities to effectively use the techniques in the prevention, treatment, and rehabilitation of injuries and conditions among patients. I would appreciate any ideas or suggestions for the improvement of this text in future editions. Please feel free to contact me with your suggestions through my publisher, F. A. Davis Company, or directly.

—JOEL W. BEAM

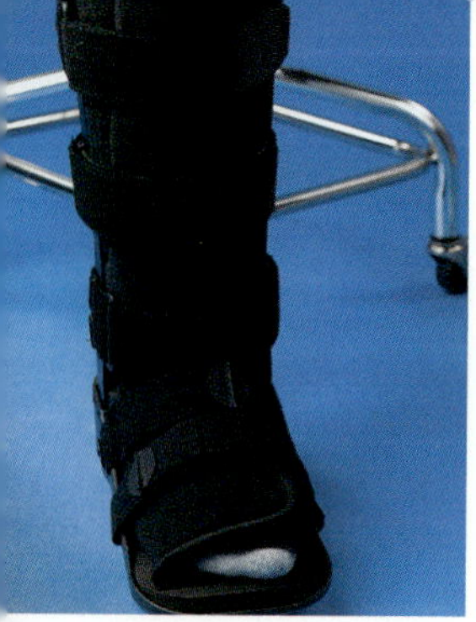

# Contents

# Part One

# Introduction

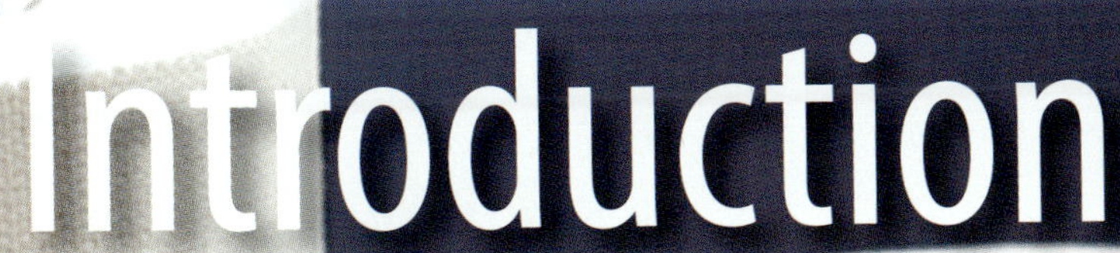

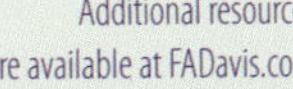

**ICON KEY**

| | |
|---|---|
| Helpful Hint | 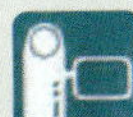 |
| Tape may be applied directionally from either left or right | |
| Additional resources are available at FADavis.com | 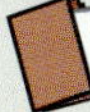 |
| A technique video is available at FADavis.com | |
| Evidence-Based Practice |  |
| Evidence Summary | |

# Tapes, Wraps, Braces, and Pads

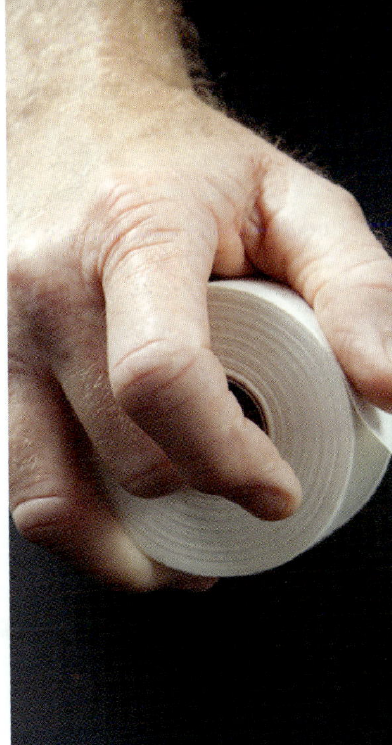



## LEARNING OBJECTIVES

1. Explain and demonstrate evidence-based practice and the process used to make clinical decisions for the implementation of taping, wrapping, bracing, and padding techniques into clinical practice.
2. Discuss and explain the types, objectives, and application recommendations for taping, wrapping, bracing, and padding techniques used when preventing, treating, and rehabilitating injuries.
3. Discuss and demonstrate the ability to select the appropriate types of tapes, wraps, braces, and pads used when preventing, treating, and rehabilitating various injuries.

Taping, wrapping, bracing, and padding techniques have been used for many years by health care professionals in the prevention, treatment, and rehabilitation of injuries. Athletic trainers, the health care professionals who typically apply the techniques, are skilled in technique application as a result of instruction and practice. For example, in a day, a typical athletic trainer (AT) may tape 20 ankles, wrap two hand contusions, apply three knee braces, and construct two protective pads. With appropriate didactic instruction in anatomy, biomechanics, injury evaluation, treatment, and rehabilitation, students can become proficient in the application of these techniques. In fact, practice may be the only hurdle to becoming proficient.

The application of taping, wrapping, bracing, and padding techniques should be implemented within the paradigm of evidence-based medicine (EBM). Evidence-based medicine is the integration of the best available research evidence with individual clinical expertise and patient goals, values, and preferences to make clinical decisions.[1] The evidence comes from patient-centered, clinically relevant research[2] on taping, wrapping, bracing, and padding interventions published in the scientific literature. Evidence is evaluated to determine its quality and value to day-to-day clinical practice. The evidence can support or refute previously accepted techniques or reveal new techniques that produce improved patient outcomes. Clinical expertise within EBM is the knowledge and proficiency in anatomy, biomechanics, injury evaluation, treatment, and rehabilitation, and taping, wrapping, bracing, and padding techniques. Clinical judgment is developed from clinical training, experience, and practice. Patient goals, values, and preferences are different among patients based on sport, occupation, lifestyle, and activity level. These must be identified and implemented into the practice of EBM.

The implementation of EBM into practice, or evidence-based practice (EBP), achieves several goals. EBP improves patient care, promotes critical thinking among clinicians, and advances the profession of athletic training.[2] EBP is a process of five progressive steps: (1) developing clinically relevant questions, (2) searching for the best evidence, (3) evaluating and appraising the evidence, (4) implementing the evidence into clinical practice with patients, and (5) evaluating the effects of interventions on patient outcomes.[1–3] Many of these steps require research training, knowledge, and skills;

"

large amounts of time; and financial and personnel resources to successfully complete. For a more detailed discussion of EBM and EBP, see the Further Reading section at the end of this chapter.

Clinical decision making and the prevention, treatment, and rehabilitation of injuries and conditions should be based on the available evidence, clinical expertise, and patient goals and values. Current research investigating the effectiveness of taping, wrapping, bracing, and padding techniques has overall produced a limited amount of evidence in the literature. While some techniques such as ankle taping and bracing and knee bracing have undergone study, many techniques lack any or sufficient investigation of their effectiveness on patient outcomes. The mere presence of evidence from studies does not necessarily mean the technique has been shown to be the gold standard as evidence differs in quality and applicability to clinical practice. Furthermore, expert opinion and clinical experience are often the only source of evidence to guide clinical decision making with taping, wrapping, bracing, and padding techniques.

Evidence, or research data, is produced from different sources, and a brief overview of the hierarchy of these sources can assist in determining the importance or strength of the findings and application to clinical practice. The highest level of evidence in the hierarchy comes from a meta-analysis followed by a systematic review. A meta-analysis uses statistical methods to combine and analyze data from clinical studies that meet pre-specified eligibility criteria to reach a conclusion as to the effectiveness of an individual treatment or technique. Systematic reviews comprehensively assess relevant studies on a topic and synthesize the findings into a qualitative summary of the evidence. Randomized controlled trials are studies that compare a randomly assigned experimental group (group that receives a treatment) with a randomly assigned control group (group that does not receive a treatment) using statistical methods to determine differences between the groups. Cohort studies compare two groups over time, a group that receives a treatment with a group that does not, to evaluate the effect of the treatment. Case-control studies look back in time and compare a group with a specific condition with a group without the condition to examine the differences among the groups. Case series are collections or reports of patients with a specific condition or who are receiving a specific treatment. Case reports are similar to case series but report on only one patient. Case series and case reports do not include a control group. Expert opinion is the lowest level of evidence and is based on opinions from authorities or expert communities, usual practice, or clinical experience.

---

### DETAILS

Here is a quick look at the evidence hierarchy with simulated examples of study types or research areas. The highest level of evidence is a meta-analysis and the lowest level is expert opinion.

- Meta-analysis: A collection of 10 well-designed, similar studies examining the effectiveness of semirigid orthotics in reducing rates of plantar fasciitis among male and female intercollegiate basketball athletes.
- Systematic review: A comprehensive literature review of 50 studies investigating the effect of epicondylitis strap braces on grip strength among recreational tennis players with lateral epicondylitis.
- Randomized controlled trial: The effects of a lower leg neoprene sleeve on vertical jump height among healthy, female high school volleyball athletes randomly assigned to an experimental group (wearing neoprene sleeve) and control group (not wearing neoprene sleeve).
- Cohort studies: The effectiveness of a video-based instructional method in teaching taping techniques in five athletic training programs compared with five similar athletic training programs with traditional instruction (lecture and lab) over a 2-year period.
- Case-control studies: The effects of functional knee braces used prophylactically on side-to-side movements among a group of healthy, intercollegiate football linemen with two seasons of brace wear during practices and competitions compared with a group of healthy intercollegiate football linemen who do not wear the braces.
- Case series: A review of all medical records from Mason County High Schools with interscholastic soccer program(s) documenting the diagnosis of osteitis pubis among male and female athletes to characterize common mechanisms of injury.
- Case reports: The use of a unique taping technique in the treatment of gamekeeper's thumb in a high school lacrosse athlete.
- Expert opinion: "Always overlap tape by ½ of the width to avoid gaps and inconsistent layering."

---

The evidence hierarchy can be useful to help establish the importance of data findings or recommendations to clinical practice. In later chapters, "Evidence Summary" boxes will present relevant data from reviews and studies and accompany specific taping, wrapping, bracing, and padding techniques. Let us now look at a fictitious example of the EBP process and how clinicians can use the information for clinical decision making.

The fourth match yesterday of the varsity female soccer season was hectic for Sigmund Bass. Sigmund is an AT at Beaver Orthopedic Clinic and performs outreach at SRT High School. The match was played in the rain at a regional park on a worn artificial turf field. The field was slick from the rain, and the athletes were having difficulty maintaining contact with their cleats on the turf. Over a span of 10 minutes in the second half, two midfielders sprinted to intercept separate passes. The midfielders attempted to stop quickly but lost their footing on the wet turf, falling on an outstretched arm and forcing their wrists into hyperextension. Just minutes later, the goalkeeper dove toward the inside post for a save and collided with an opponent, forcing her wrist into hyperextension. Several possessions later, the striker was moving toward the goal for a shot and was slide tackled by an opponent, falling to the turf, forcing her wrist into hyperflexion. Each athlete was removed from the match following her injury and evaluated and treated by Sigmund on the sidelines. The athletes did not return to the match.

Today, the team physician evaluates the athletes in her office. Radiographs demonstrate no bony pathology. The team physician diagnoses each athlete with a second-degree hyperextension or hyperflexion wrist sprain. Sigmund and the team physician develop a treatment program for each athlete and discuss various wrist taping and bracing techniques for the athletes to prevent further injury upon a return to activity.

Using their combined 40 years of experience with the application and use of wrist taping and bracing techniques among athletes, Sigmund and the team physician consider which technique to use with the soccer athletes. The development of a focused, **clinically relevant question** (Step 1) is needed to actually find an answer as to which technique is most appropriate for the athletes. Sigmund and the team physician developed the clinically relevant question, "Is taping or bracing more effective for soccer athletes with hyperextension or hyperflexion wrist sprains to provide support and protect from further injury during sport activity?" This question included the criteria of a focused, clinical question in the PICO format:[4,5]

The **P**atient population or **P**roblem: Soccer athletes with hyperextension or hyperflexion wrist sprains

The **I**ntervention: Taping techniques

A **C**omparison intervention (if relevant): Bracing techniques

The clinical **O**utcome of interest: Provide support and protect from further injury during sport activity

Sigmund returns to Beaver Orthopedic Clinic and enlists several colleagues to assist him in **searching for the best evidence** (Step 2) to answer the clinically relevant question. The group begins their search using electronic databases through the Internet in the Clinic and at the local university, which offers on-campus access to many subscription bibliographic databases. Some medical databases can be accessed free of charge while others require a subscription.

---

## DETAILS

### Electronic Databases for Evidence-Based Medicine
#### Free Access
Cochrane Library, http://www.cochrane.org/
MEDLINE/PubMed, http://www.nlm.nih.gov/bsd/pmresources.html
The Joanna Briggs Institute, http://joannabriggs.org/
PICO searching, http://pubmedhh.nlm.nih.gov/nlmd/pico/piconew.php
PubMed, https://www.ncbi.nlm.nih.gov/pubmed/
PEDro, http://www.pedro.org.au/
Centre for Evidence-Based Medicine, http://www.cebm.net/
Google Scholar, http://scholar.google.com/
Agency for Healthcare Research and Quality, http://www.ahrq.gov/

Bandolier, http://www.bandolier.org.uk
*BMJ* Evidence-Based Medicine, https://ebm.bmj.com/

#### Subscription-Based Services
CINAHL Complete, https://www.ebsco.com/products/research-databases/cinahl-complete
SPORTDiscus, https://www.ebsco.com/products/research-databases/sportdiscus
DynaMed Plus, https://dynamed.com/home/
ProQuest Health and Medicine, http://www.proquest.com/libraries/academic/health-medicine/
Taylor & Francis Online, http://www.tandfonline.com
ScienceDirect, http://www.sciencedirect.com
eBook Collection, https://www.ebscohost.com/ebooks/academic/subscriptions/academic-ebook-subscriptions

---

Based on Sigmund's clinical question, the group searches each database with specific search methods to retrieve the best matched studies and reviews. The individual search terms or combination of terms they use for the databases include wrist taping, wrist bracing, wrist support, wrist guards, wrist soccer injuries, wrist sprains, wrist injury treatment, wrist hyperflexion, wrist hyperextension, randomized controlled trials, meta-analysis, systematic review, randomized trial, clinical trial, double blind, single blind, and case report. The group uses additional criteria to further narrow the number of results obtained from the searches to those most relevant. The group limits the search to studies that are randomized controlled trials or quasi-randomized controlled trials, were published in the last 7 years, have participants 12 years of age and older, and are published in the English language.

The search is performed over several weeks and produces 30 possible references for the group to review. Most of the electronic databases only provide article citations while others include an abstract with the citation. The databases at the local university produce several full text complete articles. The group meets and discusses the retrieved citations, abstracts, and full text articles to again narrow the studies to those most relevant based on the clinical question and selection criteria. This review produces a list of 11 studies, and full text articles are obtained at the university by photocopying from journals, interlibrary loan services, and free web access to journals.

Sigmund, the team physician, and the group are now tasked with **evaluating and appraising the evidence** (Step 3). Each study is evaluated to determine its value to clinical practice. This step requires the most judgment in the EBP process.[2] Several rating scales are available to quantitatively evaluate individual studies, but many require research training and experience.

---

**DETAILS**

For more complete information on rating scales, see the Further Reading section at the end of this chapter.

---

Because of their limited training and experience with formal rating scales and quantitative methods to evaluate the evidence, the group instead asks three questions[3] of each study during the appraisal. The first question is "Are the results of the study valid?" The study results should be truthful, demonstrated through well-designed methodology of the study described in the text. Next, "What are the actual results?" The results should be reliable; when used in clinical practice, similar outcomes are produced. Last is "Are the findings clinically relevant to my patients?" The findings should be applicable and important to the patient population, high school female soccer athletes.

The group completes the evaluation and appraisal in several meetings and determines that the 11 studies are valid, reliable, and clinically relevant at different levels to the high school soccer athletes. Among the 11 studies, six are well-designed randomized controlled trials (RCTs) conducted in university research laboratories with non-athletic and athletic subjects. These studies examined the effects of various wrist taping and bracing techniques on active flexion and extension. The six studies demonstrated that taping techniques were significantly favored (reduced greater flexion and extension) over bracing techniques. Two separate studies

comparing wrist taping and bracing techniques examined injury rates among intercollegiate football athletes. The incidence of wrist injury was significantly reduced over a competitive season with the use of bracing techniques compared with taping techniques. A small study examined the cost-effectiveness of wrist taping and bracing techniques among athletes with sprains in various sports at eight high schools. Over a 2-year period, the findings revealed that the use of bracing techniques was cost-effective compared with taping techniques in the treatment of wrist sprains. Two case reports found that a novel wrist bracing technique was subjectively rated as superior by professional ice hockey athletes with a sprain for comfort, ease of use, and protection (reduction in flexion and extension) during practices.

Sigmund and the team physician meet to discuss **implementing the evidence into clinical practice with patients** (Step 4). Evidence, clinical expertise, and patient goals, values, and preferences should determine the selection of the taping or bracing intervention for the soccer athletes. The evidence from the six RCTs supported the use of taping techniques to reduce wrist flexion and extension. Other evidence from three studies demonstrated that bracing techniques reduced rates of injuries and were cost-effective compared with taping techniques. The case reports produced favorable results for patient satisfaction with a new bracing technique. Based solely on the evidence hierarchy, it appears taping techniques should be used with the athletes. Sigmund and the team physician have numerous years of experience with wrist taping and bracing techniques. The team physician has seen very positive patient outcomes with bracing techniques in treating wrist sprains, and Sigmund is proficient in the application of taping techniques. However, Sigmund will not travel to the five away matches remaining in the season, and the budget for purchasing additional taping supplies is limited. The goal of the taping or bracing intervention for the athletes is to provide stability and protection and limit excessive wrist flexion and extension. The taping or bracing intervention needs to be easy to apply, adjust, and remove, comfortable to wear, lightweight, and comply with sport association rules. Based on Sigmund's experience, he believes the soccer athletes will prefer a bracing technique. Sigmund and the team physician carefully examine the evidence, their clinical expertise, and the patient population and decide to use bracing techniques to protect the injured midfielders, goalkeeper, and striker from further injury. The athletes are progressing well in the treatment program. They are fitted with functional wrist braces and instructed on their use as they begin functional activities on the field.

Sigmund closely follows the athletes during the final stages of their treatment program as they progress back into activity, **evaluating the effects of interventions**

**on patient outcomes** (Step 5). With 2 weeks of brace wear and a full return to practices and competitions, the athletes report to Sigmund that the braces are easy to apply and adjust, comfortable to wear, and lightweight in construction. The athletes state the braces provide stability and increase their confidence in performing at pre-injury levels. The athletes continue to wear the braces and finish the soccer season without further injury.

At the conclusion of a clinical case such as the previous example, an evaluation of the EBP process should be conducted by asking if the clinical question was answered, by asking if quality evidence was located in a timely manner, by asking if the evidence was appropriately evaluated, and by asking if integration of the evidence, clinical expertise, and patient goals, values, and preferences produced an acceptable clinical decision.[4]

---

**DETAILS**

For more detailed discussion of outcomes assessment, see the Further Reading section at the end of this chapter.

---

In this case, Sigmund was able to use EBP to find and apply an appropriate intervention for the injured soccer athletes. Faced with a unique situation, Sigmund and his group created a clinically relevant question to guide the search for an answer. The evidence search was conducted with specific terms and criteria in medical databases to focus on relevant studies and reviews for the clinical question. The group evaluated the evidence to determine its usefulness and application to the clinical situation. Although the evidence demonstrated support for both taping and bracing techniques, the strongest evidence from the six RCTs suggested that taping techniques were the appropriate intervention for the soccer athletes. However, other evidence supporting bracing techniques and the clinical expertise of Sigmund and the team physician, goal of the intervention, and needs of the athletes were integrated in the clinical decision to use a bracing intervention. An evaluation at the completion of the season demonstrated that the clinical outcome, no further injury of the wrist among the athletes, was achieved.

## TAPES

The use of tape in preventing, treating, and rehabilitating injuries and conditions has been and continues to be popular with health care professionals. Intercollegiate and professional sport medical staffs often allot large proportions of their budgets to tape and associated supplies necessary for application. Many different types of tape are available. The decisions regarding which type to purchase and use should be based on the desired objective of the technique.

## Types

Tapes fall into three main categories: non-elastic, elastic, and cast (Fig. 1–1). Non-elastic and elastic tapes have an adhesive backing that can adhere directly to the skin and other materials.

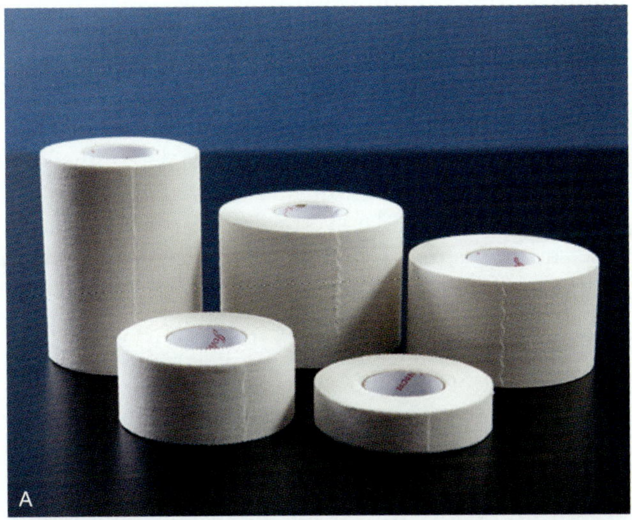

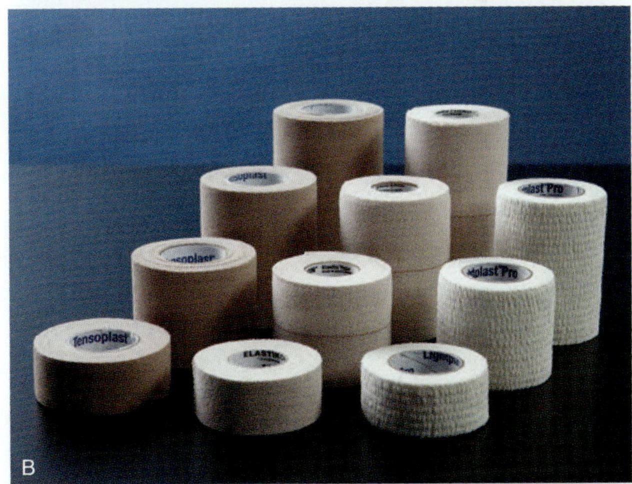

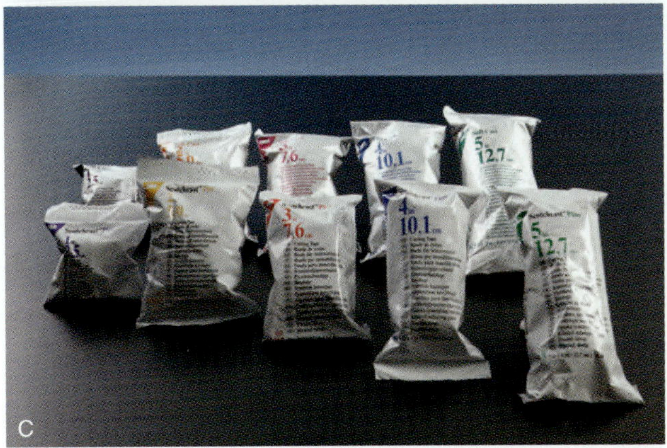

**Fig. 1–1  A** *Variety of non-elastic tape.* **B** *Variety of heavyweight and lightweight elastic tape.* **C** *Variety of semirigid and rigid cast tape.*

### Non-Elastic

As the name implies, non-elastic tape does not possess elastic properties, so conformability to body contours can be difficult. Non-elastic tape is manufactured in a variety of sizes and colors. The most commonly used is white, which is available in ½, 1, 1½, 2, and 3 inch widths by 10 to 15 yard lengths (see Fig. 1–1A).

Non-elastic tape is made of cotton and/or polyester with a zinc oxide adhesive mass backing. Some types possess a high adhesive backing designed for application directly to the skin. The number of longitudinal and vertical fibers per inch in the backing determines the quality of the tape.[6] High-quality tapes have 85 or more longitudinal fibers and 65 vertical fibers per square inch; lesser-quality tapes have 65 or fewer longitudinal fibers and 45 vertical fibers. The quality of the tape will determine the amount and durability of the adhesive backing and the roll tension. The adhesive mass should be of a quality to withstand moisture, perspiration, and body and joint movements of the patient and to allow for easy removal. High-quality tapes typically possess the greatest amount of adhesive backing. Roll tension refers to how the tape comes off the roll. The tension ideally should be even and fluid when removing the tape from the roll.

### Elastic

Elastic tape, commonly referred to as stretch tape, is manufactured in heavyweight and lightweight designs. The tape is available in 1, 1½, 2, 3, and 4 inch widths by 5 yard length in two commonly used colors: white and tan (see Fig. 1–1B).

Elastic tape is made of twisted cotton with an adhesive backing. The quality of elastic tapes is determined in a fashion similar to that for non-elastic tapes. The heavyweight tape is thicker than the lightweight design and provides more tensile strength and support when applied to the body. Several of the heavyweight designs require taping scissors to cut the tape from the roll during technique application. Elastic tapes have the ability to conform to the contour of the body while providing support.

### Cast

Unlike non-elastic and elastic tapes, cast tape is a fiberglass fabric containing a polyurethane resin that reacts to water and air, causing a chemical reaction. This reaction makes the fiberglass set, or become hard. The tape is manufactured on a roll in semirigid and rigid types and is available in 1, 2, 3, 4, and 5 inch widths by 4 yard length (see Fig. 1–1C). Semirigid tape provides support while allowing range of motion of the body parts; rigid tape provides complete immobilization. Both types conform to the contour of the body. Taping scissors are needed to cut cast tape.

## Objectives of Taping

Use taping techniques to:

- Provide support and reduce range of motion in preventing injuries
- Provide support and reduce range of motion in treating and rehabilitating existing injuries
- Secure elastic wraps when preventing, treating, and rehabilitating injuries
- Secure pads in preventing and treating injuries
- Secure dressings in treating wounds

## Recommendations for Tape Application

Applying tape is more than simply "placing the sticky side down." The following recommendations will assist in effectively applying taping techniques.

### Preparation of the Patient

Clean and dry the skin of the patient. Body oils from perspiration, lotions, and dirt/grass will lessen the adhesive properties of the tape. In some cases, shave the body hair over the area for effective application and removal of the tape. The position of the patient during application is important. As a general rule, when applying non-elastic and cast tapes, position the joint in the range of motion in which the joint will be stabilized. The position of the joint when applying elastic tape will vary because of the stretch qualities of the tape. There are exceptions to these rules, which will be illustrated in subsequent chapters.

### Tearing Tape

Learning how to tear non-elastic and elastic tapes is the first step in becoming proficient in technique application. There are many methods to tear tape, but all have two commonalities: becoming comfortable with a method and practicing it to become efficient. A description of one successful method follows; it can be altered to accommodate individual preference (Fig. 1–2).

Practice this method to become proficient at tearing all sizes of non-elastic tape. Without this skill, smooth and efficient application of non-elastic tape will not be possible. The roll of tape should remain in one hand during application in order to avoid the time it would take to set the tape down and pick it up again repeatedly.

The ability to tear most sizes of lightweight elastic tape should come with skill in tearing non-elastic tape. The ability to tear heavyweight elastic tape requires experience and variation of hand and finger positions on the roll (Fig. 1–3). Do not become overly concerned if tearing heavyweight elastic tape is difficult; most health care professionals use taping scissors to cut heavyweight elastic tape during application. If the position of the patient

**STEP 1:** Hold the roll of non-elastic tape in one hand. Place the third finger of the hand through the roll to provide stabilization (see Fig. 1–2A). The roll should rest on the **proximal** phalanx of the finger and slightly on the palm.

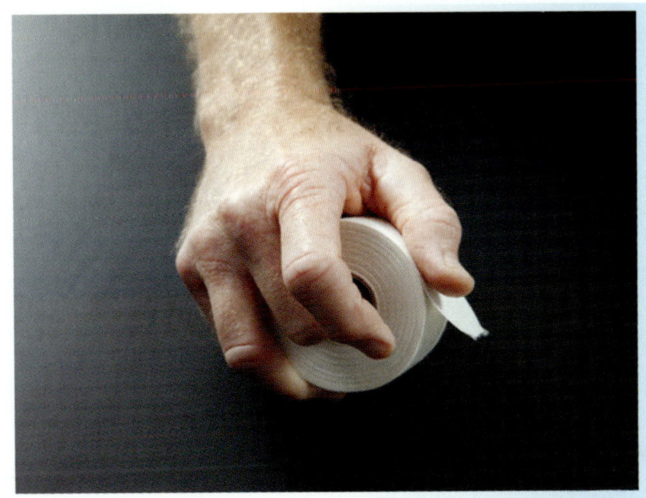

**Fig. 1–2 A**

**STEP 2:** Place the tape extending from the roll between the tips of the thumb and second finger (see Fig. 1–2B).

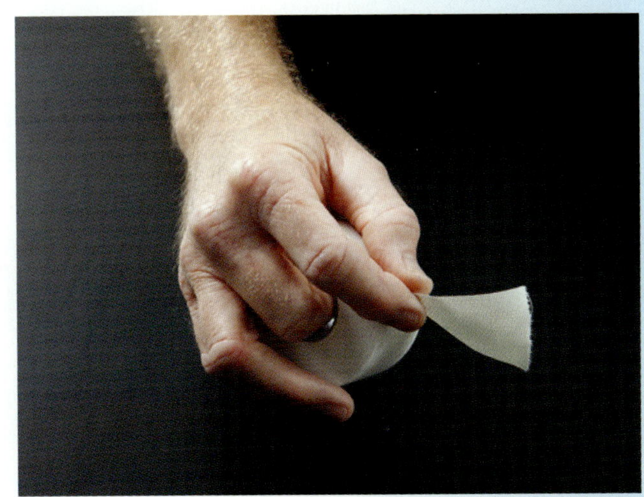

**Fig. 1–2 B**

**STEP 3:** With the thumb and second finger of the other hand, hold the extended tape between the fingertips in close proximity to the fingers of the first hand (see Fig. 1–2C).

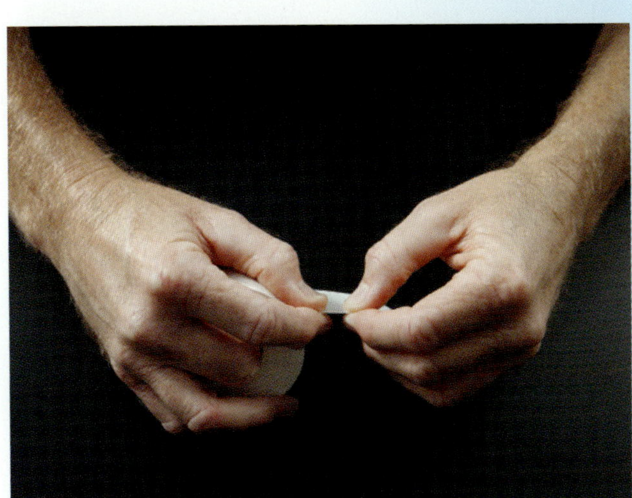

**Fig. 1–2 C**

*Steps Cont.*

**Tapes, Wraps, Braces, and Pads**

**STEP 4:** Following this placement, pull both hands in straight, opposing directions with a slight downward motion (see Fig. 1–2D). Pressure on the fingertips with this movement will begin to tear the horizontal fibers of the tape.

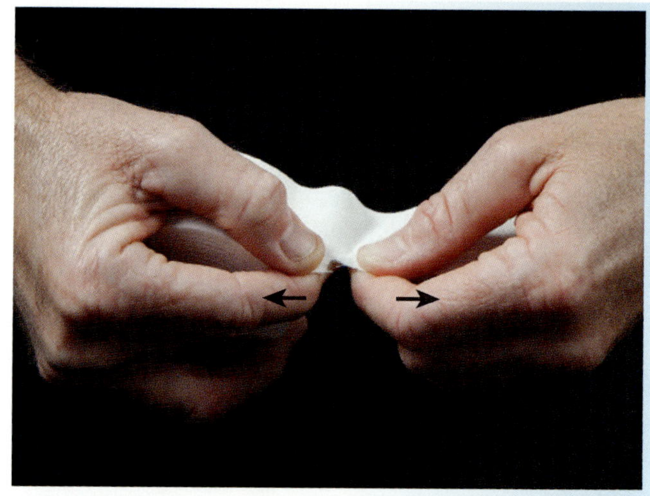

Fig. 1–2 D

**STEP 5:** As the tape begins to tear, quickly **supinate** the hand holding the roll and **pronate** the other hand in a tearing motion (see Fig. 1–2E). The hands will rotate in opposite directions. Avoid twisting or crimping the tape. With practice, these two movements become synchronized into one movement.

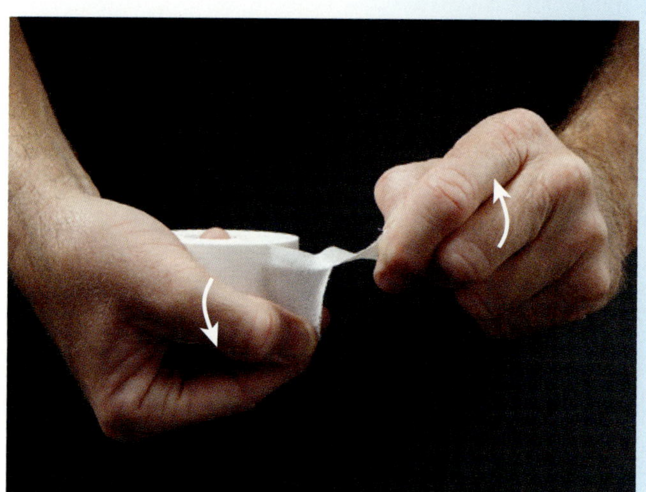

Fig. 1–2 E

allows, have him or her cut the tape with scissors during technique application. This procedure will lessen the application time and will involve the patient in the technique.

**Helpful Hint |**

Hold the roll of elastic tape in one hand without placing a finger through the roll (see Fig. 1–3A). Instead of placing the extended tape between the fingertips of the thumbs and second fingers, grasp the tape between the distal thumbs and second, third, fourth, and fifth fingers of each hand (see Fig. 1–3B). The fingers will push the tape into the palms of the hands. Pull the tape tight to remove the elastic properties and rotate the hands in opposite directions (see Fig. 1–3C). As the hands rotate, use the forearms and upper arms to assist with the rotating movement.

## *Application of Non-Elastic and Elastic Tape*

These general recommendations will guide the application of non-elastic and elastic taping techniques (Fig. 1–4). Individual variations of the techniques are presented in each chapter.

Once the patient is positioned on the taping table or bench with the skin clean and dry, begin the taping technique. Decide whether non-elastic or elastic tape will be applied directly to the skin or over pre-wrap. Applying tape directly to the skin will provide the greatest support but may cause skin irritation with daily use. Regardless of which method is used, applying adherent tape spray prior to taping should lessen migration of the tape (see Fig. 1–4A). Pre-wrap is a thin, porous foam material wrapped on 3 inch rolls (see Fig. 1–4B). Apply one layer of the wrap in an overlapping fashion, covering the body area.

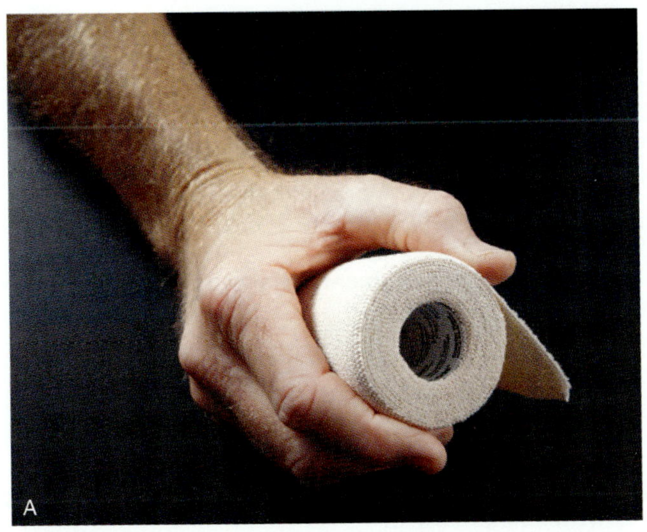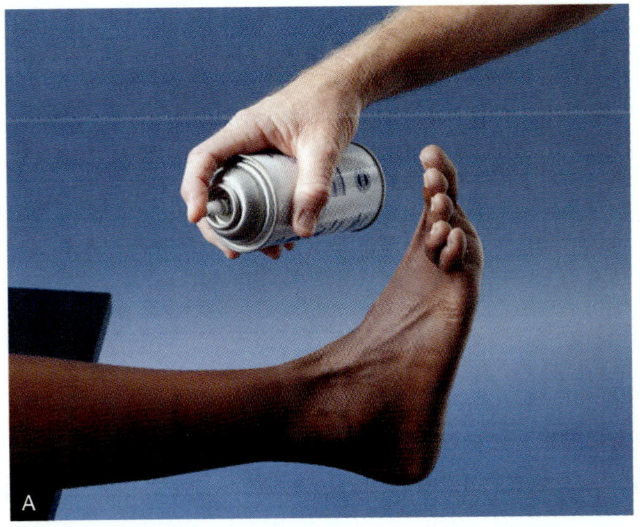





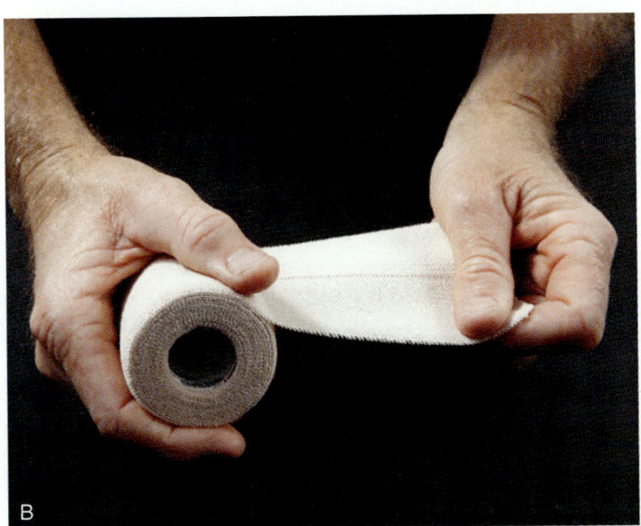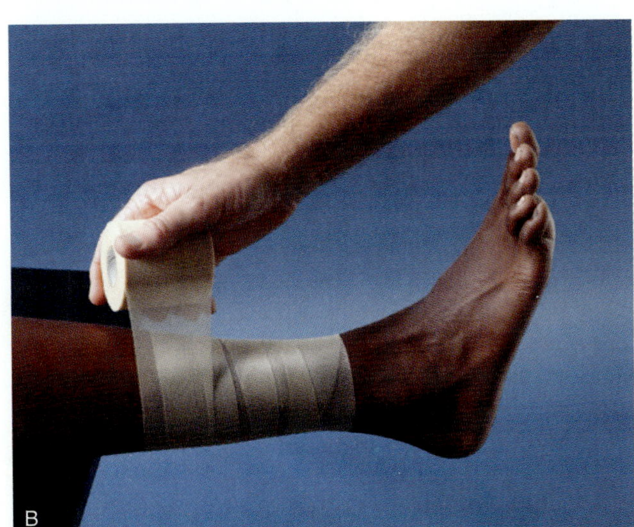

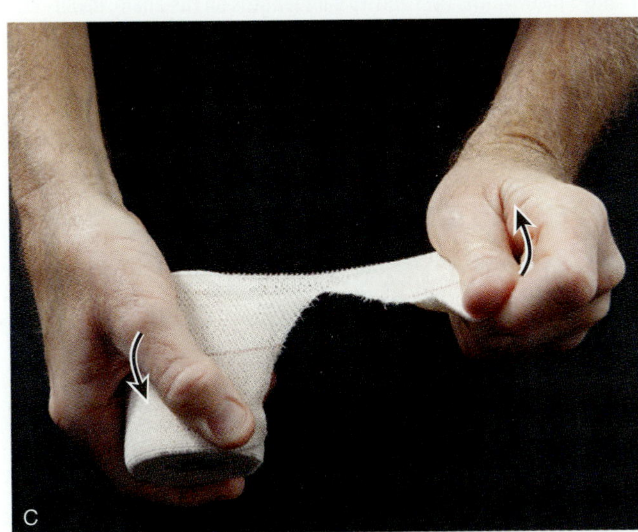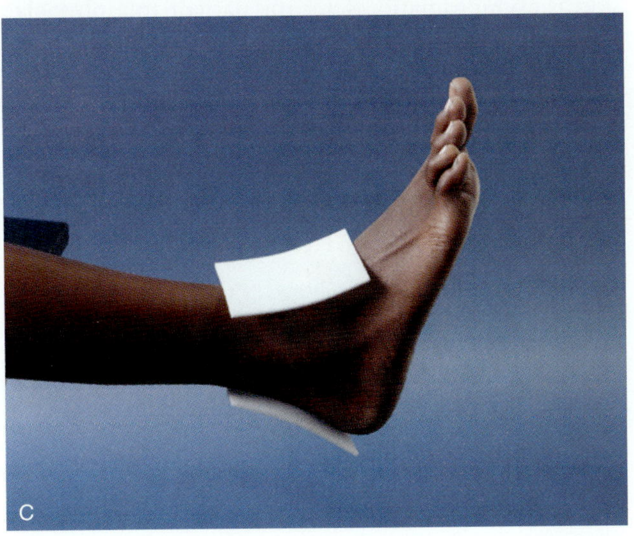

**Fig. 1–3**

**Fig. 1–4**

Tape techniques applied over bony prominences and high-friction areas should receive extra attention. Use thin foam pads on the heel and lace areas with ankle and foot techniques. For patients who require daily taping, provide additional protection by using skin lubricants and foam pads. Use thin foam pads over bony prominences and high-friction areas to reduce irritation, which can lead to cuts or blisters of the skin (see Fig. 1–4C).

As previously mentioned, the objective of the technique and the size of the patient will dictate the type of the tape to use. Non-elastic tape does not have elastic properties and will adhere to the body at the specific angle in which the tape is applied. Non-elastic tape also provides more stability than elastic tape. Applying non-elastic tape over body contours can be difficult, however, especially with small joints. With practice and experience, the correct angles of application will be obtained. Do not force non-elastic tape to fit body contours. Place non-elastic tape over the belly of a muscle carefully to avoid causing constriction. Focus attention on restricting range of motion affecting normal body movements such as gait. In these cases, use elastic tape to provide support while allowing normal body movement.

Allergic reactions and trauma to the skin can occur when tape is applied. A reaction to taping materials, such as adherents or zinc oxide, can appear immediately or days following contact. Redness, swelling, and itching may indicate an allergic reaction. In this situation, protect the area from further injury and treat accordingly. If taping materials are shown to be the cause, discontinue their use. Replace the closed basketweave technique (see Fig. 4–4), for example, with a lace-up ankle brace (see Fig. 4–15) to limit inversion, eversion, plantar flexion, and dorsiflexion until the skin is asymptomatic. Refer the patient to a physician if symptoms persist.

Blisters and lacerations are often the result of gaps, wrinkles, and inconsistent roll tension during application. Proper management of the wound includes cleansing, debridement, and dressing. If the wound is open, maintain an environment optimal for healing (moist, clean, warm).

Apply these materials over the wound dressing. Cut a felt or foam donut pad (see Fig. 3–26) to lessen the amount of stress and impact over the wound. Applying skin lubricants either under or over a donut pad to further reduce friction is possible. Hydrogel pads may also be applied to reduce friction. Use adhesive gauze material (see Fig. 3–15) to attach the pad to the skin.

Follow these recommendations when applying non-elastic and elastic tapes:

- Gather the equipment and supplies needed (which may include adherent tape spray, pre-wrap, taping scissors, and various tapes, wraps, and pads) prior to beginning technique application.
- As a general rule, each technique begins and ends with anchor strips.
- To avoid gaps, overlap each strip of tape by at least ½ of its width.
- To avoid wrinkles, smooth each strip of tape with the fingers or hands as it is applied.
- Avoid gaps, wrinkles, and inconsistent roll tension, which may lead to skin irritations such as cuts and blisters.
- Follow the sequence of strips in each technique, avoiding multiple wraps or turns around a muscle or joint.
- Exercise caution when applying tape on patients with broken skin, rashes on the skin, or known allergies to taping materials.

---

**DETAILS**

Use non-elastic and elastic tapes of ½ and 1 inch widths by 5 and 15 yard lengths on the foot, toes, hand, and fingers; 1½, 2, and 3 inch widths by 5 and 15 yard lengths on the ankle, lower leg, knee, thigh, hip/pelvis, upper arm, elbow, forearm, wrist, hand, and fingers; and 3 and 4 inch widths by 5 and 15 yard lengths on the knee, thigh, hip/pelvis, shoulder, upper arm, elbow, chest/abdomen, and spine.

---

**DETAILS**

For more complete information on the management of blisters and lacerations, see the Further Reading section at the end of this chapter.

---

Use foam, felt, lubricants, or hydrogel pads to protect a blister or laceration during tape application.

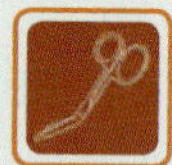

**Helpful Hint |**

If ½ inch or 1 inch non-elastic or elastic tapes are not available, create a roll from 1½ inch or 2 inch non-elastic or 2 inch elastic tape. Begin a longitudinal tear down the extended end of the tape at the desired width. Continue to tear this strip around the roll one time, leaving the other strip anchored on the roll. Strips in the same (¾ inch or 1 inch) or different (½ inch and 1 inch) widths on the same roll of non-elastic and elastic tapes may be made.

## *Application of Cast Tape*

Rigid cast tape is normally applied by an orthopedic technician or physician following acute fractures. Application guidelines for rigid casting are beyond the scope of this text and can be found elsewhere. Semirigid tape, on the other hand, is used by many health care professionals when total immobilization is not required. The objective of the technique and size of the patient will determine the type and width of tape to use. In the athletic setting, semirigid tape is often used to provide support and protection when treating various injuries. The use of semirigid tape may be restricted based on state credentialing and scope-of-practice laws. Athletic trainers should carefully review applicable state practice acts prior to applying semirigid tape.

Applying cast tape requires several pieces of equipment: gloves, taping scissors, water, self-adherent wrap, stockinet, or padding material. Position the patient on the taping table or bench.

Generally, cast tape is applied over stockinet and soft cast padding, Gore-Tex padding, or self-adherent wrap. Apply the cast tape over one layer of stockinet placed directly on the skin and covered with two to three layers of soft cast padding material. This technique is commonly used with rigid tape techniques that require extended periods of wear. Protect the padding material under the cast tape from excessive moisture to prevent skin **maceration** and itching. An alternative to use with rigid tape is a Gore-Tex cast padding, which repels water, allowing any type of water activity, including bathing. Moisture underneath the cast tape evaporates, and the skin dries completely. In the athletic setting, apply three to four layers of self-adherent wrap underneath semirigid cast tape to allow reuse of the cast on removal.

Applying semirigid cast tape requires experience and skill (see Fig. 11–17). The following recommendations apply to cast tape techniques:

- Wear examination or surgical gloves coated with petroleum jelly or silicone to protect the hands from tape resin and to prevent the tape from adhering to the gloves during application.
- Open the sealed foil pouch and remove the roll of tape. Most rigid and semirigid tapes require immersion in water of 70° to 75°F to begin the chemical reaction. Firmly squeeze the roll three times while submerged. Approximately 3–5 minutes is allowed to apply, mold, and shape the tape before setting occurs.
- Apply the tape in a spiral or circular pattern with slight roll tension.
- Overlap each layer by ⅓–⅔ of the width of the tape. The number of layers applied will determine the amount of support.
- Avoid gaps, wrinkles, inconsistent roll tension, and direct contact of the tape with the skin to lessen irritation.
- Use taping scissors to make partial cuts in the material to fit the contours of the body. Pad bony prominences to lessen the occurrence of irritation.
- Place the last 8–12 inches of tape on the body without roll tension. Smooth and mold the tape to the body part with the hands to achieve adhesion of the layers.
- Approximately 10–15 minutes after removal of the tape from its pouch, curing is complete.

---

**DETAILS**

Use cast tape of 1 inch width by 4 yard length on the toes and fingers; 2 inch width by 4 yard length on the foot, ankle, forearm, wrist, and hand; 3 inch width by 4 yard length on the ankle, lower leg, upper arm, elbow, and forearm; 4 inch width by 4 yard length on the ankle, lower leg, knee, thigh, hip/pelvis, shoulder, upper arm, elbow, chest/abdomen, and spine; and 5 inch width by 4 yard length on the ankle, knee, thigh, hip/pelvis, shoulder, chest/abdomen, and spine.

---

## *Removing Tape*

Removing tape can cause injury to the patient and should be performed in a controlled manner.

### Non-Elastic and Elastic

There are several ways to remove non-elastic and elastic tapes (Fig. 1–5).

- Manually, remove the skin from the tape in a direct line with the body.[7]
  - One hand grasps the tape and pulls it across the skin while the other hand pulls the skin in the opposite direction (see Fig. 1–5A). Do not rip the tape from the skin.
- Tape removal solvents in spray or liquid forms work as well.
  - Apply the solvent between the skin and tape to dissolve the adhesive (see Fig. 1–5B).
  - Thoroughly wash the area and monitor for possible skin reactions to the chemicals.
- Taping scissors and cutting tools used for removal allow patients to perform the task themselves. Taping scissors are designed with a blunt end to reach under the tape and reduce the chance of damage to the skin[7] (see Fig. 1–5C). Tape cutters are molded plastic tools with a single-edged metal blade located at the end (see Fig. 1–5D). These tools fit into the hand and also have a blunt end. Purchase replacement blades for tape cutters as needed.

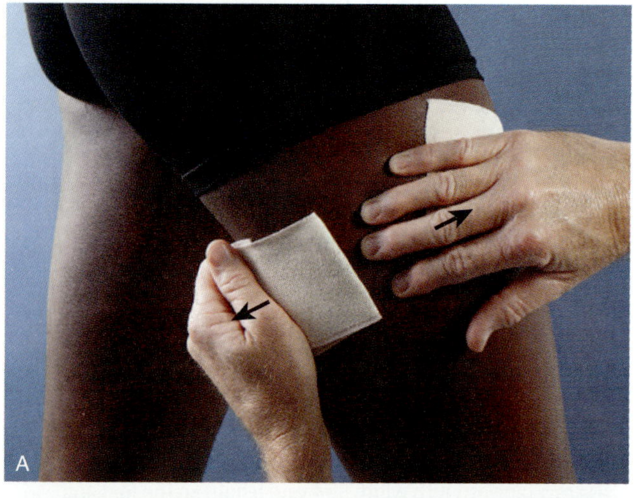

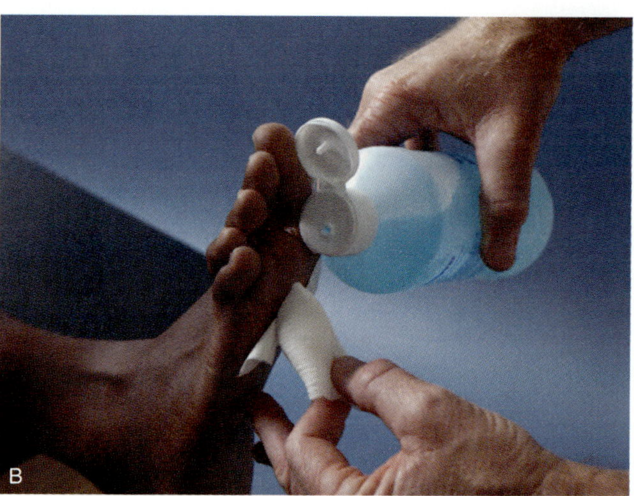

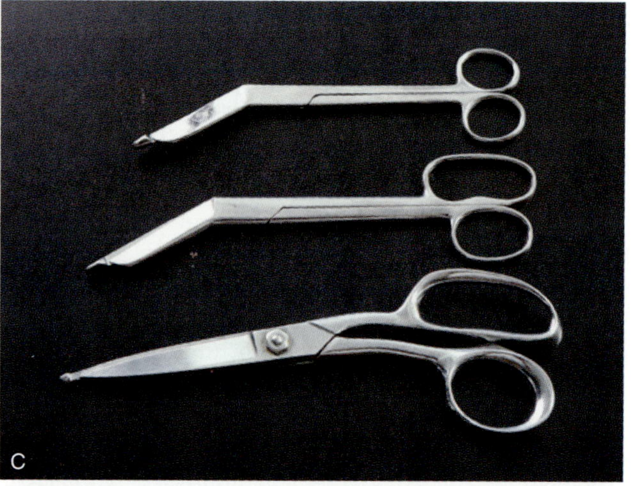

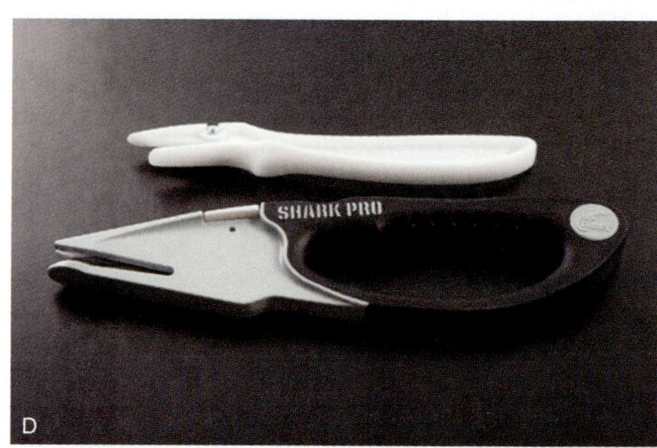


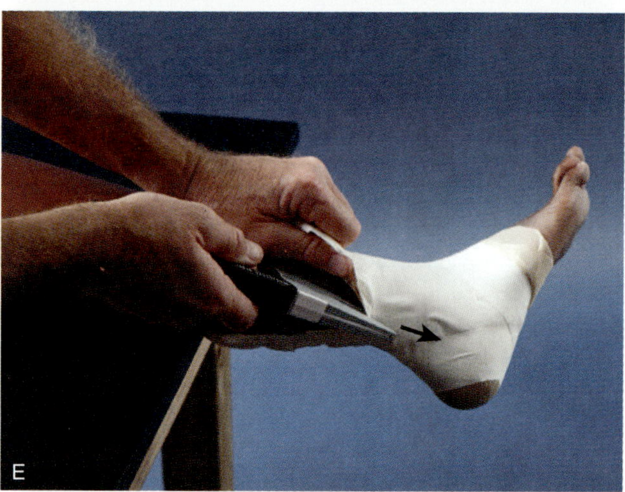

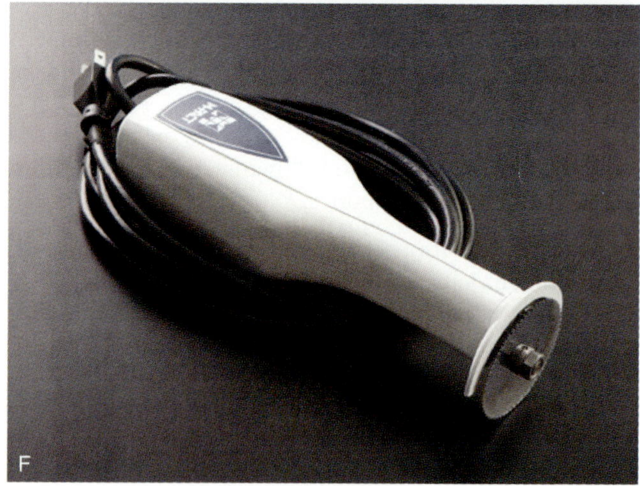

**Fig. 1–5 A** *Removing skin from tape.* **B** *Liquid tape removal solvent.* **C** *Taping scissors. (Top) Single ring. (Middle) Double ring. (Bottom) Heavy duty.* **D** *Tape cutters.* **E** *Removing tape with cutters.* **F** *Cast saw.*

- To remove tape, slip the blunt end of the scissors or cutter under the tape and cut in a **proximal-to-distal** direction away from the body. Keep the scissors or cutter parallel to the skin, following the contour of the body and avoiding bony prominences (see Fig. 1–5E).

### *Cast*

Remove semirigid cast tape with taping scissors or a cast saw and spreaders or by unwrapping. Rigid tape requires the use of a cast saw, cast spreaders, and scissors (see Fig. 1–5F). Guidelines for cast saw use can be found elsewhere. Exercise care when operating a cast saw.

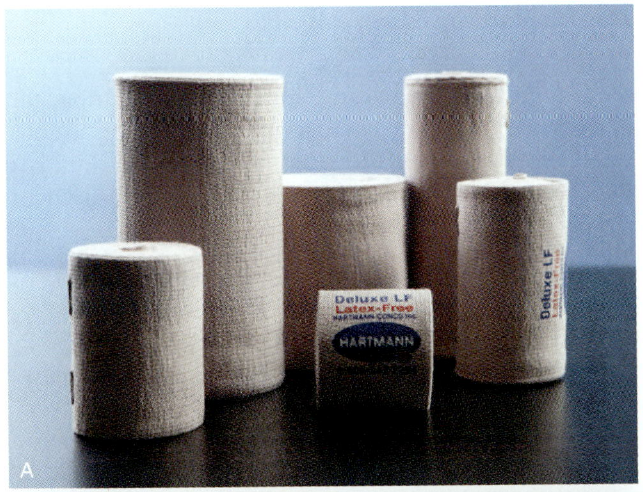

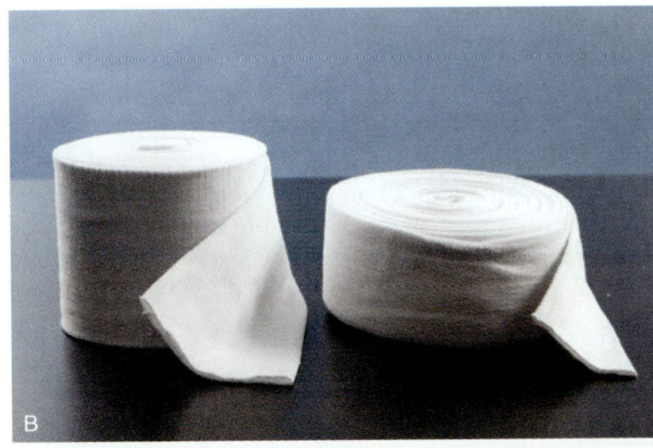

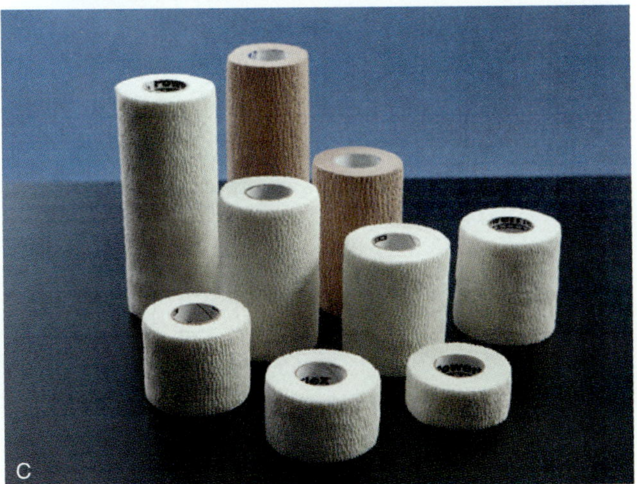

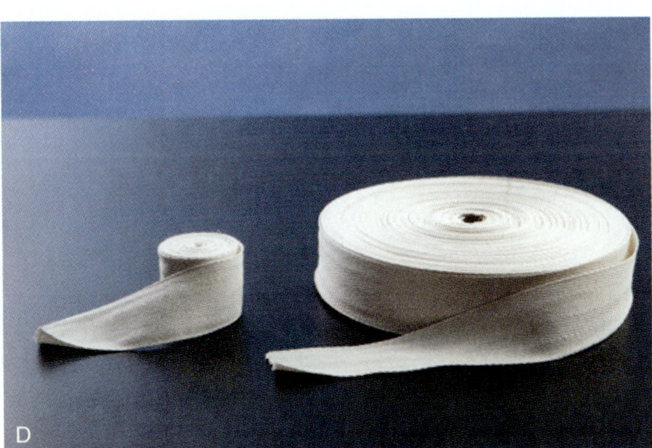

**Fig. 1–6 A** *Variety of elastic wraps.* **B** *Variety of elastic sleeves.* **C** *Variety of self-adherent wrap.* **D** *Cloth wrap. (Left) Individual wrap. (Right) Roll.*

### Clinical Application Question 1

During football practice, several players begin to complain of a burning sensation over the **posterior** heel area. Prior to practice, you applied a preventive taping technique to their ankles. You remove the tape and discover irritation of the skin over the posterior heel of each player.

➡ **Question: How can you treat and prevent skin irritation?**

### ...IF/THEN...

**IF** the scissors or cutter cannot be easily placed between the tape and skin, **THEN** apply a skin lubricant to the blunt end of the scissors or cutter to assist in cutting the tape in tight areas.

## WRAPS

Wraps are used for a variety of purposes and can be reused for multiple applications. Similar to tapes, many different types of wraps are available; their use should be based on the objective of the technique.

## Types

Wraps, similar to tape, can be divided into three basic types: elastic, self-adherent, and cloth (Fig. 1–6).

### *Elastic*

Elastic wraps allow for adjustments of compression during application. These wraps also conform well to body contours, providing multidirectional compression. Use Velcro fasteners, metal clips, or tape to anchor the wraps. Wash and dry elastic wraps after each use and reuse them. Similar to elastic wraps, elastic sleeves provide compression to the extremities. No additional anchor is required. Elastic wraps are made of cotton, rubber latex, or nylon in white and tan provided in 2, 3, 4, and 6 inch widths by 5 yard length and in 4 and 6 inch widths by 10 yard length (see Fig. 1–6A). The sleeves are made of cotton and rubber latex in 2, 2½,

**Tapes, Wraps, Braces, and Pads**

3, 3½, 4, 5, 6, 7, and 8 inch widths by 11 yard length (see Fig. 1–6B).

### Self-Adherent

Self-adherent wraps have elastic properties and the ability to adhere to themselves without irritation to hair or skin. These wraps come in a variety of colors and tear manually. Self-adherent wraps conform to body contours easily and provide adjustable compression. The wraps are intended for single use. Made of elastic yarn, they are available in 1, 1½, 2, 2¾, 3, 4, and 6 inch widths by 6 yard length (see Fig. 1–6C).

### Cloth

Cloth wraps, referred to as ankle wraps, are made of strong cotton weaves in a 2 inch width by 36 or 72 yard length roll. Cut individual wraps in 72–96 inch lengths from the roll (see Fig. 1–6D). Use cloth wraps in a **prophylactic** manner to prevent medial and lateral ankle sprains. The wraps provide mild support. Wash and dry cloth wraps after each use and reuse.

## Objectives of Wrapping

Use wrapping techniques to:

- Provide compression to reduce effusion and swelling when treating and rehabilitating injuries
- Provide support and reduce range of motion when preventing, treating, and rehabilitating injuries
- Secure pads when preventing and treating injuries
- Secure dressings when treating wounds

## Recommendations for Wrap Application

The following recommendations apply generally to all wrapping techniques.

### Preparation of the Patient

The objective of the wrapping technique will determine the position of the patient. For example, when applying a wrap over a muscular area, have the patient sustain muscular contraction during the technique to lessen the chance of constriction. To provide support and reduction in range of motion, position the joint in the range of motion in which the joint will be stabilized. Because wraps do not possess adhesive properties, wraps may be applied directly to the skin or, for cloth wraps, over socks.

After determining the technique objective and positioning the patient, choose the appropriate type of wrap.

### Application of Elastic Wraps

Elastic wraps have the potential to cause injury and should be used with care. Improper application can cause impairment in circulation, abnormal accumulation of swelling or effusion, or irritation of the skin. Use these recommendations for assistance when applying elastic wraps.

- Apply elastic wraps with firm, constant tension.
- Overlap each successive turn of the wrap by ½ its width while being careful to eliminate gaps, wrinkles, and inconsistent roll tension, which may cause skin irritation.
- Apply compression wrap techniques in a **distal-to-proximal** sequence to assist in venous return (see Fig. 3–17). Never cover the **distal** aspects of the extremities with the wrap. Keep the tips of the fingers and toes visible and monitor for impairment of circulation.
- Anchor elastic wraps with Velcro fasteners, metal clips, or non-elastic or elastic tapes.
- Place the end of the wrap and anchor on the dorsal or **anterior** aspect of the body part for comfort and easy removal.

Detailed elastic wrap application techniques are presented in individual chapters.

---

**DETAILS**

Use elastic wraps of 2 inch width by 5 yard length on the foot, toes, wrist, hand, and fingers; 3 inch width by 5 yard length on the foot, ankle, wrist, and hand; 4 inch width by 5 yard length on the foot, ankle, lower leg, upper arm, elbow, forearm, and wrist; 6 inch width by 5 yard length on the lower leg, knee, thigh, shoulder, upper arm, elbow, and chest/abdomen; 4 inch width by 10 yard length on the knee, thigh, hip/pelvis, shoulder, chest/abdomen, and spine; and 6 inch width by 10 yard length on the knee, hip/pelvis, shoulder, chest/abdomen, and spine.

---

Migration, slippage, or bunching of the elastic wrap may lessen the effectiveness of the technique (Fig. 1–7). To prevent this from occurring, use one of several methods.

- Apply adherent tape spray to the area prior to applying the wrap.
- Placing non-elastic or elastic tape strip(s) directly on the skin under the wrap is also possible.
  - Tear a 6–8 inch piece of tape and double the strip onto itself, leaving the adhesive mass exposed on both sides.

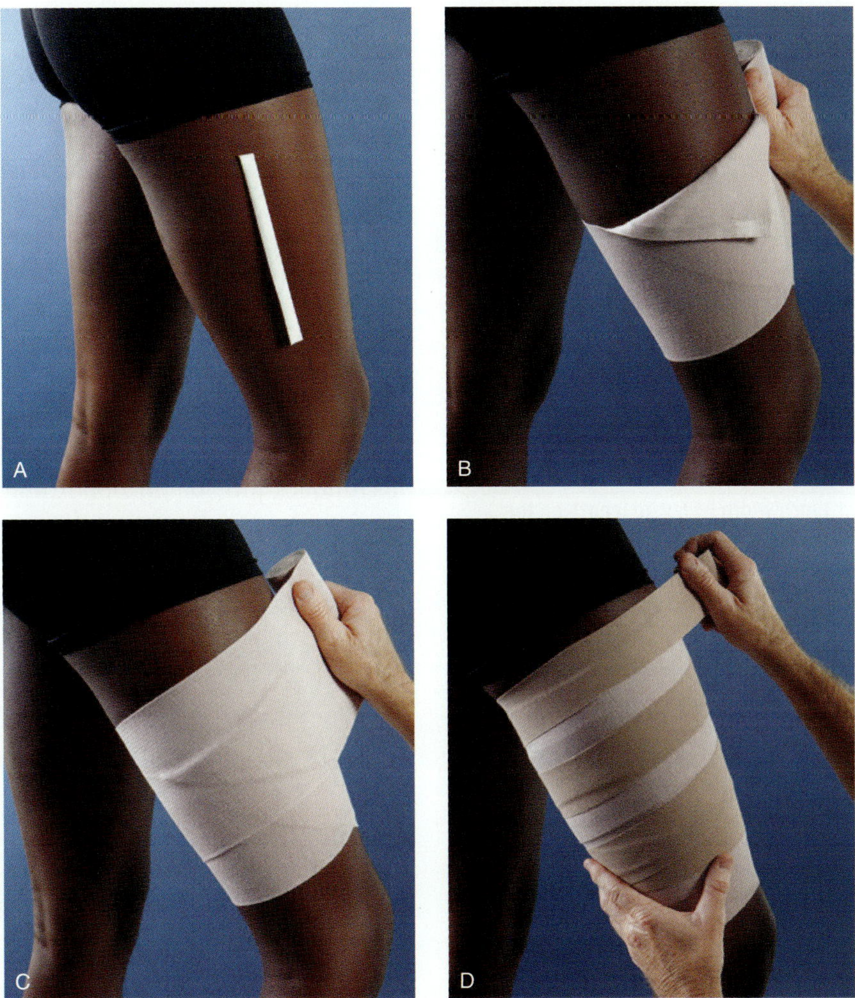

**Fig. 1–7**

- Place the strip(s) in a **longitudinal** position directly on the skin and then apply the wrap (see Fig. 1–7A).
- Adjusting anchors may also lessen migration, slippage, and bunching. Begin the wrapping technique by placing the loose end of the wrap on the skin.
  - When applying the first wrap or turn around the body part, fold the loose end over by ⅓–½ of the wrap's width (see Fig. 1–7B).
  - When applying the next wrap or turn, cover the folded end and continue with the technique (see Fig. 1–7C).
- Another method involves placing an elastic tape anchor directly on the skin.
  - When the wrapping technique is completed, apply the anchor partially on the wrap and partially on the skin in an overlapping manner (see Fig. 1–7D).

To fit different areas of the body, cut different lengths of elastic sleeves from a roll. Apply the elastic sleeve directly to the skin by simply pulling the sleeve onto the extremity (see Fig. 6–16). Use the sleeves during athletic, work, and casual activities.

> **. . . IF/THEN . . .**
> **IF** an elastic wrap loses its stretch characteristics and fails to conform to body contours, which is common with repeated use and cleaning, **THEN** use the elastic wrap only during treatment to anchor an ice bag to a body part.

### *Application of Self-Adherent Wraps*

Self-adherent wrap is manufactured on a roll and is applied with the same technique as elastic tape. The wrap has similar uses as elastic tape and wraps. In many taping techniques, the wrap may be used in place of pre-wrap to provide protection from irritation and additional support to a joint.

- Apply the wrap with firm and consistent tension, following body contours.
- Anchoring does not require fasteners, clips, or additional tape, an advantage of the wrap.
- Avoid gaps, wrinkles, and inconsistent roll tension.

The use of self-adherent wrap is discussed further in individual chapters.

---

### DETAILS

Use self-adherent wrap in 1 inch width by 6 yard length on the toes and fingers; 1½ and 2 inch widths by 6 yard length on the foot, ankle, wrist, and hand; 2¾ and 3 inch widths by 6 yard length on the foot, ankle, lower leg, upper arm, elbow, forearm, and wrist; 4 inch width by 6 yard length on the lower leg, knee, thigh, upper arm, elbow, and forearm; and 6 inch width by 6 yard length on the knee, thigh, hip/pelvis, shoulder, chest/abdomen, and spine.

---

### *Application of Cloth Wraps*

Use cloth wraps to provide support to the ankle. Apply a cloth wrap over a sock (see Fig. 4–14). Place thin foam pads over high-friction areas under the wrap to reduce irritation. Apply these wraps with firm, constant tension and keep constant pressure on the wrap as it is passed between the hands.

### *Removal of Wraps*

Remove elastic and cloth wraps by unwrapping the material after use. Use taping scissors to cut tape anchors. Remove an elastic sleeve by pulling it off the extremity in a distal direction. Use taping scissors or tape cutters to remove self-adherent wraps. Wash and dry elastic and cloth wraps after each use and reuse.

---

### Clinical Application Question 2

A professor at the local university participating in an intramural basketball league on campus sustains a first-degree **inversion sprain** of the left ankle. He is taken to the athletic training facility for treatment. After applying an ice bag, you decide to use a wrap to provide compression to reduce effusion and swelling.

➡ **Question: What type of wrap can you use?**

---

### … IF/THEN …

**IF** small amounts of non-elastic and/or elastic tape, pre-wrap, and/or self-adherent wrap are left on rolls, **THEN** collect the unused rolls in a box; soccer athletes use the tape to anchor shin guards; others use the pre-wrap and self-adherent wrap to tie their hair up; and some use tape and wrap cores to construct heel lifts (see Fig. 6–11) and tear drop thumb spica supports (see Fig. 11–14).

---

## BRACES

Advances in the research and development of bracing techniques provide an opportunity to select among a variety of types. Braces are designed to be used for specific injuries and conditions and are available for the majority of body areas and joints.

## Types

Braces can be classified according to their fit, purpose, and body area design (Fig. 1–8).

### *Fit*

The fit of a brace refers to the sizing and manufacturing, either off-the-shelf or custom-made. Off-the-shelf braces come in predetermined sizes, such as small, medium, large, and extra large (see Fig. 1–8A). Off-the-shelf braces are ready to use upon purchase and are generally less expensive than custom-made designs. Although braces are manufactured in predetermined sizes, many companies provide circumference measurements of body areas on the package to assist in proper fitting. Most off-the-shelf braces allow for small size adjustments during wear.

Custom-made braces are fitted and manufactured for specific patients. Manufacturer representatives or orthopedic technicians typically perform the fitting procedures prior to construction of the braces (see Fig. 1–8B). The type of injury, surgical procedure, and rehabilitation, as well as the limb girth, height, weight, and sport/occupation of the patient, often determine which model of brace to purchase. Because the braces are custom-fitted, increases in muscular girth from the development of strength or length of bones from growth periods may need to be considered.

### *Purpose*

Braces are used for dynamic purposes and can be grouped as prophylactic, functional, and rehabilitative.[8] A prophylactic brace is designed to protect an uninjured joint and the surrounding soft tissue structures.

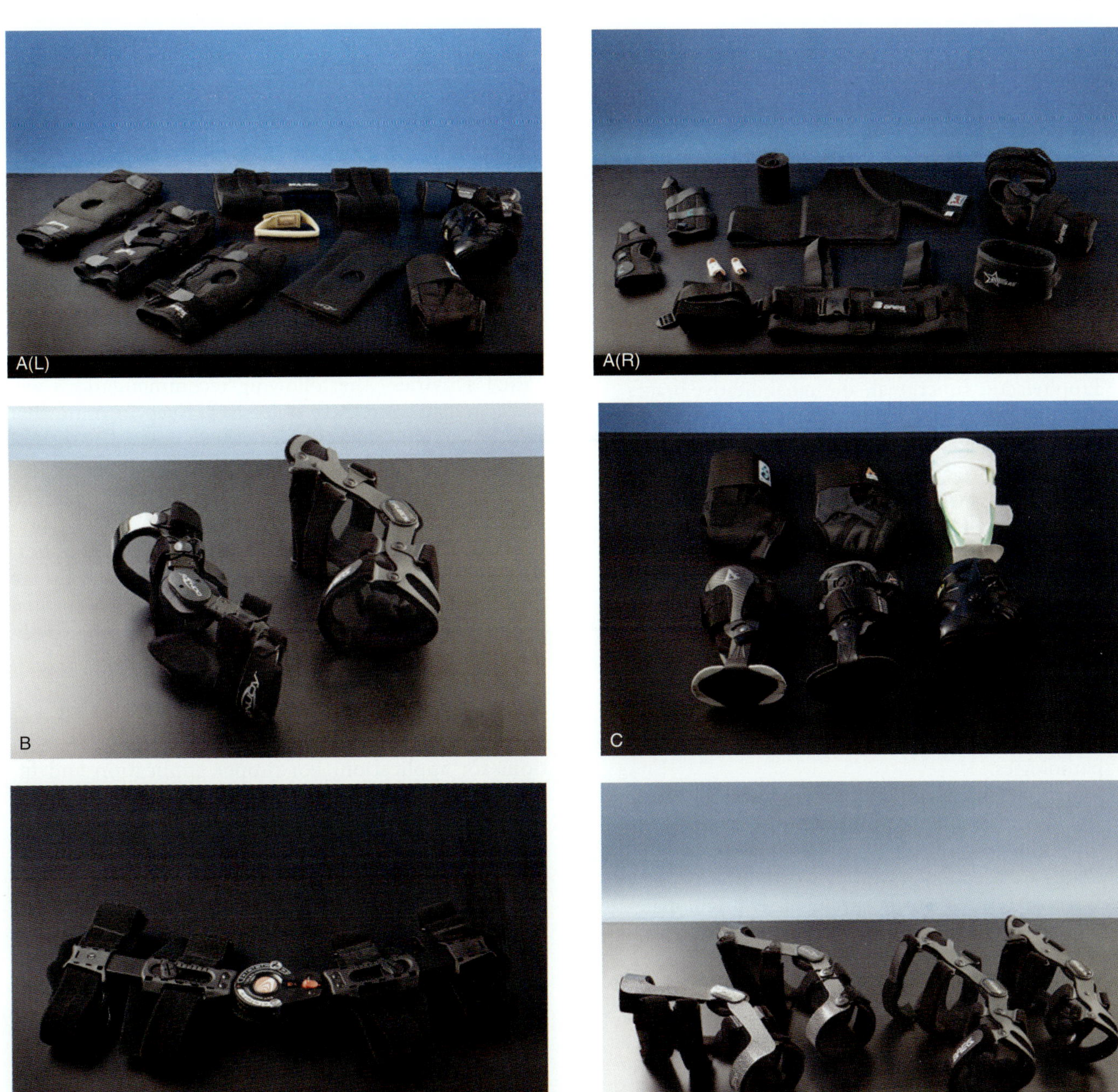

**Fig. 1–8 A** *(Left) Variety of off-the-shelf lower extremity braces. (Right) Variety of off-the-shelf upper extremity braces.* **B** *Custom-made braces. (Left) Elbow. (Right) Knee.* **C** *Variety of prophylactic ankle braces.* **D** *Rehabilitative elbow brace.* **E** *Variety of functional ACL knee braces.*

Use ankle braces, for example, as alternatives to ankle taping to protect against abnormal ranges of motion[9] (see Fig. 1–8C).

A rehabilitative brace is used to provide immobilization following a surgical procedure. Many designs allow for control of range of motion for the patient through the use of adjustable hinges. An example is the use of hinged elbow braces for the progression of passive and active **flexion** and **extension** during rehabilitation following **ulnar collateral ligament** reconstruction (see Fig. 1–8D).

Functional braces are used to provide support and protection for existing injuries or postsurgical repairs or reconstructions.[8] Use off-the-shelf and custom-made brace designs, for example, to reduce anterior translation of the tibia on the femur to protect an injured **anterior cruciate ligament (ACL)** or ACL graft following reconstruction[10] (see Fig. 1–8E).

### Body Area

Braces are designed to provide compression, protection, support, and limitations in range of motion for specific areas of the body. For example:

- Orthotics are used for many foot injuries and conditions.
- Braces commonly referred to as walking boots provide immobilization and control of range of motion for foot and ankle fractures and sprains.
- Night splints are used as nocturnal braces to assist in the treatment of plantar fasciitis by keeping the foot in dorsiflexion.
- Prophylactic, functional, and rehabilitative braces for the ankle in lace-up, semirigid, air/gel bladder, and wrap designs provide support and limit range of motion.
- Neoprene sleeves, rubber material commonly coated with elastic nylon, provide compression and support of muscular strains for the lower leg.
- Braces for the knee are available in prophylactic, functional, and rehabilitative designs.
- Neoprene sleeves and shorts support muscular strains of the thigh and hip/pelvis.
- Functional braces worn on the body or attached to football shoulder pads can reduce range of motion with glenohumeral instabilities and rotator cuff pathologies.
- Functional braces are used to lessen medial and lateral stresses and range of motion with ligamentous injuries in the elbow. Rehabilitative elbow braces are used for postsurgical conditions.
- Wrist braces made of neoprene or semirigid materials are available in prophylactic, functional, and rehabilitative designs.
- Braces for the hand and fingers can provide immobilization, support, and compression.
- Functional and rehabilitative braces for the chest/abdomen and spine can provide support and immobilization for a variety of injuries and conditions.

Illustrations and further discussions of these and other braces are found in subsequent chapters.

Braces are constructed from a variety of materials. The materials used vary as much as the types of braces. Many braces are constructed from tempered and aircraft aluminums and carbon composites. Other braces use semirigid plastic, layered nylon, polyester Lycra, and air and gel bladders. Neoprene, porous nylon, and polyester materials are also used in many brace designs.

## Objectives of Bracing

Use bracing techniques to:

- Provide support and protection when preventing injuries
- Provide support and protection when treating and rehabilitating existing injuries
- Provide compression to reduce effusion and swelling when treating and rehabilitating injuries
- Provide control of range of motion when treating and rehabilitating injuries

## Recommendations for Brace Application

Braces are designed to provide compression, support, and protection for the patient during sport, work, and casual activities. The following recommendations will assist in achieving these objectives. Keep in mind that new braces are similar to footwear in that a few days of wear are required for a break-in period.

### Preparation of the Patient

Clean and dry the skin of the patient for brace application. The position of the patient is determined by the type of brace worn. For example, place the patient in a seated position to apply an ankle brace and in a standing position to apply a shoulder brace.

### Application of Braces

When purchased, each brace will have specific instructions for application. For proper application and fit, follow the step-by-step procedure carefully. Deviation from the steps may cause injury to the patient. One advantage of bracing techniques is that it is possible to teach the patient the application procedure, which will lessen the time required for health care professionals to assist. Several brace designs allow for adjustments in the outer shell or frame, straps, inner pads, and hinges to achieve proper fit. Follow manufacturer guidelines when performing any adjustments to the brace.

Brace migration is a common problem that may occur even with proper fit. The easiest method to correct migration is to stop the activity and reapply the brace in the step-by-step procedure. Using a neoprene sleeve under the brace can also help lessen migration. However, the additional girth of the sleeve may affect the original fitting measurements of the brace. Applying adherent tape spray over the body area that makes contact with the brace can also lessen migration. If adherent tape spray is used, monitor brace straps for damage from the adherent and chemical components in the spray. This disadvantage of bracing (migration) is also one of its advantages; bracing allows for adjustability and reuse.

Intercollegiate and high school athletic associations provide rules governing the use of braces in practices and competitions. The National Collegiate Athletic Association (NCAA)[11] and the National Federation of State High School Associations (NFHS)[12] allow braces to be worn if no metal or **nonpliable** substance is exposed. If a metal or nonpliable substance is exposed, closed-cell, slow-recovery foam or similar material of at least ½ inch thickness must cover the areas. Padded covers for many braces may be purchased through the manufacturer. For a more comprehensive discussion of NCAA and NFHS rules, see Chapter 13.

### *Removal of Braces*

The majority of braces can be removed by the patient after use. Release the straps and lift the brace from the body part. Several braces, such as shoulder instability designs and designs attached directly to the skin with tape, do require assistance.

## Care of Braces

Clean braces and allow them to dry in a well-ventilated area between use. Clean and inspect braces regularly. Rinse the frames and hinges of rigid braces with clean, fresh water, then drain and air-dry them. Hinge lubrication is typically not required. If lubrication is needed, use a dry lubricant such as Teflon spray. Hand wash straps and frame liners in cold water with mild detergent, then rinse and air-dry. Wash neoprene and other soft brace materials in cold water with mild detergent, rinse, and air-dry. Do not heat straps, liners, or neoprene materials in a dryer. Monitor hinge screws and movable parts for loosening and excessive wear. Replacement straps and frame liners are available for many brace designs.

---

### Clinical Application Question 3

A metal fabricator returns to work following surgery and rehabilitation of the right knee. The surgeon has placed her in a custom-made functional knee brace for all work activities. During the past week in the afternoons, the brace gradually migrates distally.

➡ **Question: What can you do to prevent the migration?**

---

### ...IF/THEN...

**IF** a brace is no longer needed by a patient to provide protection, support, and/or immobilization, **THEN** wash and retain the brace for use in the future or use for spare parts as recommended by the manufacturer.

---

## PADS

Pads are used to provide protection from injury or further injury for the patient. Many sports require padding during play. Padding techniques range from a simple piece of felt or foam to advanced protective gear such as a football helmet.

## Types

Pads are categorized into two basic types: pads made of soft, low density materials and those of hard, high density materials[8] (Fig. 1–9). Soft, low-density materials are light and comfortable on the body because of the presence of air in the material. These materials protect the patient from impact forces only at low-intensity levels. By contrast, hard, high-density materials are less comfortable on the body but protect the patient from forces at high-impact levels. These materials have the

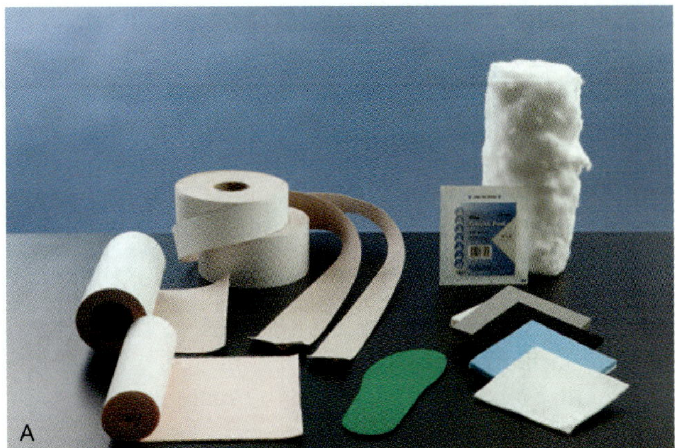

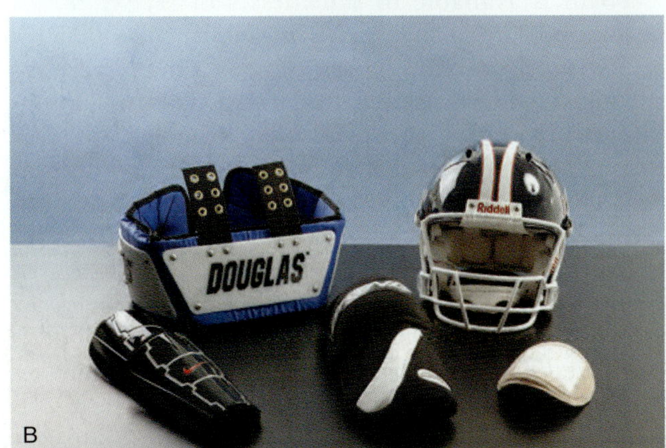


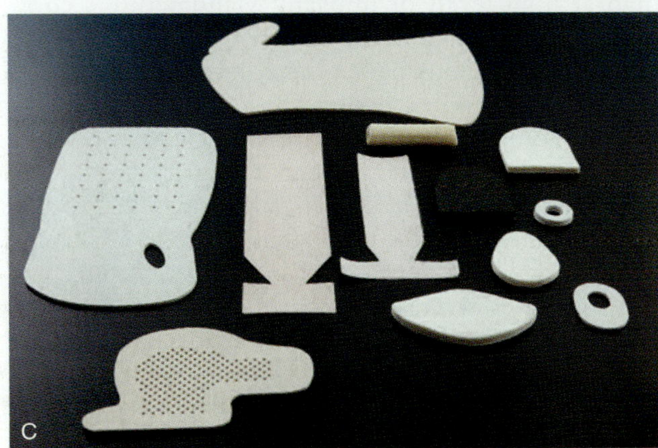

**Fig. 1–9 A** *Variety of soft, low-density pads.* **B** *Variety of hard, high-density pads.* **C** *Variety of pre-cut and pre-formed pads.*

ability to absorb energy through deformation, resulting in less force at the area of impact.

### *Soft, Low-Density Pads*

Soft, low-density materials used by health care professionals include cotton, gauze, moleskin, felt, foam, and viscoelastic polymers. These materials come in a variety of lengths, widths, and thicknesses (see Fig. 1–9A). Cotton is found in most facilities and is used to provide a mild padding effect.[7] Apply gauze in various thicknesses to lessen friction or impact forces. Use adhesive gauze material in 2, 4, and 6 inch widths and 2 and 10 yard lengths to lessen friction, cover wound dressings, and attach pads to the body. Moleskin is available in heavyweight and lightweight elastic and non-elastic designs in 1, 1½, 2, 3, 7, 9, and 12 inch widths by 1, 4, 5, and 25 yard lengths. Use the material on high-friction areas to lessen the chance of skin irritations. Moleskin may also be used with many taping techniques to provide additional support. Made from matted wool and rayon fibers, felt comes in thicknesses of ⅟16, ⅛, ¼, and ½ inch sheets and 36–108 inch rolls. Many types are available, with and without an adhesive backing, to provide support, protection, and compression. Felt has absorbent properties that allow the material to remain in place during activity.

Foam is available in thicknesses of ⅛, ¼, ⅜, ½, ⅝, ¾, and 1 inch sheets and 36–108 inch rolls, with and without an adhesive backing. Foam is perhaps the most widely used material for padding. Foam material that allows air to transfer from cell to cell is referred to as **open-cell foam**. These foams deform or compress quickly as stress is applied, providing minimal shock-absorbing qualities.[8] Open-cell foam is commonly used as a liner in the construction of custom-made pads. **Closed-cell foam** does not allow transfer of air from cell to cell. These foams are not as comfortable on the body, but the material regains its original shape quickly following impact. Closed-cell foams provide less cushioning at low levels of impact than at high levels of impact.[8] Manufacturers combine both open- and closed-cell foams in the construction of various pads. These padding techniques will be discussed in Chapter 13.

Thermomoldable foams are materials that allow custom-fitting to the patient for protection. The material is available in sheets of ⅟16, ¼, ⅜, ½, and ⅝ inch thicknesses. Heat the material first in a conventional oven and then fit to a body part. After cooling, the material retains its shape and can be reheated and remolded if necessary. These foams can be used anywhere on the body, especially as outer padding of rigid casts.

Viscoelastic polymers, used in the design of inner soles, protect against pressure and friction forces. Some of these insoles have an adhesive backing to reduce migration during activity. Use viscoelastic polymers to prevent and treat a variety of injuries and conditions.

### *Hard, High-Density Pads*

Hard, high-density pads are constructed from polycarbonate, plastic, thermoplastic, and casting materials (see Fig. 1–9B). Polycarbonate materials are used in many helmet designs for construction of the outer shell. Off-the-shelf padding designs, such as shoulder pads, use high-density plastics for the outer shell. All of these materials are available in off-the-shelf designs or can be used for custom-made padding techniques.

For custom-made pads, purchase thermoplastic materials made from plastic or rubber with varying amounts of conformability and resistance in thicknesses of ⅟16, ³⁄32, ⅛, and ³⁄16 inch sheets. Heat these materials at temperatures ranging from 150° to 170°F for 35 seconds to 1 minute for the materials to become pliable for molding to the body part. Use heating sources such as water, a conventional or microwave oven, or a heat gun. The most commonly used source of heat is a hydrocollator. Professionals have between 1 and 5 minutes to mold and shape the material before the thermoplastic cools and becomes rigid. The materials used in the manufacturing process and the material's thickness will affect heating and molding times. Use thermoplastics to protect, support, and splint multiple areas of the body.

Casting materials made from fiberglass or plaster can also be used to protect, support, and splint various areas of the body. Fiberglass material is preferred over plaster by most health care professionals because of the ease of use and less clean-up time required.

Many soft, low-density and hard, high-density pads come in off-the-shelf designs. Moleskin, felt, foam, viscoelastic polymers, and thermoplastic materials are available in pre-cut and pre-formed designs (see Fig. 1–9C). For example, moleskin plantar fascia and turf toe straps, felt heel lifts and arch pads, foam blister and corn pads, viscoelastic polymer orthotics, and thermoplastic thumb spica and wrist cock-up splints are available from manufacturers in a variety of sizes and thicknesses. These pre-cut and pre-formed materials can lessen application and fabrication time and perhaps eliminate wasted materials.

## Resilience

The resilience of soft and hard materials will determine their ability to withstand impact forces.[8] Following impact, highly resilient materials regain their shape. Use these materials over body areas that receive frequent impact. Slow-recovery, nonresilient materials provide optimal protection and are usable over body areas that receive sporadic impact.

## Objectives of Padding

Use padding techniques to:

- Provide support and protection when preventing injuries
- Provide support and protection when treating and rehabilitating existing injuries
- Provide compression to reduce effusion and swelling when treating and rehabilitating injuries

## Recommendations for Pad Application

The following recommendations will assist in applying padding techniques.

### *Preparation of the Patient*

Because most padding techniques require tapes and/or wraps to secure pads to the body, preparation of the patient should follow the guidelines for taping and wrapping applications.

### *Application of Pads*

Off-the-shelf and custom-made pads may be attached to the body with a variety of methods. The three techniques discussed briefly here are covered in more detail in later chapters. When tape is used, pads are placed over pre-wrap or self-adherent wrap. Elastic tape is used to anchor the pad to the body part in a circular or spiral pattern (see Fig. 9–12). Non-elastic tape may be applied loosely around the pad as an anchor. Elastic wraps are also used to apply pads (see Fig. 8–14). The size of the pad and body part involved will determine the width and length of the wrap. Elastic tape is used to anchor the wrap. With some techniques, apply pads directly to the skin (see Fig. 8–10). The use of adherent tape spray and heavyweight elastic tape lessens migration or slippage of the pad during activity. Exercise care with applying tape directly to the skin daily as allergic reactions and trauma to the skin can occur.

### *Custom-Made Pads* 

Custom-made pad designs may be constructed for a variety of body areas. Begin the designs with a paper pattern to avoid wasting materials (Fig. 1–10).

Some manufacturers include paper patterns with the materials to assist with construction. Pads may also be designed by outlining the body part directly on the material, then cutting the material with taping scissors. For example, position a patient on a piece of felt or foam to outline the foot.

Construction of a custom-made thermoplastic pad requires several types of materials and equipment (Fig. 1–11). Select the appropriate thermoplastic material based on conformability, resistance, and thickness. Use soft, low-density foam to line the inside of the pad. Additional equipment includes taping scissors, a heating source, 1 inch or 1½ inch non-elastic tape, 2 inch or 3 inch elastic tape, an elastic wrap, ¼ inch or ½ inch felt, and rubber cement.

---

**… IF/THEN …**

**IF** mistakes are made in the design and/or construction of custom-made, thermoplastic material pads, causing an irregular fit, **THEN** save the materials in order to use them again, potentially in the design of another pad.

---

### *Mandatory Padding*

The NCAA[11] and NFHS[12] have rules that govern the use of mandatory injury prevention and injury protection padding for practices and competitions. Sports that require the use of mandatory protective equipment include baseball, fencing, field hockey, football, ice hockey, lacrosse, rifle, soccer, skiing, softball, track and field (padding on pole vault box), water polo, and wrestling. Currently, basketball, gymnastics, swimming and diving, and volleyball do not have rules regarding mandatory protective equipment. Chapter 13 provides a more in-depth examination of protective equipment.

Rules[11,12] governing protective pads prohibit the use of fiberglass, plaster, metal, or other nonpliable materials unless they are covered by closed-cell, slow-recovery foam or similar material of at least ½ inch thickness. Moreover, these hard, unyielding materials may be used to protect an existing injury only. Written verification from a physician may be required. Protective pads cannot create a hazard for the athlete or his or her opponent. The on-site referee or official has the authority to judge whether the protective pad is allowed for use in competition. Seek out the referee or official prior to the start of the competition to obtain approval of the pad. That way, if the pad is found unacceptable, there is time available to make the necessary changes before the competition.

**STEP 1:**    Cover the area to be padded with paper (see Fig. 1–10A).

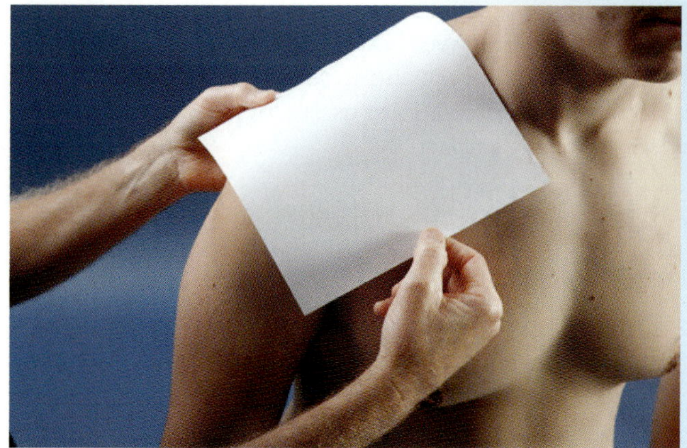

Fig. 1–10 A

**STEP 2:**    Draw, cut, and shape the pattern based on the objectives of the technique (see Fig. 1–10B).

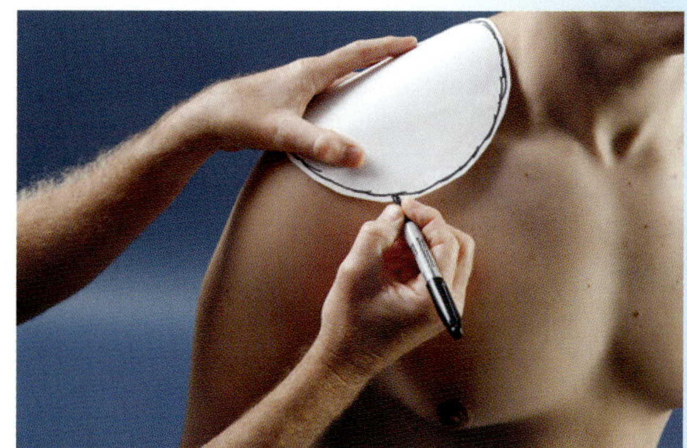

Fig. 1–10 B

**STEP 3:**    Lay the paper on the padding material and outline the pattern with a felt tip pen (see Fig. 1–10C).

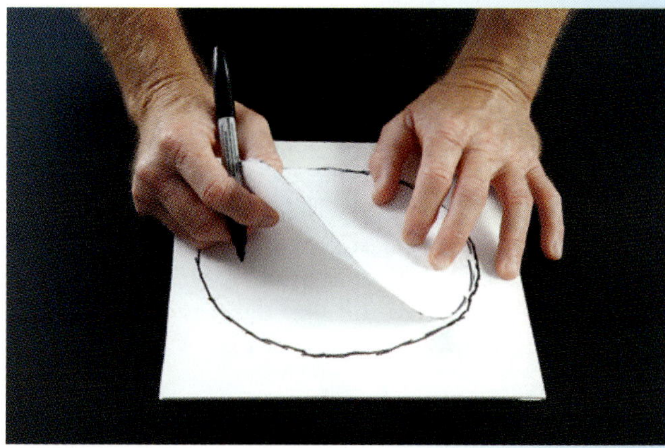

Fig. 1–10 C

**STEP 1:**  Cut a piece of ¼ inch or ½ inch felt slightly larger than the injured area (see Fig. 1–11A).

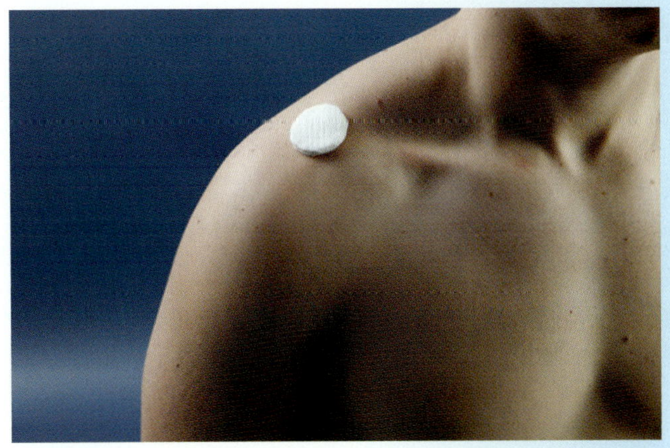

**Fig. 1–11 A**

**STEP 2:**  Attach the felt directly to the skin over the injured area with a strip of non-elastic tape (see Fig. 1–11B).

If no paper pattern is available, construct the design of the pad. Using the paper pattern, cut a piece of thermoplastic material. With partial heating of the material, cutting is made easier. Heat the material following the manufacturer's instructions. If using water as the heating source, remove the material when heated and place it on a towel to remove excess water.

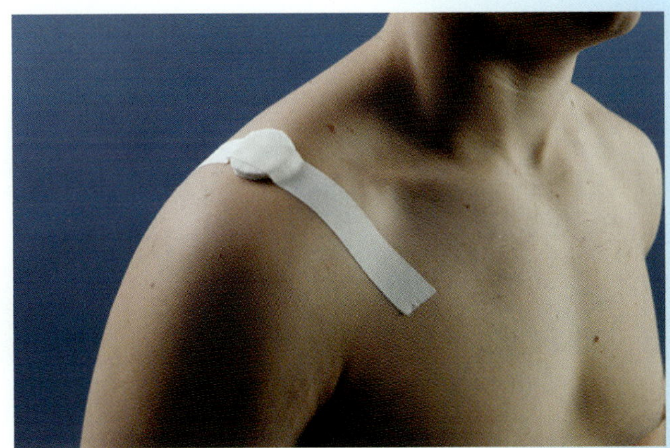

**Fig. 1–11 B**

**STEP 3:**  Apply the pliable thermoplastic material to the body part over the felt pad and lightly mold the material around the contours and felt pad with the hands (see Fig. 1–11C).

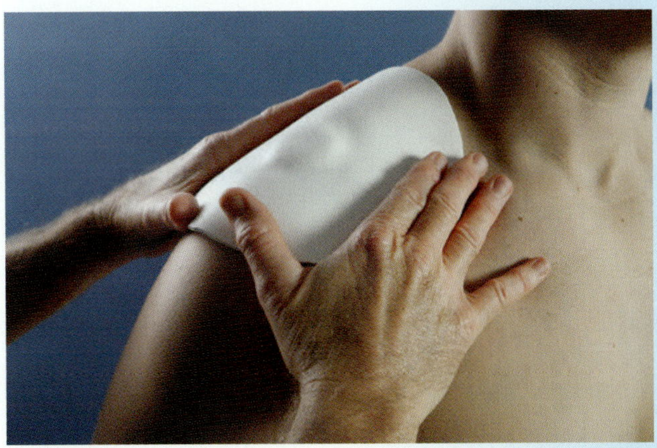

**Fig. 1–11 C**

*Steps Cont.*

**STEP 4:** Apply an elastic wrap in a circular or spiral pattern over the body part and thermoplastic material to assist with molding (see Fig. 1–11D).

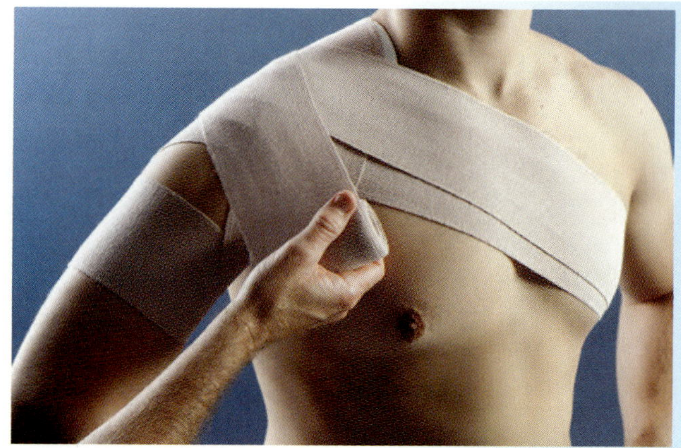

**Fig. 1–11 D**

**STEP 5:** Continue to mold the material to the body with the hands (see Fig. 1–11E).
Pay attention to the recommended amount of time available before the material cools. Apply an ice bag or pack over the material to decrease the cooling time.

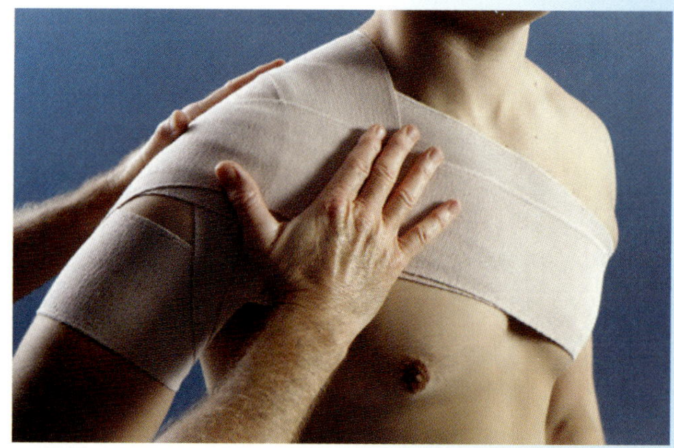

**Fig. 1–11 E**

**STEP 6:** After the material cools, carefully remove the elastic wrap. Inspect the thermoplastic material to ensure proper shape and contour before removing. Use a felt tip pen to mark on the material any areas that require trimming (see Fig. 1–11F).

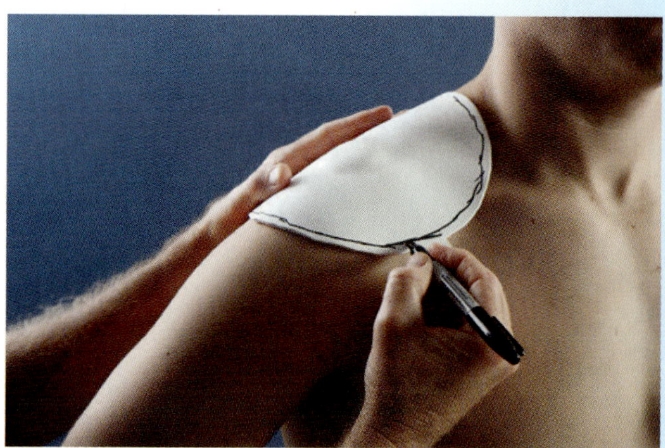

**Fig. 1–11 F**

**STEP 7:** Remove the thermoplastic material and felt from the body part. Trim the material with taping scissors to remove sharp edges (see Fig. 1–11G). Place the material once again on the body part to make certain of the fit. Additional trimming may be necessary.

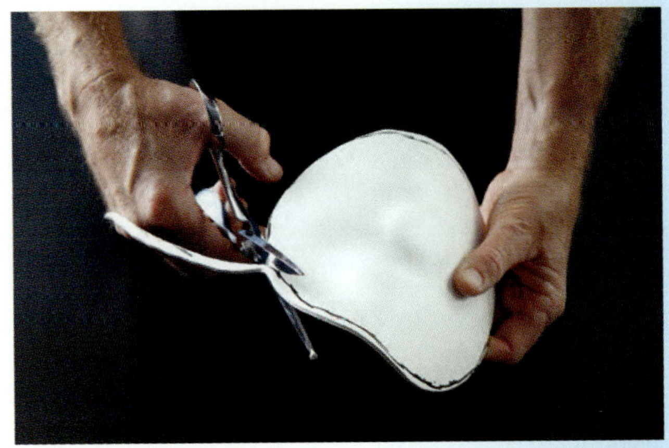

**Fig. 1–11 G**

**STEP 8:** Completely dry the inside surface of the thermoplastic material. Place the thermoplastic material on soft, low-density foam and outline an area ½ inch larger than the material (see Fig. 1–11H). Cut the piece of foam.

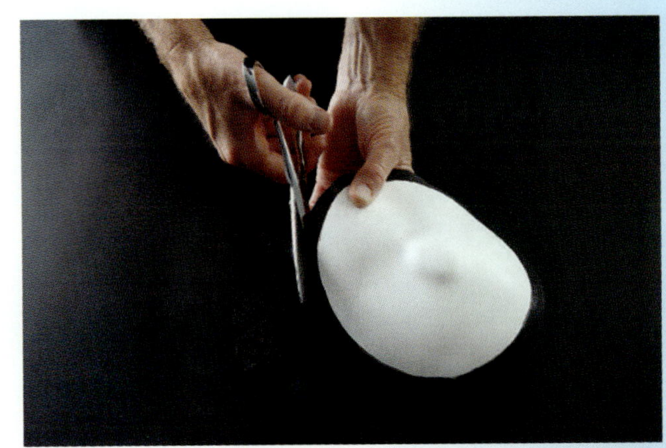

**Fig. 1–11 H**

**STEP 9:** If using adhesive foam, remove the backing and attach the foam to the inside surface of the thermoplastic material. Otherwise, apply rubber cement or another non-toxic cement on the inside surface of the thermoplastic material and on the foam side that will be in contact with the material. When the cement is ready, attach the foam to the inside surface of the material (see Fig. 1–11I). The foam should extend ½ inch from each side of the thermoplastic material. This extra padding prevents irritation and possible injury from the semirigid thermoplastic material.

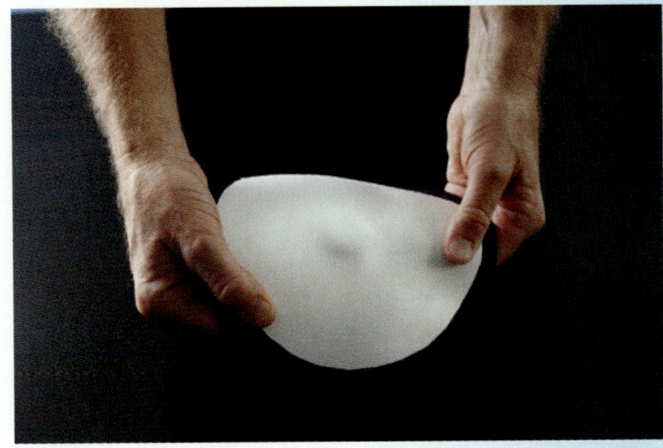

**Fig. 1–11 I**

*Steps Cont.*

**STEP 10:**  Use taping scissors to cut the foam away from the raised area shaped by the felt pad (see Fig. 1–11J). This raised area will disperse the impact force away from the injured area to the outer edges of the pad, preventing further damage.

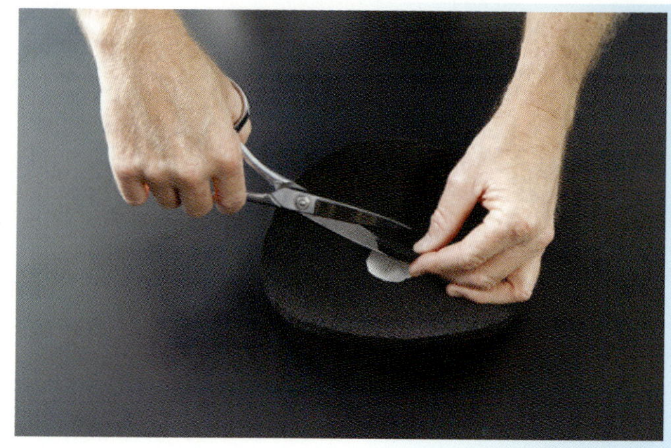

Fig. 1–11 J

**STEP 11:**  Cut strips of elastic tape to line the edges of the pad. Place strips on the top edges of the pad in a square pattern, then on the bottom edges (see Fig. 1–11K).

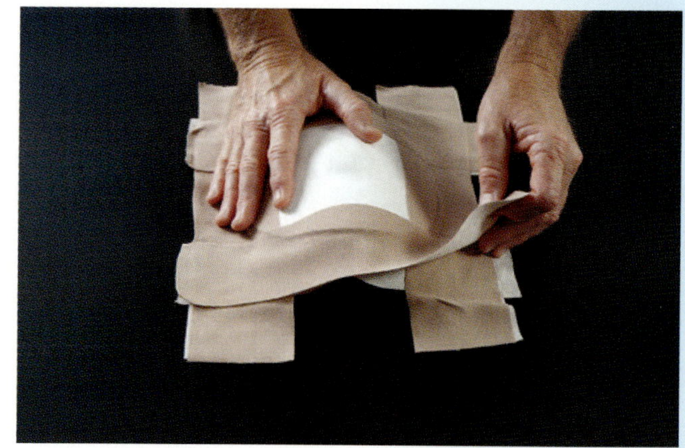

Fig. 1–11 K

**STEP 12:**  The tape strips should be applied on the thermoplastic material and extend beyond the foam by at least ¼ inch (see Fig. 1–11L). Use the fingers to adhere the top and bottom tape strips together.

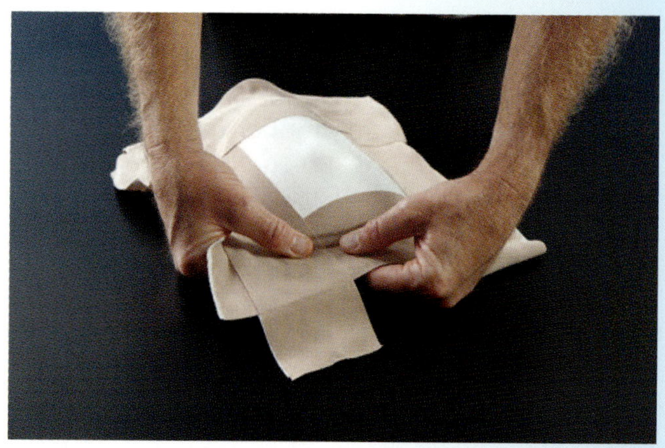

Fig. 1–11 L

**STEP 13:** Trim the edges of the tape around the pad to provide a uniform edge, leaving enough of the tape to maintain adherence (see Fig. 1–11M). The elastic tape prevents separation of the foam from the thermoplastic material following repeated use.

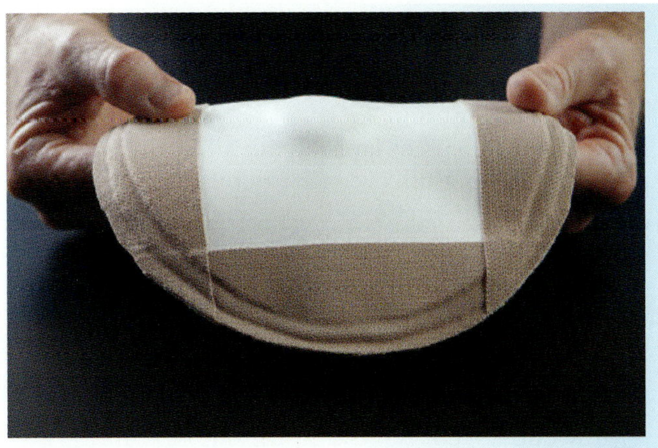

**Fig. 1–11 M**



### *Removal of Pads*

The removal of mandatory protective equipment is typically done by the athlete following use, although custom-made pads secured to the body part with tape or an elastic wrap may require assistance for removal. Use taping scissors or tape cutters to cut pads secured with tape. Unwrap elastic wraps and reuse them. Remove pads applied directly to the skin with tape as described earlier. Moleskin adheres to the skin more tightly than other materials, especially when used on weight-bearing surfaces of the body. Use particular caution when removing moleskin from the plantar surfaces of the feet. Remove moleskin in the same manner as tape. Using a tape removal solvent may prove helpful.

---

**Clinical Application Question 4**

The starting right offensive tackle on your football team has a second-degree **ulnar collateral ligament** sprain of the left thumb. Your team physician will allow him to return to play if the player is placed in a semirigid thumb spica cast.

➡ **Question: What should you do to meet NCAA and NFHS rules?**

---

## STICKING POINTS

This information focuses on "what not to do" or "things to watch out for" when applying taping, wrapping, bracing, and padding techniques. Use these pointers to avoid common mistakes.

## Tapes

- Always overlap tape by ½ of the width to avoid gaps and inconsistent layering.
  - Gaps between strips of tape can pinch the underlying skin and result in a blister or laceration. These wounds are referred to as tape cuts.
  - Inconsistent layering can allow the underlying skin to bulge through the tape and cause a blister or laceration. Generally, the application of at least two layers of tape is sufficient.
- Avoid wrinkles in the layer of tape that is applied next to the skin.
  - Wrinkles in the tape can increase the amount of tension over a small area of the skin and result in a blister or laceration.
- When applying tape, focus attention on the correct angles of application.
  - Application angles must follow the contours of the body to prevent constriction of soft tissue or abnormal restriction of range of motion.
- Continually monitor roll tension during application. Students often ask, "How tight does the tape need to be?" The finished technique should fit snugly to the body part and be comfortable to the patient given the objectives of the technique. For example, while the correct application of the elbow **hyperextension** taping technique will limit elbow extension, the elastic tape anchor placed around the proximal upper arm may cause mild constriction of the biceps.

Tapes, Wraps, Braces, and Pads

# Wraps

- Similar to tape, overlap wraps to avoid gaps and inconsistent layering.
- Gaps or inconsistent layering can affect the mechanical pressure over the injured area. As a result, swelling or effusion can accumulate in these areas, lessening the effectiveness of the technique.

# Braces

- Closely follow the manufacturer's instructions when applying braces.
  - The omission or reversal of just one step in the application process may alter the intended purpose or fit of the brace. For example, improperly applying a functional knee brace may allow range of motion beyond the limits of the healing process, possibly predisposing the patient to further injury.

- Use caution when making adjustments or alterations to braces.
  - Cutting or repositioning straps, applying tape anchors, or trimming the brace shell may affect the structural design of the brace. Consult the brace manufacturer if questions arise.

# Pads

- Use appropriate materials in the design and construction of protective pads. Select the materials based on the density, resiliency, and thickness.
  - Padding of the **acromioclavicular (AC) joint** following a sprain or **contusion** requires several types of materials. Construct the outer shell from hard, high-density thermoplastic material and line the inside of the pad with low-density foam. Using only low-density foam will not provide effective protection from high-impact forces.

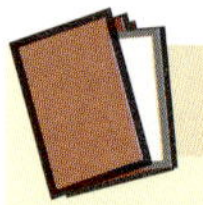

## EVIDENCE-BASED PRACTICE

As discussed in the chapter, evidence-based practice (EBP) is a five step process undertaken to incorporate the best evidence; expertise of the clinician; and patient goals, values, and preferences into clinical decisions for patients. Understanding and practicing with the steps is necessary to effectively implement your findings into clinical practice. Use this activity with your faculty and clinical preceptor to develop the knowledge and skills of EBP. At the conclusion of later chapters, "Evidence-Based Practice" activities will present a clinical case and provide the opportunity to further develop your skills in the EBP process.

The steps of EBP are (1) developing clinically relevant questions, (2) searching for the best evidence, (3) evaluating and appraising the evidence, (4) implementing the evidence into clinical practice with patients, and (5) evaluating the effects of interventions on patient outcomes.

### Clinical Question

The first step in the EBP process is developing a relevant clinical question in the PICO format to answer. At the clinical site, closely observe the taping, wrapping, bracing, and padding techniques used and applied to the athlete and patient population. Ask yourself questions such as "Which technique is the most effective to prevent inversion ankle sprains?" "Are neoprene knee sleeves beneficial for meniscal tears?" "What is the best way to protect an AC joint sprain?" or "How can I provide support to the MCP joint of an athlete with

allergies to adhesive tape and neoprene?" Develop three to five clinically relevant questions in the PICO format using these examples or specific situations or questions at the clinical site. The questions must include the patient population or problem, the intervention, a comparison intervention (if relevant), and the clinical outcome of interest. For example, "Do lateral strap braces reduce pain in racquetball players with chronic lateral epicondylitis?" Seek assistance from your faculty and clinical preceptor in the development of the questions.

### Searching for Evidence

Find the answer to the clinically relevant question by searching for the best available evidence. Choose one of the clinical questions formulated at the clinical site and develop a search strategy with assistance of your faculty and/or library staff. Based on the clinical question, the strategy should include search terms, search limitations, and electronic databases and online and print journals to search. Using the clinical question example, "Do lateral strap braces reduce pain in racquetball players with chronic lateral epicondylitis?," search terms could include lateral epicondylitis, elbow strap braces, and pain reduction. Search limitations could include randomized controlled trials, age restrictions in study participants to match your patient population, and studies published in the last 3 to 5 years. Databases and journals are those most relevant and accessible to retrieve quality evidence to answer the clinical question. Use the strategy and perform the search. The results of the search can be varied, producing numerous or limited findings. And remember, evidence from expert opinion or clinical experience occasionally guides clinical decisions. Develop a list of retrieved citations, abstracts, and articles and thoroughly review each to determine those most relevant to the clinical question. After this review, obtain full text articles of the studies and reviews selected.

### Evaluating the Evidence

A critical appraisal is needed to determine the value of the evidence to clinical practice. Choose three studies from the search and evaluate each with these questions, "Are the results of the study valid?" For example, Were the patients randomized? Was the study blinded? Was there a complete follow-up? "What are the actual results?" For example, What was the treatment effect? Were the results similar across studies? What is the clinical and/or statistical significance of the results? "Are the findings clinically relevant to my patients?" For example, Were the study participants similar to my patient population? Is the intervention cost-effective? Will my patients benefit from the intervention? Seek assistance from your faculty as this step requires the most judgment and experience in the EBP process. Prepare a summary of the answers to the questions for each study. Synthesize the study findings and appraisal to determine the implications for clinical practice.

### Implementing the Evidence

Following the appraisal, you must determine whether and how the evidence is implemented into the clinical situation. Involve your faculty and clinical preceptor and critically examine and integrate the available evidence, your clinical experience, and the patient goals, values, and preferences to determine the clinical course of action at the clinical site. For example, a new taping, wrapping, bracing, or padding technique is supported by evidence, but the subjects in the studies do not match your patient population for age and physical conditioning; as a result, the new technique is not implemented and other interventions are considered. In another clinical situation, a taping, wrapping, bracing, or padding technique not previously studied continues to be used with patients based on the past experiences of the clinician and successful patient outcomes.

### Evaluating the Outcomes

The last step in the EBP process is evaluating the effects of interventions on patient outcomes. For example, how well did the EBP process work? Was the clinical question answered? Did the search produce quality evidence and was the evidence critically appraised? Did the integration of the available evidence, clinician expertise, and patient goals and preferences produce a rational clinical decision? Did the clinical decision result in successful outcomes for the patient(s)? What was your experience with the EBP process? Use these questions and develop others specific to the patient(s) in the clinical site. Develop answers to each question, evaluating your performance and the clinical outcomes. Involve your faculty and clinical preceptor in a discussion of the answers and how EBP can enhance your skills for improved patient care.

---

### WRAP-UP

- The best available evidence, clinician expertise, and patient goals and values should guide clinical decisions for patient care.
- Apply non-elastic, elastic, and cast tapes to support and reduce range of motion, and secure wraps, pads, and dressings.
- Tapes are torn manually or cut with taping scissors.
- Tapes are commonly applied directly to the skin or over pre-wrap, self-adherent wrap, or cast padding.
- Remove tape from the body manually or with taping scissors or cutting tools.
- Use wraps to provide compression and support, reduce range of motion, and secure pads and dressings.
- Several methods may be used to prevent migration, slippage, or bunching of wraps.
- Wraps are rolled onto the body and removed by unwrapping or cutting.
- Off-the-shelf and custom-made braces provide support, protection, and compression, and control range of motion.
- Follow the manufacturer's step-by-step procedures when applying braces.
- Soft, low-density and hard, high-density padding materials provide support, protection, and compression.
- Pads may be applied to the body in a variety of methods.
- NCAA and NFHS rules mandate padding of all exposed nonpliable materials for practices and competitions.

Tapes, Wraps, Braces, and Pads

- Before applying tapes, wraps, braces, and pads, clean and dry the skin of the patient, then position the body part according to the technique objective.
- Overlap tapes and wraps and avoid gaps, wrinkles, and inconsistent roll tension during application.

## WEB REFERENCES

### Active Ankle Systems
http://www.activeankle.com
- This website is an online catalog for the brace manufacturer and provides injury prevention and care, fitting, and ordering information.

### Andover
https://andoverhealthcare.com/sports-medicine-products/
- This site provides information about a variety of tapes and self-adherent wraps, presentations, and demonstrations, as well as resources for college professors and students.

### Breg
http://www.breg.com
- This website is an online catalog for the manufacturer and provides sizing information on prophylactic, rehabilitative, and functional braces.

### BSN Medical
http://www.bsnmedical.com/
- This site allows you access to information on tapes, wraps, braces, pads, and wound care products.

### DJO
http://www.djoglobal.com/
- This site is an online catalog for the manufacturer and provides research and development and fitting information about prophylactic, rehabilitative, and functional braces, and pads.

### Hartmann
https://hartmann.info/en-US
- This website is an online catalog for the manufacturer and provides information about a variety of tapes, wraps, braces, pads, and wound care products.

### Henry Schein
https://www.henryschein.com/us-en/medical/default.aspx?did=medical&stay=1
- This site is an online catalog for sports medicine products, including tapes, wraps, braces, and pads.

### Johnson & Johnson
http://www.jnj.com/
- This site provides access to information on tapes, wraps, pads, and wound care products and educational resources for patients and students.

### Medco
http://www.medco-athletics.com/
- This website is an online catalog for sports medicine products, including tapes, wraps, braces, and pads.

### MedSpec
http://www.medspec.com
- This site is an online catalog for the brace manufacturer and provides fitting and ordering information.

### Sports Health
http://www.sportshealth.com/
- This website is an online catalog for sports medicine products and provides fitting and ordering information and educational materials and resources.

### 3M
http://www.3m.com
- This site provides access to information on tapes, wraps, pads, and wound care products and educational materials and resources.

### Ultra Ankle
http://www.ultraankle.com
- This website is an online catalog for the brace manufacturer and provides fitting and ordering information.

## FURTHER READING

### Additional Information on Evidence-Based Medicine
- Straus, SE, Glasziou, P, Richardson, WS, and Haynes, RB: Evidence-Based Medicine: How to Practice and Teach It, ed 4. Elsevier Churchill Livingstone, Philadelphia, 2011.
- Greenhalgh, T: How to Read a Paper: The Basics of Evidence-Based Medicine, ed 5. BMJ Books, UK, 2014.
- Duke University Medical Center Library & Archives, Evidence-Based Practice, http://guides.mclibrary.duke.edu/ebm

### Additional Information on Rating Scales
- Ebell, MH, Siwek, J, Weiss, BD, Woolf, SH, Susman, J, Ewigman, B, and Bowman, M: Strength of recommendation taxonomy (SORT): A patient-centered approach to grading evidence in the medical literature. Am Fam Physician 69:548–556, 2004.
- Jadad, AR, Cook, DJ, Jones, A, Klassen, TP, Tugwell, P, Moher, M, and Moher, D: Methodology and reports of systematic reviews and meta-analyses. JAMA 280:278–280, 1998.
- Moher, D, Cook, DJ, Jadad, AR, Tugwell, P, Moher, M, Jones, A, Pham, B, and Klassen, TP: Assessing the quality of reports of randomized trials: Implications for the conduct of meta-analyses. Health Technol Assess 3:i–iv, 1999.
- Jadad, AR, Moher, D, and Klassen, TP: Guides for reading and interpreting systematic reviews, II: How did the authors find the studies and assess

their quality? Arch Pediatr Adolesc Med 152:812–817, 1998.

### Additional Information on Outcomes Assessment

- Snyder, AR, Parsons, JT, Valovich McLeod, TC, Bay, RC, Michener, LA, and Sauers, EL: Using disablement models and clinical outcomes assessment to enable evidence-based athletic training practice, part I: Disablement models. J Athl Train 43:428–436, 2008.
- Valovich McLeod, TC, Snyder, AR, Parsons, JT, Bay, RC, Michener, LA, and Sauers, EL: Using disablement models and clinical outcomes assessment to enable evidence-based athletic training practice, part II: Clinical outcomes assessment. J Athl Train 43:437–445, 2008.

Beam, JW, Buckley, B, Holcomb, W, and Ciocca, M: National Athletic Trainers' Association position statement: Management of acute skin trauma. J Athl Train 51:1053–1070, 2016.

## REFERENCES


1. Sackett, DL, Rosenberg, WM, Gray, JA, Haynes, RB, and Richardson, WS: Evidence based medicine: What it is and what it isn't. BMJ 312:71–72, 1996.
2. Steves, R, and Hootman, JM: Evidence-based medicine: What is it and how does it apply to athletic training? J Athl Train 39:83–87, 2004.
3. Fineout-Overholt, E, Melnyk, BM, and Schultz, A: Transforming health care from the inside out: Advancing evidence-based practice in the 21st century. J Prof Nurs 21:335–344, 2005.
4. Straus, SE, and Sackett, DL: Using research findings in clinical practice. BMJ 317:339–342, 1998.
5. Centre for Evidence-Based Medicine: Asking focused questions. https://www.cebm.net/2014/06/asking-focused-questions/, 2018.
6. Bragg, RW, Macmahon, JM, Overom, EK, Yerby, SA, Matheson, GO, Carter, DR, and Andriacchi, TP: Failure and fatigue characteristics of adhesive athletic tape. Med Sci Sports Exerc 34:403–410, 2002.
7. Prentice, WE: Principles of Athletic Training: A Guide to Evidence-Based Clinical Practice, ed 16. McGraw-Hill, New York, 2017.
8. Anderson, MK: Foundations of Athletic Training: Prevention, Assessment, and Management, ed 6. Wolters Kluwer, Philadelphia, 2017.
9. Wilkerson, GB: Biomechanical and neuromuscular effects of ankle taping and bracing. J Athl Train 37:436–445, 2002.
10. Fleming, BC, Renstrom, PA, Beynnon, BD, Engstrom, B, and Peura, G: The influence of functional knee bracing on the anterior cruciate ligament strain biomechanics in weightbearing and nonweightbearing knees. Am J Sports Med 28:815–824, 2000.
11. National Collegiate Athletic Association: 2014–15 Sports Medicine Handbook, ed 25. NCAA, Indianapolis, 2014. http://www.ncaapublications.com/productdownloads/MD15.pdf.
12. National Federation of State High School Associations: 2018 Football Rules Book. National Federation of State High School Associations, Indianapolis, IN, 2019.

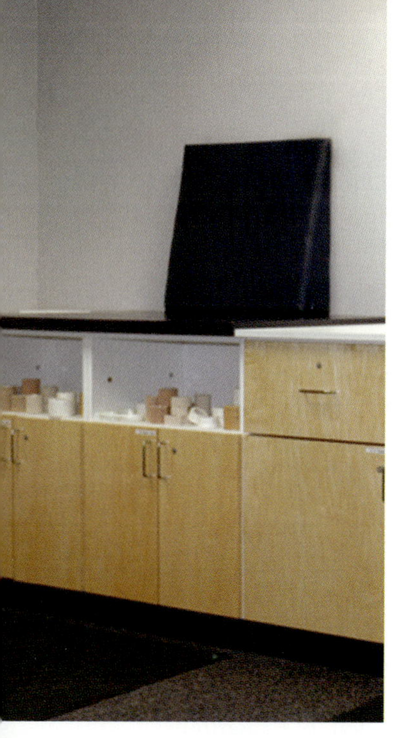

# 2

# Facility Design for Taping, Wrapping, Bracing, and Padding



In a health care facility, the space designated for taping, wrapping, bracing, and padding techniques should receive careful consideration. Whether the space is developed within new or existing structures, several design aspects need to be addressed. In scholastic, intercollegiate, and professional sport facilities, this space is commonly referred to as the **taping area**. Other health care facilities, such as clinics, typically do not have dedicated space for a taping area because of a lower patient demand for technique application. For our discussion, **application area** will refer to the facility space dedicated to taping, wrapping, bracing, and padding techniques.

The design of the application area should be based on evidence-based practice, specifically ergonomic principles. Ergonomics is defined by *Taber's Cyclopedic Medical Dictionary* (p. 837)[1] as "the science concerned with fitting a job to a person's anatomical, physiological, and psychological characteristics in a way that enhances human efficiency and well-being." Health care professionals who are responsible for applying taping, wrapping, bracing, and padding techniques come in many different sizes and shapes. Accordingly, spaces and tables should be designed to accommodate these differences. The goal of ergonomics is to provide an efficient, healthful, and safe working environment. This goal can be achieved with careful planning of new facility construction or existing facility renovations.

Planning for new construction or renovation of a facility's application area should also direct thought to current and future program needs as well as structural considerations. Program needs, such as the number of patients requiring daily technique application, available time and staff, and long-range plans, will assist in deciding on furniture and space. Application areas in scholastic, intercollegiate, and professional sport facilities are typically the most congested spaces, especially during peak periods prior to practices and competitions. Application areas in these facilities should be located close to an entrance and exit for easy access. The time available to complete taping, wrapping, bracing, and padding techniques is often influenced by predetermined practice, competition, and appointment schedules. Note that adequate staffing of health care professionals who are proficient in applying the techniques is also an important consideration.

After determining current needs, attempt to make long-range projections based on the organization's strategic plan, such as future renovations to the facility or the addition of staff or sport teams. As interest in the health care of the active population continues to grow, the space required to apply taping, wrapping, bracing, and padding techniques will also increase.

After assessing program needs, consider structural needs in the application area. Structural factors include table design; storage areas; benches; seating; floor, wall, and ceiling coverings; and the design of electrical, plumbing, ventilation, and lighting systems.

## TABLES/BENCHES

Tables and benches used in the application area can be purchased or constructed in a variety of sizes and shapes to accommodate individual differences and space restrictions (Fig. 2–1).

- Use multiple individual tables or benches in areas without space constraints (see Fig. 2–1A).
- Use custom-made tables or benches in areas with irregular or limited spaces to fit into corners between walls or as an island around a support beam in a multi-floor facility (see Fig. 2–1B).

When applying ergonomic principles, vary the height of the tables and benches between 30 and 40 inches to accommodate the different heights of health care professionals and positions of patients. Some taping, wrapping, bracing, and padding techniques require the patient to be placed in a seated position, while other techniques mandate a standing position on a table or bench. Vary the width of the tables and benches between 2 and 3 feet with individual and custom-made designs. The table and bench tops should be constructed of durable, easy-to-clean material such as Formica. Many facilities use vinyl material with padding for added comfort.

### ... IF/THEN ...

**IF** individual table heights need to be adjusted to accommodate different heights of a staff, **THEN** consider placing wood blocks or boards underneath the legs or table to form a stable base for the desired height.

An important feature to include with tables and benches is storage space for taping, wrapping, bracing, and padding supplies (Fig. 2–2).

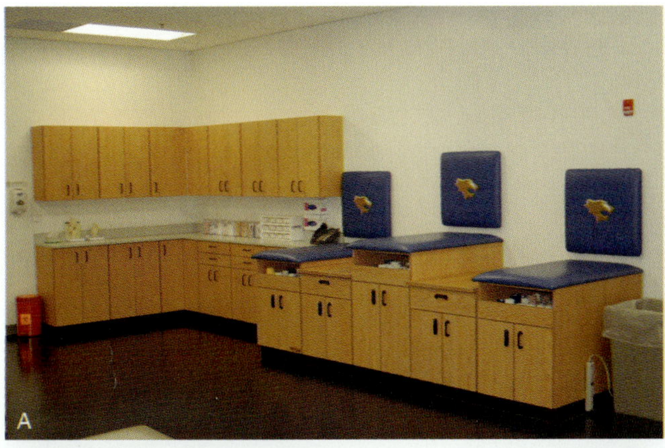

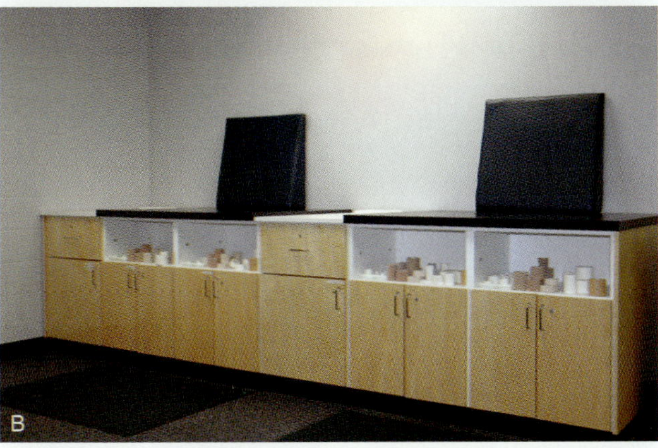

**Fig. 2–1 A** *Multiple taping tables in an athletic training facility. (Courtesy of Georgian Court University, Lakewood, NJ, and Hausmann Industries, Northvale, NJ.).* **B** *Custom-made taping bench positioned between two walls.*

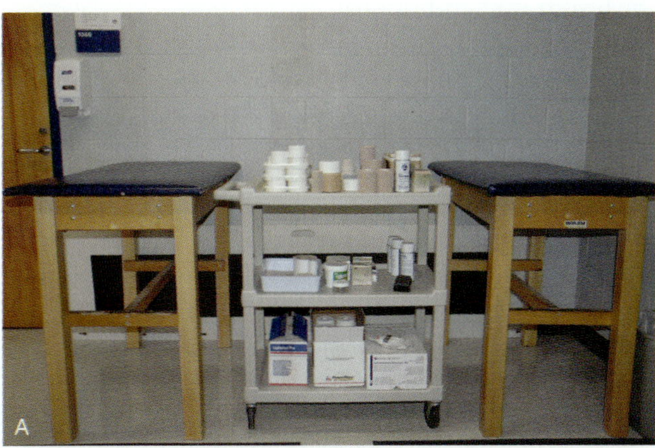

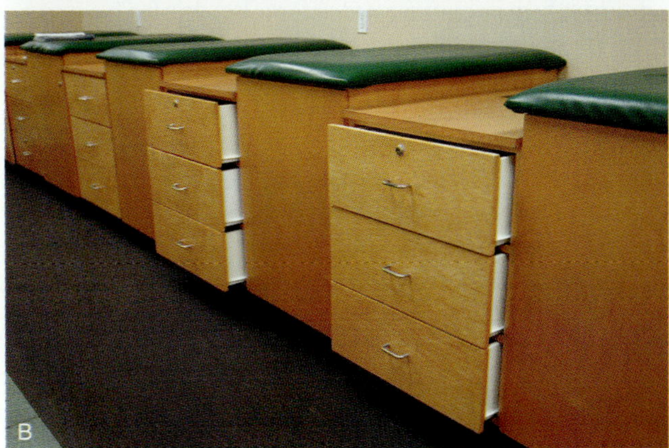

**Fig. 2–2 A** *Cart positioned between two individual taping tables.* **B** *Drawers in a taping bench.*

- When using individual tables and benches, built-in storage underneath or carts placed between the tables provide easy access to materials (see Fig. 2–2A).
- Countertops with drawers positioned between individual tables and benches present another option (see Fig. 2–2B).

Adequate countertop space allows supplies to be arranged and readied prior to daily technique application. Custom-made tables and benches are commonly built with storage space. Design these storage spaces with features that allow for storage of specific sizes or types of tapes, wraps, braces, and pads to assist with timely, efficient technique application. Design all storage spaces in tables and benches with easy access in mind.

Clean and disinfect tables and benches immediately after completing application of taping, wrapping, bracing, and padding techniques. Use **disinfectant** agents to clean the tables, benches, and countertops. While most facilities do not use the application area to treat open wounds, exposure to **bloodborne pathogens** should be a consideration. The Occupational Safety and Health Administration (OSHA)[2] has developed standards for bloodborne pathogens, and facilities should develop and adhere to a plan of universal precautions to protect the health care professional and patients.

---

### DETAILS

OSHA[2] Guidelines state, "Employers shall ensure that the worksite is maintained in a clean and sanitary condition. The employer shall determine and implement an appropriate written schedule for cleaning and method of decontamination based upon the location within the facility, type of surface to be cleaned, type of soil present, and tasks or procedures being performed in the area. . . . Contaminated work surfaces shall be decontaminated with an appropriate disinfectant after completion of procedures; immediately or as soon as feasible when surfaces are overtly contaminated or after any spill of blood or other potentially infectious materials; and at the end of the work shift if the surface may have become contaminated since the last cleaning."

---

### Clinical Application Question 1

You are developing plans for the renovation of the application area in your facility. The available space allows you to consider using multiple individual taping tables.

⟹ **Question: What evidence-based practice and ergonomic principles should you consider in the design of the tables?**

---

## STORAGE

The following recommendations should assist in the proper storage of tapes, wraps, braces, and pads.

## Tape

Intercollegiate and professional sport teams may purchase 100–500 cases of tape per year, which requires a large amount of storage space. The type of storage space is key. The storage and handling of non-elastic and elastic tapes can determine their effectiveness when they are ready to be used (Fig. 2–3). Store tape in a cool, moisture-free environment. The room or area used for storage should also have an adequate ventilation system, as discussed later in this chapter. Tape is normally purchased by the box or case—depending on the type and size—and packaged 16–24 rolls per box or case. Store tape in its original box or case and stack the boxes or cases with the tops facing up and the bottoms facing down. Stacking boxes or cases on their sides or down side up may cause indentations in the rolls. These indentations can be thought of as "bruises" and may affect roll tension during application. Many manufacturers place tape dividers or roll holders in boxes or cases to protect individual rolls from damage during storage (see Fig. 2–3A). When removing tape from boxes or cases, handling prior to application can also cause damage. Squeezing or haphazard storage can

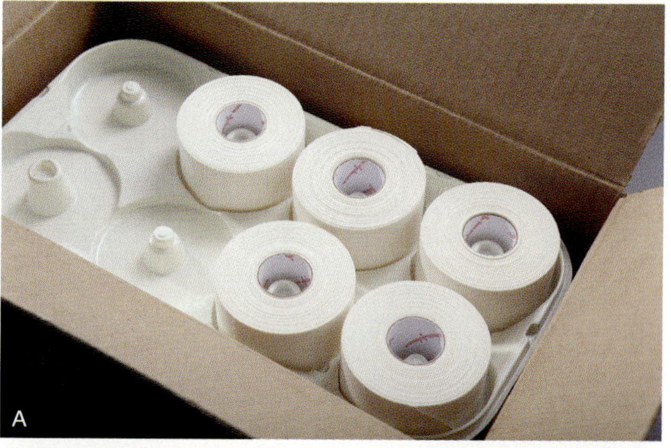

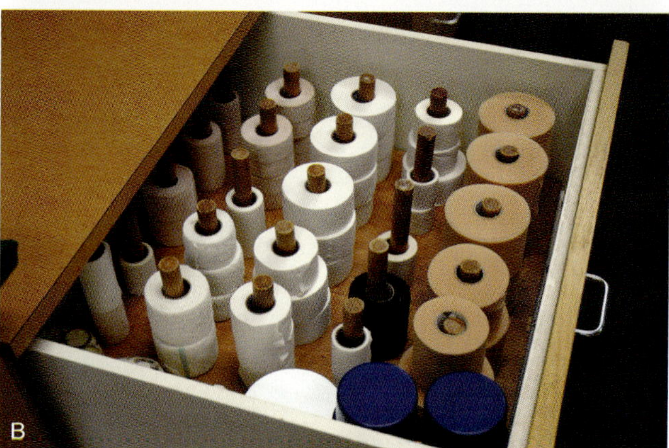

**Fig. 2–3 A** *Case of non-elastic tape with dividers/holders.* **B** *Taping bench drawer with wooden dowels.*

cause excessive pressure on the side of the roll and produce indentations. Stack tape stored in taping tables and benches individually or place onto custom-made wooden dowels (see Fig. 2–3B).

When traveling with tape, store it in its original box or case or in an area protected from excessive pressure and heat. Many intercollegiate and professional teams use trunks that are designed to store tape in compartments. Protect tape carried in personal medical kits from direct sunlight. Heat and humidity will also damage the tape.

Limit the storage of non-elastic and elastic tapes to a 1-year period. While tape does not have an expiration date, time can adversely affect the adhesive mass and roll tension, resulting in difficult application. Inventory regularly and rotate the tape stock when necessary.

Store rolls of cast tape in the original sealed pouch in a cool, dry area. Unlike non-elastic and elastic tapes, cast tape does have an expiration date. Using cast tape after the expiration date may result in shortened setting times, incomplete curing, or premature hardening of the fiberglass material on the roll.

## Wraps

Elastic and cloth wraps are typically stored in taping tables and benches in the application area. Drawers in the tables or benches may be divided to store wraps by different sizes or lengths, allowing for easy access. Store and handle self-adherent wrap in the same manner as non-elastic and elastic tapes.

Clean elastic and cloth wraps by following OSHA[2] Standards for bloodborne pathogens. After proper washing and drying, roll the wraps for the next application. Hand-driven devices can be purchased to roll the wraps and are recommended for cloth wraps to prevent wrinkles. Manually roll elastic wraps and be sure the wraps are completely dry before rolling. If multiple wraps are to be cleaned, either tie the wraps together or place them in a mesh bag to prevent tangling.

---

**Helpful Hint |**

After collecting the used wraps, lay them lengthwise on a table or bench top. Using 1 inch non-elastic tape, gather one end of the bundle and tightly encircle the wraps. At 24–36 inch increments, continue to encircle the wraps with the tape. Because the wraps will most likely be different lengths, continue with taping as far as possible to include the majority of them. Wash and dry the bundle together. Near the completion of the drying cycle, cut the tape to allow the taped areas to dry.

Using a mesh bag, place the wraps in a small to medium-size bag. Securely tie the end and wash and dry with other items such as towels.

---

## Braces

Braces are normally kept in a storage room or cabinet and brought to the application area for use. The storage area should be ventilated and free of moisture to prevent damage to the braces. The size of many designs prohibits storage in taping tables and benches.

## Pads

Soft, low-density pads can be stored in taping tables and benches in the application area. Arrange the pads in drawers by thickness and length. Hard, high-density materials of thermoplastics and cast tapes should be stored in a cool, dry area. It may be a good idea to store small pieces of thermoplastic material in tables and benches for easy access during application sessions.

---

**Clinical Application Question 2**

You have a limited storage area in your facility, and only a portion of this area is well-ventilated.

➡ **Question: What taping, wrapping, bracing, and padding materials will you store in this area?**

---

**. . . IF/THEN . . .**

**IF** the storage space allows, **THEN** place wooden pallets directly on the floor and stack tape on the pallets to allow cool, dry air to circulate freely around the boxes/cases.

---

## SEATING

If space is available in the application area, use benches or chairs for patients as they wait, which should lessen the flow of traffic. The lower traffic flow also allows additional space in which to move during technique application. Construct benches with hinged tops to provide storage underneath for supplies. Use Formica or another durable, easy-to-clean material for construction of the benches or chairs.

## FLOORS

The floor of the application area is both a cosmetic and sanitary concern (Fig. 2–4). High traffic and use of adherent tape spray, fiberglass casting tape, and water can quickly stain and damage floor coverings. At the same time, continuous technique application for 1 to 2 hour periods can cause back and lower body fatigue. If the facility has pre-existing carpet in the area, use non-slip plastic, rubber, or carpet runners or mats to

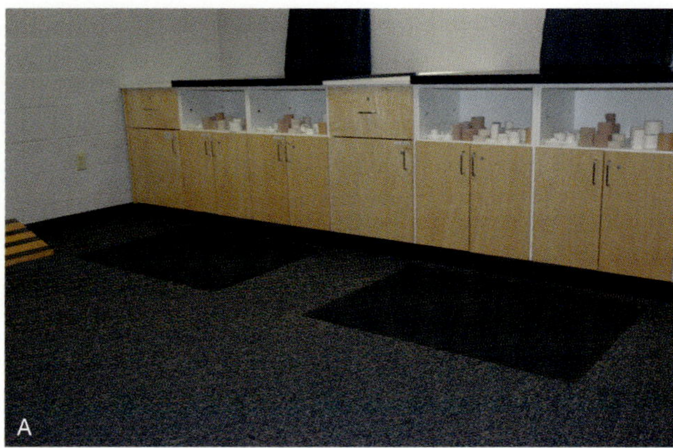

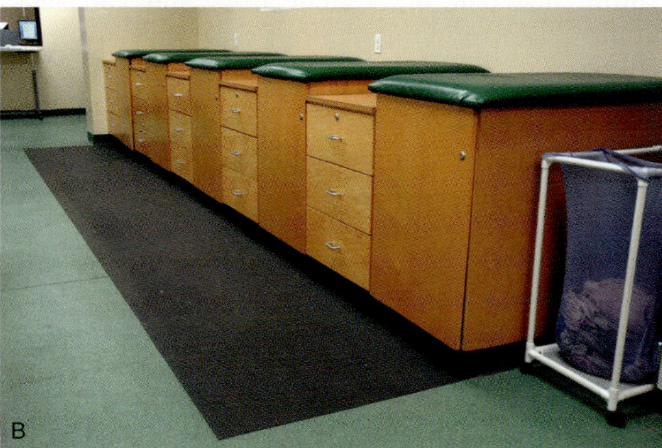

**Fig. 2–4 A** *Non-slip carpet mats placed over carpet.* **B** *Non-slip rubber runner placed over tile.*

lessen soiling and damage and provide some cushion (see Fig. 2–4A). Using non-slip runners or mats over tile or vinyl is also possible (see Fig. 2–4B).

As the runners or mats become soiled or damaged, clean or replace them with new ones. Remove the runners or mats to clean the carpet, tile, or vinyl floor. Clean plastic and rubber runners and mats with a mild dish soap and warm water. Rinse completely to remove any sticky residue. A bristle brush will lift dirt from any grooves. Carpets can be cleaned by a wet or dry process with electric shampoo machines. Clean tile with an electric floor washer or polisher-scrubber with ¼ cup of low-sudsing detergent in 1 gallon of water. Rinse completely. Vinyl can be cleaned with a mild dish soap and mop. Rinse with a towel.

Tape and adhesive residue attracts additional dirt and debris and can build up quickly. Removing this residue from the runners, mats, and floor often requires commercial cleansing products and solvents. Several of these products contain harsh chemicals and can damage these surfaces. Before using a commercial product, always test a spot for damage, such as color fastness.



## WALLS

Walls can be constructed with a variety of materials, such as cinder block, drywall, or tile. Use paint that will resist moisture and allow for easy cleaning. Many facilities with high traffic loads attach Plexiglas or similar material to the wall directly behind taping tables and benches. When a patient is sitting on the table or bench, her or his back rests against the material on the wall. The material protects the wall from dirt and may be cleaned and disinfected daily without damage to the actual wall surface.

## CEILING

The application area ceiling should be easy to clean and resistant to moisture. The ceiling must be at a height to provide clearance for patients in standing positions on tables and benches. For example, a standing position is required for applying an adductor strain wrapping technique. Exposed plumbing pipes or ventilation ducts may reduce ceiling heights. Adjust the position of tables and benches in the application area to find ceiling heights that allow clearance for patients in standing positions. The prescribed ceiling height depends on the height of the tables and benches and the patient.

## ELECTRICAL

The demand for electrical outlets in the application area may be less than in other specialized areas in a health care facility (Fig. 2–5). Outlets are required when using cast cutters, heat guns, supplemental lighting, and cleaning equipment. Referring to the facility as a whole, Secor[3] suggested placement of electrical outlets every 4 feet. Outlets are normally placed approximately 3 to 4 feet off the floor so that they are safe in the event of accidental spills. If involved in the pre-design of new construction or renovations of a facility, plan for exact placement of outlets between tables and benches. Equip all outlets in a health care facility with **ground**

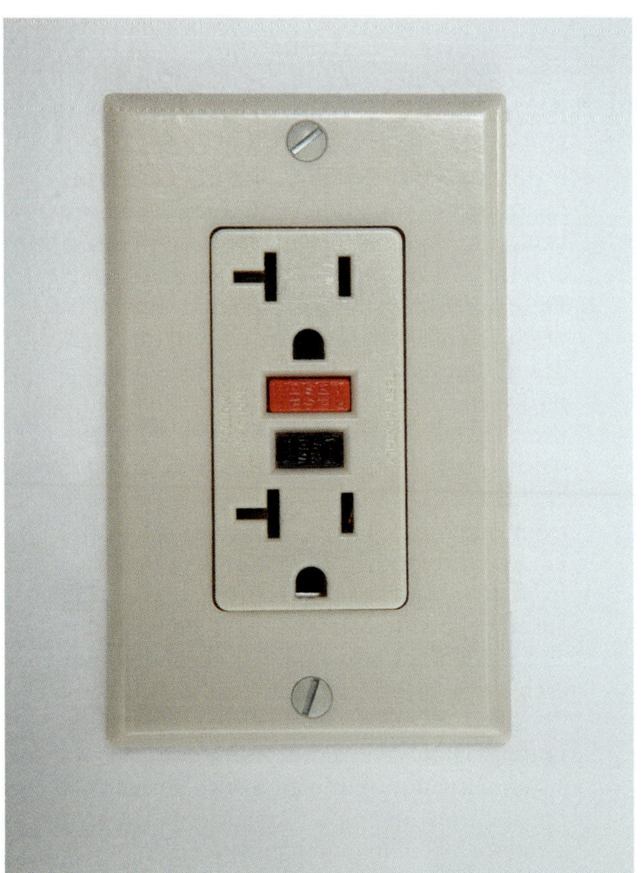

**Fig. 2–5** *GFI breaker on wall.*

**fault interrupter (GFI)** breakers (see Fig. 2–5). GFI breakers and hospital-grade plugs protect patients, health care professionals, and equipment from electrical damage.

# PLUMBING

The plumbing system is perhaps one of the most expensive components of a health care facility. Attention to current and future water needs is important in the pre-design process. A supply of hot and cold water in the application area is convenient but not required. Water is required for constructing thermoplastic materials, applying casting tapes, and hand cleansing after using adherent tape sprays and adhesive tapes. A hand-washing station with hot and cold water is ideal. Fixtures that allow control of water with foot pedals, along with soap and paper towel dispensers, should meet the demands of the application area.

# VENTILATION

Because the application area often has high traffic and because the area often serves as the storage facility for supplies, proper ventilation is a major concern. Konin and Ray[4] stated that temperature and humidity are the two most important ventilation concerns. Separate thermostat controls for the athletic training facility or outpatient clinic allow for ventilation adjustments during periods of high traffic and seasonal environmental changes. Placing thermostats in each room or specialized area in a facility is optimal to control temperature and humidity. Penman and Penman[5] recommend a humidity level between 40% and 50%. High levels of humidity not only can result in uncomfortable working conditions but also may promote the growth of bacteria and fungi and may damage supplies. Taping, wrapping, bracing, and padding supplies require storage in cool, dry places. Supplemental or portable air conditioners or fans assist with temperature and humidity control during high traffic periods.

---

### ... IF/THEN ...

**IF** footwear, school textbooks or bags, and athletic equipment constantly clutter the application area, **THEN** have athletes leave these items in the locker room or outside the door of the athletic training facility to lessen congestion during technique application.

---

# LIGHTING

The application area does not require the most intense illumination in a health care facility. While the area should be lit better than storage rooms, examination and treatment areas typically require more illumination. Recessed lighting commonly found in health care facilities is sufficient for the application area. Use mounted or floor lamps of various intensities if additional lighting is desired. Natural light from windows or skylights can enhance illumination in the application area. However, many health care facilities are located within buildings, well away from natural lighting. Such internal locations are often chosen for patient privacy and equipment and supply security.

---

### Clinical Application Question 3

Each day, your application area becomes congested because several sport teams practice at the same time. The coaches are unwilling to change practice times to lessen the congestion.

➡ **Question: How can you manage this situation?**

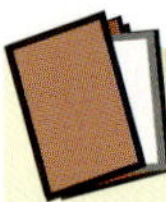

## EVIDENCE-BASED PRACTICE

Facility Design for Taping, Wrapping, Bracing, and Padding

Heather Jones, a PT/AT, works in the town's Boone Orthopedic Clinic, which has just started an outreach program with Mogol High School. For the past 3 years, a teacher/AT has been employed at the high school. Recently, the teacher/AT left the high school to accept another position. Although Mogol High School is known for its modern facilities, the school is planning renovations. The athletic booster organization at the high school has raised substantial private funds for the project and supports the health care services provided to the athletes. The high school administrators approach Heather in hopes that she will assist them in the renovation of their facility, specifically the athletic training facility. Heather tours the building with the administrators. The high school administrators tell Heather that the new facility will be greatly expanded into separate treatment, rehabilitation, hydrotherapy, taping, wrapping, bracing, padding, physician examination, and office areas. Because of the original construction of the plumbing and ventilation systems, the new facility must remain on the second floor. Heather and the school administrators complete the tour and begin to discuss ideas for the renovations. Heather has previous experience with the design, traffic flow, and ergonomics of an athletic training facility and outlines her initial plans with the administrators. The administrators also tell Heather about the future plans and goals of the Mogol High School athletic program, which include the addition of three new sports next year. Heather returns to the clinic and begins to prepare schematic drawings of the new athletic training facility. She carefully considers the advantages and disadvantages of the placement of individual areas in previous facilities and discusses these with her colleagues. The group decides to focus first on the location of the taping, wrapping, bracing, and padding application area in the facility. Heather and the group will consider the structural and various system needs for the placement of the application area to effectively provide prevention and treatment interventions to the high school athletes throughout the year. Heather begins to explore to find the most appropriate location and design of the application area.

1. Develop a clinically relevant question from the case in the PICO format to generate answers for the selection of an appropriate location for the taping, wrapping, bracing, and padding application area in the facility. The question should include the population or problem, the intervention, a comparison intervention (if relevant), and the clinical outcome of interest.

2. Design a search strategy and search to find the best evidence to answer the clinical question. The strategy should include relevant search terms, electronic databases, online journals, and print journals to use for the search. Discussions with your faculty, clinical preceptor, and other health care professionals can provide evidence from expert opinion.

3. Choose three to five full text studies or articles from your search or the chapter references. Evaluate and appraise each article to determine its value and usefulness to the case. Ask these questions for each study: (1) Are the results of the study valid? (2) What are the actual results? and (3) Are the findings clinically relevant to my patients? Prepare a summary of the evaluation with answers to the questions and rank the articles based on the evidence hierarchy in Chapter 1.

4. Integrate findings from the evidence, your clinical experience, and goals of the application area for the athletes into the clinical decision. Consider which location may be the most appropriate for the taping, wrapping, bracing, and padding application area.

5. Evaluate the EBP process and your experience within the case. Consider these questions in the evaluation.

Was the clinical question answered?
Did the search generate quality evidence?
Was the evidence evaluated appropriately?
Was the evidence, your clinical experience, and goals of the application area integrated to make the clinical decision?
Did the intervention (location of the application area) produce successful outcomes for Heather and the athletes?
Was the EBP experience positive for Heather and the high school?

**Facility Design for Taping, Wrapping, Bracing, and Padding**

## WRAP-UP

- Design and construction of the application area should be based on ergonomic principles.
- The design of the application area should include current and future program needs and structural considerations.
- Use taping tables and benches in varying heights with storage areas for technique application.
- Store taping, wrapping, bracing, and padding materials in a well-ventilated area.
- Use additional seating to lower the flow of traffic.
- Non-slip plastic, rubber, or carpet runners or mats protect the floor and may reduce lower body fatigue.
- Use moisture-resistant paint on the wall and ceilings.
- Ceiling heights should allow patients to stand on taping tables and benches.
- Place electrical outlets equipped with GFI breakers 3 to 4 feet off the floor.
- A hand-washing station should provide the water needs for the application area.
- Control temperature and humidity with a separate thermostat located in the application area.
- Illumination in the application area can be supplied with standard recessed lighting.
- Clean and disinfect tables, benches, and countertops with appropriate agents following use.

## WEB REFERENCES

**U.S. Department of Labor Occupational Safety and Health Administration: Ergonomics**
http://www.osha.gov/SLTC/ergonomics/
- This website provides ergonomic guidelines and solutions for health care facilities.

**U.S. Department of Labor Occupational Safety and Health Administration: Bloodborne Pathogens**
http://www.osha.gov/SLTC/bloodbornepathogens/index.html
- This site contains OSHA Standards and safety and health topics related to bloodborne pathogens.

**Athletic Business**
http://www.athleticbusiness.com
- This site provides access to a monthly print and digital magazine that contains information about facility planning.

**Hausmann Industries**
http://www.hausmann.com
- This website is an online catalog for the manufacturer and provides information on a variety of sports medicine equipment, including taping tables and benches.

## REFERENCES

1. Taber's Cyclopedic Medical Dictionary, ed 23. F.A. Davis, Philadelphia, 2017.
2. U.S. Department of Labor Occupational Safety and Health Administration: Bloodborne Pathogens, 2019. https://www.osha.gov/SLTC/bloodbornepathogens/
3. Secor, MR: Designing athletic training facilities or "Where do you want the outlets?" Athl Train J Natl Athl Train Assoc 19:19–21, 1984.
4. Konin, JG, and Ray, R: Management Strategies in Athletic Training, ed 5. Human Kinetics, Champaign, IL, 2019.
5. Penman, KA, and Penman, TM: Training rooms aren't just for colleges. Athletic Purchasing and Facilities 6:34–37, 1982.

# Injuries and Conditions of the Lower Body

# Foot and Toes

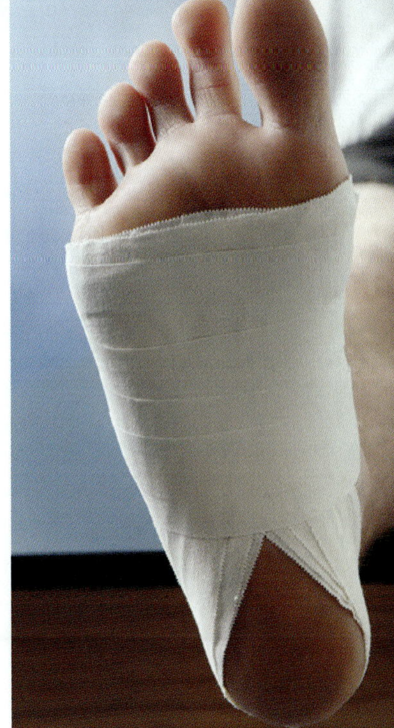



## INJURIES AND CONDITIONS

During athletic, work, and casual activities, the foot and toes must react to acute and chronic forces. As a result, injuries and overuse conditions often occur. Walking produces constant shearing forces between the foot and toes and the ground in anteroposterior, lateral-to-medial, and vertical directions. During running, these same forces increase as speeds increase. In sports, sudden cutting, twisting, and deceleration movements further increase the stresses. A contusion, sprain, or fracture can occur when a football wide receiver decelerates and plants his right foot to make a cut or quick turn to his left, placing anteroposterior, lateral-to-medial, and rotational stresses on the foot and toes. Common injuries to the foot and toes include the following:

- Contusions
- Sprains
- Strains
- Fractures
- Overuse injuries and conditions
- Blisters

## Contusions

Contusions to the foot and toes are caused by compressive forces and weight-bearing activities. A contusion is trauma to the soft tissue. Compression on the **dorsal** or **plantar** surface of the area can cause inflammation and pain. For example, activities that require jumping and sudden change of direction can lead to contusion of the calcaneus, referred to as a heel bruise (Fig. 3–1). Training errors and the use of poorly designed shoes may contribute to such injuries.

## Sprains

Sprains to the toes are typically caused by contact with an unmovable object, producing abnormal joint range of motion. A sprain involves trauma to ligaments and may result in only mild pain or complete loss of function. Sprains are commonly categorized as Grade I, II, or III, with III being the most severe. Forced hyperextension of the **metatarsophalangeal (MTP) joint** of the great toe (turf toe) is associated with excessive flexibility of athletic shoes and sport activities on artificial grass surfaces (see Figs. 3–1 and 3–2). Another sprain to the great toe MTP joint is caused by forced **hyperflexion** (soccer toe) and may occur with instep ball strike of a soccer ball.[1] Sprains to the MTP and **interphalangeal (IP) joints** of the toes are caused by **valgus** and **varus** stresses and result in injury to the collateral ligaments (see Fig. 3–1). Midfoot sprains occur through excessive

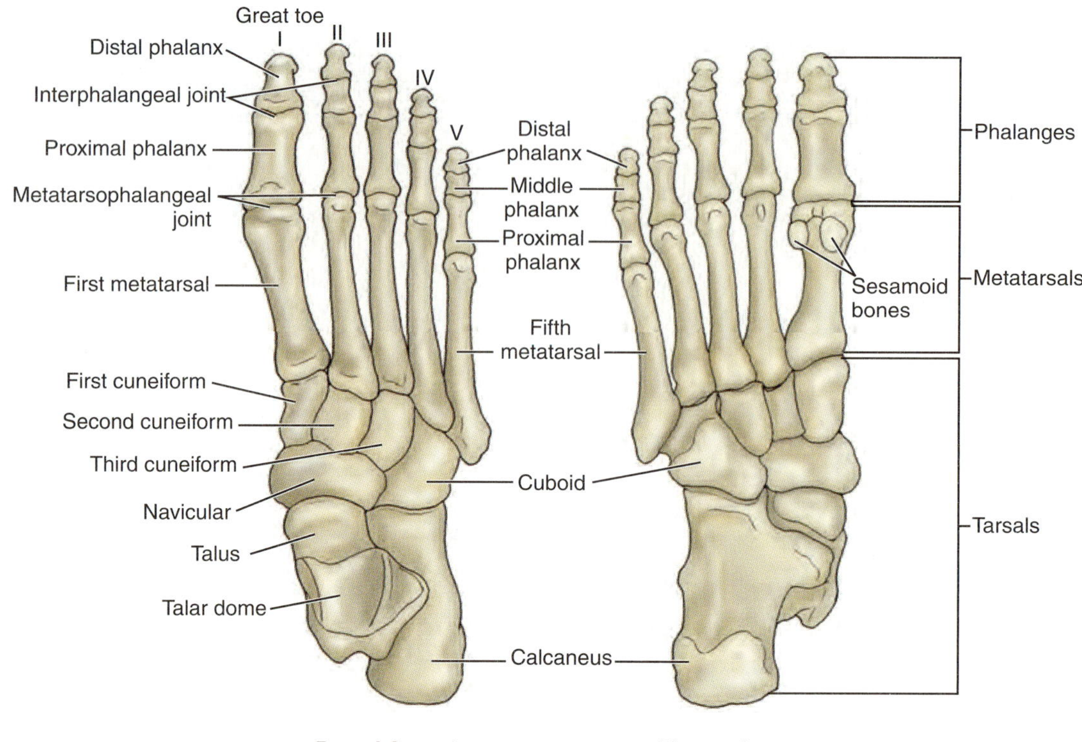



**Fig. 3–1** *Bones and joints of the foot and toes.*

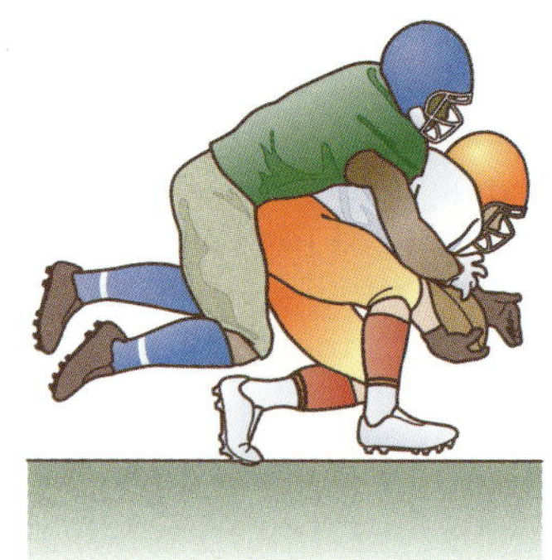

**Fig. 3–2** *Great toe metatarsophalangeal (MTP) joint sprain. Note forced hyperextension at the MTP joint (turf toe).*

**plantar flexion, dorsiflexion,** or rotational stress that can occur with stepping on an opponent's foot or stepping into a hole.

## Strains

Strains to the foot commonly affect the **longitudinal, metatarsal,** or **transverse arch** (Fig. 3–3). Strains involve trauma to a muscle and/or tendon. Injury can be caused by overloads of the musculature and ligamentous support through activity on rigid surfaces.[2]

Repetitive activity on asphalt or concrete surfaces in footwear without arch support can contribute to a strain. **Pes cavus,** or high arches, may also contribute to an arch strain.

## Fractures

Fractures to the foot and toes may involve the tarsals, metatarsals, or phalanges (see Figs. 3–1 and 3–4). Mechanisms of injury commonly include excessive **inversion, eversion**, dorsiflexion, plantar flexion, rotation, and axial loading.[1,2] For example, a fracture can occur as a basketball player jumps to rebound the ball, either landing directly on the calcaneus or on an opponent's foot, causing excessive inversion or eversion. If there is a possibility of a fracture, refer the patient to a physician.

## Overuse

**Overuse** injuries and conditions are caused by excessive, repetitive stress to the foot and toes. Pressure from the heel box of a shoe may lead to **retrocalcaneal bursitis.** Medial heel pain, commonly **plantar fasciitis,** may result from poor running technique and inflexible

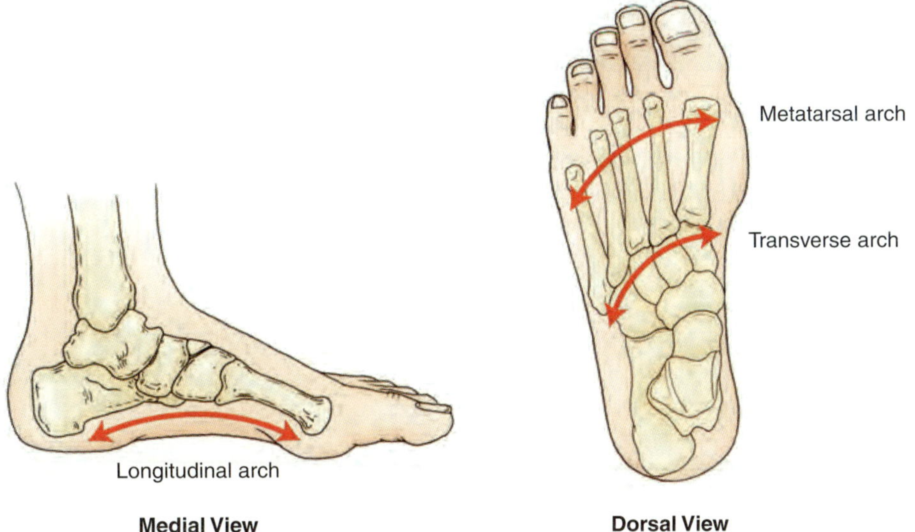


**Fig. 3–3** *Arches of the foot.*

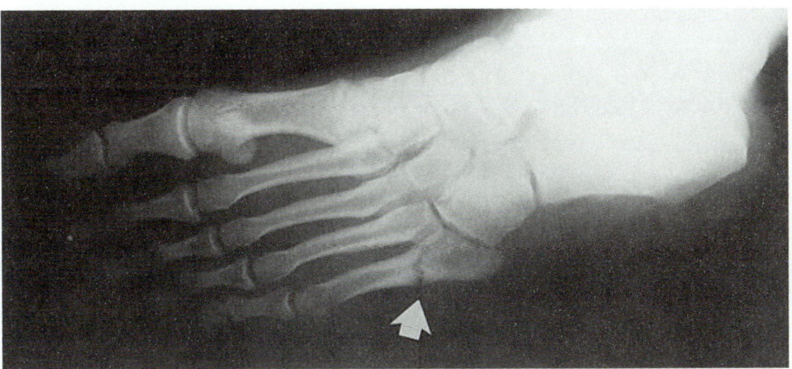

**Fig. 3–4** *Oblique view of the foot showing a complete fracture at the proximal diaphysis of the 5th metatarsal. (Courtesy of McKinnis, LN. Fundamentals of Musculoskeletal Imaging, 4th ed. Philadelphia, PA: F.A. Davis Company: 2014.)*

musculature (Fig. 3–5). Repetitive hyperextension of the great toe may cause **sesamoiditis**[2] (see Fig. 3–1). **Metatarsalgia** may follow injury to the transverse arch. Ill-fitting shoes and foot pronation can lead to plantar **interdigital neuroma. Bunions** and **bunionettes** may be the result of ill-fitting shoes.

## Blisters

Because the majority of athletic, work, and everyday activities require some type of footwear, blisters caused by shearing forces are common. Blisters are particularly common during the beginning of competitive sport seasons or when wearing new shoes or orthotics. Use a break-in period, gradually increasing the wear time with new shoes and semirigid and rigid orthotics to lessen shearing forces and the development of blisters.

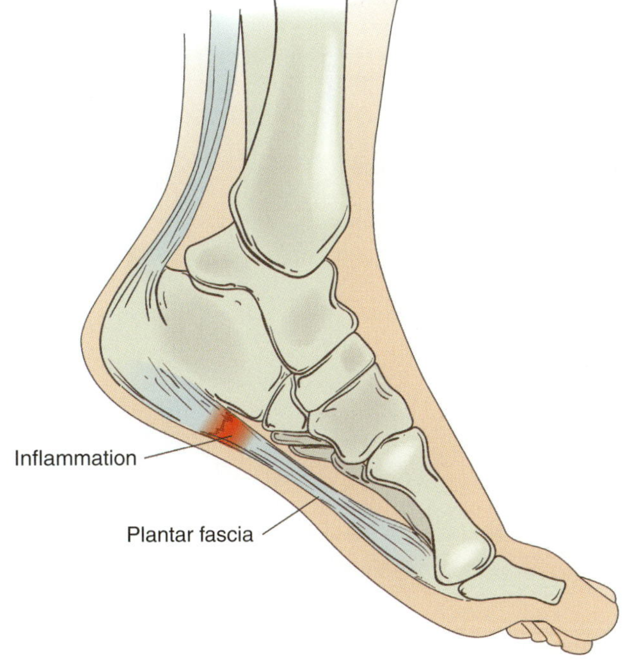


**Fig. 3–5** *Plantar fasciitis.*

# Taping Techniques

Several arch taping techniques will provide support to the arch and forefoot areas. While one technique may provide adequate support for one patient, applying the same technique on another patient with a similar injury may be ineffective because of the mechanism of injury, foot structure, or sport or activity. When deciding on a technique, consider the intended purposes of the technique, the injury, the patient, and the activity; then select the appropriate technique and monitor the outcomes. Note that many of these techniques may be used for lower leg injuries and conditions as indicated.

## CIRCULAR ARCH    Figure 3–6

- **Purpose:** The circular arch technique provides mild support to the longitudinal arch (Fig. 3–6). Use this straightforward technique for longitudinal arch strains and pes cavus and **pes planus** conditions.
- **Materials:**
  - 1½ inch non-elastic tape
  *Options:*
  - Pre-wrap or self-adherent wrap, adherent tape spray
  - ⅛ inch or ¼ inch foam or felt, taping scissors
  - 2 inch or 3 inch elastic tape
- **Position of the patient:** Sitting on a taping table or bench with the leg extended off the edge and the foot placed at a 90 degree angle.
- **Preparation:** Apply the technique directly to the skin.
  *Options:*
  Apply adherent tape spray, then apply pre-wrap or self-adherent wrap around the midfoot area to provide additional adherence and lessen irritation.
  Incorporate a foam or felt pad with the circular arch to provide additional support. This technique is illustrated in the Padding Techniques section (see Fig. 3–25).
- **Application:**

**STEP 1:** Anchor 1½ inch non-elastic tape on the **medial** aspect of the foot, just proximal to the MTP joint of the great toe (Fig. 3–6A).

*Option:* *Use 2 inch or 3 inch elastic tape instead of non-elastic tape for added comfort and conformability.*

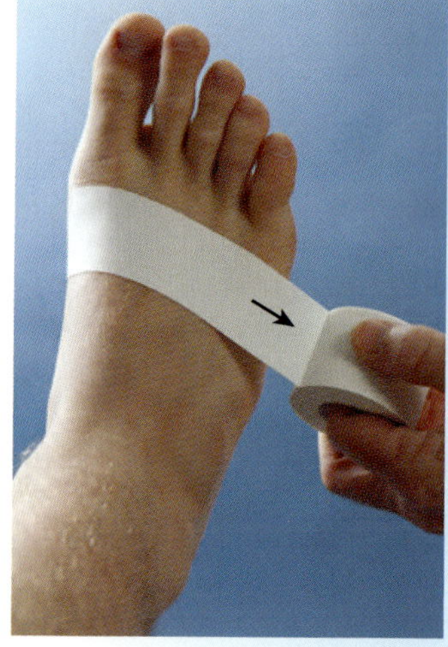

**Fig. 3–6 A**

**STEP 2:** Pull the tape in a **lateral** direction across the dorsum of the foot and continue across the plantar surface. Anchor the strip on the dorsal aspect of the foot (Fig. 3–6B). Avoid excessive roll tension that may cause constriction of the foot on weight-bearing.

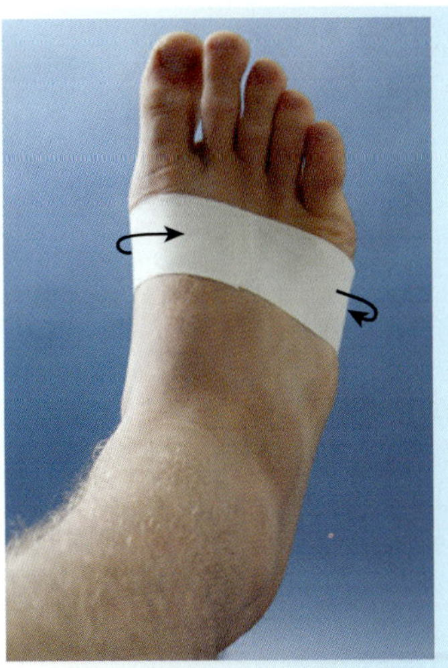

**Fig. 3–6 B**

**STEP 3:** Continue with three to five additional strips in a proximal direction (Fig. 3–6C). Overlap each strip by ½ of the width of the tape. These strips should not cause constriction of the proximal dorsal foot during dorsiflexion.

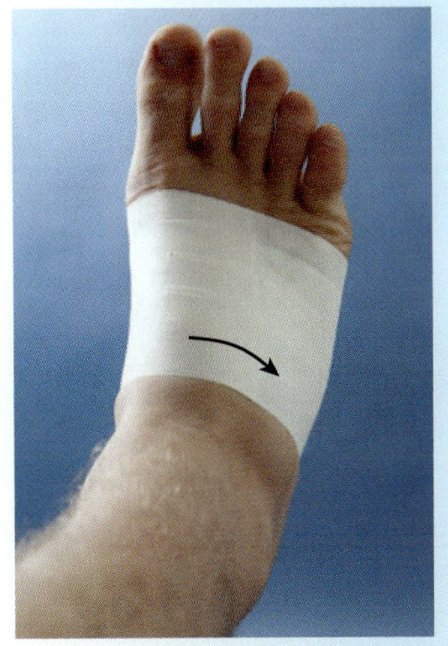

**Fig. 3–6 C**

## "X" ARCH    Figure 3–7

➠ **Purpose:** Use the "X" arch technique to provide mild to moderate support for the longitudinal arch and forefoot in the treatment of arch strains, plantar fasciitis, pes cavus, and pes planus (Fig. 3–7).

➠ **Materials:**
  • 1 inch and 1½ inch non-elastic tape, adherent tape spray

➠ **Position of the patient:** Sitting on a taping table or bench with the leg extended off the edge and the foot placed at a 90 degree angle.

➠ **Preparation:** Apply adherent tape spray on the plantar forefoot area.

➠ **Application:**

**STEP 1:** Place a 1 inch non-elastic tape anchor directly on the skin over the base of the metatarsal heads (Fig. 3–7A). This anchor may encircle the foot, but this is not necessary.

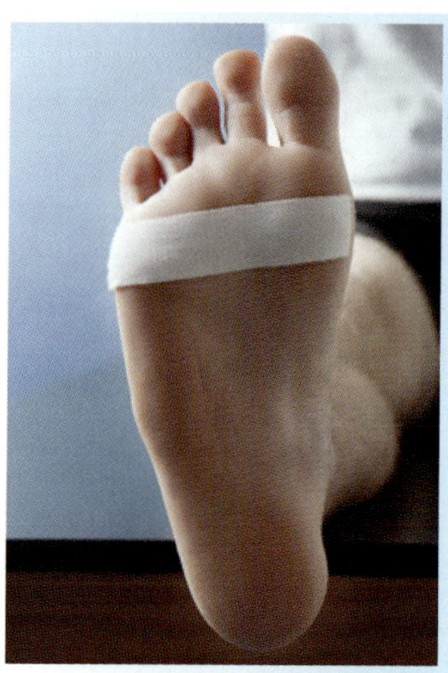

Fig. 3–7 A

**STEP 2:** Anchor the first "X" strip of 1 inch non-elastic tape under the base of the fifth toe, proceed at an angle around the medial heel with moderate roll tension, and finish at the base of the great toe (see Fig. 3–7B).

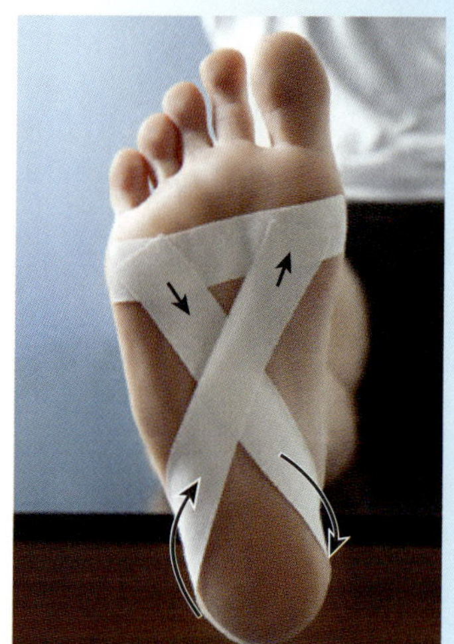

Fig. 3–7 B

**STEP 3:** Anchor the next "X" strip at the base of the great toe, angle around the lateral heel with moderate roll tension, and finish at the base of the fifth toe (see Fig. 3–7C).

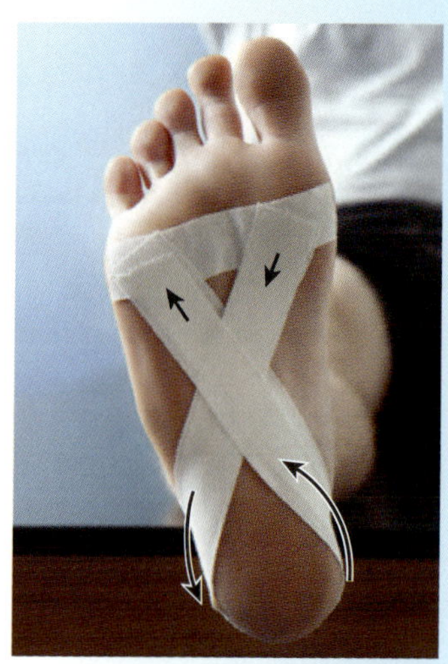

Fig. 3–7 C

**STEP 4:** Continue with each strip two to three additional times, overlapping each on the plantar surface of the foot by ⅓ to ½ of the tape width (see Fig. 3–7D). These strips will overlap minimally as they cross the heel.

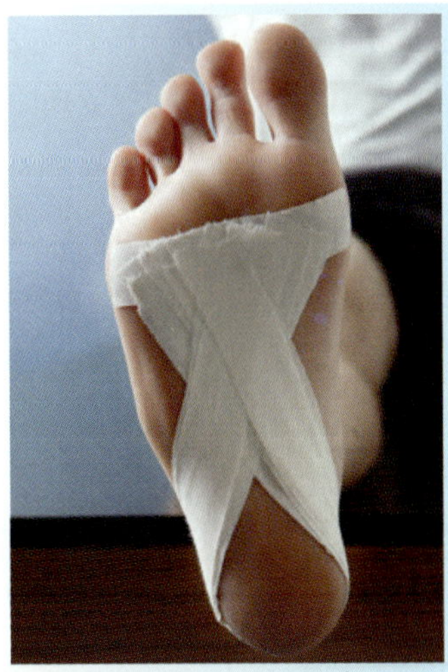

**Fig. 3–7 D**

**STEP 5:** Finish by applying an anchor strip over the MTP joints, covering the ends of the tape (see Fig. 3–7E).

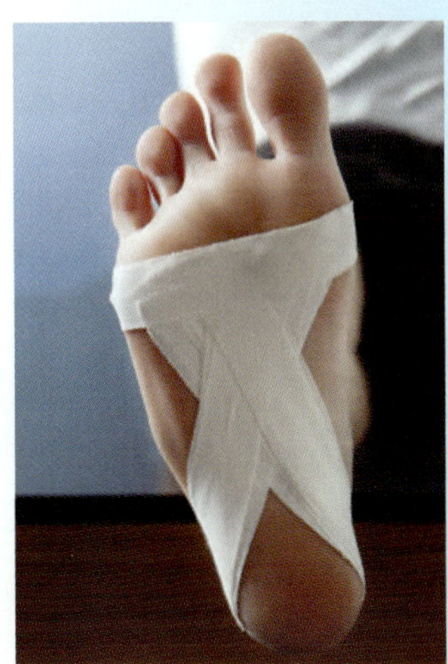

**Fig. 3–7 E**

**STEP 6:** Apply four to five circular strips with 1½ inch non-elastic tape, as illustrated in Figure 3–6, to cover the arch (see Fig. 3–7F).

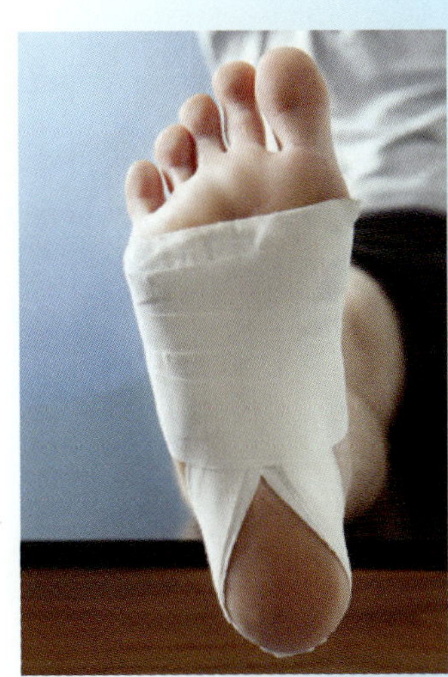

**Fig. 3–7 F**

## LOOP ARCH    Figure 3–8

➡ **Purpose:** The loop arch technique also provides mild to moderate support to the longitudinal arch and forefoot (Fig. 3–8).

➡ **Materials:**
  • 1 inch and 1½ inch non-elastic tape, adherent tape spray

➡ **Position of the patient:** Sitting on a taping table or bench with the leg extended off the edge and the foot placed at a 90 degree angle.

➡ **Preparation:** Apply adherent tape spray to the plantar forefoot area.

➡ **Application:**

**STEP 1:**  Apply a 1 inch non-elastic tape anchor over the base of the metatarsal heads. Begin the first loop strip of 1 inch non-elastic tape at the base of the fifth toe, proceed around the lateral heel with moderate roll tension, and finish at the base of the fifth toe (Fig. 3–8A).

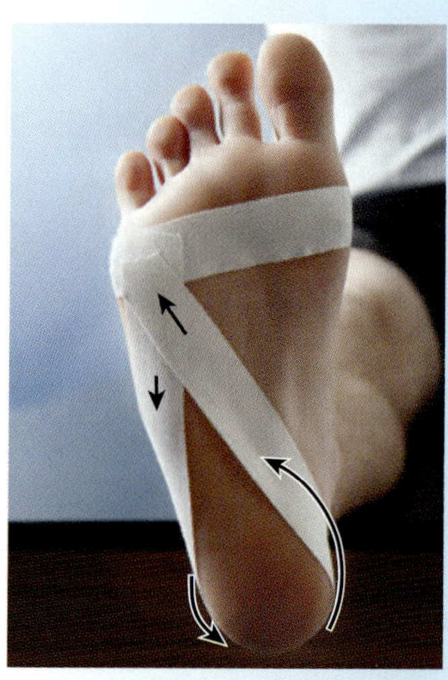

**Fig. 3–8 A**

**STEP 2:**  Anchor the next loop strip at the base of the great toe, continue around the medial heel with moderate roll tension, and finish at the base of the great toe (Fig. 3–8B).

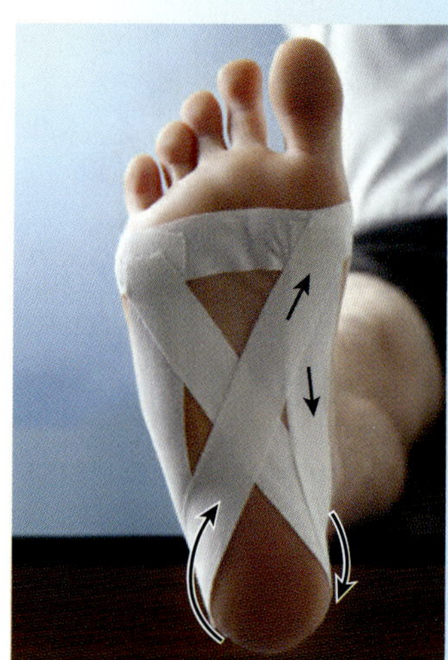

**Fig. 3–8 B**

**STEP 3:**   Repeat each loop strip two to three times, overlapping each by ⅓ to ½ of the tape width on the plantar foot (Fig. 3–8C). Overlapping of the strips on the heel will be minimal.

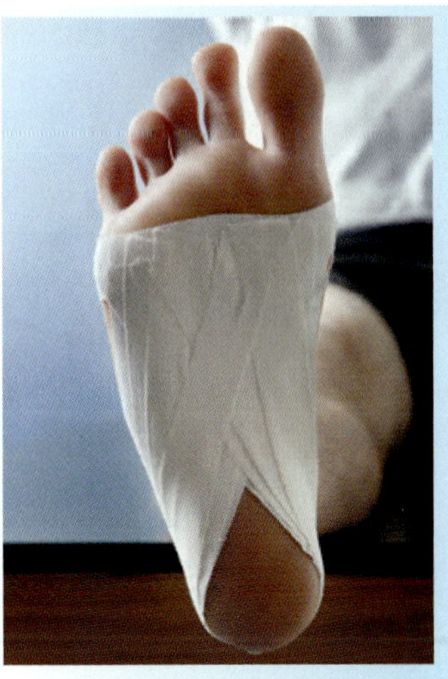

**Fig. 3–8 C**

**STEP 4:**   Apply a 1 inch non-elastic anchor strip over the tape ends on the plantar foot. Use 1½ inch non-elastic tape circular strips to cover the arch (Fig. 3–8D).

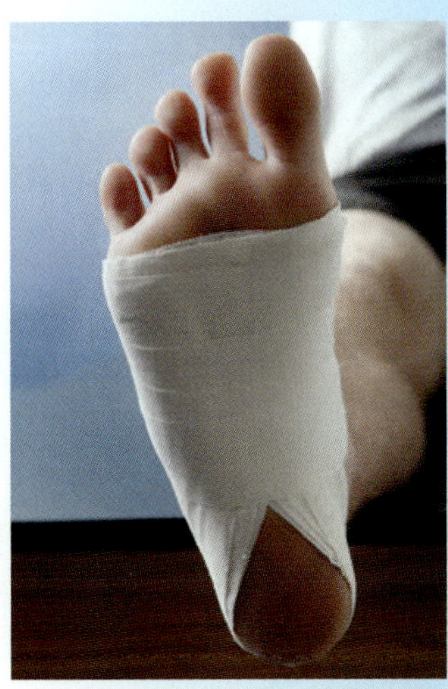

**Fig. 3–8 D**

**DETAILS**

The "X" and loop arch taping techniques are interchangeable as both provide mild to moderate support for the longitudinal arch and forefoot. The health care professional's and patient's preferences commonly determine which technique is applied.

## WEAVE ARCH   Figure 3–9

⟹ **Purpose:** The weave arch technique is perhaps the most supportive of the arch techniques, providing moderate support to the longitudinal arch and forefoot (Fig. 3–9).
⟹ **Materials:**
  • 1 inch and 1½ inch non-elastic tape, adherent tape spray

➠ **Position of the patient:** Sitting on a taping table or bench with the leg extended off the edge and the foot placed at a 90 degree angle.
➠ **Preparation:** Apply adherent tape spray to the plantar forefoot.
➠ **Application:**

**STEP 1:**  Place a 1 inch non-elastic tape anchor over the metatarsal heads. Anchor a strip of 1 inch non-elastic tape over the third metatarsal head, proceed at an angle around the lateral heel, and finish just lateral to the starting point near the third metatarsal head (Fig. 3–9A).

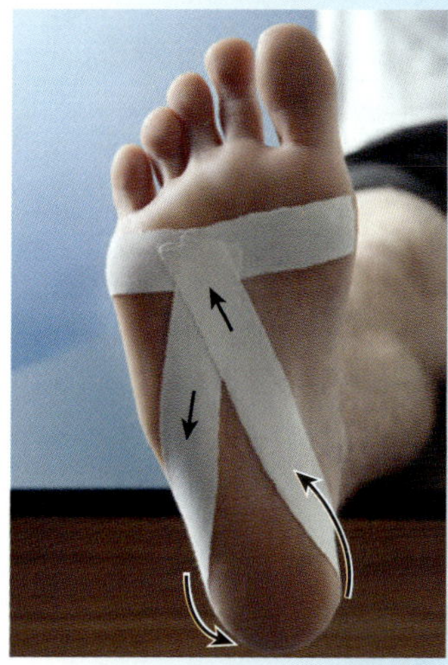

Fig. 3–9 A

**STEP 2:**  Anchor the next strip on the second metatarsal head, continue around the lateral heel, and finish on the fourth metatarsal head (Fig. 3–9B).

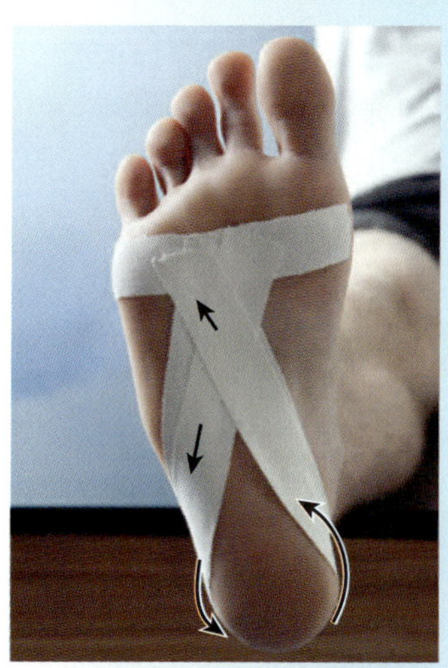

Fig. 3–9 B

**STEP 3:**  Begin the next strip on the fourth metatarsal head, continue around the lateral heel, and finish on the fifth metatarsal head (Fig. 3–9C).

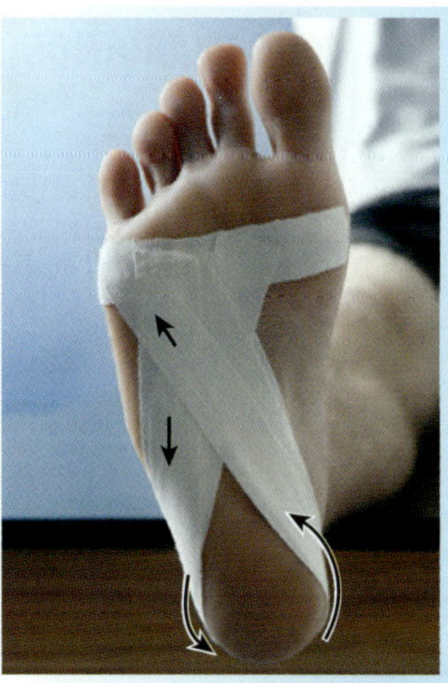

**Fig. 3–9 C**

**STEP 4:**  Begin the last strip on the great toe metatarsal head, continue around the lateral heel, and finish on the great toe metatarsal head (Fig. 3–9D). Apply the strips with a moderate amount of roll tension. The strips should resemble a weave pattern on the plantar surface of the foot. These strips will overlap minimally across the heel.

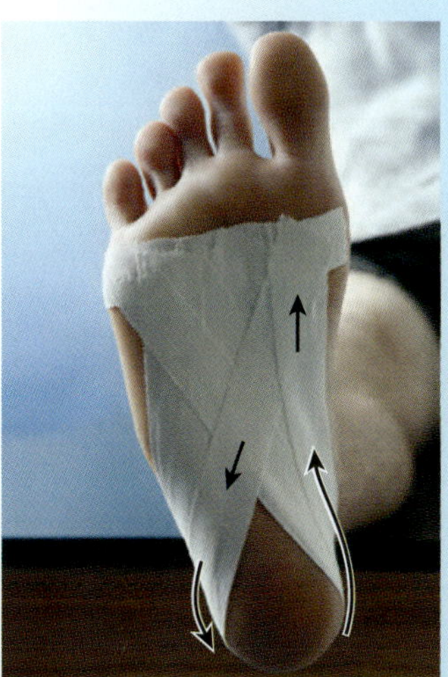

**Fig. 3–9 D**

**STEP 5:**  Apply supportive 1½ inch non-elastic tape anchor strips over the pattern, as illustrated in the circular arch technique (Fig. 3–9E).

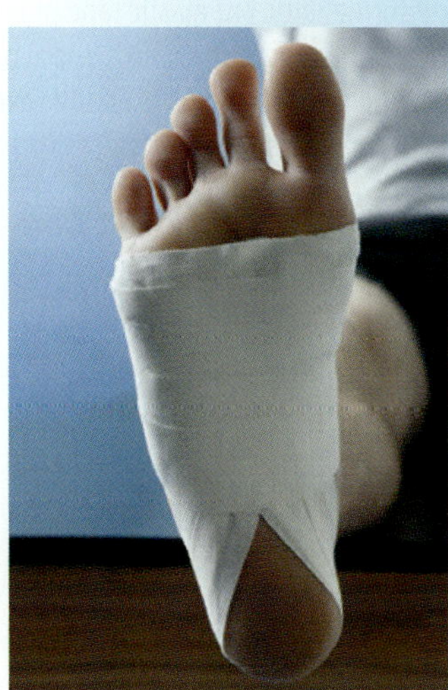

**Fig. 3–9 E**

## ANCHOR VARIATION TO THE "X," LOOP, AND WEAVE ARCH TECHNIQUES

➠ **Purpose:** A variation to anchor the "X," loop, or weave arch techniques entails applying a series of tape strips across the plantar foot. Consider using these strips to provide additional support to the plantar foot when treating arch strains, plantar fasciitis, pes cavus, and pes planus.

➠ **Materials:**
  • 1 inch non-elastic tape

➠ **Position of the patient:** Sitting on a taping table or bench with the leg extended off the edge and the foot placed at a 90 degree angle.

➠ **Preparation:** Application of "X," loop, or weave arch technique, excluding the circular strips.

➠ **Application:**

**STEP 1:** Tear individual strips of 1 inch non-elastic tape and apply with equal tension inward toward the plantar foot. Anchor each strip on the medial and lateral borders of the foot. Begin on the proximal foot and continue with additional strips in a distal direction, overlapping by ½ of the tape width to cover the entire arch (Fig. 3–9F).

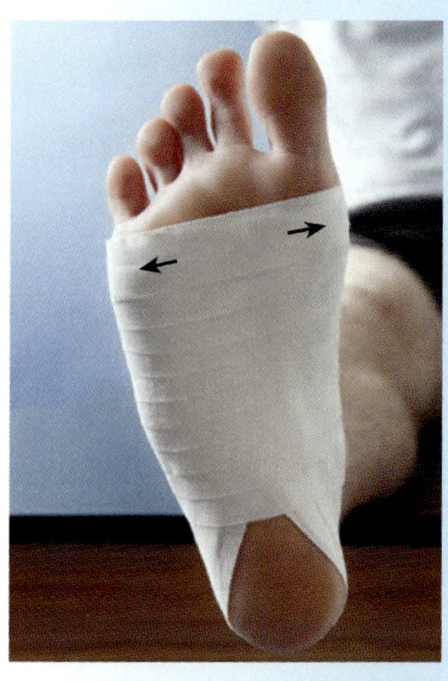

**Fig. 3–9 F**

**STEP 2:** Apply the circular arch technique, as illustrated in Figure 3–6, to cover the arch.

### DETAILS

For the circular, "X," loop, and weave techniques, elastic tape of 1 inch width may be used in place of non-elastic tape for comfort and conformability, but elastic tape provides less support to the arch and forefoot. Non-elastic tape of 1 inch width is most commonly used for the techniques, but 1½ inch width may be required for large feet. If one of these techniques is applied daily, monitor the heel area for skin irritation. Thin foam pads or adhesive gauze material placed directly on the heel prior to applying the tape should lessen irritation.

## LOW-DYE        Figure 3–10

➠ **Purpose:** The Low-Dye technique is commonly used in treating arch strains, plantar fasciitis, and lower leg injuries and conditions to provide moderate support and correct structural abnormalities, such as excessive pronation. Two methods are interchangeable in applying the Low-Dye technique; the first is illustrated here (Fig. 3–10) and the second is online at FADavis.com.

### *Low-Dye Technique One*

➤ **Materials:**
  • 1 inch and 2 inch non-elastic and 2 inch elastic tape, adherent tape spray
➤ **Position of the patient:** Sitting on a taping table or bench with the leg extended off the edge and the foot in a neutral position.
➤ **Preparation:** Apply adherent tape spray to the lateral and medial surfaces of the foot.
➤ **Application:**

**STEP 1:**  Anchor 1 inch non-elastic tape directly to the skin over the lateral surface of the fifth MTP joint, continue around the heel, and finish on the medial surface of the first MTP joint (Fig. 3–10A).

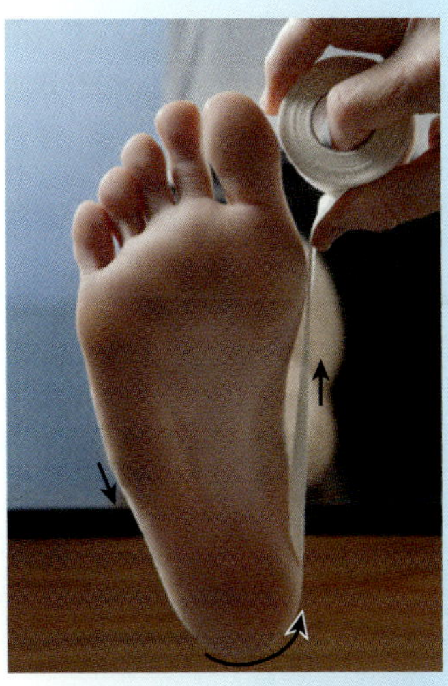

**Fig. 3–10 A**

**STEP 2:**  Repeat this step twice, overlapping by ½ of the tape width (Fig. 3–10B). Apply the tape with moderate roll tension **inferior** to the medial and lateral malleoli.

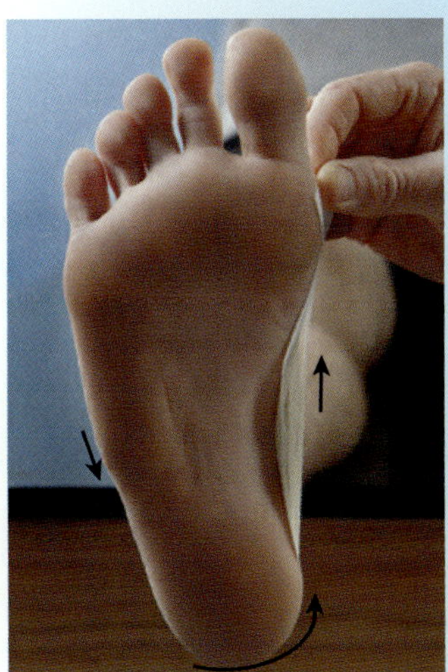

**Fig. 3–10 B**

*Steps Cont.*

**Foot and Toes**

**STEP 3:** Anchor a strip of 2 inch non-elastic tape on the lateral dorsum of the proximal foot, continue across the plantar aspect, and finish on the medial dorsum (Fig. 3–10C).

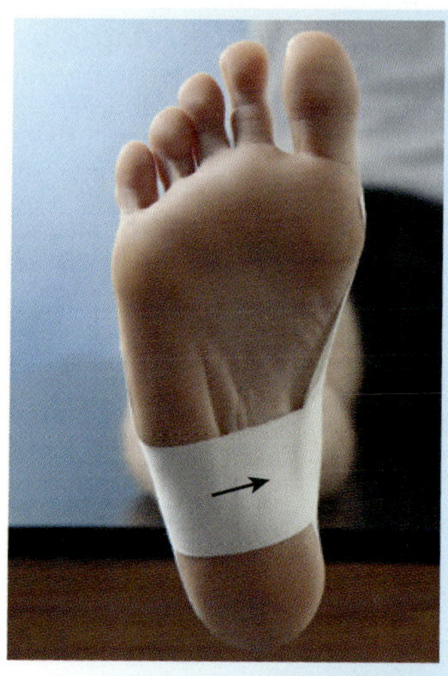

**Fig. 3–10 C**

**STEP 4:** Apply two additional strips in the same manner, overlapping each by ½ of the tape width with moderate roll tension (Fig. 3–10D). These strips, C and D, should cover the 1 inch tape strips (see Figs. 3–10A and B) but not encircle the foot. Next, apply a 1 inch non-elastic strip as illustrated in Figure 3–10A.

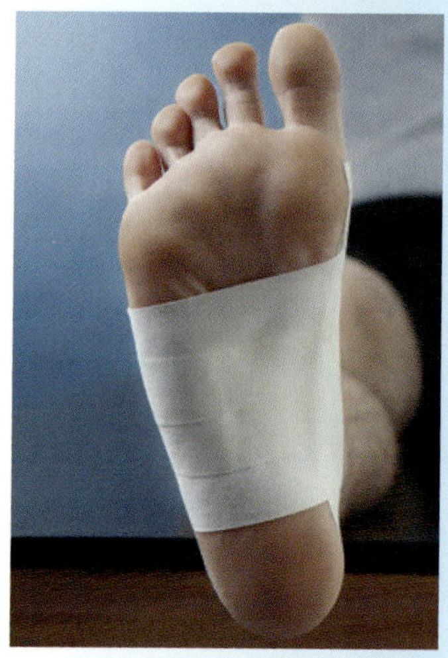

**Fig. 3–10 D**

**STEP 5:** Finish by applying an anchor strip of 2 inch elastic tape on the lateral dorsum, continue across the plantar surface, and finish on the lateral dorsum to encircle the arch with mild to moderate roll tension (see Fig. 3–10E).

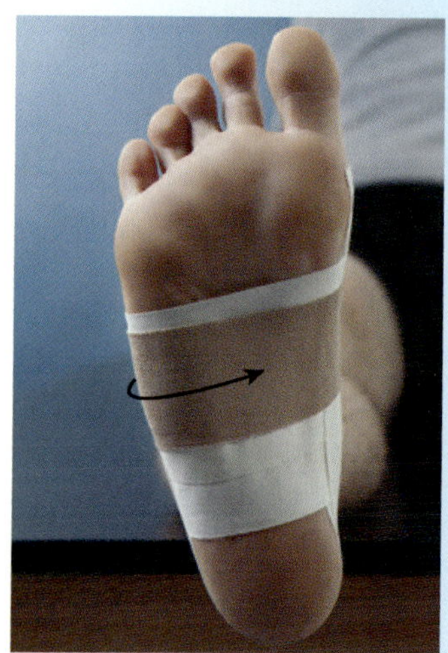

**Fig. 3–10 E**

## EVIDENCE SUMMARY

Arch taping techniques are designed to support the longitudinal arch and forefoot and correct structural abnormalities in the prevention and treatment of lower extremity injuries and conditions. A 2011 evidence-based review[3] revealed that therapeutic taping was more effective in controlling foot pronation than motion control footwear and custom-made and off-the-shelf orthotics during treadmill and overground running, walking, and static standing conditions. However, the differences in pronation among taping, footwear, and orthotic interventions was small and may not be clinically meaningful.[3] Among the taping techniques in the review—Low-Dye, high-Dye, and stirrup—the Low-Dye was found to be the least effective in controlling pronation. The high-Dye and stirrup techniques extended onto the lower leg, which may provide greater leverage to control pronation than the Low-Dye.[3]

Research focusing on the biomechanical effects of various arch taping techniques during walking and running has demonstrated consistent findings. Past investigations revealed that the navicular-sling, Low-Dye, high-Dye, and X-arch techniques immediately raised the height of the navicular[4–9] but lost their supportive qualities in a short time during exercise.[4–8] Researchers[5,10–16] have demonstrated that the modified reverse-6 and modified reverse-6 with Low-Dye techniques increased the height of the dorsal arch and decreased the width of the midfoot, with support lasting for hours. Other researchers have found that the Low-Dye, navicular-sling, and augmented Low-Dye (Low-Dye, calcaneal slings, reverse-6 strips) techniques increased plantar pressure in the lateral midfoot[4,17–22] and decreased plantar pressure in the medial and lateral forefoot.[4] These results appear to support the theory that taping assists in maintaining the shape and height of the longitudinal arch, restricting subtalar and midtarsal joint motion, and affecting plantar pressures in the foot by reducing pressures in the forefoot and shifting pressures to the lateral midfoot region to prevent or reduce excessive pronation.[4]

Several electromyographic investigations of the lower leg have shown reductions in muscle activity with arch taping techniques. Researchers[23] found when examining individuals with a flat-arched foot posture that the augmented Low-Dye technique reduced activity of the tibialis anterior, tibialis posterior, and peroneus longus. Other researchers[24,25] found a reduction in tibialis anterior and tibialis posterior activity among individuals with various foot types with the augmented Low-Dye. Increased activity of the tibialis anterior and tibialis posterior has been associated with excessive pronation,[26–29] and the use of the augmented Low-Dye may be effective in reducing pronation.

Overall, some evidence supports the use of arch taping techniques to temporarily lessen excessive pronation. The findings suggest that more complex taping techniques, such as the augmented Low-Dye involving application onto the lower leg, and use of heavyweight elastic tape may provide greater support than lower profile taping techniques with non-elastic tape. (See "Further Reading" for the steps of application of the augmented Low-Dye.[21]) Further research is needed to examine the differences among the individual techniques and the biomechanical effects on the foot during activity to provide health care professionals additional evidence for implementation of the most effective techniques into clinical practice.

## PLANTAR FASCIA STRAP    Figure 3–11

- **Purpose:** Use the plantar fascia strap technique to provide moderate support to the longitudinal arch and lessen the symptoms associated with plantar fasciitis (Fig. 3–11).
  This technique requires fewer supplies than the Low-Dye techniques in treating plantar fasciitis.
- **Materials:**
  • 2 inch or 3 inch width heavyweight moleskin (pre-cut straps or from roll), taping scissors
  *Options:*
  • Adherent tape spray
  • 2 inch elastic tape
- **Position of the patient:** Sitting on a taping table or bench with the leg extended off the edge and the foot placed in a neutral position.

⟹ **Preparation:** To make a strap, cut a piece of 2 inch or 3 inch width moleskin in a 9–11 inch length strip. Determine the length of the strap by the size of the foot. Measure approximately 1–1½ inches from one end and draw a line. From this line, measure another 1–1½ inches and draw a second line.
***Option:***
Apply adherent tape spray to the plantar forefoot to provide additional adherence.

⟹ **Application:**

**STEP 1:** On each side of the strip beginning at the second line, make an angled cut toward the first line, leaving at least 1 inch between the cuts at the first line (Fig. 3–11A).

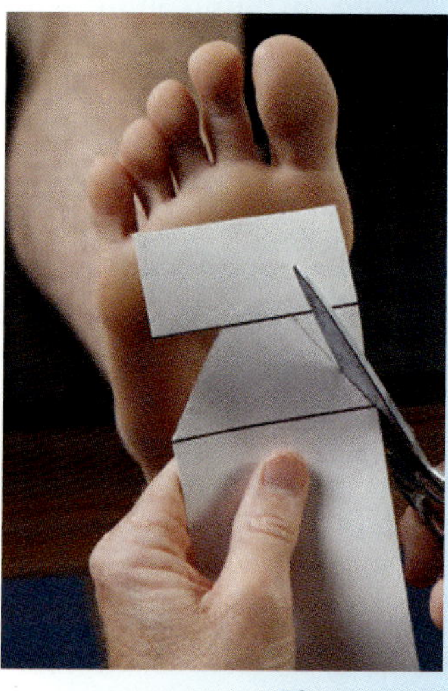

**Fig. 3–11 A**

**STEP 2:** Anchor the cross bar end of the strap directly to the skin over the posterior heel (Fig. 3–11B). Position the cut in the strap just **superior** to the plantar surface of the foot.

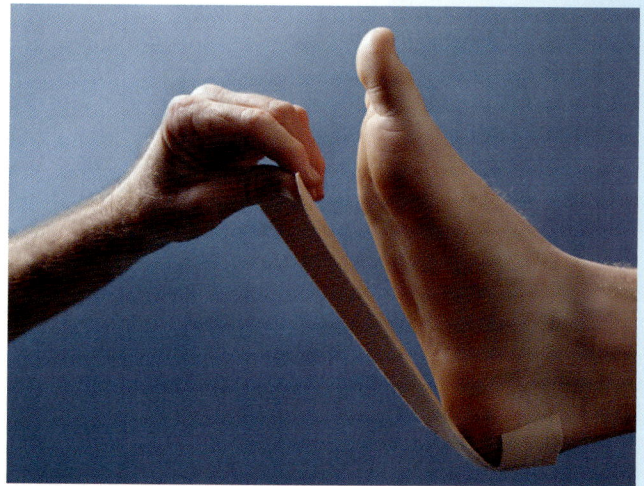

**Fig. 3–11 B**

**STEP 3:** Pull the strap with slight tension toward the metatarsal heads and anchor (Fig. 3–11C). Check the tension of the strap by allowing the patient to step down and take a few steps. Appropriate tension should support the longitudinal arch and lessen pain with weight-bearing movements. If necessary, reposition the strap by removing the end at the metatarsal heads and reanchor.

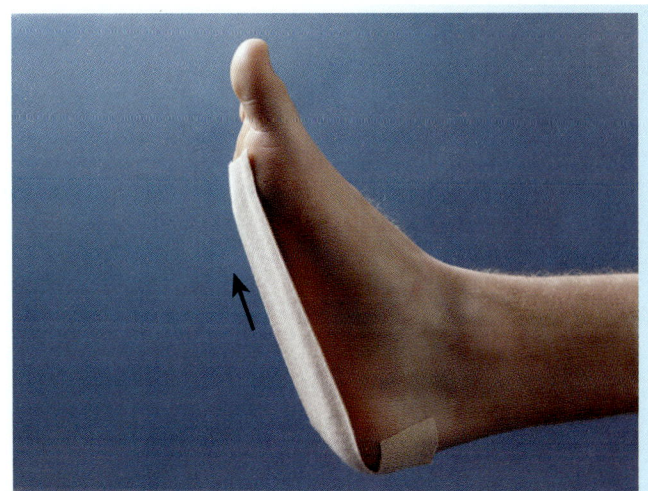

**Fig. 3–11 C**

**STEP 4:** Smooth the strap directly to the skin with your hands and cut any excess moleskin from the metatarsal heads (Fig. 3–11D).

*Option:* *An anchor of 2 inch elastic tape may be applied around the metatarsal heads in a lateral-to-medial direction to anchor the strap, but this is not required.*

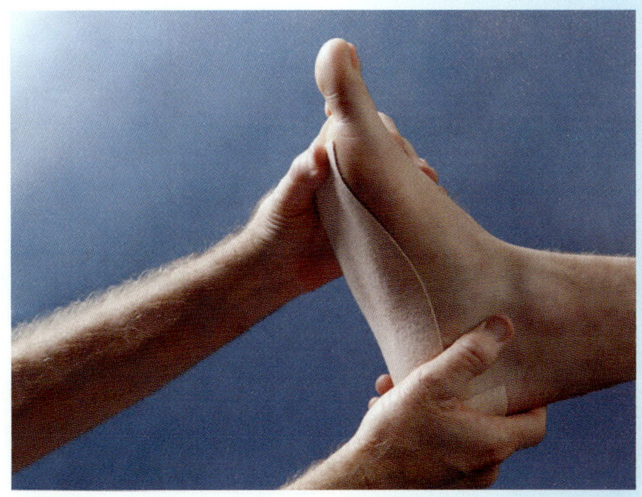

**Fig. 3–11 D**

---

**...IF/THEN...**

**IF** application of the circular, "X," and/or loop arch taping technique does not provide adequate support for a longitudinal arch strain, **THEN** consider using the weave, Low-Dye, or plantar fascia strap taping or orthotic technique, which may provide greater support to the longitudinal arch.

---

**Clinical Application Question 1**

Late in the season, an intercollegiate softball outfielder begins to demonstrate pain over the medial heel. You suspect plantar fasciitis and are proficient in applying several taping techniques to treat the injury. However, your supply inventory is low, leaving only non-elastic tape available for use.

➡ **Question: What taping techniques can you use to treat plantar fasciitis?**

## BUDDY TAPE    Figure 3–12

➤ **Purpose:** Use the buddy tape technique following sprains, dislocations, and fractures of the toes to provide mild to moderate stability for the collateral ligaments. The injured toe is taped together with the largest adjacent toe (Fig. 3–12). The buddy tape technique is commonly used with the toe wedge technique to lessen medial deviation of the great toe at the MTP joint in the treatment of bunions or hallux valgus. The toe wedge technique and steps of application can be found on FADavis.com. 💲

➤ **Materials:**
• ½ inch non-elastic tape, ⅛ inch foam or felt, adherent tape spray, taping scissors
  *Option:*
• 1 inch non-elastic or elastic tape or self-adherent wrap

➤ **Position of the patient:** Sitting on a taping table or bench with the leg extended off the edge and the foot placed in a neutral position.

➤ **Preparation:** Apply adherent tape spray to the involved toes. To maintain anatomical alignment, cut a piece of ⅛ inch foam or felt the length of the shortest toe to be taped. Do not apply tape directly over the joints. When applying tape to the toes, monitor for skin irritation of adjacent toes.

> **Helpful Hint |**
> Apply a skin lubricant such as petroleum jelly over the tape and to adjacent toes. The lubricant will reduce friction between the tape and skin to prevent blisters and abrasions.

➤ **Application:**

**STEP 1:**    Apply a strip of ½ inch non-elastic tape around the proximal end of the foam or felt and place between the toes (Fig. 3–12A).

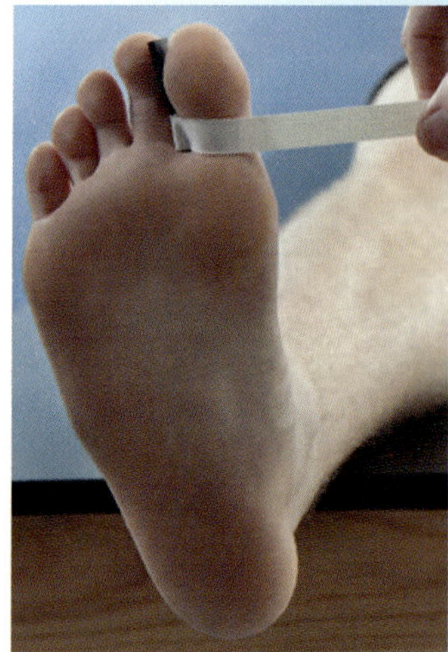

**Fig. 3–12 A**

**STEP 2:**   Encircle the toes between the MTP and proximal interphalangeal (PIP) joints with the tape lock-in strip (Fig. 3–12B). The direction of the tape does not matter (hereinafter symbolized by ◂▦▸).

**Helpful Hint |**
The lock-in strip will prevent the foam or felt from dislodging and loosening during activity as perspiration and moisture begin to affect the tape adhesive.

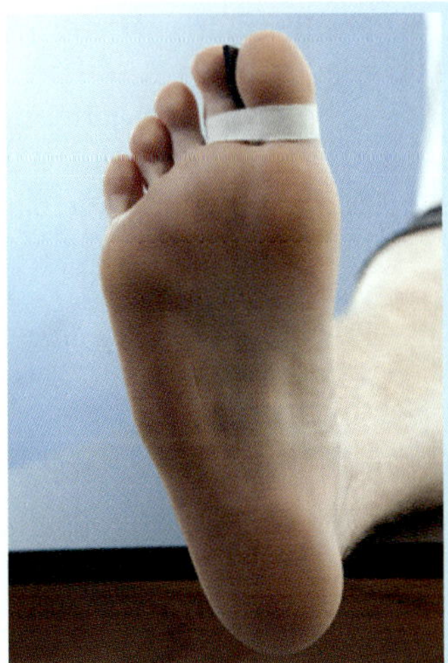

**Fig. 3–12 B**

**STEP 3:**   Maintain alignment of the toes and apply three to five circular strips of ½ inch non-elastic tape with mild to moderate roll tension between the MTP and PIP joints and the PIP and distal interphalangeal (DIP) joints ◂▦▸ (Fig. 3–12C). End the strips on the dorsal aspect of the toes to lessen unraveling due to contact with clothing during activity.

*Option:*   *Use 1 inch non-elastic or elastic tape or self-adherent wrap on large toes to provide adequate support.*

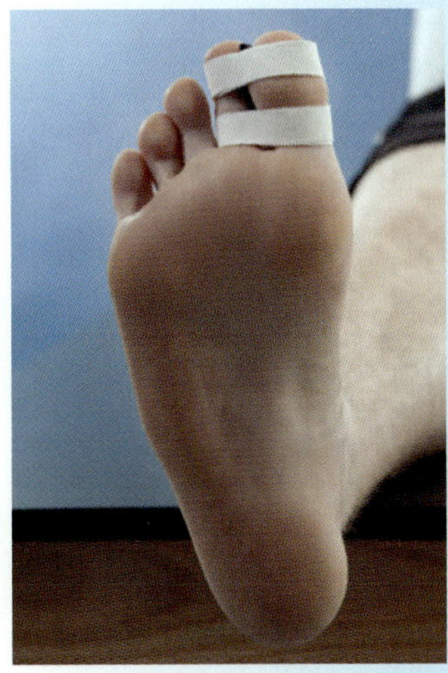

**Fig. 3–12 C**

## TOE STRIPS          Figure 3–13

▸ **Purpose:** Use the toe strips technique following a hyperextension (turf toe) or hyperflexion (soccer toe) sprain to provide mild to moderate support and reduce range of motion at the MTP joint (Fig. 3–13). Depending on the specific injury (turf or soccer toe) hyperextension, hyperflexion, or multidirectional range of motion can be reduced.

▸ **Materials:**
   • 1 inch non-elastic or elastic tape, 2 inch elastic tape or self-adherent wrap, adherent tape spray

➡ **Position of the patient:** Sitting on a taping table or bench with the leg extended off the edge and the foot placed in a neutral position. Determine painful range(s) of motion by stabilizing the midfoot, proximal to the metatarsal heads. To determine painful flexion, place a finger on the proximal dorsal phalanx of the great toe and slowly move the toe into flexion until pain occurs. Place a finger on the proximal plantar phalanx and slowly move the toe into extension to determine painful extension. Once painful range of motion is determined, place the great toe in a pain-free range and maintain this position during application.

➡ **Preparation:** Apply adherent tape spray to the midfoot and great toe.

➡ **Application:**

**STEP 1:**    Place a 1 inch non-elastic or elastic tape anchor directly to the skin around the mid-to-distal great toe and a 2 inch elastic tape or self-adherent wrap anchor around the midfoot with mild roll tension ◀▬▬▶ (Fig. 3–13A).

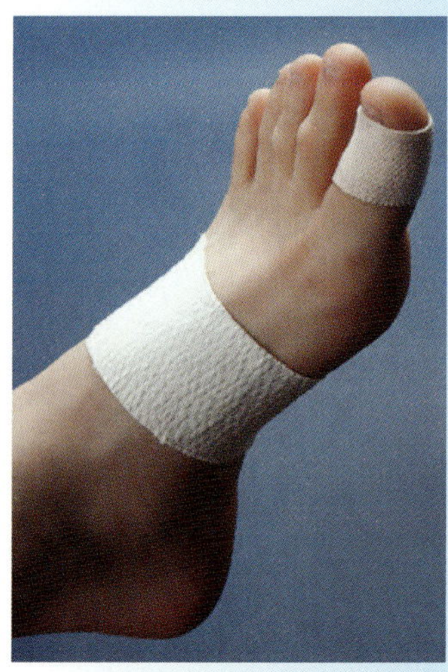

**Fig. 3–13 A**

**STEP 2:**    To limit hyperextension, anchor a 1 inch non-elastic tape strip on the lateral plantar surface of the toe and continue to the midfoot anchor (Fig. 3–13B).

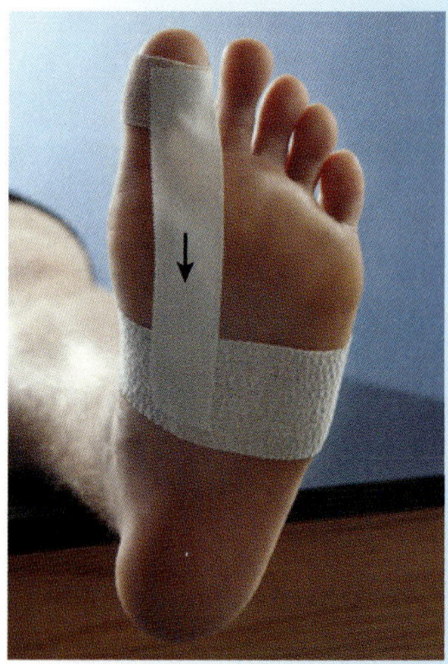

**Fig. 3–13 B**

**STEP 3:**   Apply three to four additional strips, overlapping by ½ of the tape width (Fig. 3–13C).

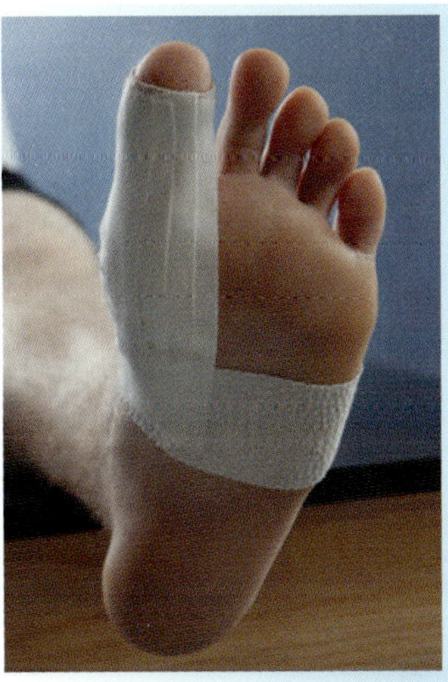

**Fig. 3–13 C**

**STEP 4:**   To limit hyperflexion, anchor a 1 inch non-elastic strip on the lateral dorsal surface of the toe and continue to the midfoot anchor (Fig. 3–13D).

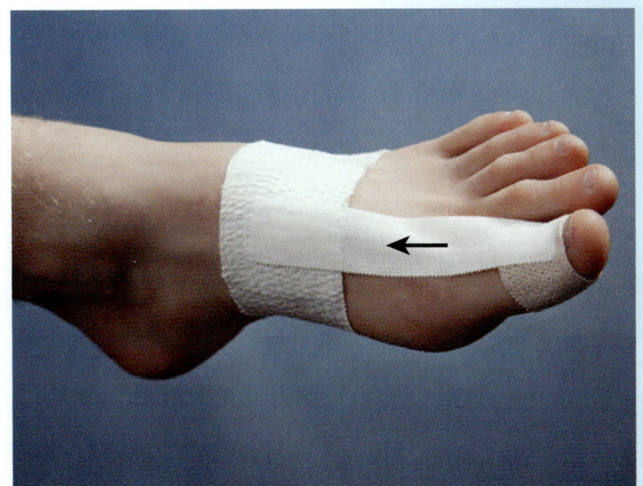

**Fig. 3–13 D**

**STEP 5:**   Apply three to four additional strips, overlapping each one (Fig. 3–13E).

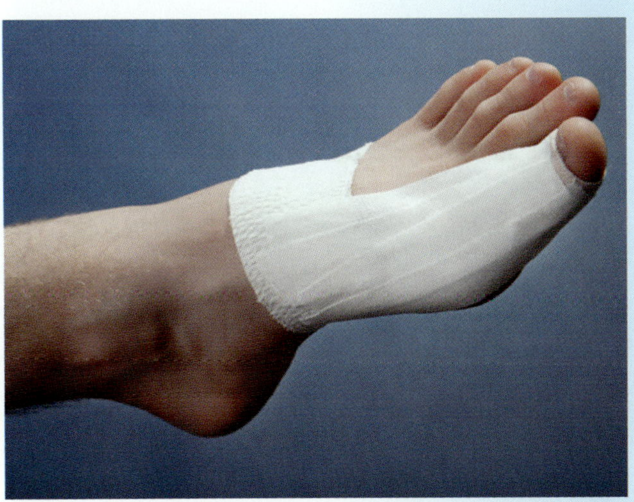

**Fig. 3–13 E**

*Steps Cont.*

Foot and Toes

**STEP 6:** To limit multidirectional motion, anchor a 1 inch non-elastic tape strip on the lateral plantar toe, proceed at an angle over the medial foot, and finish on the dorsal midfoot anchor (Fig. 3–13F).

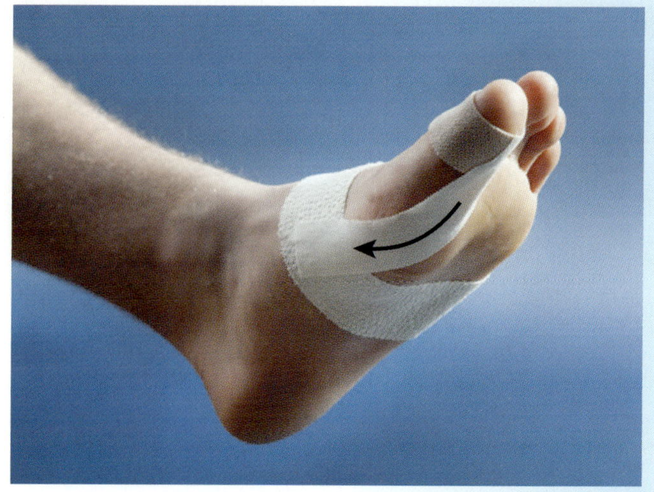

Fig. 3–13 F

**STEP 7:** Next, anchor a strip on the lateral dorsal toe, proceed at an angle over the medial foot, and finish on the plantar midfoot anchor (Fig. 3–13G).

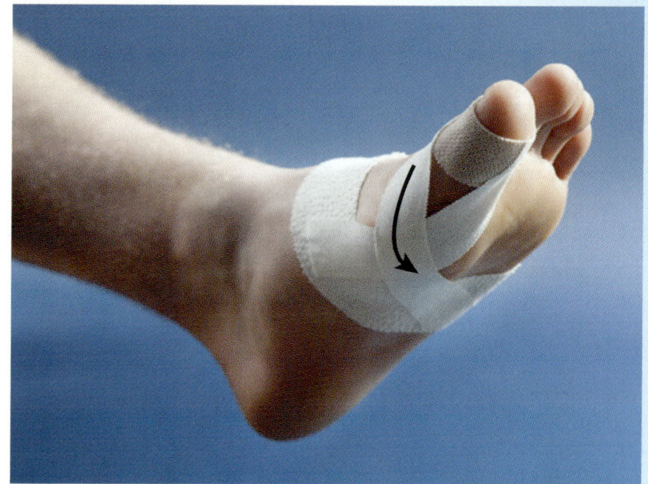

Fig. 3–13 G

**STEP 8:** Place three to four additional strips, alternating anchor points on the toe, to produce a weave-type pattern (Fig. 3–13H).

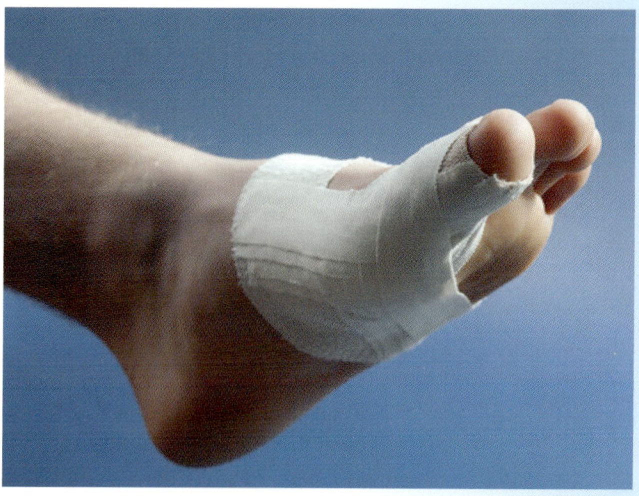

Fig. 3–13 H

**STEP 9:** Place a 1 inch non-elastic or elastic tape anchor around the mid-to-distal great toe and a 2 inch elastic tape anchor around the midfoot with mild roll tension ◀▦▶ (Fig. 3–13I). End the tape on the dorsal aspect of the toe and foot.

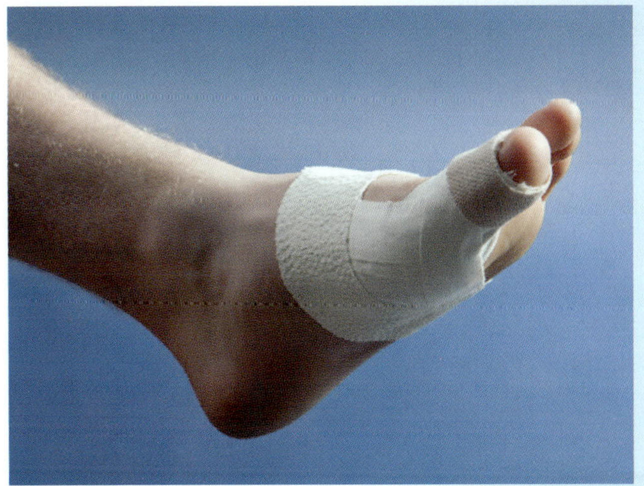

**Fig. 3–13 I**

### Toe Strip Variation

➠ **Purpose:** A variation to the toe strips technique to limit multidirectional motion involves applying tape strips that enclose the great toe. Use this technique with painful hyperflexion and hyperextension associated with an MTP joint sprain.

➠ **Materials:**
   • 1 inch non-elastic or elastic tape, 2 inch elastic tape or self-adherent wrap, adherent tape spray

➠ **Position of the patient:** Sitting on a taping table or bench with the leg extended off the edge and the foot placed in a neutral position. Determine painful range(s) of motion. Once determined, place the great toe in a pain-free range and maintain this position during application.

➠ **Preparation:** Apply adherent tape spray to the midfoot and great toe.

➠ **Application:**

**STEP 1:** Place a 1 inch non-elastic or elastic tape anchor directly to the skin around the mid-to-distal great toe and a 2 inch elastic tape or self-adherent wrap anchor around the midfoot with mild roll tension ◀▦▶. Beginning on the lateral plantar toe, apply individual 1 inch non-elastic tape strips, anchoring on the midfoot. Continue to place individual strips in the same manner around the toe, overlapping by ½ of the tape width. Place the last strip on the lateral dorsal surface of the great toe (Fig. 3–13J).

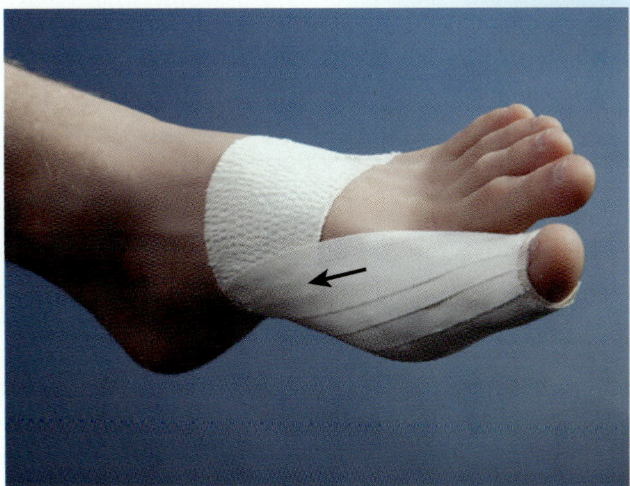

**Fig. 3–13 J**

*Steps Cont.*

Foot and Toes

**STEP 2:** Place a 1 inch non-elastic or elastic tape anchor around the mid-to-distal great toe and a 2 inch elastic tape anchor around the midfoot ◄▬▬► (Fig. 3–13K). End the tape on the dorsal aspect of the toe and foot.

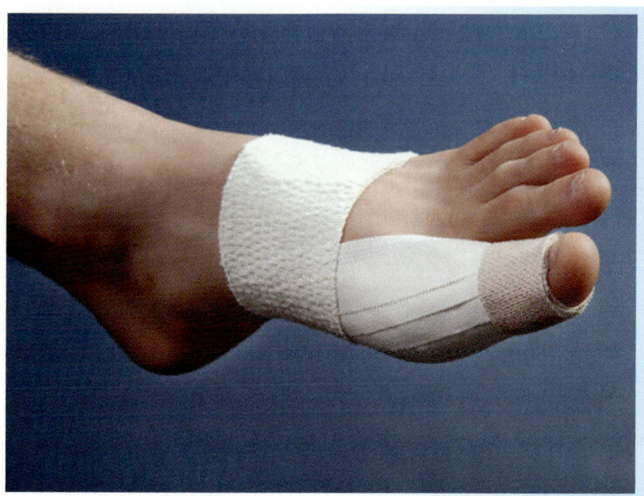

**Fig. 3–13 K**

## ⊕ TOE SPICA

▸ **Purpose:** The toe spica technique provides mild support to the MTP joint of the great toe in the treatment of great toe sprains. This technique and steps of application can be found on FADavis.com.

## TURF TOE STRAP    Figure 3–14

▸ **Purpose:** The turf toe strap technique provides moderate support to the great toe and limits excessive range of motion, typically hyperextension (Fig. 3–14). This technique requires fewer supplies than the toe strips technique in treating MTP joint sprains. 

▸ **Materials:**
- 2 inch or 3 inch width heavyweight moleskin (pre-cut straps or from roll), 1 inch non-elastic or elastic tape, taping scissors

   *Options:*
   - Adherent tape spray
   - 2 inch elastic tape

▸ **Position of the patient:** Sitting on a taping table or bench with the leg extended off the edge and the foot placed in a neutral position. Determine painful range(s) of motion. Once determined, place the great toe in a pain-free range and maintain this position during application.

▸ **Preparation:** Cut individual straps in the shape of an uppercase "T" from a roll of 2 inch or 3 inch heavyweight moleskin by following the technique illustrated in Figure 3–11 but leaving only ½–¾ inch for the cross bar.

   *Option:*
   Apply adherent tape spray to the toe and plantar forefoot to provide additional adherence.

▸ **Application:**

**STEP 1:**  Anchor the strap directly to the skin on the plantar surface of the mid-to-distal great toe (Fig. 3–14A).

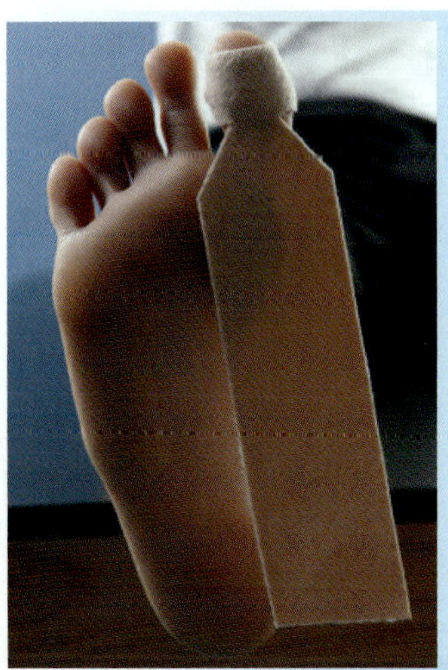

**Fig. 3–14 A**

**STEP 2:**  Check the position of the toe and apply slight tension to the strap and anchor on the plantar surface of the foot near the calcaneus (Fig. 3–14B). Check for appropriate strap tension by allowing the patient to step down and walk. Appropriate tension should limit excessive hyperextension and reduce pain with weight-bearing movements. Reposition the plantar foot anchor if necessary. Smooth the moleskin to the skin.

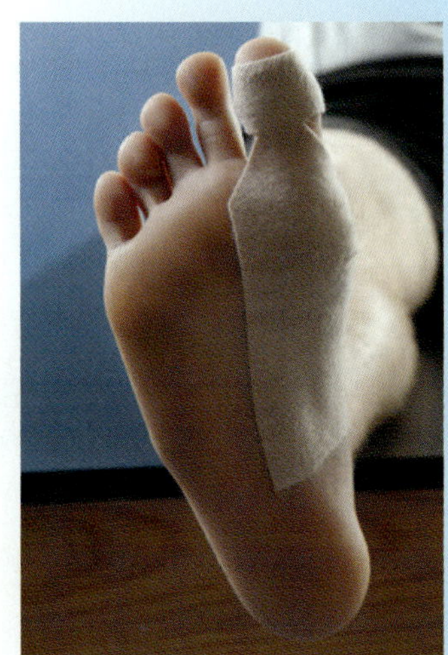

**Fig. 3–14 B**

**STEP 3:**  Apply a 1 inch non-elastic or elastic tape anchor with mild roll tension around the strap on the mid-to-distal toe ◂▭▸ (Fig. 3–14C). End the tape on the dorsal aspect of the toe.

*Option:*  *An anchor of 2 inch elastic tape can be applied around the midfoot to anchor the strap, but this is not required* ◂▭▸.

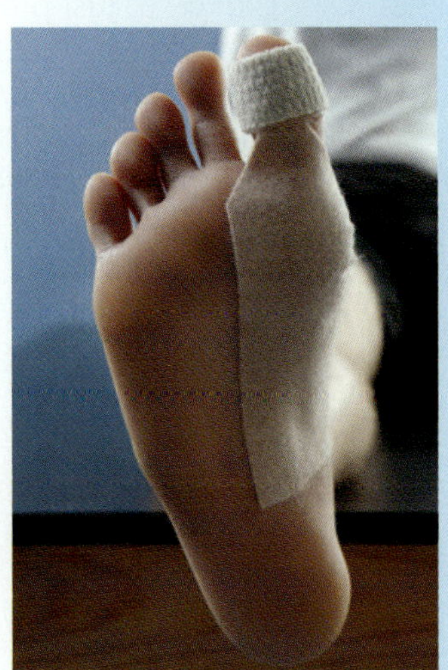

**Fig. 3–14 C**

## ELASTIC MATERIAL     Figures 3–15 and 3–16

➡ **Purpose:** Use elastic materials to cover wound dressings and attach pads to the foot (Fig. 3–15) and toes (Fig. 3–16) in treating wounds, contusions, and blisters. The material should be lightweight and not restrict range of motion. Because of the elastic material's thin profile and great adhesive strength, use the material in place of tape.

➡ **Materials:**
• Adhesive gauze material, ½ inch non-elastic tape, taping scissors
*Option:*
• 2 inch or 3 inch lightweight elastic tape

➡ **Position of the patient:** Sitting, prone, or supine on a taping table or bench with the leg extended off the edge and the foot in a neutral position.

➡ **Preparation:** Apply adhesive gauze material directly to the skin and use without adherent tape spray.

➡ **Application:**

**STEP 1:**   After applying a sterile wound dressing or pad, cut a piece of the material. The piece of adhesive gauze material should extend from ½–1 inch beyond the dressing or pad to adhere properly to the skin (Fig. 3–15). Smooth the material to the foot.

**Helpful Hint |**
Round all corners of the material to prevent the edges from rolling on contact with clothing.

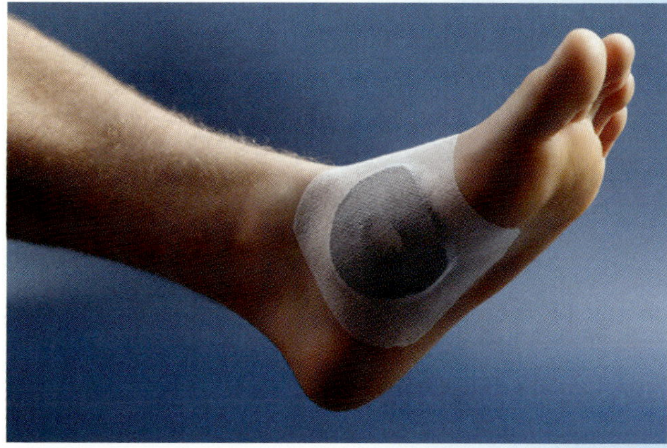

**Fig. 3–15**

**STEP 2:**   For the toes, cut a piece of the elastic material to cover an area from the tip of the toe to just proximal to the DIP or PIP joint. Place the center of the material over the toe (Fig. 3–16A).

*Option:*   *If adhesive gauze material is not available, use 2 inch or 3 inch lightweight elastic tape.*

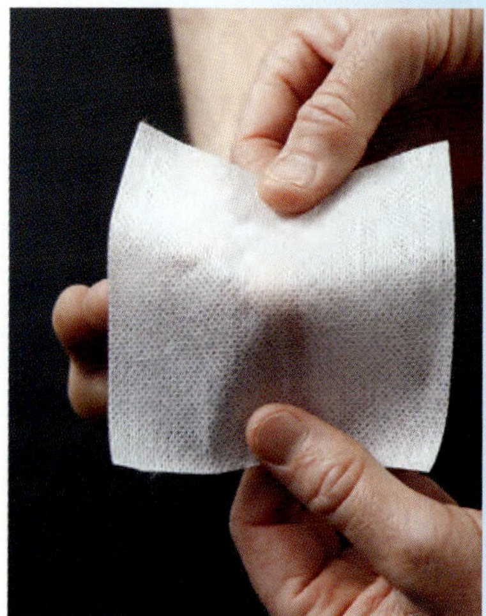

**Fig. 3–16 A**

**STEP 3:** Fold the sides over the toe, avoiding wrinkles. Press the sides of the material together against the toe (Fig. 3–16B).

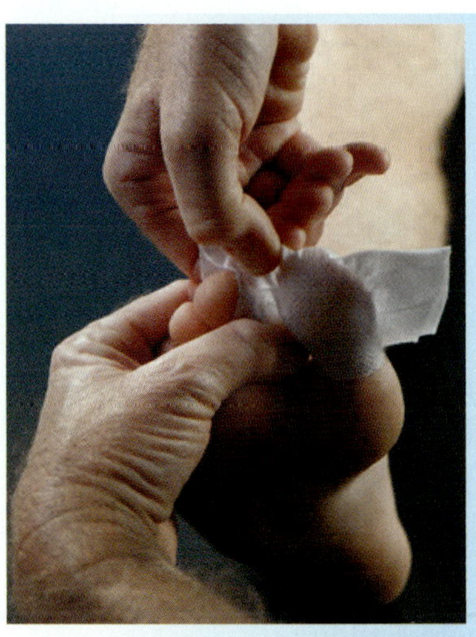

**Fig. 3–16 B**

**STEP 4:** Cut the excess material away from the sides, leaving enough of the material to maintain adherence (Fig. 3–16C). If the toe is large enough, place anchors with ½ inch non-elastic tape around the distal, middle, or proximal phalanx ◄━━━►. End the tape on the dorsal aspect of the toe.

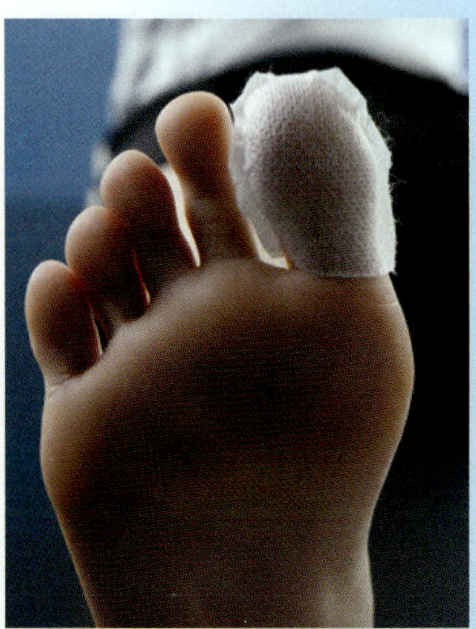

**Fig. 3–16 C**

---

### Clinical Application Question 2

You are treating a recreational runner for a distal third phalanx fracture with the buddy tape technique. After applying the technique several times, the adjacent toes become abraded.

➡ **Question: How can you treat the abrasion and prevent future blisters and abrasions from occurring?**

---

# Wrapping Techniques

By applying mechanical pressure around the injured site, compression wraps assist in reducing the amount of space available for swelling.[30] Use elastic and self-adherent wraps and elastic tape on the foot and toes to treat inflammation that accompanies contusions, sprains, strains, and overuse injuries and conditions (Fig. 3–17).

## FOOT AND ANKLE COMPRESSION WRAP    Figure 3–17

➡ **Purpose:** The foot and ankle or toe compression wrap technique aids in reducing mild, moderate, or severe swelling. 

➡ **Materials:**
  • 2 inch, 3 inch, or 4 inch width by 5 yard length elastic wrap determined by the size of the foot, metal clips, 1½ inch non-elastic or 2 inch elastic tape, taping scissors
  • 1 inch elastic tape or self-adherent wrap for the toes

*Options:*
  • ⅛ inch or ¼ inch foam or felt
  • 2 inch, 3 inch, or 4 inch width self-adherent wrap or elastic tape, pre-wrap, thin foam pads

➡ **Position of the patient:** Sitting on a taping table or bench with the leg extended off the edge and the foot in pain-free dorsiflexion.

➡ **Preparation:** Apply the technique directly to the skin.

*Option:*
Cut a ⅛ inch or ¼ inch foam or felt pad and place it over the inflamed area directly to the skin to assist in venous return.

Using tape, apply one layer of pre-wrap directly to the skin and use thin foam pads over the heel and lace areas to prevent irritation (see Fig. 4–4A).

➡ **Application:**

**STEP 1:**    Holding the elastic wrap, anchor the extended end on the distal plantar surface of the foot and proceed around to encircle the anchor ◀▦▶ (Fig. 3–17A).

*Option:*    *2 inch, 3 inch, or 4 inch width self-adherent wrap or elastic tape can also be used when an elastic wrap is not available.*

> **Helpful Hint |**
> Anchoring of the elastic or self-adherent wrap or elastic tape on the plantar surface of the foot may perhaps lessen migration of the wrap or tape, particularly with weight-bearing movements.

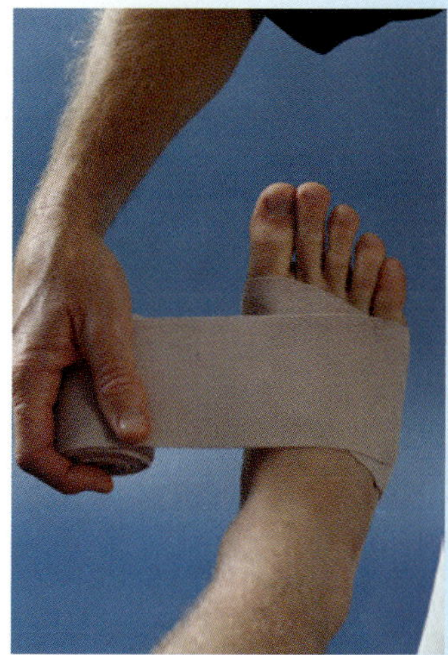

**Fig. 3–17 A**

**STEP 2:**    Continue to apply the wrap in a spiral pattern, overlapping by ½ of the width, changing angles of the wrap, and moving in a proximal direction (Fig. 3–17B).

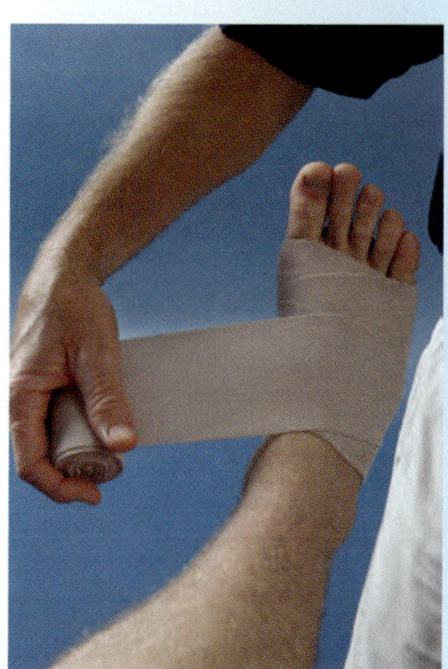

**Fig. 3–17 B**

**STEP 3:**  Incorporate the heel lock technique (see Fig. 4–5) with the spiral pattern to enclose the heel ◀▦▶ (Fig. 3–17C). Avoid gaps, wrinkles, and inconsistent roll tension in the distal-to-proximal application.

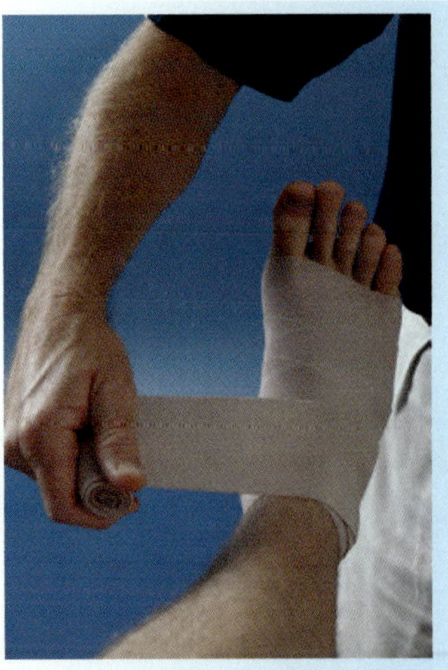

**Fig. 3–17 C**

**STEP 4:**  Continue with the spiral pattern and anchor over the distal lower leg with Velcro, metal clips, or loosely applied 1½ inch non-elastic or 2 inch elastic tape ◀▦▶ (Fig. 3–17D). With practice, apply the greatest amount of roll tension distally and lessen tension as the wrap continues proximally.

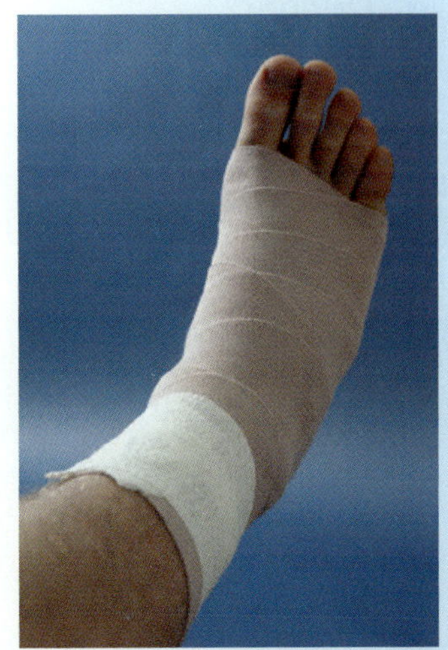

**Fig. 3–17 D**

**STEP 5:**  For the toes, apply 1 inch elastic tape or self-adherent wrap in a distal-to-proximal circular pattern over the toe ◀▦▶ (Fig. 3–17E). End the tape or wrap on the dorsal aspect of the toe. Apply pressure greatest at the distal end and less toward the proximal end. The tip of the toe should remain exposed to monitor circulation. No additional anchor is required.

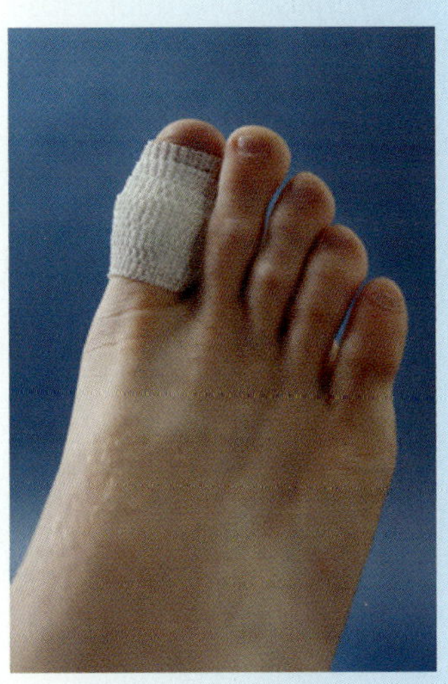

**Fig. 3–17 E**

### ...IF/THEN...

**IF** an elastic wrap compression technique does not provide adequate pressure around the foot, allowing swelling to migrate distally following a dorsal midfoot contusion, **THEN** consider using self-adherent wrap or pre-wrap and elastic tape, which possess greater ability to conform to the contours of the foot, to provide adequate pressure.

# Bracing Techniques

Bracing techniques provide immobilization or support, or they correct structural abnormalities in preventing and treating injuries and conditions of the foot and toes. Many of these techniques also work for other lower extremity injuries and conditions.

### Orthotics

The use and construction of orthotics have been and continue to be a common practice in the health care setting. Orthotics are designed to correct and support structural abnormalities of the foot, such as excessive supination and pronation and pes cavus, and can be purchased off-the-shelf or individually fabricated in a variety of shapes with many different types of materials. Generally, orthotics can be categorized as three types: soft, semirigid, and rigid.

### Soft Orthotics

Soft orthotics are designed to absorb shock and reduce friction and stress of the foot. They are constructed of a variety of materials such as felt, foam, plastic, rubber, silicone, and viscoelastic polymers (Fig. 3–18). Many of these orthotics can be purchased off-the-shelf and do not require cast molds or fabrication.

Felt and foam are frequently used to construct soft orthotics. For our purposes, the construction and application of felt and foam orthotics in treating sesamoiditis, metatarsalgia, interdigital neuroma, heel contusions, and bunions are discussed in the Padding Techniques section of this chapter. The types of soft orthotics are discussed next.

## HEEL CUPS    Figure 3–18 A

➡ **Purpose:** Use heel cups for heel pain associated with contusions, spurs, plantar fasciitis, and lower leg, knee, and back injuries and conditions.

➡ **Design:**
- Hard heel cups are made from plastic to provide support; soft cups are constructed of latex rubber, silicone, and viscoelastic polymers to provide support and shock absorption.
- Heel cups come according to the foot size or weight of the patient.
- Some designs have adjustable inserts to provide individual fit and support.
- To prevent adaptive changes with the use of one heel cup, place a cup in each shoe. Clean heel cups with soap and water and reuse them.

➡ **Application:**

**STEP 1:**   Insert the cups into the heel box of each shoe over the insole. Additional adhesive to prevent migration is normally not required (Fig. 3–18A).

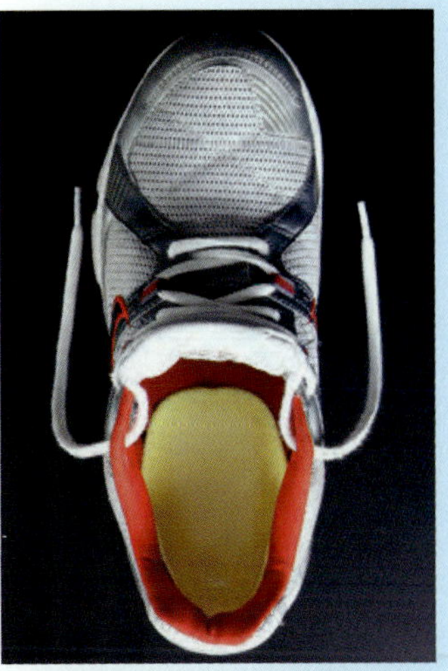

**Fig. 3–18 A** *Heel cup inserted into a shoe.*

## SOFT INSOLES    Figure 3–18 B

- **Purpose:** Full-length neoprene, silicone, thermoplastic rubber, polyurethane foam, and viscoelastic polymer insoles provide shock absorption for the entire plantar surface of the foot.
- **Design:**
  - Purchase the insoles off-the-shelf in specific shoe sizes or cut them from a large roll of the soft material.
  - Some designs allow for custom molding and fitting.
  - Use the insoles over the existing insoles or as replacements.
- **Application:**

**STEP 1:**   Trimming the insole with taping scissors may help in finding the best fit. Additional adhesive is typically not required to hold the insole in place. Loosen the shoe laces and slide the soft insole toward the toe box (Fig. 3–18B).

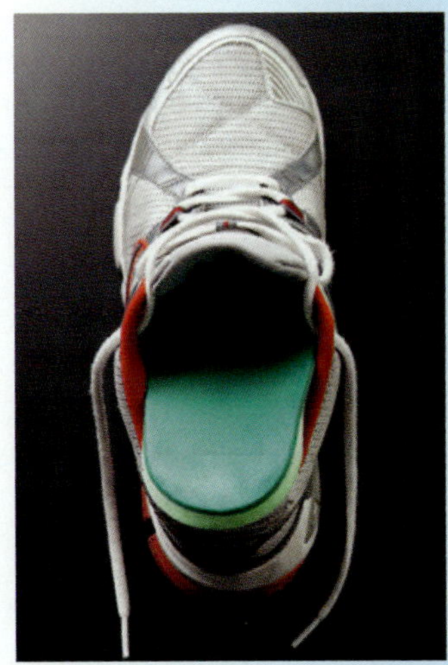

**Fig. 3–18 B** *Soft insole partially inserted into a shoe.*

### Semirigid Orthotics

Semirigid orthotics are constructed from thermoplastic, cork, leather, and foam materials. These orthotics are designed to absorb shock, reduce friction and stress, and support and correct structural abnormalities of the forefoot and/or rearfoot[31] (Fig. 3–19). Because of the adaptability, support, control, and flexible construction, semirigid orthotics are perhaps the most widely used type with the athletic population.[30] Purchase the orthotics in off-the-shelf designs or have them custom-made in a health care facility or orthotic laboratory.

- **Purpose:** Use semirigid orthotics in preventing and treating many rearfoot and forefoot injuries and conditions such as MTP sprains, arch strains, interdigital neuroma, sesamoid fractures, metatarsalgia, bunions, and plantar fasciitis.

➠ **Design:**
- These orthotics typically consist of a semirigid outer shell with a soft, durable covering.
- Off-the-shelf designs are manufactured according to shoe size to provide cushion and support to the longitudinal and metatarsal arches (Fig. 3–19A). Some designs allow for custom molding and fitting.
- Other off-the-shelf designs consist of a steel, graphite, carbon fiber, or thermoplastic material insert to restrict forefoot and toe range of motion, such as hyperextension with turf toe injuries (Fig. 3–19B).
- Custom-made designs are fabricated after foot impressions or casts are taken (Fig. 3–19C).

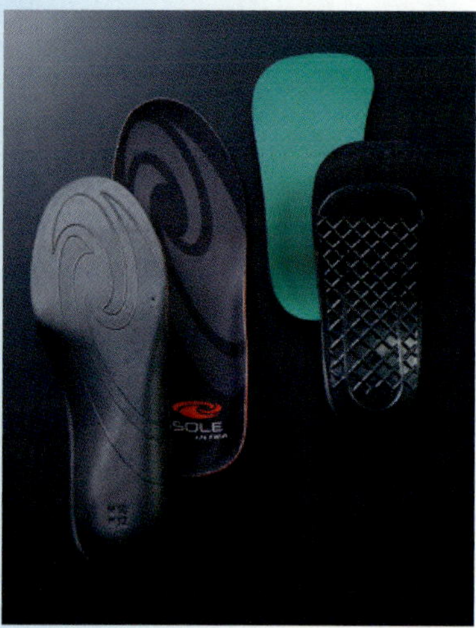

**Fig. 3–19 A** *Off-the-shelf semirigid orthotics. (Left) Full length. (Right) ¾ length.*

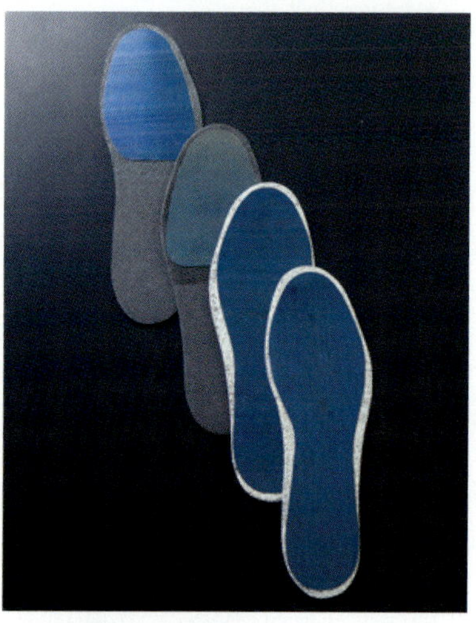

**Fig. 3–19 B** *Off-the-shelf steel semirigid orthotics. (Left) ½ length. (Right) Full length.*

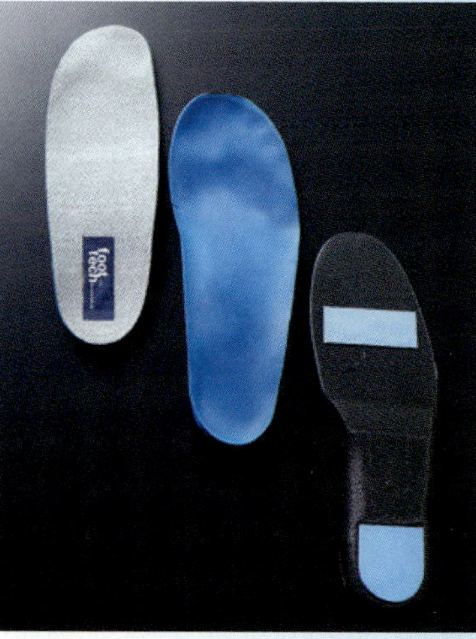

**Fig. 3–19 C** *Custom-made semirigid orthotics.*

## DETAILS

With custom-made semirigid designs, posts are used to correct structural abnormalities and are either intrinsic or extrinsic.[31] Intrinsic posts are built into the orthotic mold, and extrinsic posts are applied on the orthotic shell. Extrinsic posts, constructed of foam or cork material, are used more often with semirigid orthotics and can be modified easily by adding or removing the material.

### Rigid Orthotics

Rigid orthotics are used when the injury or condition warrants absolute biomechanical control of structural abnormalities[31] (Fig. 3–20). The rigid properties of the materials make fabrication time consuming and do not allow for errors. Many health care professionals send casts or molds to orthotic laboratories for construction. Intrinsic posts are commonly used with rigid designs.

Important facts to be familiar with regarding the use of rigid orthotics include the following:
- Because of the inflexibility of the materials, fewer athletes use rigid orthotics.[30]
- The designs have frequently been used with limited success in treating structural abnormalities in adolescents.[32]
- Use rigid orthotics in preventing and treating MTP sprains, arch strains, and excessive pronation or supination.
- The orthotics are constructed from a foot cast and made of rigid acrylic plastic or graphite materials (Fig. 3–20).

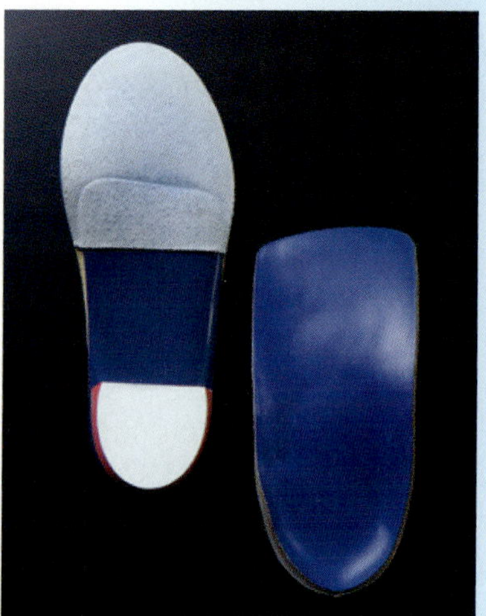

**Fig. 3–20** *Custom-made rigid orthotics.*

## EVIDENCE SUMMARY

Orthotics are prescribed and used in the treatment and prevention of numerous injuries and conditions. Several evidence-based reviews have investigated the efficacy of orthotics in the treatment of lower extremity and back injuries and conditions. A 2007 review[33] found insufficient data to determine the effectiveness of semirigid and soft orthotics in the prevention and treatment of back pain among a mixed population. The review also revealed that the use of semirigid and soft orthotics did not prevent back pain among military recruits. A 2014 review[34] examined the efficacy of off-the-shelf and custom-made semirigid and soft orthotics in the prevention and treatment of low back pain among adult subjects. The findings demonstrated insufficient evidence to support the use of these orthotic designs in the prevention and treatment of low back pain.

Other reviews have focused on orthotics and lower extremity injuries and conditions. Examining interventions for Morton's neuroma, a review[35] demonstrated no evidence to support the use of orthotics designed to pronate the foot to lessen levels of pain in adults. A 2008 review[36] examined the effects of orthotics on the reduction of plantar pain associated with several foot conditions. Among a mixed population with pes cavus, semirigid orthotics reduced greater amounts of pain than sham orthotics. Semirigid orthotics were shown to reduce greater amounts of pain associated with hallux valgus compared to no treatment, but surgery was more effective than the orthotic. Investigations of the effects of orthotics on the reduction of plantar heel pain associated with plantar fasciitis have produced conflicting results among various populations. Semirigid orthotics were found to be more effective than sham orthotics in the improvement of function scores, but no more effective than night splints, lower leg stretching, and mobilization in lessening pain scores.[36] Among more recent reviews, two investigated the use of orthotics in the treatment of plantar heel pain. Findings from a 2018 review[37] included 20 trials and found no evidence to support the use of off-the-shelf and custom-made orthotics to reduce patient-reported pain scores and improve function outcome measures at 3, 3 to 12, and 12 month or longer periods. A separate 2018 review[38] included 19 trials and demonstrated that off-the-shelf and custom-made orthotics were more effective in the reduction of patient-reported pain scores at 7 to 12 week periods compared to sham orthotics. However, no differences in pain and function scores were found between off-the-shelf, custom-made, and sham orthotics at 0 to 6 and 13 to 52 week periods. In the treatment of lower extremity overuse injuries and conditions, a review[39] revealed no differences in levels of pain between the use of custom-made and off-the-shelf orthotics and no orthotic. Additionally, no differences in efficacy were found between custom-made and off-the-shelf designs.

The use of orthotics in the prevention of lower extremity injuries and conditions has been examined in several evidence-based reviews. A 2011 review[40] revealed minimal evidence to support the use of custom-made and off-the-shelf designs. Findings from individual trials in the review among military recruits showed custom-made orthotics worn in boots significantly reduced the incidence of medial tibial stress syndrome (MTSS) compared to no orthotic. However, custom-made orthotics had no effect on lessening rates of soft tissue injury in the ankle, Achilles tendon, and knee. Among soccer referees, soft heel inserts worn during a 5 day tournament resulted in a significant reduction in lower extremity soreness compared to no heel insert. In contrast to these findings, foam rubber heel pads worn in tennis shoes did not reduce the incidence of MTSS in a separate military recruit population. Other trials revealed no differences in the incidence of ankle sprains and foot injuries with the use of custom-made and off-the-shelf semirigid orthotics among military recruits. Three trials among military recruits investigated the effect of soft orthotics and found no significant differences in lower extremity soft tissue injuries compared to non-soft orthotics. A separate review[39] investigated the effects of custom-made and off-the-shelf orthotics versus no orthotic and found a significant reduction in lower extremity overuse conditions with the use of orthotics among military recruits. Examining orthotic designs, this review demonstrated no differences between custom-made and off-the-shelf orthotics in the reduction of overuse conditions. A 2013 review[41] investigated risk factors for the development of MTSS in runners. Among three studies, the findings showed prior use of orthotics was a significant risk factor for MTSS. However, specific orthotic designs and materials were not fully described in the studies included in the review. Findings from a 2017 review[42] examining off-the-shelf and custom-made orthotics versus no orthotic found some evidence for the orthotic designs in the prevention of lower extremity injuries and conditions. Pooled data among 10 trials showed off-the-shelf and custom-made orthotics reduced the incidence of overall lower extremity injuries. Examining specific injuries and conditions, the designs lessened the incidence of metatarsal, tibial, and femoral stress fractures and shin pain. However, off-the-shelf and custom-made orthotics had no effect on lessening rates of Achilles tendon or knee pain. The findings from pooled data among seven trials[42] examining soft orthotics demonstrated no reduction in overall, lower leg stress fracture, and soft tissue injury rates.

The effects of orthotics on foot structure and mechanics may assist health care professionals in making sound clinical decisions in regard to design. An evidence-based review[3] comparing interventions to reduce foot pronation found custom-made and off-the-shelf orthotics effective in treadmill and overground walking, running, and static standing conditions but less effective than taping and control footwear. The findings suggested that custom-made designs were more effective in controlling pronation than off-the-shelf designs. An additional review[43] demonstrated off-the-shelf orthotics with posting reduced rearfoot eversion and tibial internal rotation greater than controls in non-injured subjects during jogging. Among non-injured subjects, custom-made orthotics with and without posting produced a significantly greater reduction in loading rate than off-the-shelf designs with posting and controls. Custom-made designs with posting also resulted in a significantly greater reduction in vertical impact force compared with off-the-shelf designs with posting. A 2018 review[44] found that off-the-shelf and custom-made orthotics with medial posting at the forefoot and forefoot and rearfoot reduced rearfoot eversion during walking in controlling foot pronation among subjects with pes planus. Orthotics with neutral posting at the rearfoot and designs with an arch support had no effect on the control of excessive foot pronation. Other researchers[45] have examined plantar pressures with orthotic use and found off-the-shelf designs significantly decreased pressures in the toes, medial forefoot, and lateral midfoot and custom-made beneath the hallux, medial forefoot, and lateral midfoot compared with the original shoe insole among recreational runners. The findings also showed custom-made orthotics decreased pressure in the medial heel greater than off-the-shelf designs. Evaluating the effects of orthotics on foot kinematics among subjects with low-mobile foot posture, researchers[46] revealed that custom-made designs increased rearfoot complex dorsiflexion during midstance, perhaps providing correction of the structural abnormality. Other researchers[47] demonstrated a significant increase in pre-activity of the peroneal longus, from onset of activity to initial touchdown, following an 8 week intervention with custom-made semirigid orthotics in runners with lower extremity overuse injury symptoms. The researchers[47] suggested this pre-activity may result in enhanced dynamic control of ankle stability.

Although Nigg, Nurse, and Stefanyshyn[48] have stated that the idea of orthotics aligning the skeleton is based on a substantial amount of uncertainty, orthotics continue to be used by health care professionals. The evidence to support or refute the use of orthotics in the treatment and prevention of injuries and conditions is inconsistent in the literature. Several evidence-based reviews have been conducted investigating orthotics and provide the best available evidence. Despite variations in study participants, settings, outcome measures, intervention durations, and definitions of injury and orthotic designs, health care professionals can implement evidence-based practice to guide clinical decisions and care of the patient. Additional research is needed with well-designed randomized controlled trials using longer intervention durations and standard definitions of orthotics among various populations to provide stronger evidence for the implementation of orthotics into clinical practice.

## Clinical Application Question 3

A construction worker is experiencing general pain along the entire plantar surface of both feet during work. His boots have a steel shank sole.

➡ **Question: What bracing technique would you use to treat his condition?**

## OFF-THE-SHELF NIGHT SPLINTS　　Figure 3–21

➡ **Purpose:** Night splints are designed to keep the ankle and foot in 5 degrees of dorsiflexion and the toes in slight dorsiflexion to provide a static stretch of the plantar fascia and Achilles tendon while the patient is sleeping to reduce pain in treating plantar fasciitis (Fig. 3–21).

➡ **Design:**
- Off-the-shelf splints are designed in predetermined sizes that correspond to shoe size.
- These splints are contoured to the lower leg and foot and made of rigid plastic covered with soft foam material.
- Some designs extend from the anterior lower leg to the toes; others from the posterior lower leg to the toes.
- Many designs include a removable foam wedge used to place the foot and toes into additional dorsiflexion. Other designs use straps to adjust the ankle and toes in varying degrees of dorsiflexion.
- Velcro straps are typically used to attach the splint to the lower leg and foot.

➡ **Position of the patient:** Sitting on a taping table or bench or chair.
➡ **Application:**

**STEP 1:**  To apply most designs, release the straps, place on the lower leg and foot, and fasten the straps (Fig. 3–21).

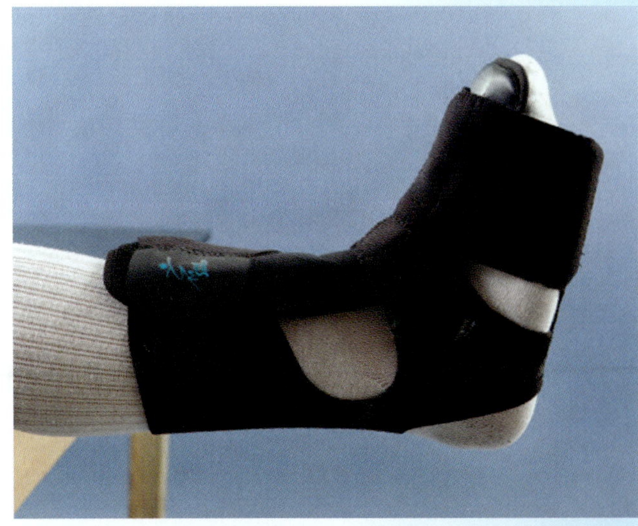

**Fig. 3–21**

## ⚕ CUSTOM-MADE NIGHT SPLINTS

➡ **Purpose:** Thermoplastic material also is useful for the construction of a night splint when an off-the-shelf design is unavailable. The splint covers the posterior aspect of the lower leg and foot, including the gastrocnemius-soleus, calcaneus, plantar surface of the foot, and distal toes. This technique and steps of application can be found on FADavis.com.

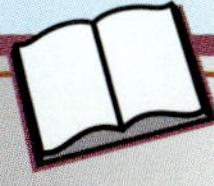

# EVIDENCE SUMMARY

Night splints, used alone or in combination with other conservative interventions, are used for the reduction of pain and improvement of functional outcomes in the treatment of plantar fasciitis. Two separate evidence-based reviews[37,38] examined the efficacy of various interventions for the treatment of plantar heel pain. Examining pain, the reviews found no significant differences in visual analogue scales of pain perception between off-the-shelf semirigid orthotics and night splints at 12 weeks and between custom-made semirigid orthotics and night splints at 12 and 26 week periods. However, a significant reduction in pain was produced at 52 weeks following the use of custom-made semirigid orthotics compared with night splints. Examining patient-reported functional outcomes, the reviews[37,38] demonstrated no significant differences in daily and sport activity scores at 12 and 52 week periods between custom-made semirigid orthotics and night splints. In contrast, custom-made semirigid orthotics produced significantly greater sport activity scores at 26 weeks compared to night splints. These limited findings and the suggestion that plantar fasciitis is self-limiting[49] with spontaneous improvement over time indicate the need for more evidence to guide clinical decisions and treatment interventions.

## DETAILS

Perhaps not as effective as off-the-shelf and thermoplastic night splints, lace-up ankle braces provide some static stretch to the plantar fascia and Achilles tendon (see Fig. 4–15). Properly fitted ankle braces do not incorporate the toes, which is a disadvantage of using this technique as a night splint. However, lace-up ankle braces are commonly found in health care settings and may be used if other splints are not available. A complete discussion of lace-up ankle braces is found in Chapter 4.

## WALKING BOOT    Figure 3–22

➡ **Purpose:** Walking boots or walkers provide complete support and immobilization in treating sprains, strains, and stable acute and stress fractures and in postoperative procedures involving the foot and toes (Fig. 3–22). Boots can replace a traditional plaster or fiberglass cast. The advantages of boots over traditional casting include lightweight design, lower cost, removal to allow for treatment and rehabilitation, adjustable range of motion, and lower adverse effects on gait kinematic and kinetic patterns.[50]

➡ **Design:**
- The boots are manufactured in predetermined sizes according to shoe size.
- The shell and medial and lateral upper arms and struts of the boots are constructed of aluminum, molded plastic, or lightweight steel materials.
- The soles consist of soft or hard rubber with a flat or rocker-shaped bottom.
- Inside the shell, a nylon foam liner or adjustable air bladder system wraps around the lower leg and foot to provide cushioning.
- Velcro straps or buckles incorporated through the shell secure the boot to the lower leg and foot.
- Boots come in a tall design that extends to the upper portion of the lower leg and a short design that extends to the middle portion of the lower leg (Fig. 3–22A).
- Several boot designs contain dials that allow for adjustments in range of motion (Fig. 3–22B).

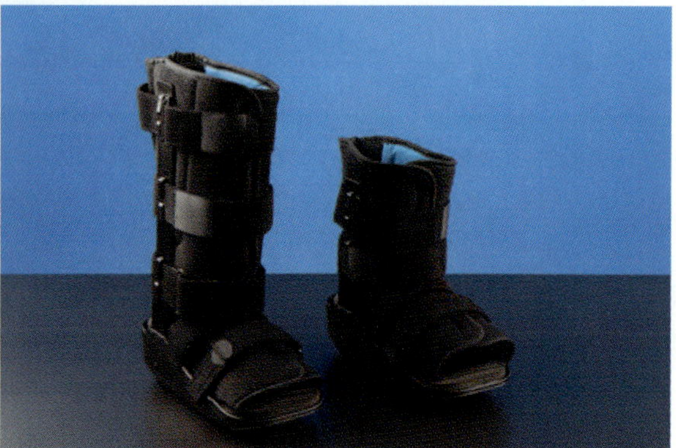

**Fig. 3–22 A** *Walking boots. (Left) Tall. (Right) Short.*

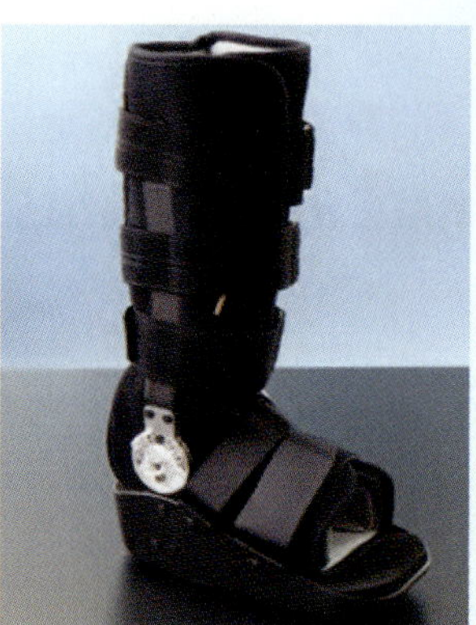

**Fig. 3–22 B** *Walking boot with an adjustable range of motion dial.*

➡ **Position of the patient:** Sitting on a taping table or bench or chair.
➡ **Application:**

**STEP 1:** Application begins with loosening the straps and separating the liner. Place the foot into the boot, moving the heel against the heel box (Fig. 3–22C).

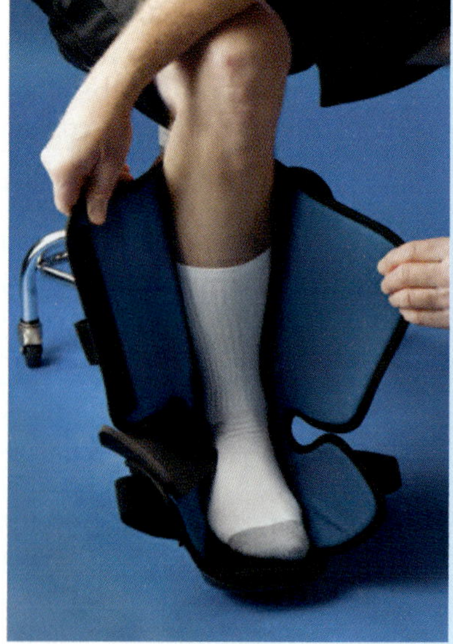

**Fig. 3–22 C**

**STEP 2:** Wrap the liner around the foot and lower leg. At the proximal foot, pull the strap tight and anchor. Next, anchor the distal foot strap. Continue to anchor the lower leg straps (Fig. 3–22D). Adjust the fit by tightening or loosening the straps.

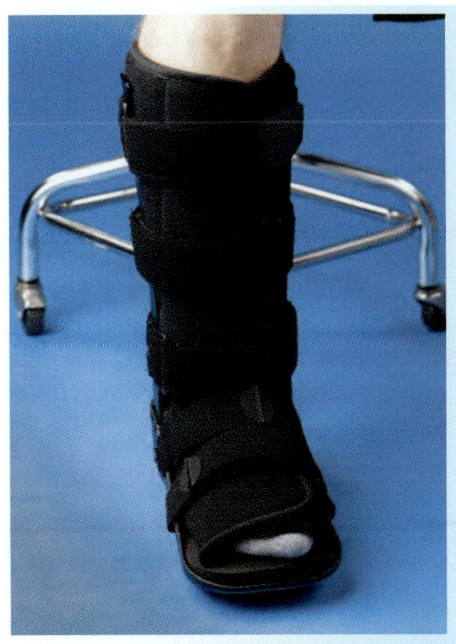

**Fig. 3–22 D**

## CAST BOOT  Figure 3–23

➠ **Purpose:** Cast boots are used as a sandal with lower leg casting or alone with postoperative procedures to absorb shock and provide mild support, allowing for a normal gait (Fig. 3–23).

➠ **Design:**
- The boots are constructed of a canvas upper and ethylene vinyl acetate (EVA) rocker-bottom with forefoot and heel Velcro straps. EVA is a thermoplastic material used in the construction of orthotics and soles of running shoes.
- The boots may be purchased in predetermined sizes according to shoe size.

➠ **Position of the patient:** Sitting on a taping table or bench or chair.

➠ **Application:**

**STEP 1:** To use, simply loosen the straps, place on the plantar surface of the cast or foot, then fasten the straps (Fig. 3–23).

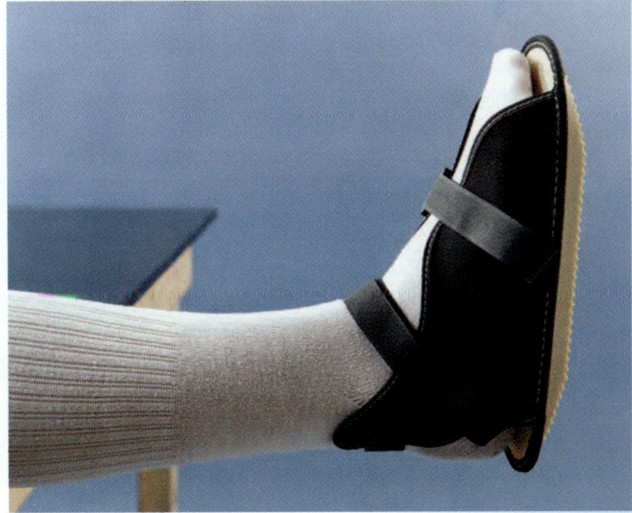

**Fig. 3–23**

## POSTOPERATIVE SHOE    Figure 3–24

➡ **Purpose:** The postoperative shoe is similar in design to the cast boot but has a wooden or rigid EVA rocker-bottom (Fig. 3–24). The stiffness of the sole reduces range of motion in the foot and toes. The shoe is used to treat metatarsal, calcaneus, and sesamoid stress fractures, foot and toe sprains, and postoperative conditions.

➡ **Position of the patient:** Sitting on a taping table or bench or chair.

➡ **Application:**

**STEP 1:**    Apply the shoe in the same manner as the cast boot (Fig. 3–24).

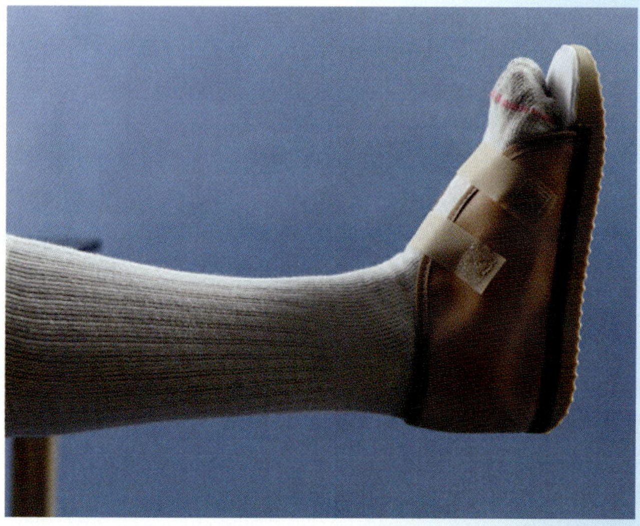

**Fig. 3–24**

---

**Clinical Application Question 4**

A police officer returns to work in the communications center after a surgical procedure to the left foot. The surgeon allows weight-bearing activities with an emphasis on a normal preoperative gait if support is provided to his foot.

➡ **Question: What type of brace could you apply to treat his foot while allowing for a normal gait?**

---

**. . . IF/THEN . . .**

**IF** off-the-shelf semirigid orthotics are effective in correcting a rear or forefoot abnormality but lose their structure and support after a short period of use, **THEN** consider a custom-made design, which will likely retain structure and support for a longer period of time because of the more durable materials used in the construction process.

# Padding Techniques

Felt and foam provide support, shock absorption, and protection and lessen stress for foot and toe injuries and conditions. Because felt and foam are readily available, many health care professionals use these materials to construct soft orthotic designs in the treatment of sesamoiditis, metatarsalgia, interdigital neuroma, heel contusions, and bunions.

## LONGITUDINAL ARCH    Figure 3–25

➠ **Purpose:** Use the longitudinal arch pad technique to provide mild to moderate support of the longitudinal arch in the treatment of arch strains, plantar fasciitis, and pes planus and cavus conditions (Fig. 3–25).

➠ **Materials:**
• ⅛ inch or ¼ inch foam or felt (pre-cut or from roll), taping scissors

➠ **Position of the patient:** Sitting on a taping table or bench with the leg extended off the edge and the foot in a dorsiflexed position.

➠ **Preparation:** Construct the pad from ⅛ inch or ¼ inch foam or felt or purchase pre-cut with an adhesive backing.

➠ **Application:**

**STEP 1:**  Cut the pad to fit from the base of the first metatarsal head to the third metatarsal head, extending to the distal calcaneus, and along the medial aspect of the foot (Fig. 3–25A).

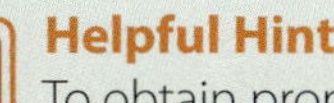

**Helpful Hint |**
To obtain proper fit, outline the longitudinal arch on the patient with a felt tip marker (Fig. 3–25B). Apply adherent tape spray over the outline. Press the selected foam or felt against the outline and hold for 5–10 seconds. The outline will transfer to the foam/felt (Fig. 3–25C). Remove the foam/felt and cut as outlined (Fig. 3–25D). This procedure is helpful with many of the techniques in this section.

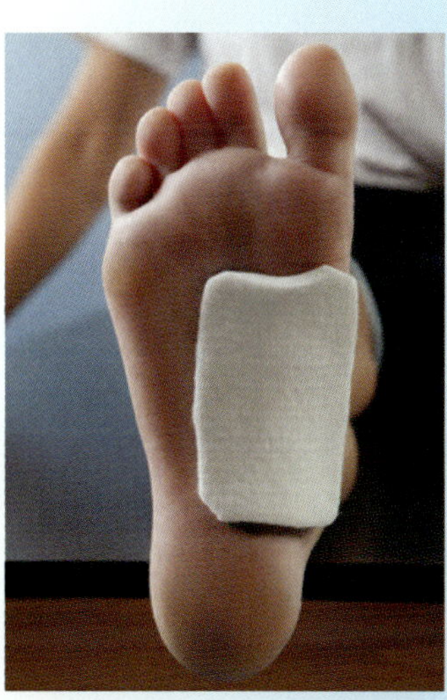

**Fig. 3–25 A**

**STEP 2:**  Attach the pad to the foot using the circular arch technique (see Figs. 3–6 and 3–25E).

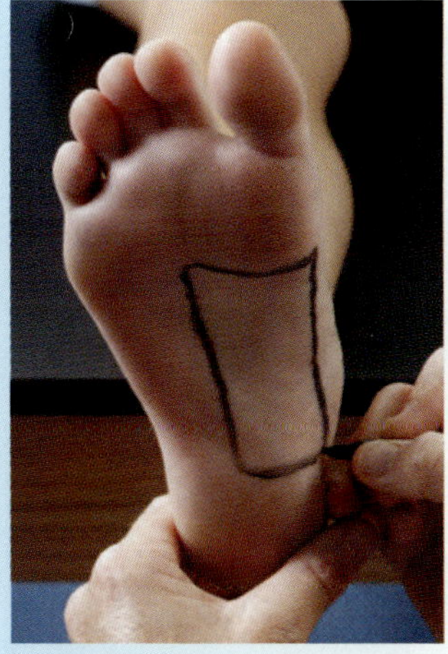

**Fig. 3–25 B**

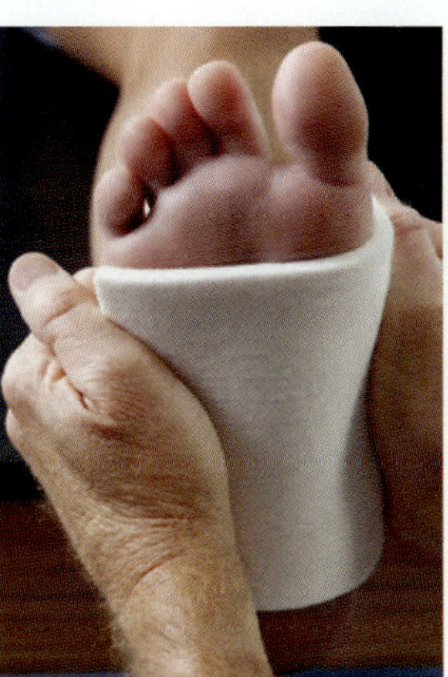

**Fig. 3–25 C**

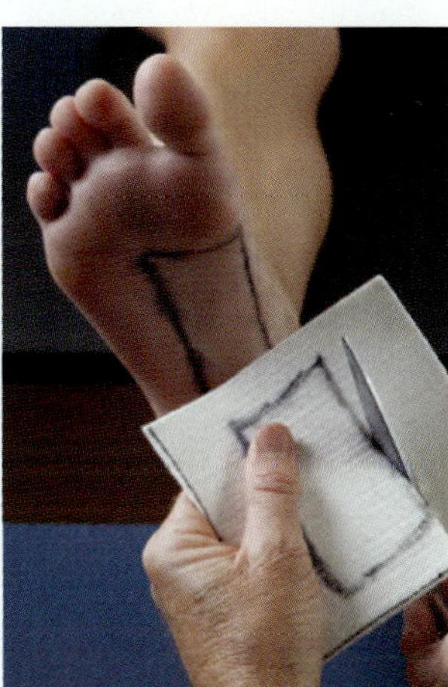

**Fig. 3–25 D**

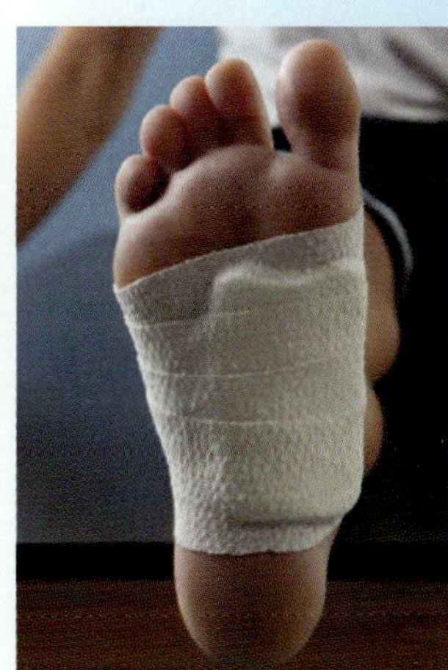

**Fig. 3–25 E**

## DONUT PADS    Figure 3–26

➡ **Purpose:** Use a donut pad to lessen the amount of stress and impact over a painful area by dispersing the stress/impact outward in the treatment of foot and toe blisters, retrocalcaneal bursitis, bunions, corns, calluses, and heel contusions (Fig. 3–26).

➡ **Materials:**
- ⅛ inch or ¼ inch foam or felt (pre-cut or from roll), taping scissors

➡ **Position of the patient:** Sitting, prone, or supine on a taping table or bench with the leg extended off the edge and the foot in a dorsiflexed position.

➡ **Preparation:** Either make the pads from ⅛ inch or ¼ inch foam or felt or purchase pre-cut with adhesive backing. Construction of the pad begins with determining the painful area. If the area of the foot or toes allows, cut the pad to extend in all directions ½ inch to 1 inch beyond the painful area. Apply adherent tape spray if necessary.

➡ **Application:**

**STEP 1:** Cut a piece of foam/felt to the appropriate size. Mark the painful area on the piece of foam/felt and cut out the area with taping scissors, creating a hole (Fig. 3–26A). This hole protects the painful area from stress/impact.

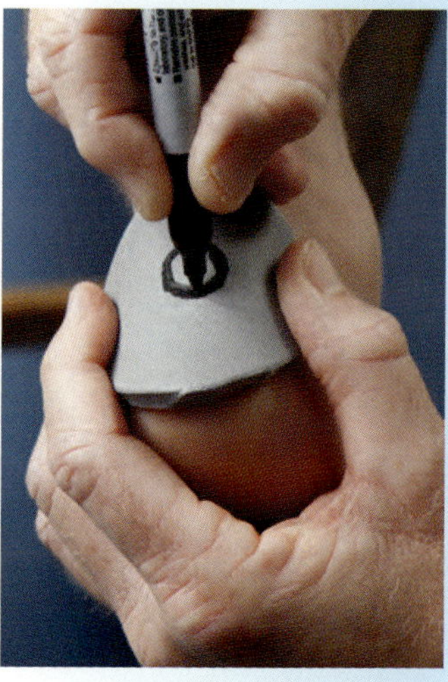

**Fig. 3–26 A**

**STEP 2:** Folding the foam/felt over into one piece and cutting in a semicircle pattern is helpful (Fig. 3–26B).

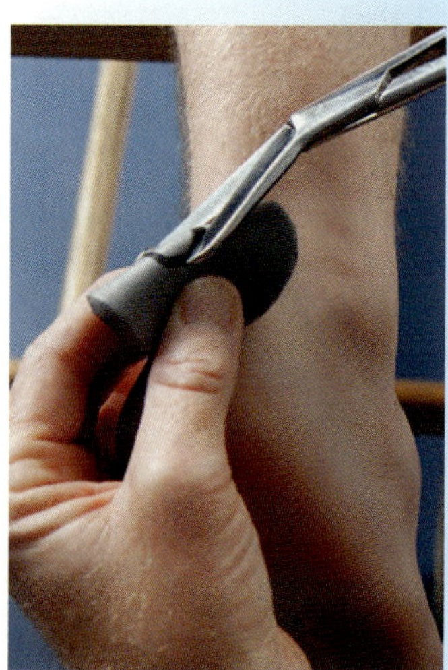

**Fig. 3–26 B**

**STEP 3:** Place the pad on the foot or toe with the hole over the painful area, such as the retrocalcaneal bursa, bunion, corn, callus, or heel and attach with adhesive gauze material or 2 inch self-adherent wrap or elastic tape using the heel lock technique (see Figs. 4–5 and 3–26C).

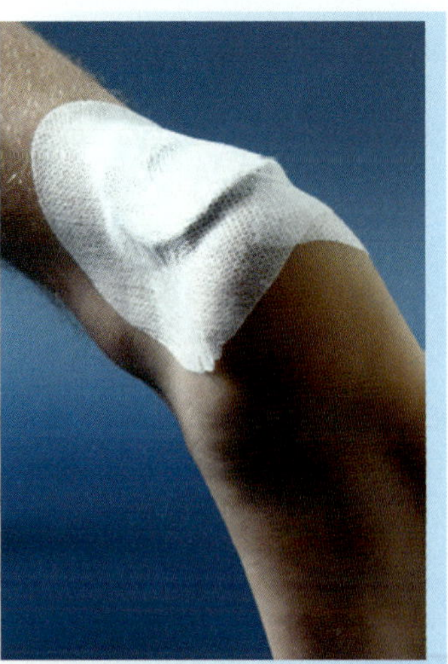

**Fig. 3–26 C**

## HEEL PADS　　Figure 3–27

➡ **Purpose:** Use heel pads in treating plantar fasciitis to provide shock absorption and relief of pain by compressing the fat pad under the calcaneus[2] (Fig. 3–27). Also use heel pads or lifts to lessen stress on the Achilles tendon in treating retrocalcaneal bursitis. The pads are commonly used when soft heel cups are not available.

➡ **Materials:**
- ¼ inch or ½ inch soft, closed-cell foam (pre-cut or from roll) or ¼ inch or ½ inch felt (pre-cut or from roll), taping scissors

  ***Option:***
- Rubber cement

➡ **Position of the patient:** Sitting on a taping table or bench with the leg extended off the edge and the foot in a dorsiflexed position.

➡ **Preparation:** Construct the pads from ¼ inch or ½ inch soft, closed-cell foam or ¼ inch or ½ inch felt or purchase in pre-cut designs with adhesive backing. Place a pad on each heel or in each shoe to prevent adaptive changes. Apply adherent tape spray if necessary.

➡ **Application:**

**STEP 1:** Cut the pad to cover the entire heel area or to the dimensions of the shoe liner (see Fig. 3–27A). Taper the distal end of the pad with taping scissors.

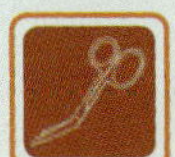

**Helpful Hint |**
Taper a foam heel pad by cutting the distal edge at an angle toward the toes (Fig. 3–27B). Taper a felt pad by separating the distal edge into sections. With your hands, pull apart the felt into three equal sections (Fig. 3–27C). Separate the sections approximately ¾–1 inch toward the curved end of the pad. Cut out the middle section (Fig. 3–27D). Press together the upper and lower sections, producing a tapered edge (Fig. 3–27E).

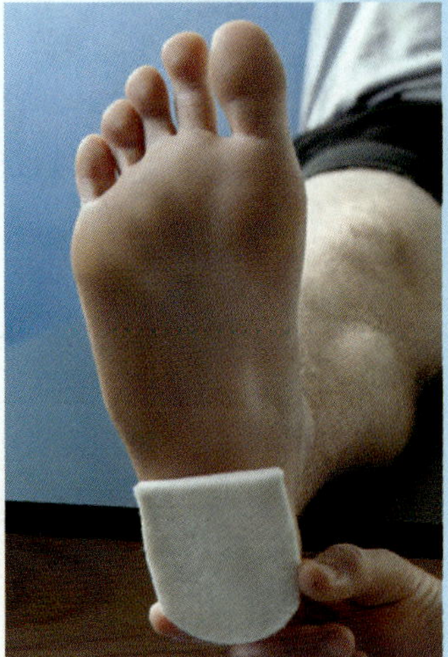

**Fig. 3–27 A**

*Steps Cont.*

**STEP 2:** Either attach the pad to the heel with adhesive gauze material or with 2 inch self-adherent wrap or elastic tape with the heel lock technique (see Figs. 4–5 and 3–27F).

*Option:* Rubber cement may be used to permanently anchor the pad to the shoe liner. Additional anchors are not required.

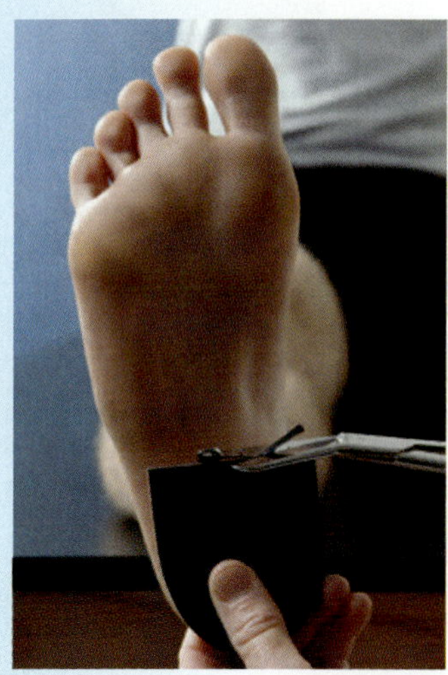

**Fig. 3–27 B**

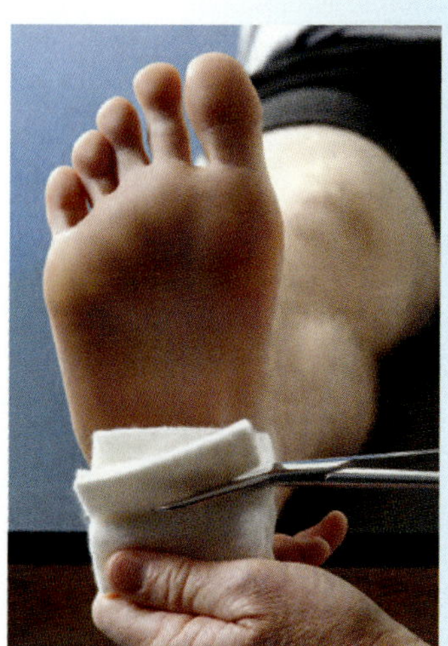

**Fig. 3–27 C**

**Fig. 3–27 D**

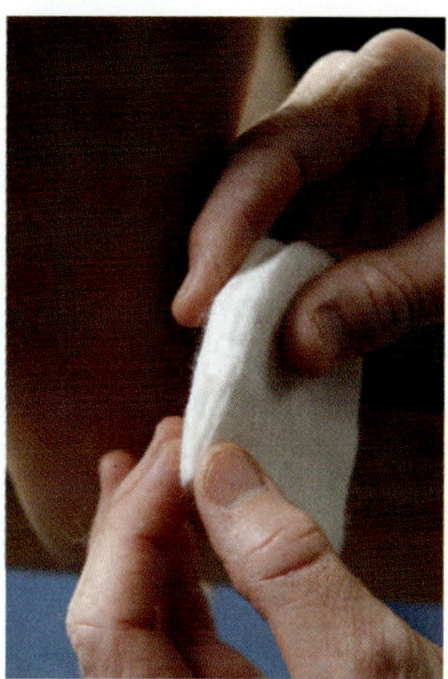

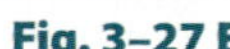

**Fig. 3–27 E**

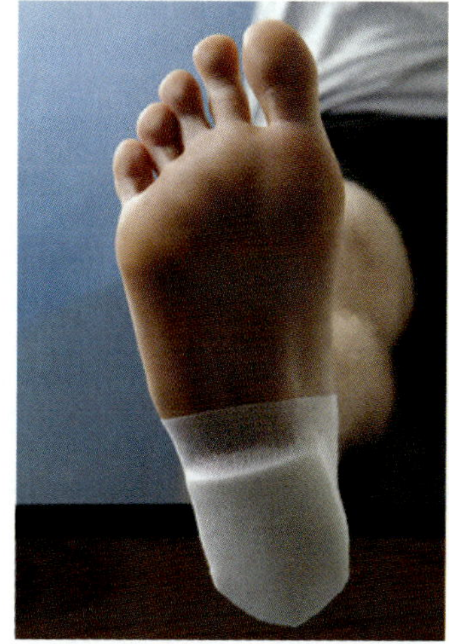

**Fig. 3–27 F**

## METATARSAL BAR     Figure 3–28

➠ **Purpose:** Metatarsal bar pads reduce stress and load on the metatarsal heads in treating sesamoiditis and metatarsalgia (Fig. 3–28).

➠ **Materials:**
  • ⅛ inch or ¼ inch felt (from roll), 1 inch non-elastic tape, 2 inch self-adherent wrap or elastic tape, pre-wrap, taping scissors

➠ **Position of the patient:** Sitting on a taping table or bench with the leg extended off the edge and the foot in a dorsiflexed position.

➠ **Preparation:** Cut the bar from ⅛ inch or ¼ inch felt. The length of the bar measures across the plantar surface of the metatarsal heads and is approximately ¾–1 inch wide.

➠ **Application:**

**STEP 1:** Temporarily attach the bar just proximal to the metatarsal heads with 1 inch non-elastic tape and allow the patient to walk to ensure proper alignment, indicated by a reduction in pain (Fig. 3–28A). Reposition the pad if necessary.

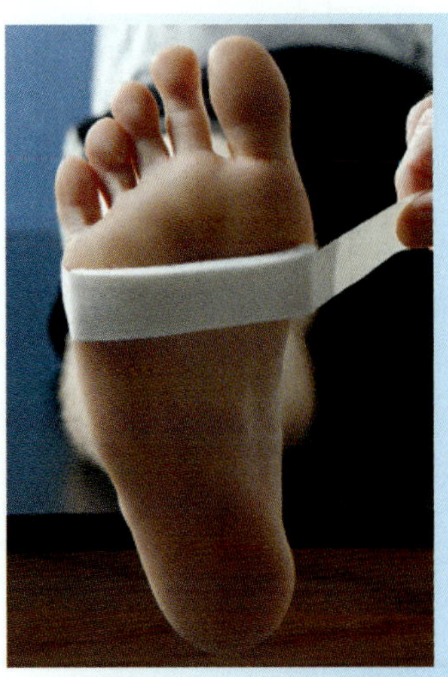

**Fig. 3–28 A**

**STEP 2:** Apply the pad with adhesive gauze material or with one to two strips of 2 inch self-adherent wrap or elastic tape directly to the skin or over pre-wrap. Anchor a strip of self-adherent wrap or elastic tape over the pad on the plantar surface of the foot. Proceed around the dorsal foot and anchor on the plantar or dorsal surface, encircling the foot ◀▬▬▶ (Fig. 3–28B).

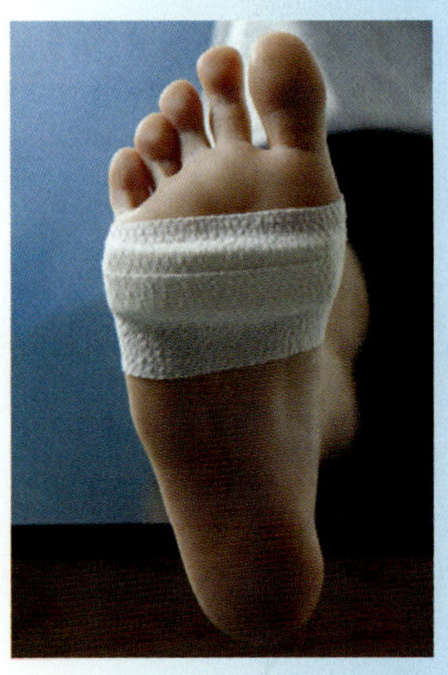

**Fig. 3–28 B**

## TEAR DROP — Figure 3–29

➡ **Purpose:** The tear drop pad technique provides mild to moderate support to the metatarsal arch in treating interdigital neuroma (Fig. 3–29). The most common location is between the third and fourth metatarsals and is referred to as Morton's neuroma.[2,51] With alignment of the metatarsal arch, a decrease in inflammation and pain should occur with the use of the pad.

➡ **Materials:**
  • ⅛ inch or ¼ inch felt (pre-cut or from roll), 1 inch non-elastic tape, taping scissors

➡ **Position of the patient:** Sitting on a taping table or bench with the leg extended off the edge and the foot in a dorsiflexed position.

➡ **Preparation:** Either cut tear drop pads from ⅛ inch or ¼ inch felt or purchase pre-cut with adhesive backing.

➡ **Application:**

**STEP 1:** Cut the pad in a tear drop shape and apply between the heads of the third and fourth metatarsals on the plantar surface of the foot (Fig. 3–29A). Temporarily apply the pad with 1 inch non-elastic tape and have the patient walk.

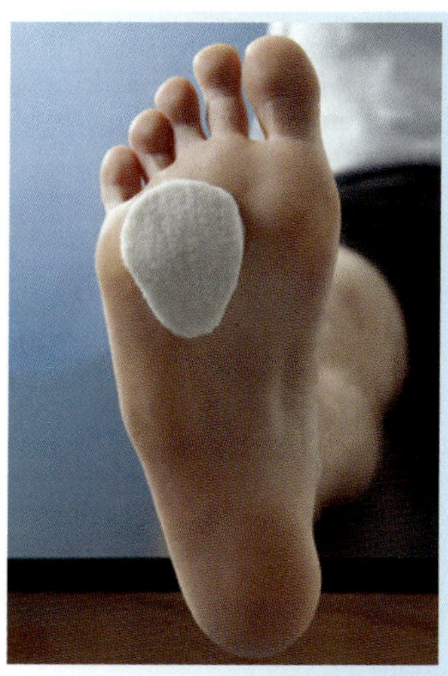

**Fig. 3–29 A**

**STEP 2:** After ensuring proper placement, indicated by a reduction in pain, apply the pad with adhesive gauze material or one to two strips of 2 inch self-adherent wrap or elastic tape directly to the skin or over pre-wrap (Fig. 3–29B).

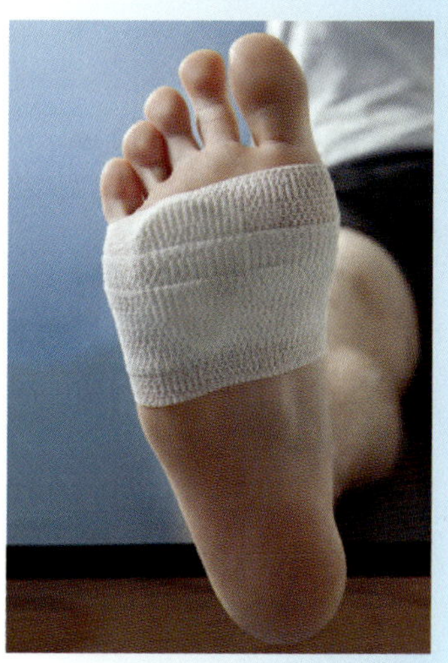

**Fig. 3–29 B**

## OVAL        Figure 3–30

➠ **Purpose:** The oval metatarsal pad is similar to the tear drop pad in design and function (Fig. 3–30). Use the pad in treating metatarsalgia and pain caused by inflexibility of the Achilles tendon, pes cavus, Morton's toe, and metatarsal arch strains. The most common site of pain is under the second or third metatarsal head. The oval pad functions to lessen stress by aligning the metatarsal heads into a correct structural position.

➠ **Materials:**
  • ⅛ inch or ¼ inch felt (pre-cut or from roll), 1 inch non-elastic tape, taping scissors

➠ **Position of the patient:** Sitting on a taping table or bench with the leg extended off the edge and the foot in a dorsiflexed position.

➠ **Preparation:** Construct the pad in an oval shape from ⅛ inch or ¼ inch felt or purchase pre-cut.

➠ **Application:**

**STEP 1:** Place the pad just proximal to the metatarsal head on the plantar surface of the foot (Fig. 3–30A). Temporarily apply the pad with 1 inch non-elastic tape and have the patient walk.

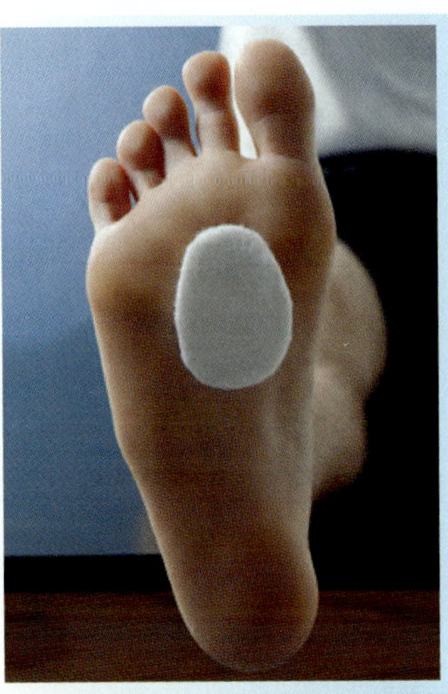

Fig. 3–30 A

**STEP 2:** After proper placement and a reduction in pain, attach the pad with adhesive gauze material or one to two strips of 2 inch self-adherent wrap or elastic tape directly to the skin or over pre-wrap (Fig. 3–30B).

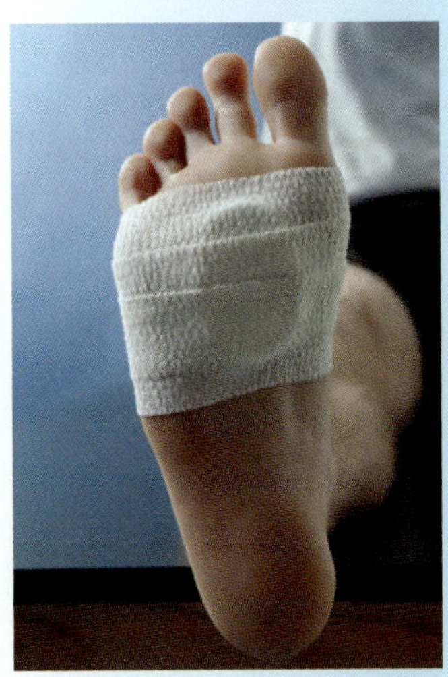

Fig. 3–30 B

| **"J"** | Figure 3–31 |

➡ **Purpose:** Use the "J" pad technique in treating sesamoiditis and sesamoid fractures to unload or lessen stress to the area[31,52] (Fig. 3–31).
➡ **Materials:**
  • ⅛ inch or ¼ inch felt (pre-cut or from roll), taping scissors
➡ **Position of the patient:** Sitting on a taping table or bench with the leg extended off the edge and the foot in a dorsiflexed position.

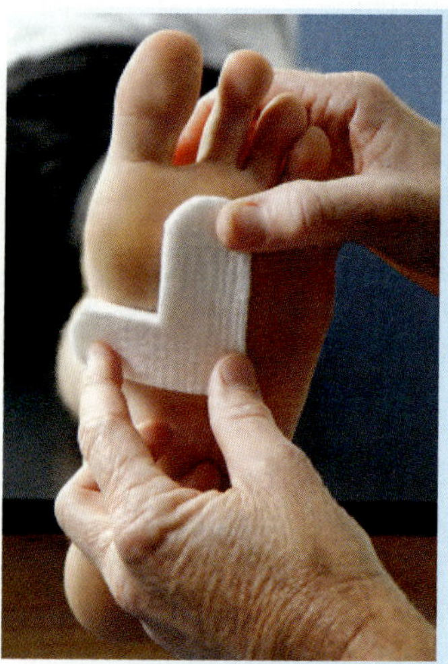

**Fig. 3–31 A**

**Preparation:** Make the pad from ⅛ inch or ¼ inch felt in the shape of an uppercase "J." Pre-cut designs are also available. Extend the pad from the second and third metatarsals, continue proximal, and turn in a medial direction proximal to the sesamoids. The pad is approximately 1–1½ inches wide (Fig. 3–31A).

**Application:**

**STEP 1:** Apply the pad with adhesive gauze material or two to three strips of 2 inch self-adherent wrap or elastic tape directly to the skin or over pre-wrap (Fig. 3–31B).

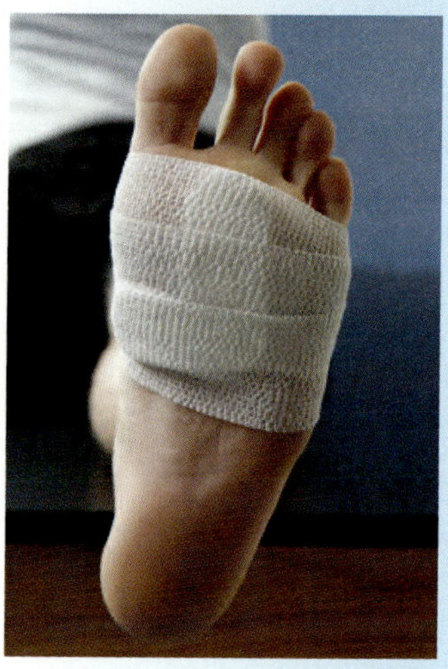

**Fig. 3–31 B**

## 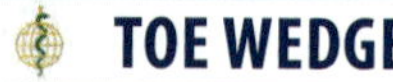 TOE WEDGE

**Purpose:** Use the toe wedge technique in the treatment of bunions or hallux valgus as a spacer to lessen medial deviation of the great toe at the MTP joint. This technique is similar to the buddy tape technique, but adequate spacing between the toes is critical. This technique and steps of application can be found on FADavis.com.

### Clinical Application Question 5

After practice, a high school football tight end removes his cleats and walks to the locker room with bare feet. He steps on a rock and suffers a contusion to the right calcaneus. The next day, he experiences moderate pain with weight-bearing activities.

**Question: What bracing or padding techniques can you use to treat his heel?**

### . . . IF/THEN . . .

**IF** a foam or felt donut padding technique anchored to the great toe with non-elastic or elastic tape and/or self-adherent wrap is too bulky and uncomfortable in the attempt to lessen friction, **THEN** consider using a low-profile hydrogel pad anchored with adhesive gauze material.

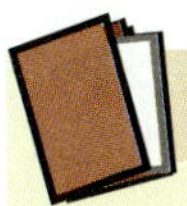

## EVIDENCE-BASED PRACTICE

The end of the second week of basketball practice has not brought any relief for Tony Krantz. Tony is a forward on the team, and he has bilateral heel pain. He first reported the pain during preseason conditioning 3 weeks ago. Jason Heideman, the PT/AT at Leigh University, has been treating Tony for the past 3 weeks with ice, massage, electrical stimulation, ultrasound, over-the-counter nonsteroidal anti-inflammatory drugs for anti-inflammatory effects, lower leg stretching, and strengthening exercises.

The treatments have allowed Tony to participate in most conditioning and practice sessions, but his pain is increasing. Tony complains of pain over the anterior/medial aspect of each calcaneus and reports that the greatest pain is present during initial weight-bearing in the morning and following team film meetings. Through his evaluation, Jason elicits pain in both feet with palpation of the anterior/medial calcaneus and passive dorsiflexion of the distal foot and toes. Jason refers Tony to the team physician for an evaluation of suspected plantar fasciitis. During the evaluation, the physician finds that point tenderness is present over the calcaneus but finds no crepitus, deformity, or neurological symptoms. The physician also notes the presence of hyperhidrosis on the plantar surfaces of both feet. Radiographs demonstrate no bony pathology, and the physician recommends that Jason continue with symptomatic treatment of bilateral plantar fasciitis.

Jason believes that Tony could benefit from the use of taping and/or bracing techniques in the treatment program but is uncertain which techniques would be best in this situation. Jason's goal for Tony is a pain-free return to all conditioning sessions, practices, and competitions.

1. Develop a clinically relevant question from the case in the PICO format to generate answers for the selection of taping and/or bracing techniques for Tony. The question should include the population or problem, the intervention, a comparison intervention (if relevant), and the clinical outcome of interest.

2. Design a search strategy and search to find the best evidence to answer the clinical question. The strategy should include relevant search terms, electronic databases, online journals, and print journals to use for the search. Discussions with your faculty, preceptor, and other health care professionals can provide evidence from expert opinion.

3. Choose three to five full text studies or reviews from your search or the chapter references. Evaluate and appraise each article to determine its value and usefulness to the case. Ask these questions for each study: (1) Are the results of the study valid? (2) What are the actual results? and (3) Are the findings clinically relevant to my patients? Prepare a summary of the evaluation with answers to the questions and rank the articles based on the evidence hierarchy in Chapter 1.

4. Integrate findings from the evidence, your clinical experience, and Tony's goals and preferences into the treatment program for Tony. Consider which taping and/or bracing techniques may be appropriate for Tony.

5. Evaluate the EBP process and your experience within the case. Consider these questions in the evaluation.

Was the clinical question answered?
Did the search generate quality evidence?
Was the evidence evaluated appropriately?
Was the evidence, your clinical experience, and Tony's goals and values integrated to make the clinical decision?
Did the intervention produce successful clinical outcomes for Tony?
Was the EBP experience positive for Jason and Tony?

## WRAP-UP

- Acute and chronic injuries to the foot and toes can be the result of compressive forces, abnormal ranges of motion, and excessive and repetitive stresses.
- The circular, "X," loop, weave, Low-Dye, and plantar fascia strap taping techniques support the longitudinal arch and forefoot.
- The buddy tape, toe spica, toe strip, and turf toe taping techniques provide support and reduce range of motion of the toes.
- Compression wrap techniques applied in a distal-to-proximal spiral pattern assist in reducing swelling and inflammation.
- Orthotics can be categorized into three types: soft, semirigid, and rigid.
- Soft, semirigid, and rigid orthotics can be used in preventing and treating acute and chronic injuries and conditions.
- Orthotics are fabricated in-house or in a laboratory from foot impressions or directly to the foot.

- Night splints, postoperative shoes, and walking and cast boots provide support and restrict range of motion.
- The longitudinal arch, metatarsal bar, tear drop, oval, "J," and toe wedge pad techniques provide support in correcting structural abnormalities.
- Donut and heel padding techniques serve as shock absorbers and reduce stress and friction.

## FADAVIS ONLINE RESOURCES

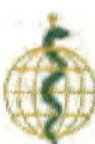

Go to the online resource center at http://Fadavis.com/ to view these additional techniques for the foot and toes.

- Low-Dye taping technique two
- Toe spica taping technique
- Custom-made night splints
- Toe wedge padding technique

## WEB REFERENCES

**American Academy of Orthotists and Prosthetists**
https://www.oandp.org
- This site provides access to the *Journal of Prosthetics and Orthotics* and *State-of-the-Science Conference Findings*, which contain clinical and educational manuscripts.

**American College of Foot and Ankle Surgeons**
https://www.acfas.org/
- This website allows the reader to search for information on the causes and treatment of foot and ankle injuries and conditions.

**American Podiatric Medical Association**
https://www.apma.org/
- This site provides general foot health information on a variety of injuries and conditions.

## FURTHER READING

Hunter, S, Dolan, MG, and Davis, JM: Foot Orthotics in Therapy and Sport. Human Kinetics, Champaign, IL, 1995. Detailed examination of the indications for orthotics and step-by-step fabrication techniques.

Vicenzino, B, McPoil, T, and Buckland, S: Plantar foot pressures after the augmented low dye taping technique. J Athl Train 42:374–380, 2007. Detailed steps for application of the augmented Low-Dye taping technique.

## REFERENCES


1. Anderson, MK: Foundations of Athletic Training: Prevention, Assessment, and Management, ed 6. Wolters Kluwer, Philadelphia, 2017.
2. Prentice, WE: Principles of Athletic Training: A Guide to Evidence-Based Clinical Practice, ed 16. McGraw-Hill, New York, 2017.
3. Cheung, RTH, Chung, RCK, and Ng, GYF: Efficacies of different external controls for excessive foot pronation: A meta-analysis. Br J Sports Med 45:743–751, 2011.
4. Newell, T, Simon, J, and Docherty, CL: Arch-taping techniques for altering navicular height and plantar pressures during activity. J Athl Train 50:825–832, 2015.
5. Ator, R, Gunn, K, McPoil, TG, and Knecht, HG: The effect of adhesive strapping on medial longitudinal arch support before and after exercise. J Orthop Sports Phys Ther 14:18–23, 1991.
6. Del Rossi, G, Fiolkowski, P, Horodyski, MB, Bishop, M, and Trimble, M: For how long do temporary techniques maintain the height of the medial longitudinal arch? Phys Ther Sport 5:84–89, 2004.
7. Vicenzino, B, Franettovich, M, McPoil, T, Russell, T, and Skardoon, G: Initial effects of anti-pronation tape on the medial longitudinal arch during walking and running. Br J Sports Med 39:939–943, 2005.
8. Yoho, R, Rivera, JJ, Renschler, R, Vardaxis, VG, and Dikis, J: A biomechanical analysis of the effects of low-Dye taping on arch deformation during gait. Foot 22:283–286, 2012.
9. Kim, T, and Park, JC: Short-term effects of sports taping on navicular height, navicular drop and peak plantar pressure in healthy elite athletes. Medicine, 2017. doi: 10.1097/MD.0000000000008714.
10. Cornwall, MW, McPoil, TG, and Fair, A: The effect of exercise and time on the height and width of the medial longitudinal arch following the modified reverse-6 and the modified augmented low-dye taping procedures. Int J Sports Phys Ther 9:635–643, 2014.
11. Cornwall, MW, Lebec, M, DeGeyter, J, and McPoil, TG: The reliability of the modified reverse-6 taping procedure with elastic tape to alter the height and width of the medial longitudinal arch. Int J Sports Phys Ther 8:381–392, 2013.
12. Jamali, B, Walker, M, and Hoke, B: Windlass taping technique for symptomatic relief of plantar fasciitis. J Sport Rehabil 13:228–243, 2004.
13. Holmes, CF, Wilcox, D, and Fletcher, JP: Effect of a modified, low-dye medial longitudinal arch taping procedure on the subtalar joint neutral position before and after light exercise. J Orthop Sports Phys Ther 32:194–201, 2002.
14. Radford, JA, Burns, J, Buchbinder, R, Landorf, KB, and Cook, C: Does stretching increase ankle dorsiflexion range of motion? A systematic review. Br J Sports Med 40:870–875, discussion 875, 2006.
15. Whitaker, JM, Augustus, K, and Ishii, S: Effect of the low-Dye strap on pronation-sensitive mechanical attributes of the foot. J Am Pod Med Assoc 93:118–123, 2003.
16. Franettovich, M, Chapman, A, Blanch, P, and Vicenzino, B: Continual use of augmented low-Dye taping

increases arch height in standing but does not influence neuromotor control of gait. Gait Posture 31:247–250, 2010

17. Lange, B, Chipchase, L, and Evans, A: The effect of low-dye taping on plantar pressures, during gait, in subjects with navicular drop exceeding 10 mm. J Orthop Sports Phys Ther 34:201–209, 2004.

18. O'Sullivan, K, Kennedy, N, O'Neill, E, and Ni Mhainin, U: The effect of low-dye taping on rearfoot motion and plantar pressure during the stance phase of gait. BMC Musculoskelet Disord 9:111–119, 2008.

19. Nolan, D, and Kennedy, N: Effects of low-dye taping on plantar pressure pre and post exercise: An exploratory study. BMC Musculoskelet Disord 10:40, 2009.

20. Russo, SJ, and Chipchase, LS: The effect of low-Dye taping on peak plantar pressures of normal feet during gait. Austral J Physiotherapy 47:239–244, 2001.

21. Vicenzino, B, McPoil, T, and Buckland, S: Plantar foot pressures after the augmented low dye taping technique. J Athl Train 42:374–380, 2007.

22. Kelly, LA, Racinais, S, Tanner, CM, Grantham, J, and Chalabi, H: Augmented low dye taping changes muscle activation patterns and plantar pressure during treadmill running. J Orthop Sports Phys Ther 40:648–655, 2010.

23. Franettovich, MM, Murley, GS, David, BS, and Bird, AR: A comparison of augmented low-Dye taping and ankle bracing on lower limb muscle activity during walking in adults with flat-arched foot posture. J Sci Med Sport 15:8–13, 2012.

24. Franettovich, M, Chapman, A, and Vicenzino, B: Tape that increases medial longitudinal arch height also reduces leg muscle activity: A preliminary study. Med Sci Sports Exerc 40:593–600, 2008.

25. Franettovich, M, Chapman, AR, Blanch, P, and Vicenzino, B: Augmented low-Dye tape alters foot mobility and neuromotor control of gait in individuals with and without exercise related leg pain. J Foot Ankle Res 3:5, 2010.

26. Gray, EG, and Basmajian, JV: Electromyography and cinematography of leg and foot ("normal" and flat) during walking. Anat Rec 161:1–15, 1968.

27. Gray, ER: The role of leg muscles in variations of the arches in normal and flat feet. Phys Ther 49:1084–1088, 1969.

28. Hunt, AE, and Smith, RM: Mechanics and control of the flat versus normal foot during the stance phase of walking. Clin Biomech 19:391–397, 2004.

29. Murley, GS, Menz, HB, and Landorf, KB: Foot posture influences the electromyographic activity of selected lower limb muscles during gait. J Foot Ankle Res 2:1–9, 2009.

30. Prentice, WE: Rehabilitation Techniques for Sports Medicine and Athletic Training, ed 6. SLACK, New Jersey, 2015.

31. Hunter, S, Dolan, MG, and Davis, JM: Foot Orthotics in Therapy and Sport. Human Kinetics, Champaign, IL, 1995.

32. Penneau, K, Lutter, LD, and Winter, RD: Pes planus: Radiographic changes with foot orthoses and shoes. Foot Ankle 2:299–302, 1982.

33. Sahrai, T, Cohen, MJ, Ne'eman, V, Kandel, L, Odebiyi, DO, Lev, I, Brezis, M, and Lahad, A: Insoles for prevention and treatment of back pain. Cochrane Database Syst Rev (4);CD005275, 2007.

34. Chuter, V, Spink, M, Searle, A, and Ho, A: The effectiveness of shoe insoles for the prevention and treatment of low back pain: A systematic review and meta-analysis of randomized controlled trials. BMC Musculoskelet Disord 15:140, 2014. doi: 10.1186/1471-2474-15-140.

35. Thomson, CE, Gibson, JNA, and Martin, D: Interventions for the treatment of Morton's neuroma. Cochrane Database Syst Rev (3);CD003118, 2004.

36. Hawke, F, Burns, J, Radford, JA, and du Toit, V: Custom-made foot orthoses for the treatment of foot pain. Cochrane Database Syst Rev (3);CD006801, 2008.

37. Rasenberg, N, Riel, H, Rathleff, MS, Bierma-Zeinstra, SMA, and van Middelkoop, M: Efficacy of foot orthoses for the treatment of plantar heel pain: A systematic review and meta-analysis. Br J Sports Med 52:1040–1046, 2018.

38. Whittaker, GA, Munteanu, SE, Menz, HB, Tan, JM, Rabusin, CL, and Landorf, KB: Foot orthoses for plantar heel pain: A systematic review and meta-analysis. Br J Sports Med 52:322–328, 2018.

39. Collins, N, Bisset, L, McPoil, T, and Vicenzino, B: Foot orthoses in lower limb overuse conditions: A systematic review and meta-analysis. Foot Ankle Int 28:396–412, 2007.

40. Yeung, SS, Yeung, EW, and Gillespie, LD: Interventions for preventing lower limb soft-tissue running injuries. Cochrane Database Syst Rev (7);CD001256, 2011.

41. Newman, P, Witchalls, J, Waddington, G, and Adams, R: Risk factors associated with medial tibial stress syndrome in runners: A systematic review and meta-analysis. Open Access J Sports Med 4:229–241, 2013.

42. Bonanno, DR, Landorf, KB, Munteanu, SE, Murley, GS, and Menz, HB: Effectiveness of foot orthoses and shock-absorbing insoles for the prevention of injury: A systematic review and meta-analysis. Br J Sports Med 51:86–96, 2017.

43. Mills, K, Blanch, P, Chapman, AR, McPoil, TG, and Vicenzino, B: Foot orthoses and gait: A systematic review and meta-analysis of literature pertaining to potential mechanisms. Br J Sports Med 44:1035–1046, 2010.

44. Desmyttere, G, Hajizadeh, M, Bleau, J, and Begon, M: Effect of foot orthosis design on lower limb joint kinematics and kinetics during walking in flexible per planovalgus: A systematic review and meta-analysis. Clin Biomech 59:117–129, 2018.

45. Lucas-Cuevas, AG, Pérez-Soriano, P, Llana-Belloch, S, Macián-Romero, C, and Sánchez-Zuriaga, D: Effect of custom-made and prefabricated insoles on plantar loading parameters during running with and without fatigue. J Sports Sci 32:1712–1721, 2014.

46. Cobb, SC, Tis, LL, Johnson, JT, Wang, Y, and Geil, MD: Custom-molded foot-orthosis intervention and multisegment medial foot kinematics during walking. J Athl Train 46:358–365, 2011.

47. Baur, H, Hirschmüller, A, Müller, S, and Mayer, F: Neuromuscular activity of the peroneal muscle after foot orthoses therapy in runners. Med Sci Sports Exerc 43:1500–1506, 2011.

48. Nigg, BM, Nurse, MA, and Stefanyshyn, DJ: Shoe inserts and orthotics for sport and physical activities. Med Sci Sports Exerc 31:S421–S428, 1999.

49. Singh, D, Angel, J, Bentley, G, and Trevino, SG: Plantar fasciitis. BMJ 315:172–175, 1997.

50. Fabian, EP, Gowling, TL, and Jackson, RW: Walking boot design: A gait analysis study. Orthopedics 22:503–508, 1999.

51. Wu, KK: Morton's interdigital neuroma: A clinical review of its etiology, treatment, and results. J Foot Ankle Surg 35:112–119, 1996.

52. Hockenbury, RT: Forefoot problems in athletes. Med Sci Sports Exerc 31:S448–S458, 1999.

# Ankle

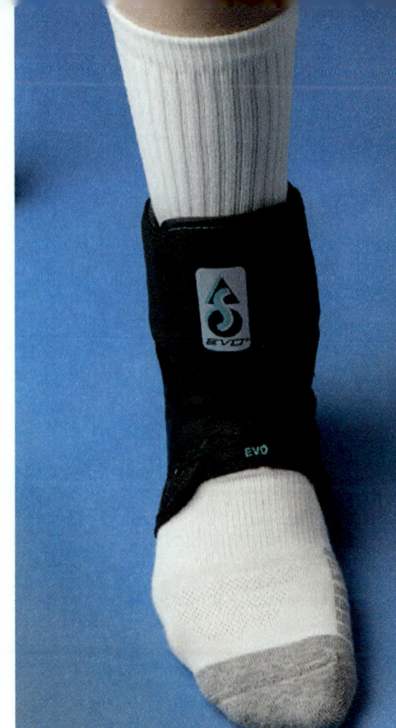




**LEARNING OBJECTIVES**

1. Discuss common injuries that occur to the ankle.
2. Demonstrate taping, wrapping, bracing, and padding techniques for the ankle when preventing, treating, and rehabilitating injuries.
3. Explain and demonstrate evidence-based practice for the implementation of taping, wrapping, bracing, and padding techniques for the ankle within a clinical case.


## INJURIES AND CONDITIONS

Injury to the ankle can occur during any weight-bearing activity due to excessive range of motion and repetitive stress. Injury to the bony and ligamentous structures of the ankle can occur from excessive range of motion caused by stepping off a curb while walking or sudden changes of direction during athletic activities. Casual and athletic activities on uneven or poorly maintained surfaces may also contribute to injury. Common injuries to the ankle include:

- Sprains
- Fractures
- Blisters

### Sprains

Ankle sprains are one of the most common sport-related injuries.[1] Injuries are caused by excessive, sudden inversion or eversion at the **subtalar joint** and can be associated with plantar flexion or dorsiflexion at the **talocrural joint** (Figs. 4–1 and 4–2). **Rotation** of the foot, either **internal** or **external**, can also contribute to injury. An inversion or eversion sprain can result, for instance, when a baseball batter steps on the corner of first base while running straight ahead to beat a throw from the second baseman, causing excessive inversion, eversion, rotation, and/or dorsiflexion. Inversion sprains are more common and can lead to damage of the **anterior talofibular, calcaneofibular**, and/or **posterior talofibular ligaments. Eversion sprains** can result in injury to the **deltoid ligament** and are often accompanied by an **avulsion fracture** of the distal tibia with severe eversion force. Excessive dorsiflexion and external rotation can cause a **syndesmosis sprain** involving the **anterior** and **posterior tibiofibular ligaments.** A syndesmosis sprain can occur, for example, during a fumble recovery in football, as the ankle of a player on the ground is forced into dorsiflexion and external rotation by others diving for the ball.

### Fractures

Fractures of the distal tibia or fibula can occur in combination with ankle sprains. A severe inversion mechanism can cause an avulsion fracture of the **lateral (fibular) malleolus** and sometimes an accompanying fracture of the **medial (tibial) malleolus**, known as a **bimalleolar fracture** (Fig. 4–3). With eversion sprains,

"

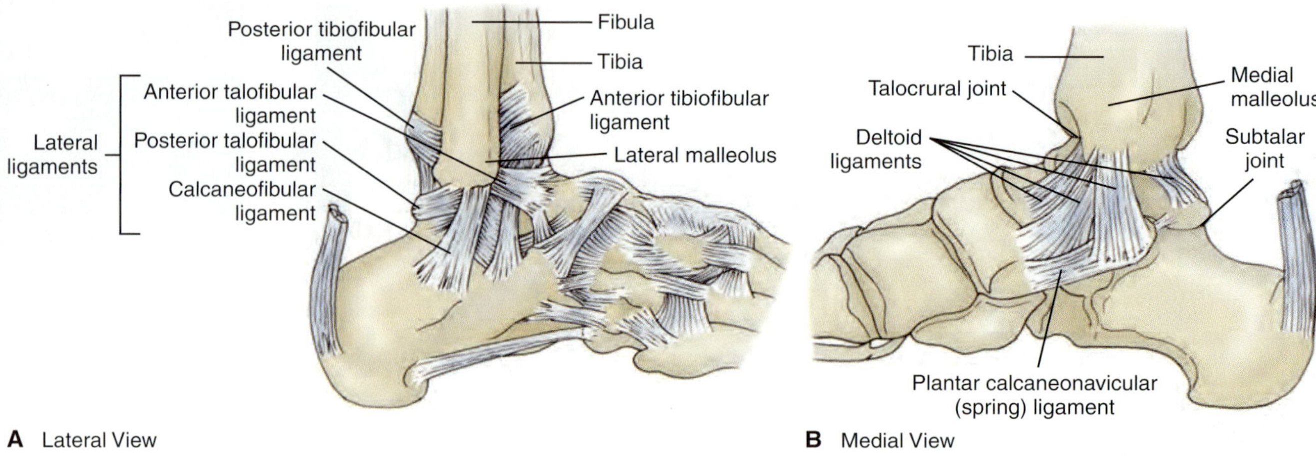


**Fig. 4–1** *Ligaments of the subtalar and talocrural joints.*

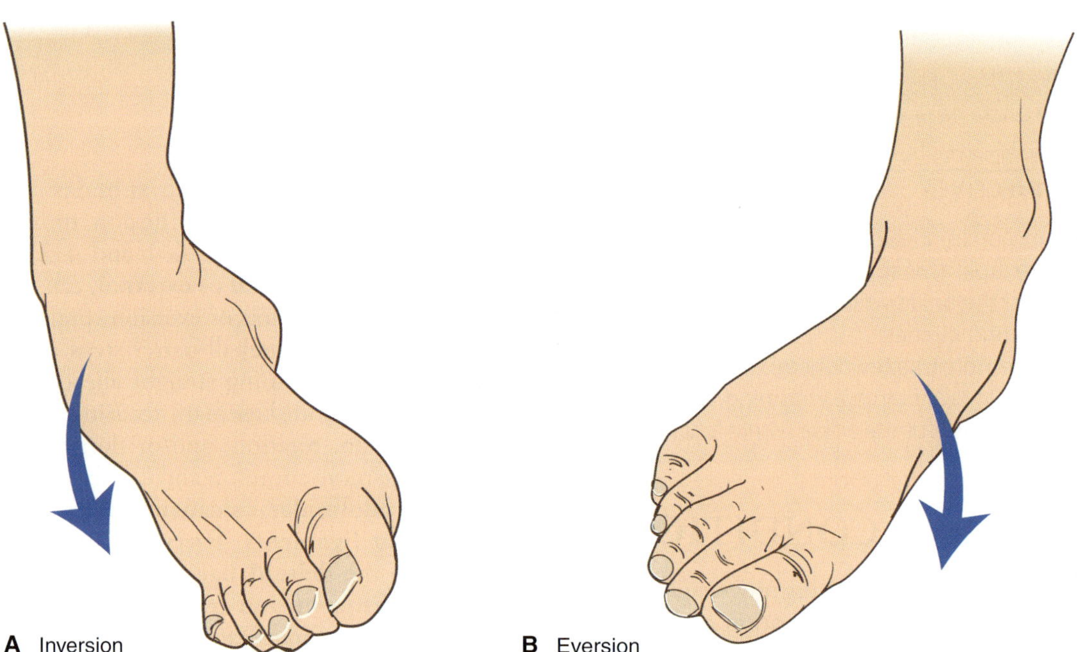


**Fig. 4–2** *Ankle sprain mechanism of injury.*

the longer fibular malleolus can be fractured as the talus is forced into the distal end. If the eversion mechanism continues, an avulsion fracture of the tibial malleolus can occur, resulting in a bimalleolar fracture. Mechanisms of injury for distal tibia and fibula fractures include forcible inversion, eversion, dorsiflexion, and internal rotation.

## Blisters

Athletic, work, and casual footwear can cause irritation of the skin. Application of taping, wrapping, and bracing techniques themselves can cause blisters from shearing forces over the heel, lace, and bony prominence areas such as the medial and lateral malleoli.

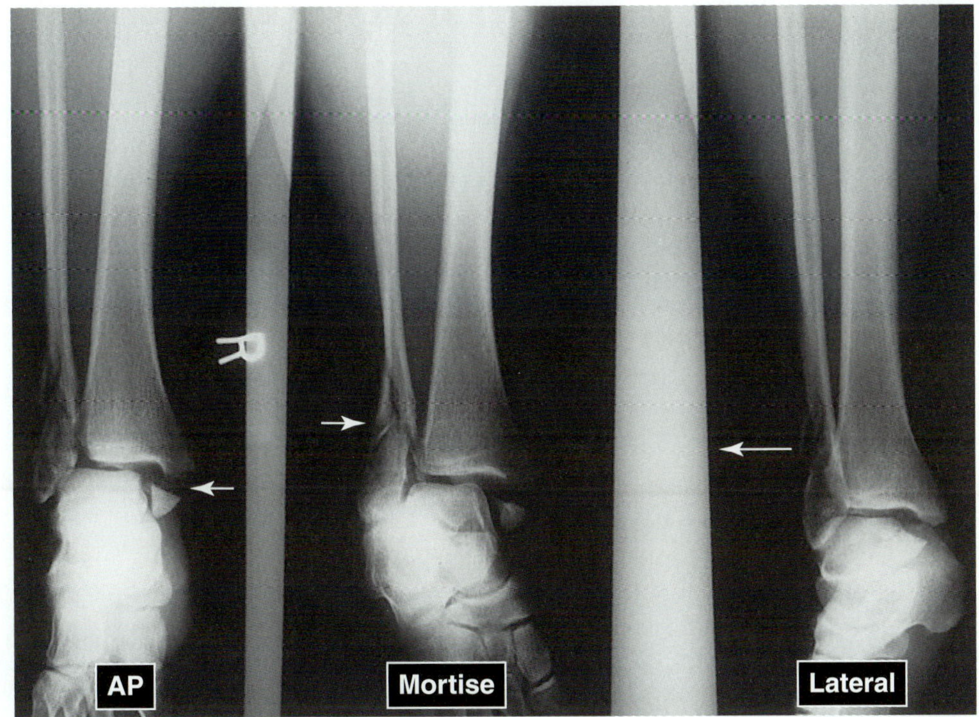



**Fig. 4–3** *Bimalleolar fracture. Note the comminuted fracture at the distal fibula, avulsion fracture of the tibial malleolus, and anterior dislocation of the fibula seen on the lateral view, inferring a torn tibiofibular syndesmosis. (Courtesy of McKinnis, LN. Fundamentals of Musculoskeletal Imaging, 4th ed. Philadelphia, PA: F.A. Davis Company: 2014.)*

# Taping Techniques

Several taping techniques reduce inversion and eversion at the subtalar joint and reduce plantar flexion and dorsiflexion at the talocrural joint, protecting against excessive range of motion. Some techniques are used to prevent sprains and others to provide support to the injured ankle during a return to activities. Several techniques are used specifically in the acute treatment of sprains and fractures to immobilize the ankle. The appropriate technique to use should be based on the intended purpose, the injury, the patient, and the activity.

## CLOSED BASKETWEAVE    Figures 4–4, 4–5, 4–6

➠ **Purpose:** The closed basketweave technique is used both to prevent and to treat inversion and eversion sprains (Fig. 4–4). It provides moderate support to the subtalar and talocrural joints and reduces range of motion. For our purposes, we first review a basic closed basketweave and then illustrate several variations used to provide additional support.

### DETAILS
There may be as many different basketweave techniques as there are health care professionals applying them, but the majority of the techniques contain some of the procedures described by Gibney[2] more than 100 years ago.

➠ **Materials:**
• 1½ inch or 2 inch non-elastic tape, taping scissors
*Option:*
• Pre-wrap or self-adherent wrap, adherent tape spray, thin foam pads, skin lubricant

➠ **Position of the patient:** Sitting on a taping table or bench with the leg extended off the edge with the foot in 90 degrees of dorsiflexion.

➠ **Preparation:** Apply the basketweave technique directly to the skin.
**Option:** Apply pre-wrap or self-adherent wrap, adherent tape spray, thin foam pads, and skin lubricant over the heel and lace areas to provide additional adherence and lessen irritation. Using self-adherent wrap appears to provide some additional support to the ankle.[3]

➠ **Application:**

**STEP 1:**   In this example, apply one layer of pre-wrap ◀▦▶ (Fig. 4–4A).

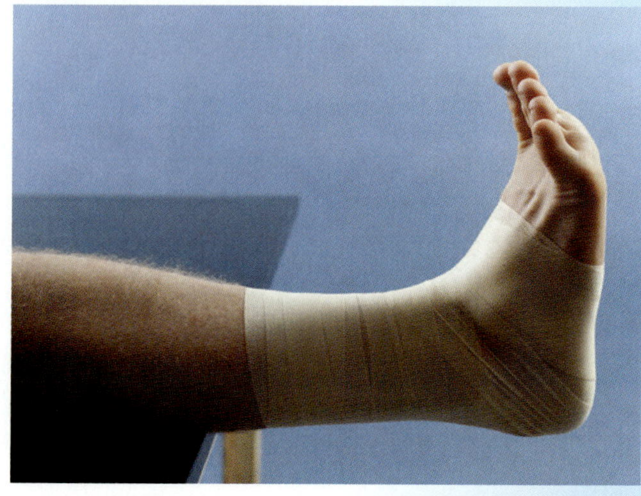

Fig. 4–4 A

**STEP 2:**   Using 1½ inch or 2 inch non-elastic tape, apply two anchor strips at a slight angle around the distal lower leg, just inferior to the gastrocnemius belly with moderate roll tension ◀▦▶ (Fig. 4–4B). An anchor strip can be placed around the midfoot ◀▦▶, proximal to the fifth metatarsal head, but this is not required. If this anchor strip is applied, monitor roll tension to prevent constriction as the foot expands on weight-bearing.

*Option:*   *Use self-adherent wrap of 1½ inch or 2 inch width for these anchors to prevent constriction.*

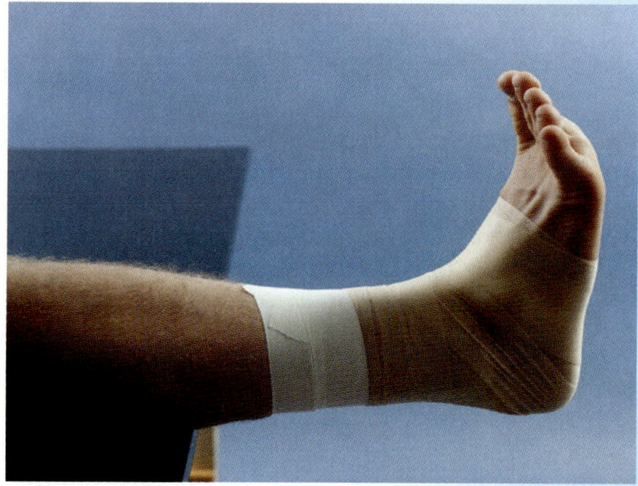

Fig. 4–4 B

**STEP 3:**  When preventing and treating inversion sprains, start the first stirrup on the medial lower leg anchor. Proceed down over the posterior medial malleolus (Fig. 4–4C), across the plantar surface of the foot, and continue up and over the posterior lateral malleolus with moderate roll tension (Fig. 4–4D).

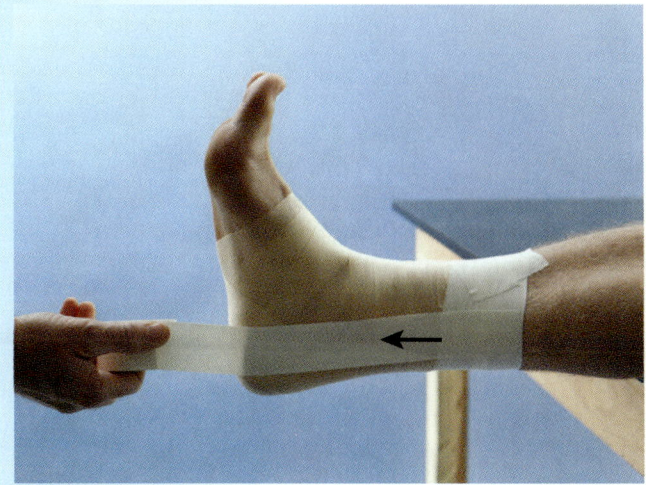

**Fig. 4–4 C**

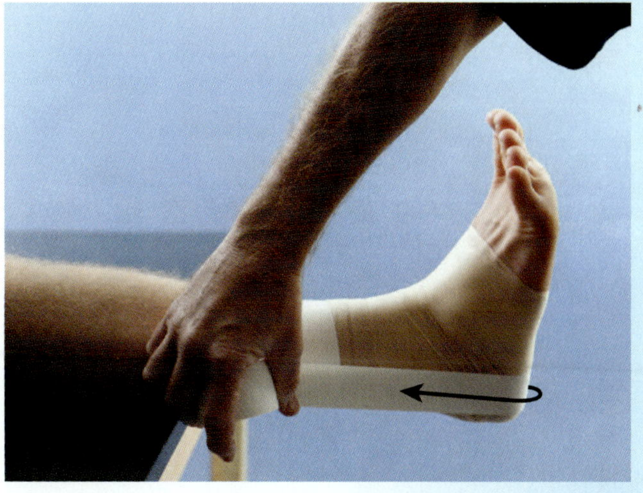

**Fig. 4–4 D**

**STEP 4:**  Finish on the lateral lower leg anchor (Fig. 4–4E).

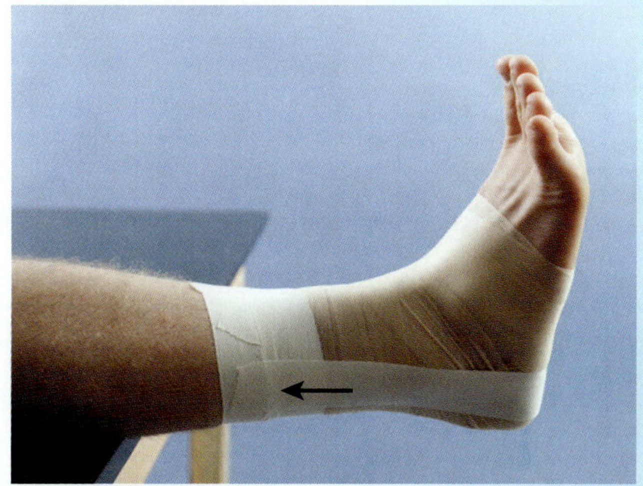

**Fig. 4–4 E**

**STEP 5:**  When preventing and treating eversion sprains, apply the stirrups on the lateral lower leg anchor and follow the same steps, finishing on the medial lower leg anchor (Fig. 4–4F). Avoid excessive roll tension that may cause inversion at the subtalar joint.

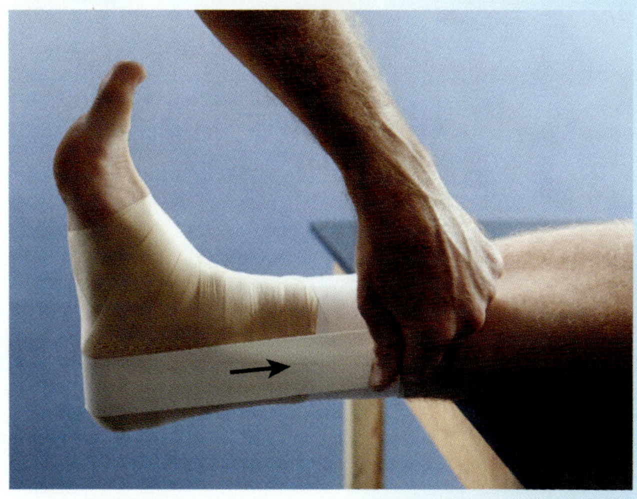

**Fig. 4–4 F**

*Steps Cont.*

**Ankle**

**STEP 6:** Begin the first horseshoe strip on the medial aspect of the midfoot (Fig. 4–4G), continue around the distal Achilles tendon, across the distal lateral malleolus, and finish on the lateral midfoot with moderate roll tension, proximal to the fifth metatarsal head (Fig. 4–4H).

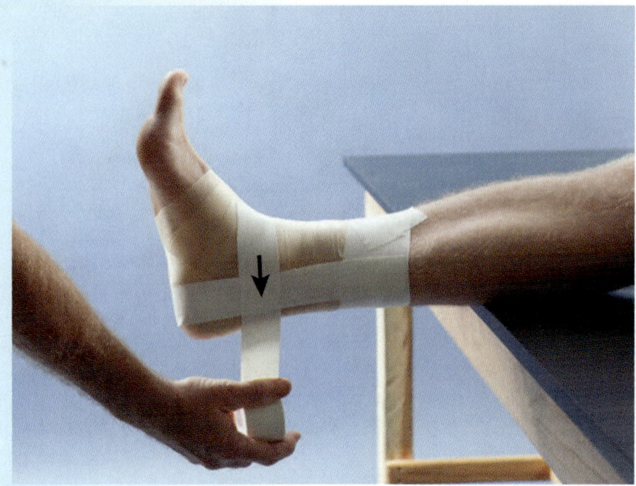

Fig. 4–4 G

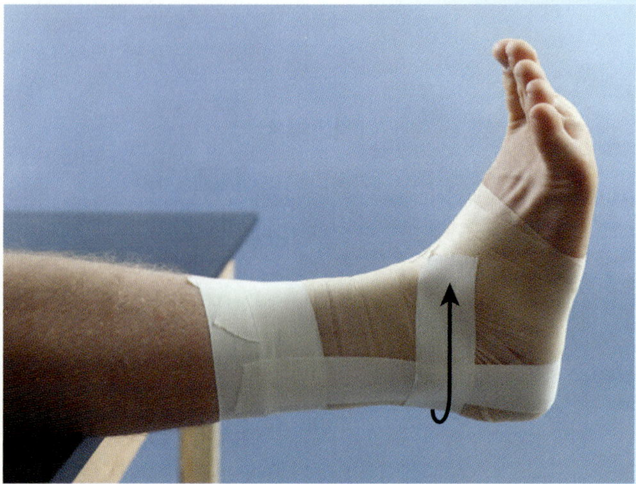

Fig. 4–4 H

**STEP 7:** Start the second stirrup on the medial lower leg by overlapping the first by ½ of the tape width, continue down over the medial malleolus (Fig. 4–4I), across the plantar foot, up and over the lateral malleolus, and anchor on the lateral lower leg (Fig. 4–4J).

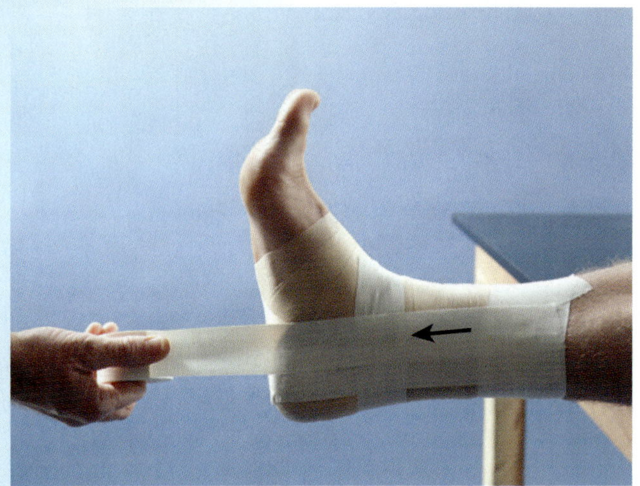

Fig. 4–4 I

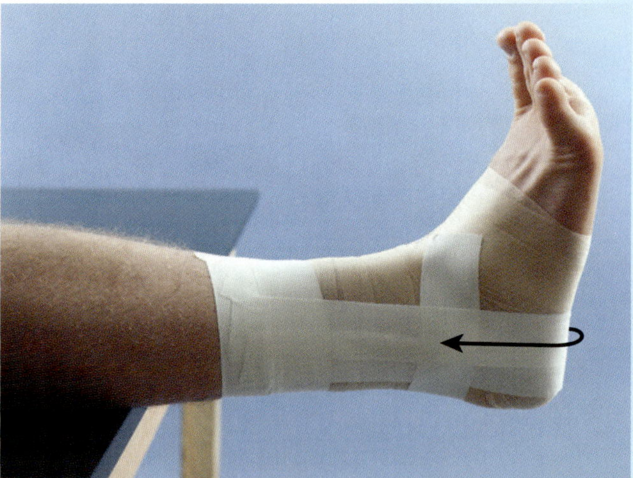

Fig. 4–4 J

**STEP 8:** The second horseshoe begins on the medial rearfoot and overlaps the first by ½ of the tape width (Fig. 4–4K).

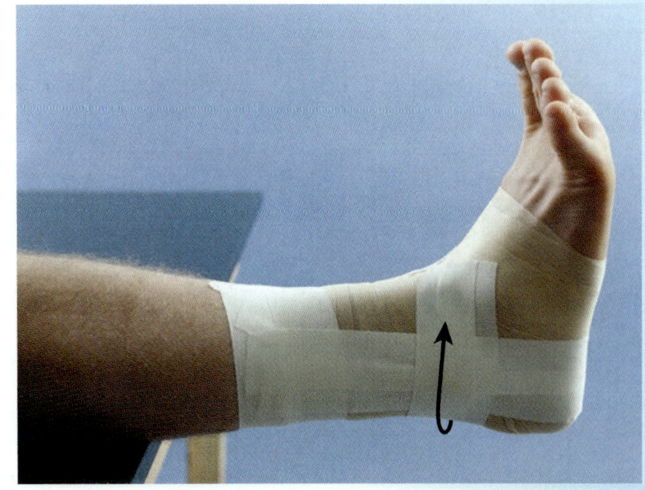

**Fig. 4–4 K**

**STEP 9:** The third stirrup, beginning on the medial lower leg, overlaps the second and covers the anterior medial and lateral malleoli (Fig. 4–4L).

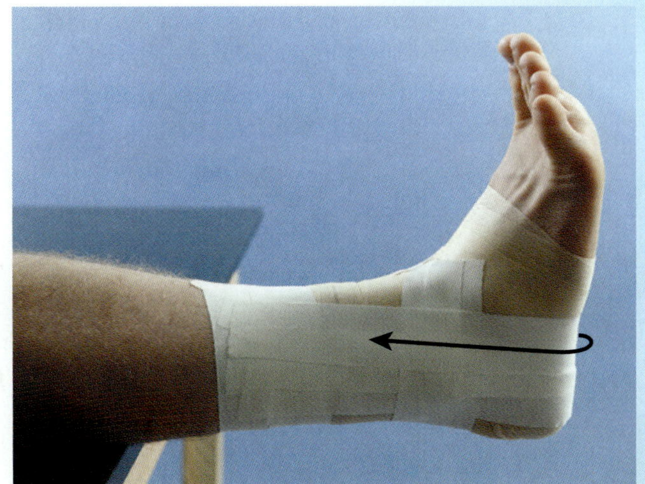

**Fig. 4–4 L**

**STEP 10:** Starting on the medial rearfoot, apply the third horseshoe, overlapping the second (Fig. 4–4M).

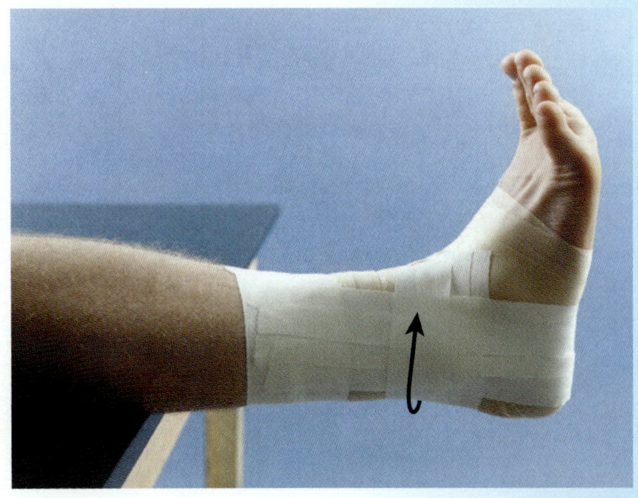

**Fig. 4–4 M**

*Steps Cont.*

Ankle

**STEP 11:** Beginning at the third horseshoe, apply closure strips in a proximal direction with moderate roll tension, overlapping each ◄▦► (Fig. 4–4N). Apply the last closure strip over the distal lower leg anchors. Progress proximally, and angle the tape to prevent gaps or wrinkles.

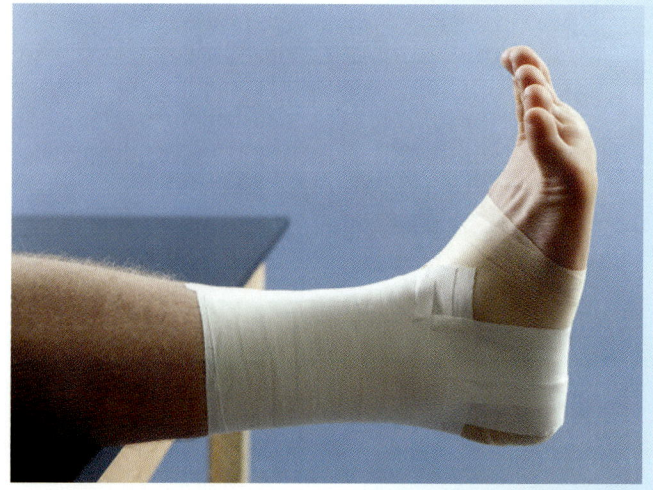

Fig. 4–4 N

**STEP 12:** Apply two to three closure strips around the midfoot in a medial-to-lateral direction with mild to moderate roll tension, remaining proximal to the fifth metatarsal head (Fig. 4–4O).

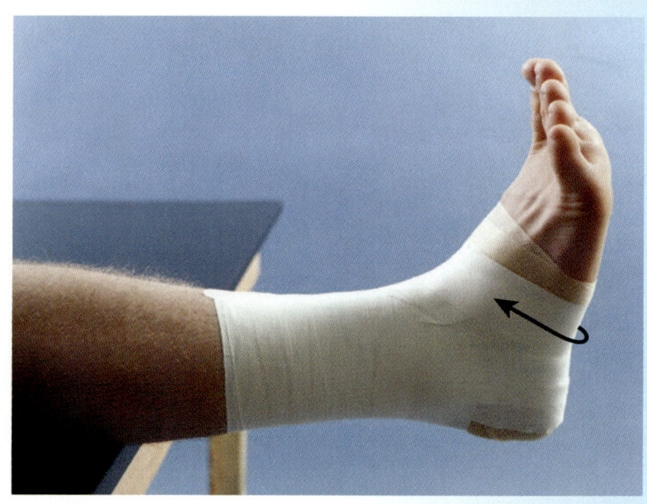

Fig. 4–4 O

### Heel Locks

➠ **Purpose:** Use heel locks to provide additional support to the subtalar and talocrural joints and secure the closed basketweave technique (Fig. 4–5). Based on patient preferences, apply heel locks in either an individual or continuous pattern. Many health care professionals apply the continuous heel lock to conserve time when applying the basketweave technique.

➠ **Materials:**
  • 1½ inch or 2 inch non-elastic tape

➠ **Position of the patient:** Sitting on a taping table or bench with the leg extended off the edge with the foot in 90 degrees of dorsiflexion.

➠ **Preparation:** Application of the closed basketweave taping technique.

### Individual Heel Locks

➠ **Application:**

**STEP 1:** Using the individual technique, anchor the lateral heel lock with 1½ inch or 2 inch non-elastic tape across the lateral lace area at an angle toward the longitudinal arch (Fig. 4–5A).

**STEP 2:** Continue across the arch, then angle the tape upward and pull across the lateral calcaneus with moderate roll tension (Fig. 4–5B), around the posterior heel, and finish on the lateral lace area (Fig. 4–5C).

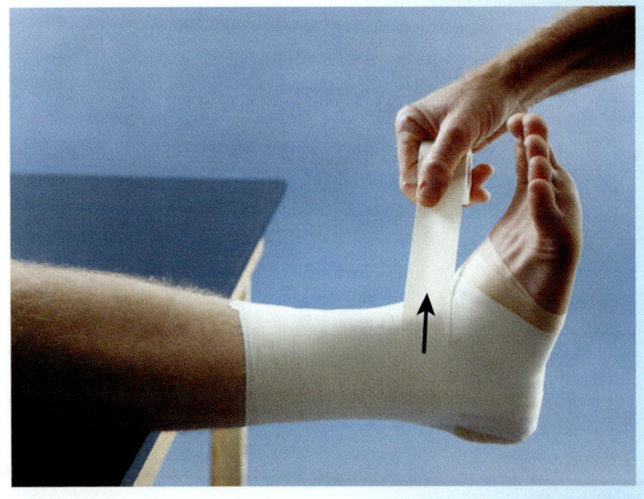

**Fig. 4–5 A**

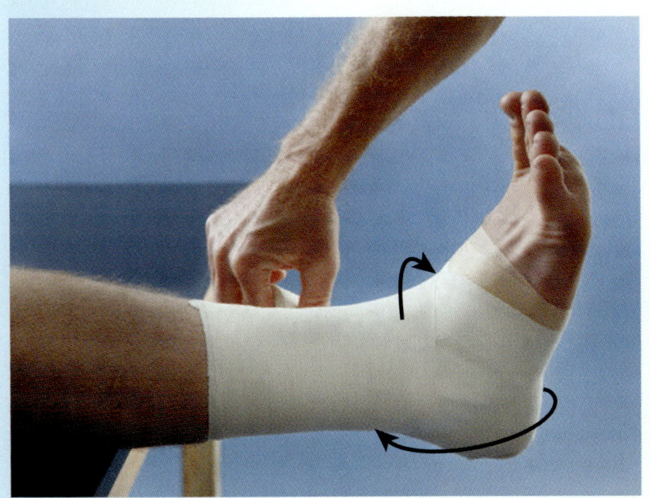

**Fig. 4–5 B**

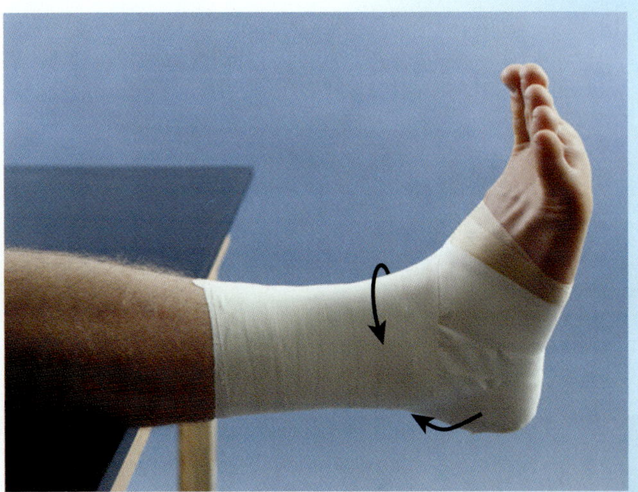

**Fig. 4–5 C**

**STEP 3:** The medial heel lock begins over the medial lace area at an angle toward the lateral malleolus (Fig. 4–5D) and continues across the posterior heel.

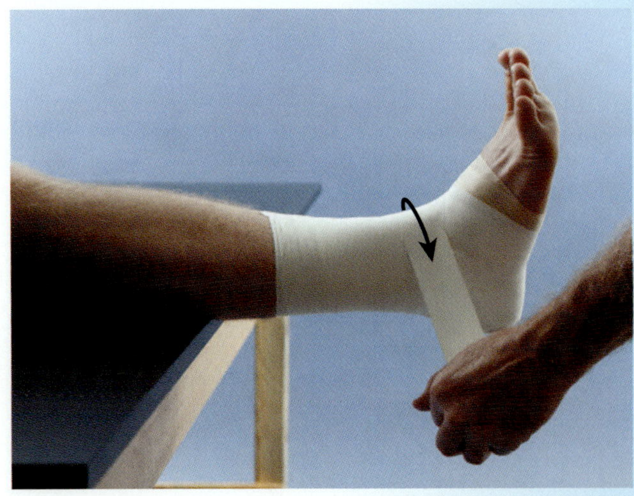

**Fig. 4–5 D**

*Steps Cont.*

**STEP 4:**   Angle the tape downward and pull across the medial calcaneus with moderate roll tension (Fig. 4–5E), under the heel, and finish on the medial lace area (Fig. 4–5F). Typically, the lateral and medial heel locks are repeated.

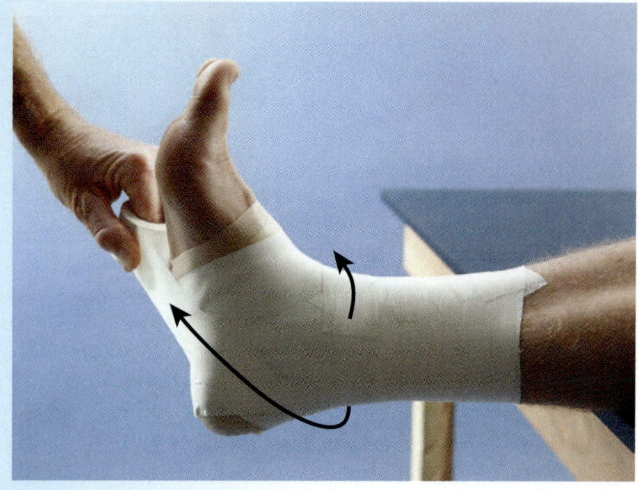

Fig. 4–5 E

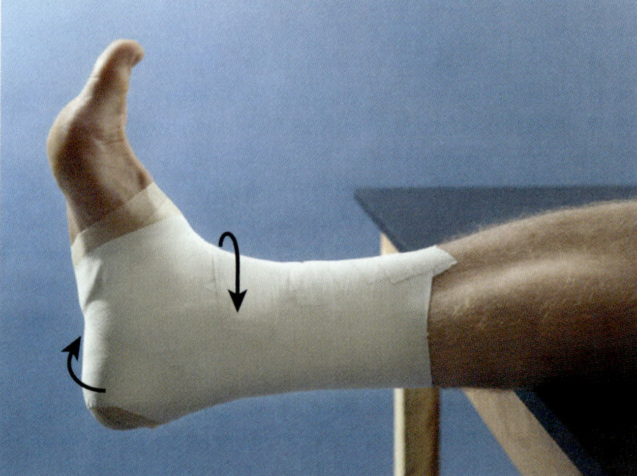

Fig. 4–5 F

### Continuous Heel Locks

**➡ Application:**

**STEP 1:**   The continuous heel lock technique combines the individual locks and is applied within a figure-of-eight pattern with moderate roll tension. Apply a lateral heel lock as shown in Figure 4–5A–C.

**STEP 2:**   Instead of tearing the tape when finished, continue around the distal Achilles tendon (Fig. 4–5G).

**STEP 3:**   Angle downward and pull the tape across the medial calcaneus (Fig. 4–5H).

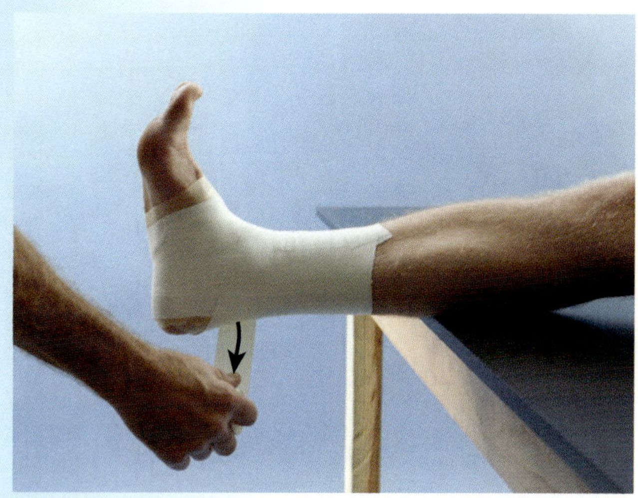

Fig. 4–5 G

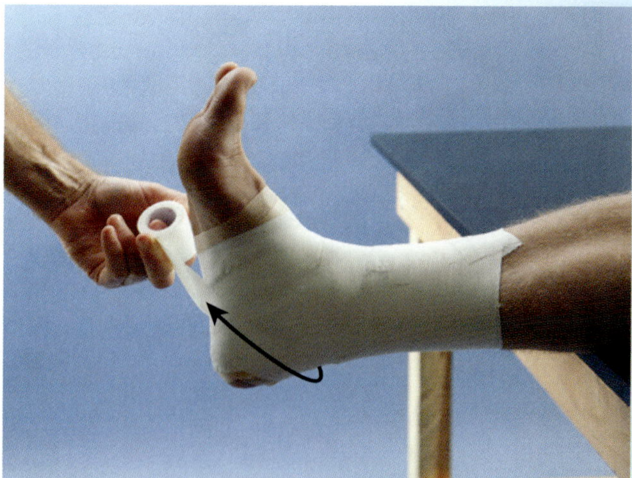

Fig. 4–5 H

**STEP 4:** Continue across the plantar foot, then up and over the dorsum of the foot toward the superior medial malleolus (Fig. 4–5I), around the posterior lower leg, and finish on the anterior lower leg (Fig. 4–5J). The continuous technique is also often repeated.

Because non-elastic tape does not possess elastic properties, starting with and maintaining the proper angles of the body contours is important.

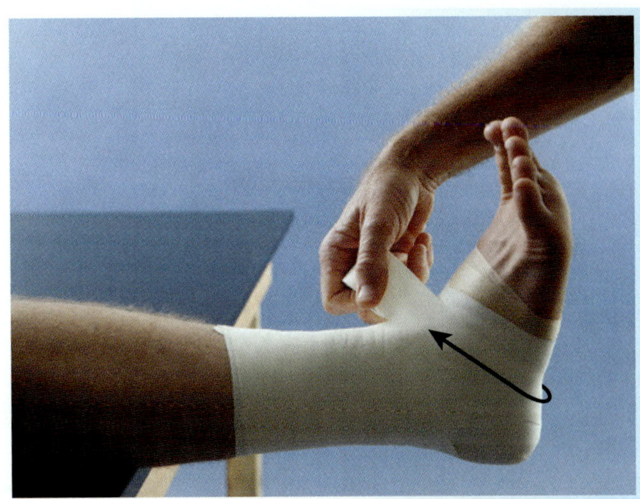

**Fig. 4–5 I**

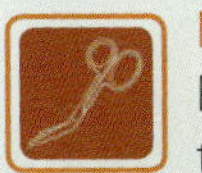
**Helpful Hint |**
Proper angles will be created if the center of the tape width covers the lateral and medial malleoli. Begin the continuous technique by anchoring the center of the tape directly over the lateral malleolus at an angle toward the longitudinal arch. Center tape placement over the lateral malleolus guides the tape toward a correct lateral heel lock and medial malleolus center placement guides toward a correct medial heel lock.

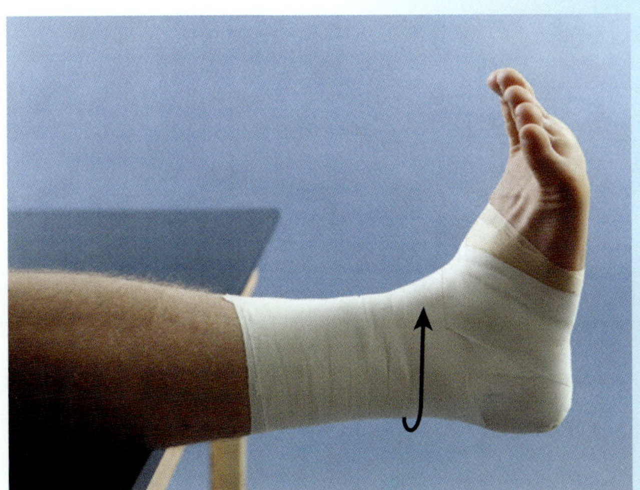

**Fig. 4–5 J**

**. . . IF/THEN . . .**
**IF** applying the continuous heel lock taping technique and the correct angles remain problematic, **THEN** apply pre-wrap or self-adherent wrap in the same pattern at the start of a taping technique for additional practice.

### *Basketweave Variation One*

➡ **Purpose:** Several variations to the basic closed basketweave technique provide additional support to the subtalar and talocrural joints and reduce range of motion (Fig. 4–6). These variations are used when patients are returning to activity or work while treating inversion, eversion, and syndesmosis sprains, and fractures.
➡ **Materials:**
  • 1½ inch or 2 inch elastic tape, taping scissors
  • 2 inch or 3 inch semirigid cast tape, gloves, water, taping scissors
➡ **Position of the patient:** Sitting on a taping table or bench with the leg extended off the edge with the foot in 90 degrees of dorsiflexion.
➡ **Preparation:** Application of the closed basketweave taping technique.
➡ **Application:**

**STEP 1:** After applying the closed basketweave, use elastic tape in 1½ inch or 2 inch widths for heel locks (Fig. 4–6A). Apply the elastic tape with the individual or continuous technique. Non-elastic tape heel locks can be applied over the elastic tape to provide additional support.

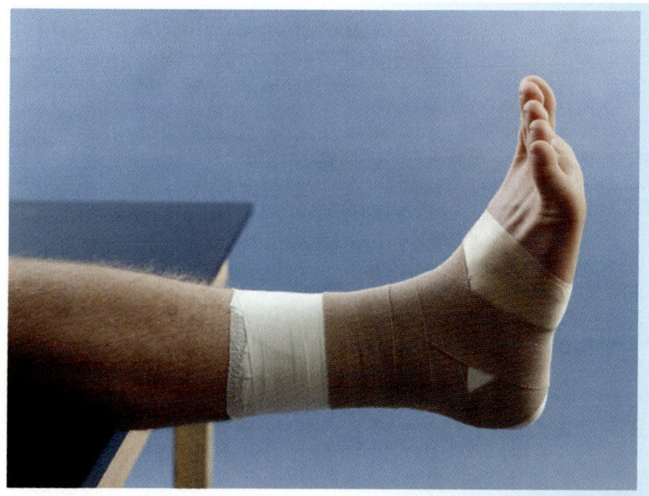

Fig. 4–6 A

**STEP 2:** If greater support is required, use semi-rigid cast tape in 2 inch or 3 inch widths for heel locks (Fig. 4–6B). Apply the basketweave technique with heel locks of non-elastic or elastic tape. Anchor the cast tape around the distal lower leg and continue with the continuous heel lock technique with mild to moderate roll tension. Smooth, mold, and shape the cast tape to the ankle. Allow 10–15 minutes for the tape to cure. Additional anchors over the cast tape are not required.

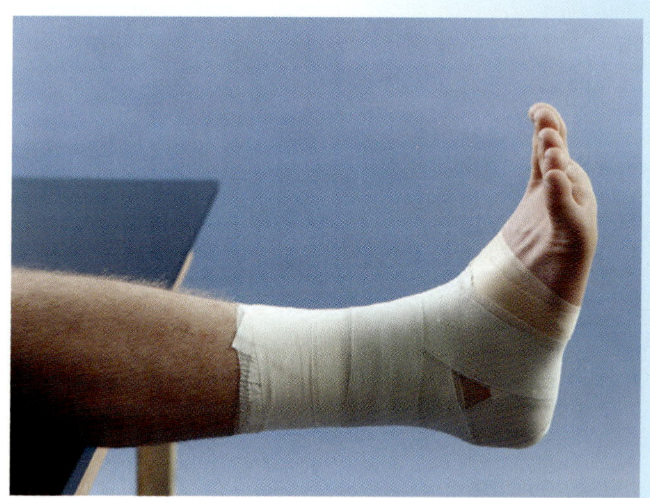

Fig. 4–6 B

### Basketweave Variation Two

➡ **Purpose:** Another variation is the application of moleskin or thermoplastic material stirrups with the closed basketweave technique. This variation, using semirigid materials, provides maximal support to the subtalar and talocrural joints, specifically inversion and eversion.

➡ **Materials:**
- 2 inch or 3 inch moleskin, taping scissors
- Paper, felt tip pen, ⅛ inch thermoplastic material, taping scissors, a heating source, an elastic wrap, 2 inch or 3 inch moleskin

➡ **Position of the patient:** Sitting on a taping table or bench with the leg extended off the edge with the foot in 90 degrees of dorsiflexion.

➡ **Preparation:** Application of the closed basketweave taping technique.

➡ **Application:**

**STEP 1:** Cut moleskin stirrups from 2 inch or 3 inch width material into 25–30 inch length straps.

**STEP 2:** Fold and cut the middle of the strap at an angle to achieve better fit over the plantar calcaneus (Fig. 4–6C).

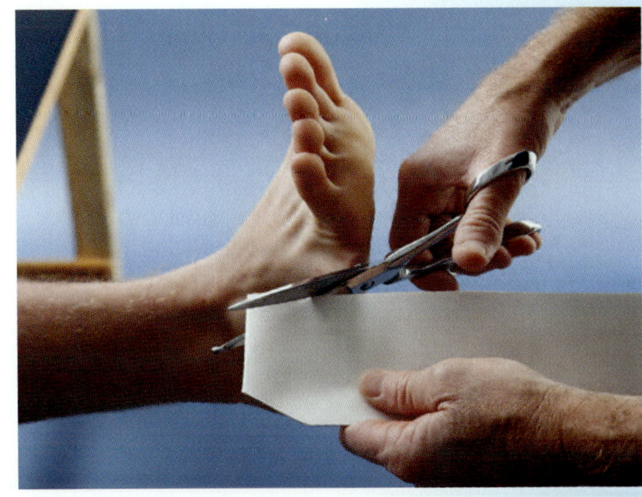

**Fig. 4–6 C**

**STEP 3:** After applying tape anchors, grasp the ends of the strap and anchor the stirrup on the plantar surface of the calcaneus (Fig. 4–6D).

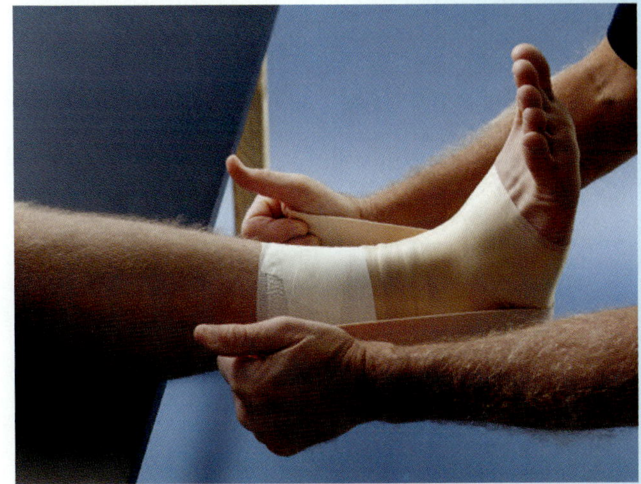

**Fig. 4–6 D**

**STEP 4:** Pull the ends toward the lower leg anchors with equal tension (Fig. 4–6E). The center of the stirrup should be located over the medial and lateral malleoli. The stirrup may also be anchored directly to the skin. Continue applying the closed basketweave and heel lock techniques.

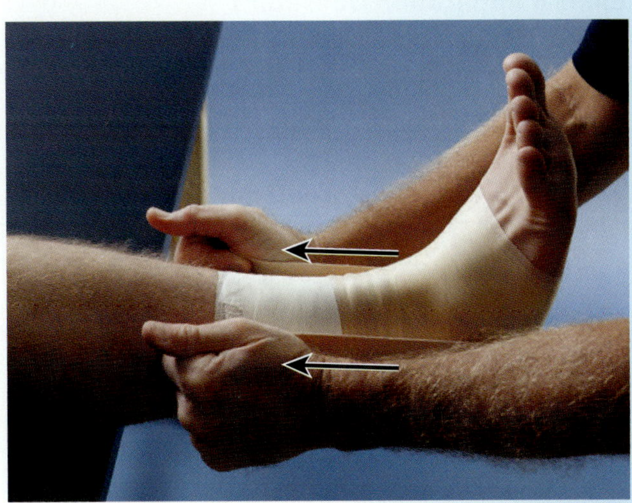

**Fig. 4–6 E**

*Steps Cont.*

**Ankle**

**STEP 5:** Thermoplastic material of ⅛ inch thickness may also be cut into a 3–4 inch width stirrup and fitted to the patient. Design, cut, heat, and mold the material (see Figs. 1–10 and 1–11C–G) over the area from the lateral lower leg anchor, over the lateral malleolus, under the calcaneus, across the medial malleolus, and finish at the medial lower leg anchor. The stirrup can be lined with moleskin (Fig. 4–6F). Apply the closed basketweave and heel lock techniques.

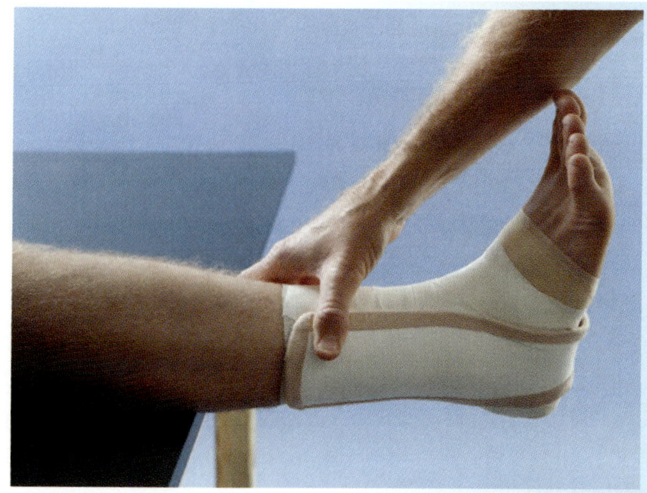

Fig. 4–6 F

**STEP 6:** Place the thermoplastic stirrup on the ankle and apply 1½ inch or 2 inch elastic tape heel locks and elastic anchor strips around the distal lower leg with moderate roll tension to attach the stirrup ◀▬▬▶ (Fig. 4–6G).

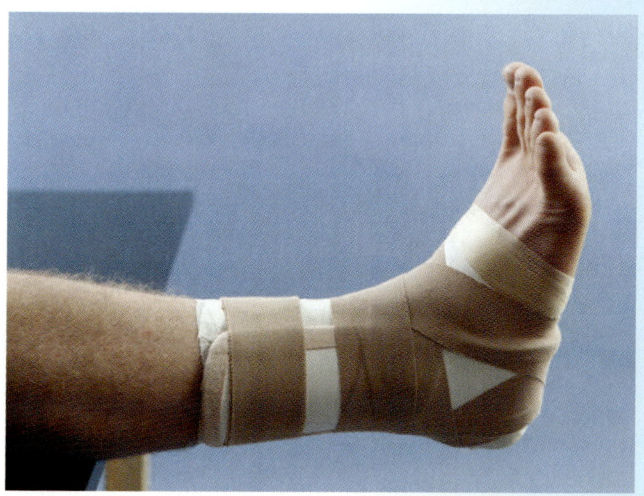

Fig. 4–6 G

## Clinical Application Question 1

A center on the basketball team is currently in phase III of a rehabilitation program for a second-degree eversion ankle sprain. This phase includes position-specific shooting, rebounding, and agility exercises. A closed basketweave technique was applied for support and protection. During the exercises, the center asks whether additional support can be provided. The entire inventory of ankle braces is being used by other members of the team, leaving only taping supplies available for use.

➠ **Question: What can be done in this situation?**

## | **ELASTIC**    Figure 4–7

➠ **Purpose:** The elastic technique is an alternative to the closed basketweave and can be applied quickly (Fig. 4–7). Because this technique offers mild support to the subtalar and talocrural joints, the elastic technique is typically used only when preventing inversion and eversion sprains for non-injured patients.

➠ **Materials:**
   • 1½ inch or 2 inch non-elastic tape, 1½ inch or 2 inch elastic tape, pre-wrap or self-adherent wrap, thin foam pads, skin lubricant, taping scissors
   ***Option:***
   • Adherent tape spray

➠ **Position of the patient:** Sitting on a taping table or bench with the leg extended off the edge with the foot in 90 degrees of dorsiflexion.

➠ **Preparation:** Apply pre-wrap or self-adherent wrap and thin foam pads and skin lubricant over the heel and lace areas.
   ***Option:*** Apply adherent tape spray under the pre-wrap or self-adherent wrap for additional adherence.

➠ **Application:**

| **STEP 1:** | Begin by placing 1½ inch or 2 inch non-elastic tape distal lower leg anchors directly to the skin or over pre-wrap or self-adherent wrap. |

| **STEP 2:** | Apply three consecutive stirrups with 1½ inch or 2 inch non-elastic tape in a medial-to-lateral direction, beginning the first over the posterior medial and lateral malleolus, overlapping each by ½ of the tape width (Fig. 4–7A). |

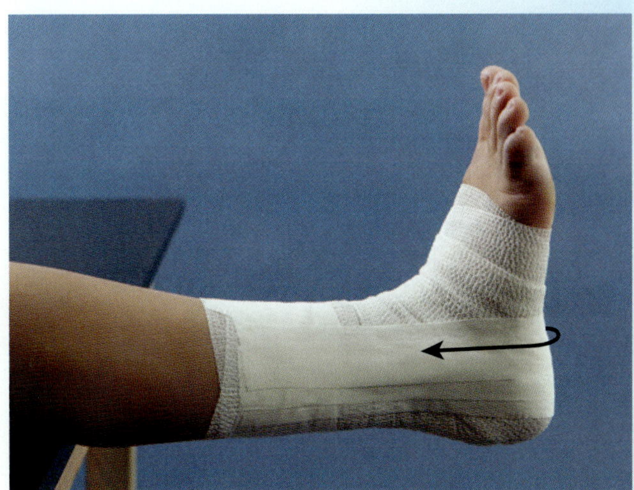

**Fig. 4–7 A**

| **STEP 3:** | Using 1½ inch or 2 inch elastic tape, anchor on the lateral lace area and apply two continuous heel locks (Fig. 4–7B). |

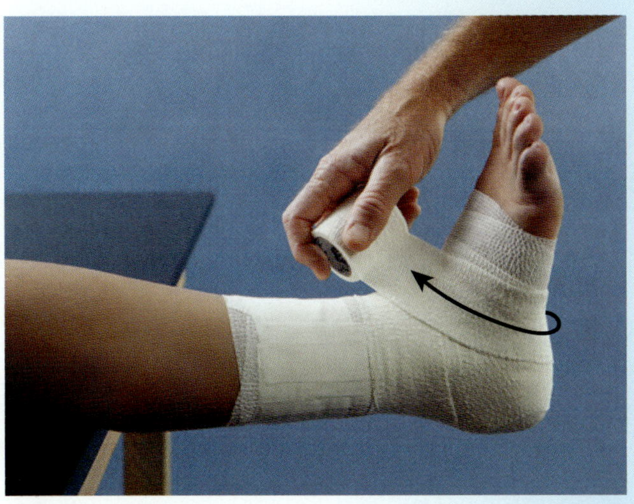

**Fig. 4–7 B**

*Steps Cont.*

**STEP 4:** From the anterior lower leg, continue to apply the elastic tape in a circular or spiral pattern with moderate roll tension (Fig. 4–7C), overlapping by ½ of the tape width, and finish on the lower leg anchor (Fig. 4–7D).

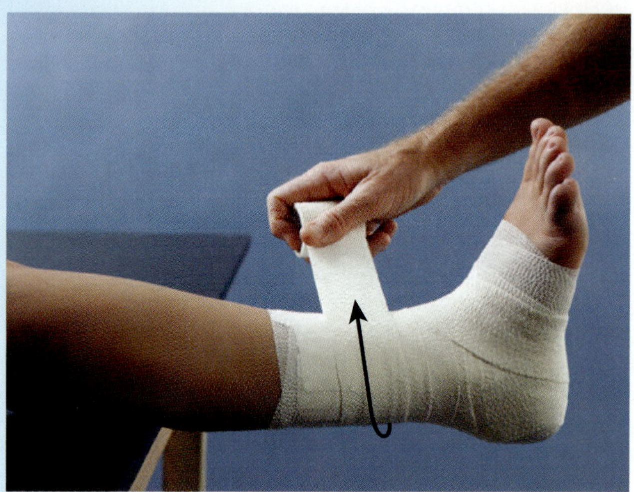

Fig. 4–7 C

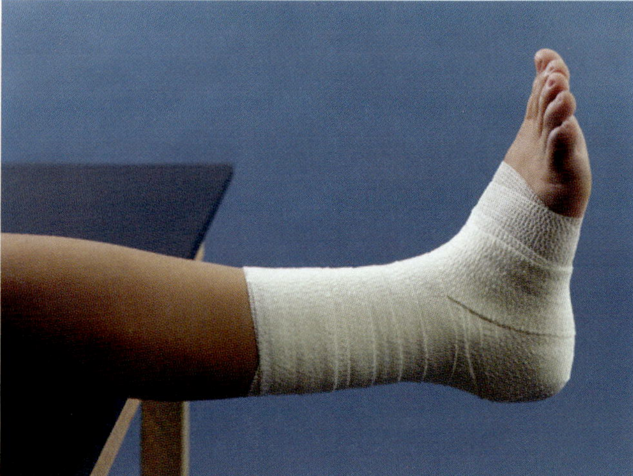

Fig. 4–7 D

**STEP 5:** Apply a heel lock with 1½ inch or 2 inch non-elastic tape with moderate roll tension (Fig. 4–7E).

*Option:* *Anchor the elastic tape at the distal lower leg with 1½ inch or 2 inch non-elastic tape.*

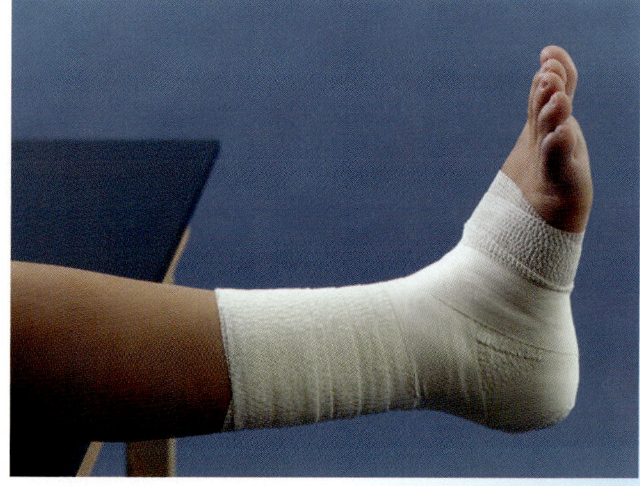

Fig. 4–7 E

**...IF/THEN...**

**IF** choosing a taping technique to support the subtalar and talocrural joints of a non-injured patient, and time is limited, **THEN** consider using the elastic technique, which involves fewer steps and can be applied more quickly than the closed basketweave.

## SPARTAN SLIPPER    Figure 4–8

➠ **Purpose:** The Spartan Slipper technique is used in combination with the closed basketweave in treating inversion, eversion, and syndesmosis sprains to provide additional support during return to activity and/or work (Fig. 4–8).

➠ **Materials:**
  • 1½ inch, 2 inch, and 3 inch non-elastic tape
  *Option:*
  • Pre-wrap or self-adherent wrap, adherent tape spray, thin foam pads, skin lubricant

➠ **Position of the patient:** Sitting on a taping table or bench with the leg extended off the edge with the foot in 90 degrees of dorsiflexion.

➠ **Preparation:** Apply directly to the skin.
  *Option:* Apply pre-wrap or self-adherent wrap, adherent tape spray, and thin foam pads and skin lubricant over the heel and lace areas to provide adherence and to lessen irritation.

➠ **Application:**

**STEP 1:**  Start the technique by placing anchors on the distal lower leg with 1½ inch or 2 inch non-elastic tape.

**STEP 2:**  With 3 inch non-elastic tape, measure and tear a strip to serve as a stirrup. Holding the ends of the stirrup, anchor on the plantar surface of the calcaneus (Fig. 4–8A).

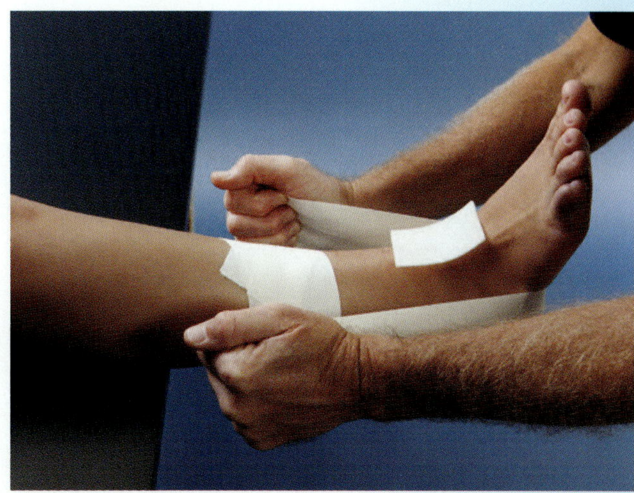

**Fig. 4–8 A**

**STEP 3:**  Pull, with equal tension, the ends of the stirrup toward the distal lower leg, and anchor (Fig. 4–8B). The center of the stirrup should cover the medial and lateral malleoli.

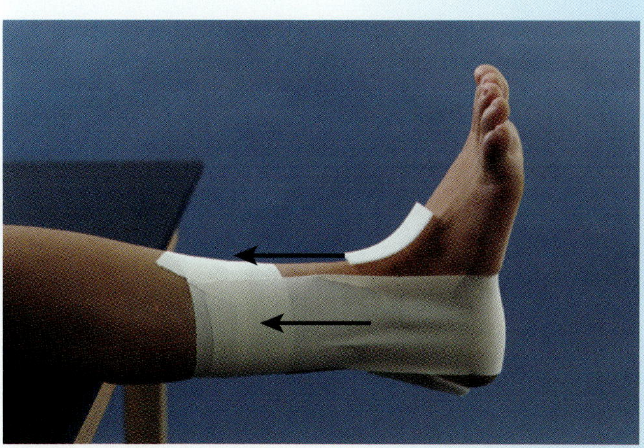

**Fig. 4–8 B**

*Steps Cont.*

**STEP 4:** Tear another stirrup strip of 3 inch non-elastic tape slightly longer than the first one. Anchor the strip on the plantar surface of the calcaneus over the previous stirrup. Starting at the ends, tear or cut lengthwise down the middle of the stirrup to the inferior medial and lateral malleoli (Fig. 4–8C).

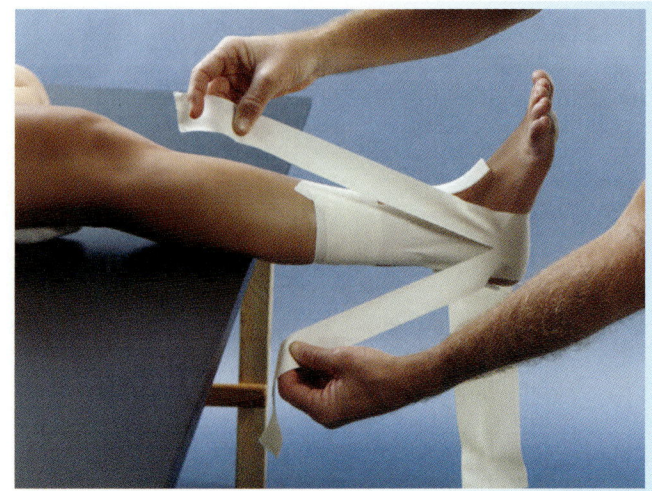

Fig. 4–8 C

**STEP 5:** Wrap the lateral stirrup ends individually around the lower leg in a spiral pattern with moderate tension (Fig. 4–8D), finishing on the distal lower leg anchor.

**Helpful Hint |**
As the stirrup ends progress from the plantar foot, crease or pinch the tape, if needed, to allow for smooth contact on the rearfoot.

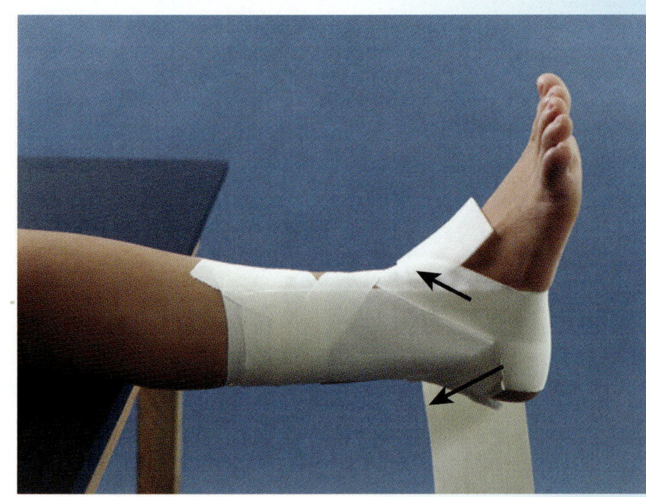

Fig. 4–8 D

**STEP 6:** Wrap the medial stirrup ends around the lower leg with moderate tension in a spiral pattern, finishing on the distal lower leg anchor, to form a slipper (Fig. 4–8E).

**STEP 7:** Continue the Spartan Slipper technique by applying a closed basketweave, with heel locks of non-elastic, elastic, or semi-rigid cast tape. Another option is to use additional stirrups of moleskin or thermoplastic materials.

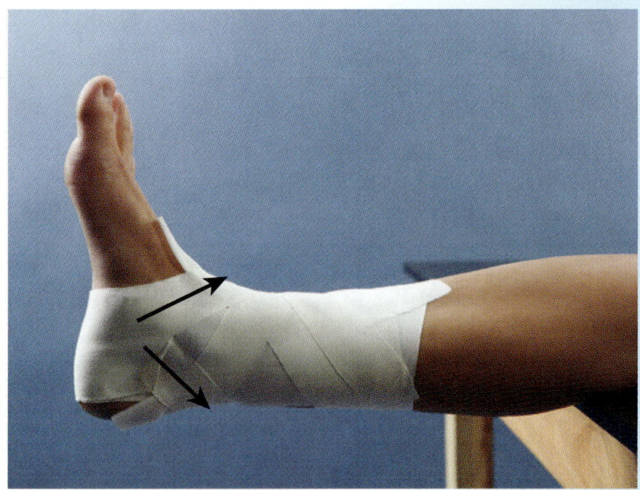

Fig. 4–8 E

## SUBTALAR SLING   Figure 4–9

➠ **Purpose:** The subtalar sling technique is also used in combination with the closed basketweave to provide additional support to the subtalar joint in treating inversion, eversion, and syndesmosis sprains[4-6] (Fig. 4–9).

➠ **Materials:**
• 2 inch heavyweight elastic tape, taping scissors
*Option:*
• Pre-wrap or self-adherent wrap, adherent tape spray, thin foam pads, skin lubricant

➠ **Position of the patient:** Sitting on a taping table or bench with the leg extended off the edge with the foot in 90 degrees of dorsiflexion.

➠ **Preparation:** Apply directly to the skin.
*Option:* Apply pre-wrap or self-adherent wrap, adherent tape spray, and thin foam pads and skin lubricant over the heel and lace areas to provide adherence and to lessen irritation.

➠ **Application:**

**STEP 1:** Apply the anchors, stirrups, and horse-shoes of the closed basketweave technique with 1½ inch or 2 inch non-elastic tape.

**STEP 2:** To prevent subtalar inversion, use a lateral sling. Anchor 2 inch heavyweight elastic tape on the medial plantar forefoot at an angle toward the distal fifth metatarsal (Fig. 4–9A).

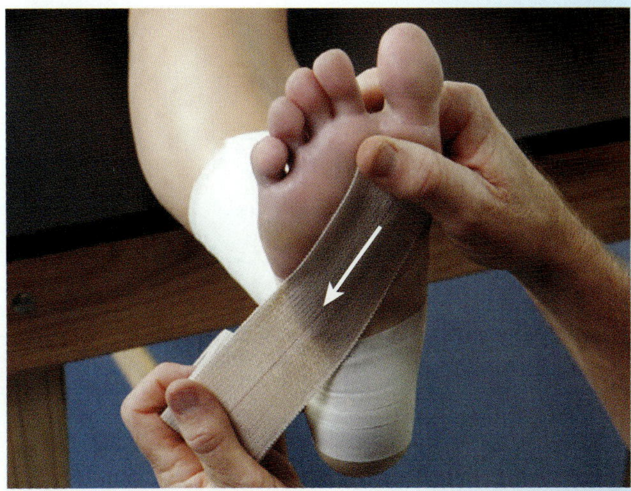

Fig. 4–9 A

**STEP 3:** Continue with moderate roll tension up and over the lateral midfoot toward the lateral malleolus (Fig. 4–9B), around the posterior lower leg, and anchor on the lateral lower leg (Fig. 4–9C). Monitor roll tension to prevent irritation of the midfoot lateral border.

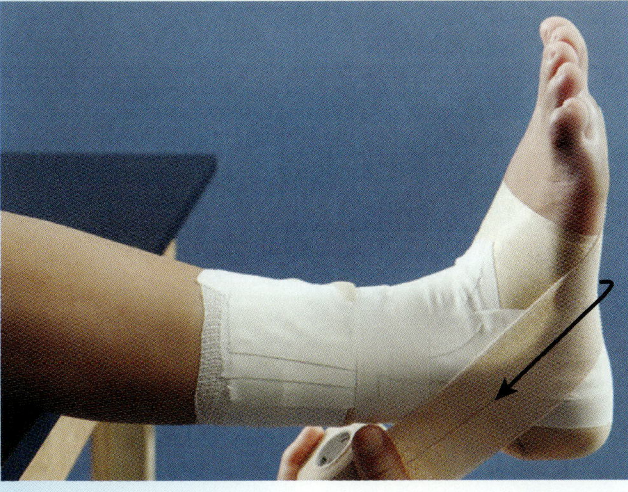
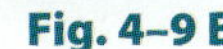

Fig. 4–9 B

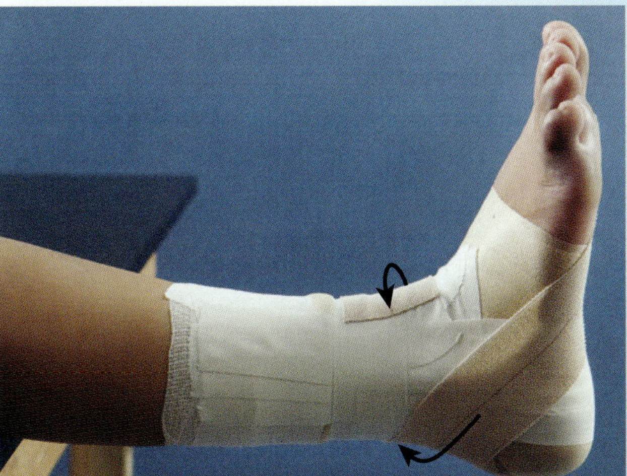

Fig. 4–9 C

*Steps Cont.*

**STEP 4:** A medial sling is used to prevent subtalar eversion. The medial sling also can be used when treating syndesmosis sprains. Anchor 2 inch heavyweight elastic tape on the lateral plantar forefoot at an angle toward the longitudinal arch (Fig. 4–9D).

**STEP 5:** Proceed up and across the arch, with moderate roll tension toward the medial malleolus (Fig. 4–9E), around the posterior lower leg, and anchor on the medial lower leg (Fig. 4–9F).

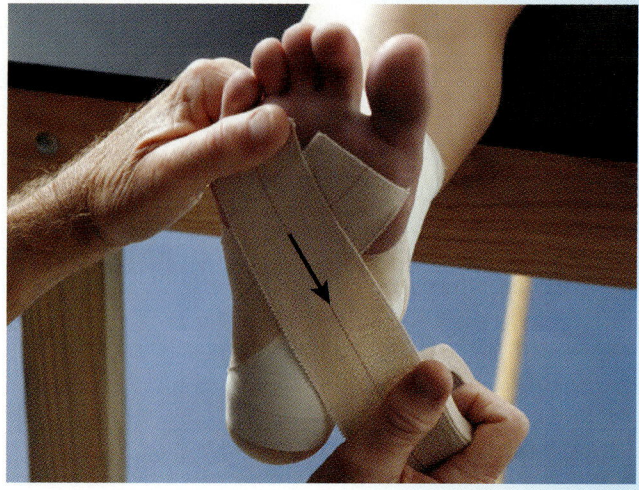

Fig. 4–9 D

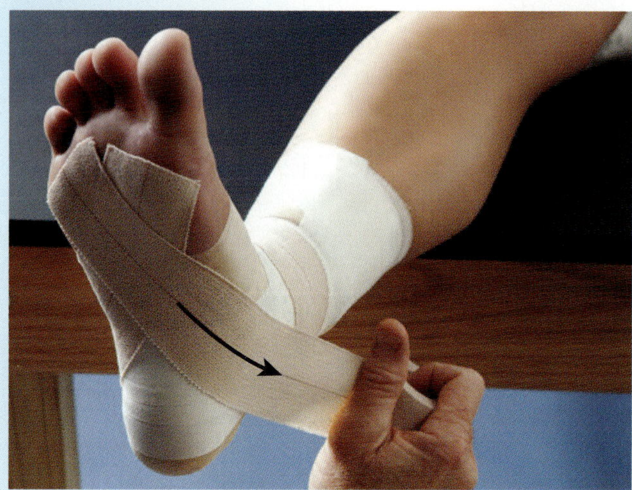

Fig. 4–9 E

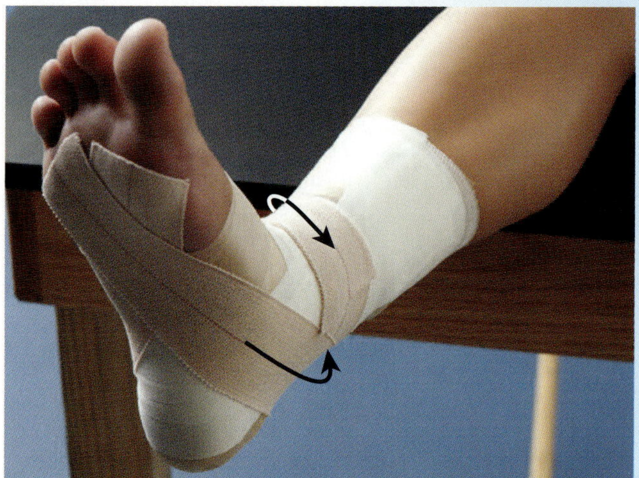

Fig. 4–9 F

**STEP 6:** An additional lateral and/or medial sling may be applied, anchoring in a more distal position on the medial or lateral forefoot (Fig. 4–9G).

**STEP 7:** After applying the subtalar sling(s), continue with closed basketweave closure strips and heel locks with 1½ inch or 2 inch non-elastic tape. Additional anchors over the distal forefoot are not required.

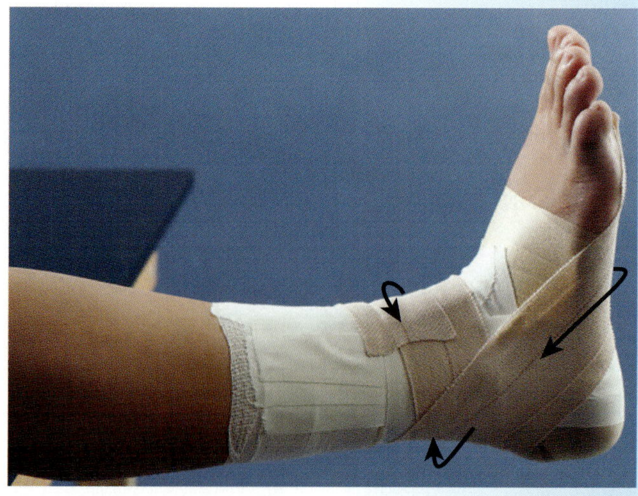

Fig. 4–9 G

**DETAILS**

Because of the high incidence of inversion sprains, apply a lateral sling when using the medial sling technique to compensate for the inversion tension of the medial sling.[4]

**. . . IF/THEN . . .**

**IF** application of the basic closed basketweave taping technique is not effective in supporting the ankle during the return to activity following a sprain, **THEN** consider using elastic or cast tape heel locks, moleskin or thermoplastic stirrups, the Spartan Slipper, and/or the subtalar sling in combination with the closed basketweave to provide greater support to the subtalar and talocrural joints.

## SPATTING

**➥ Purpose:** The spatting technique entails applying tape over athletic shoes to provide support and reduce range of motion to the subtalar and talocrural joints. Spatting is performed in sports that utilize cleats, such as rugby and American football, and can be used alone or in combination with other ankle taping and bracing techniques. Tapes in team or shoe colors are often used for the technique. This technique and steps of application can be found on FADavis.com.

## EVIDENCE SUMMARY

Several small studies have investigated the effectiveness of ankle taping, ankle taping and spatting, spatting, and no tape on ankle range of motion in pre-exercise and postexercise conditions and functional performance among various healthy populations. Examining range of motion in pre-exercise conditions, researchers demonstrated significant reductions in weight-bearing sudden ankle inversion,[7] and active and passive ankle inversion,[8–10] eversion,[8] plantar flexion,[8–10] and dorsiflexion[8] with taping, taping and spatting, and spatting compared with no tape. Findings from two studies showed taping and spatting used in combination resulted in the greatest reduction on ankle inversion[7] and plantar flexion[10] range of motion. In postexercise conditions, researchers[7] found taping, taping and spatting, and spatting provided significantly greater reductions in ankle inversion than no tape after 30 minutes of exercise. The combination of taping and spatting was again the most effective in reducing ankle inversion and there was no significant differences between taping and spatting when used alone.[7] Other researchers[9] revealed significantly greater reductions in ankle inversion with spatting at 20, 40, and 60 minutes postexercise compared with taping alone. Researchers[9] have also shown that spatting produced significantly greater reductions in ankle plantar flexion at 40 and 60 minutes postexercise compared to taping alone. However, one study[8] found no significant reductions in ankle inversion, eversion, dorsiflexion, and plantar flexion among taping, taping and spatting, and spatting compared with no tape following 15 minutes of exercise.

The effects of taping, taping and spatting, and spatting on functional performance have produced mixed results. Researchers[8,11] have demonstrated no significant effects on speed and agility performance with taping, taping and spatting, and spatting compared to no tape. Others[10] found taping and spatting significantly decreased agility performance as compared with no tape and taping, taping and spatting, and spatting produced a significant decrease in maximum vertical jump height when compared with a no tape situation. Further research is required to determine the efficacy and cost-benefit of spatting and the combination of taping and spatting on the reduction of ankle injuries among athletes who participate with cleated footwear.

**Ankle**

## POSTERIOR SPLINT | Figure 4–10

➧ **Purpose:** The posterior splint technique is used to immobilize the subtalar and talocrural joints in the acute treatment of fractures and severe inversion, eversion, and syndesmosis sprains (Fig. 4–10). Use the splint as temporary immobilization prior to further evaluation by a physician. Temporary immobilization may be required while waiting overnight for a physician appointment or returning home with an athletic team from an away competition. Two methods are interchangeable in applying the posterior splint technique; the first is illustrated here (Fig. 4–10), and the second is online at FADavis.com.

### DETAILS

Periods of immobilization are normally determined by a physician following evaluation of the patient. To provide complete immobilization, rigid cast tape is applied over stockinet and cast padding by cast technicians and physicians.

➧ **Design:**
  * Rigid splints available off-the-shelf in pre-cut and padded designs provide temporary immobilization in the treatment of fractures and sprains. The splints are constructed of several layers of rigid fiberglass material, which are covered with fabric and foam padding in 2, 3, 4, and 5 inch widths by 10, 12, 15, 30, 35, and 45 inch lengths.

### *Posterior Splint Technique One*

➧ **Materials:**
  * Off-the-shelf rigid, padded splint, gloves, water, towel, two 4 inch width by 10 yard length elastic wraps, metal clips, 1½ inch non-elastic tape or 2 inch self-adherent wrap
➧ **Position of the patient:** Prone on a taping table or bench with the leg extended off the edge. If pain and swelling allow, place the ankle in subtalar neutral.
➧ **Preparation:** Mold and apply the padded splint directly to the skin.
➧ **Application:**

**STEP 1:** Remove the splint from the package and immerse in water of 70° to 75°F to begin the chemical reaction. Submerge the splint the length of time it takes to squeeze the splint once or twice. Remove the splint and place lengthwise on a towel.

**STEP 2:** Quickly roll the splint and towel together to remove excess water (Fig. 4–10A).

**STEP 3:** Apply the splint from just inferior to the posterior knee, across the plantar foot to the distal toes (Fig. 4–10B).

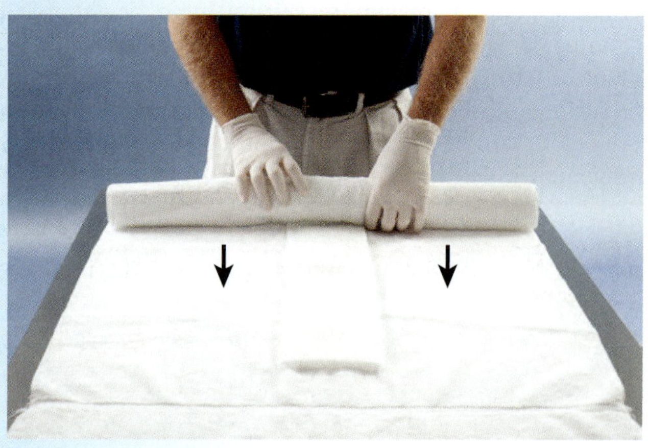

**Fig. 4–10 A**

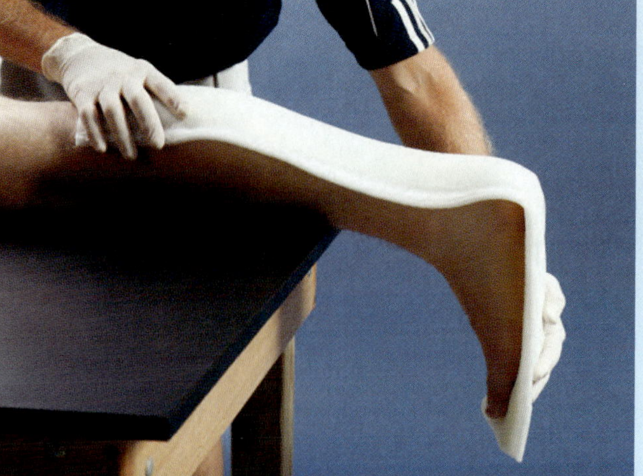

**Fig. 4–10 B

**STEP 4:** Mold the splint to the body contours with the application of a 4 inch width by 10 yard length elastic wrap in a spiral pattern with moderate roll tension ◀▬▬▶ (Fig. 4–10C). Continue to mold and shape the splint with the hands. Monitor the pain-free position of the ankle. After 10–15 minutes, the fiberglass should be cured; remove the elastic wrap.

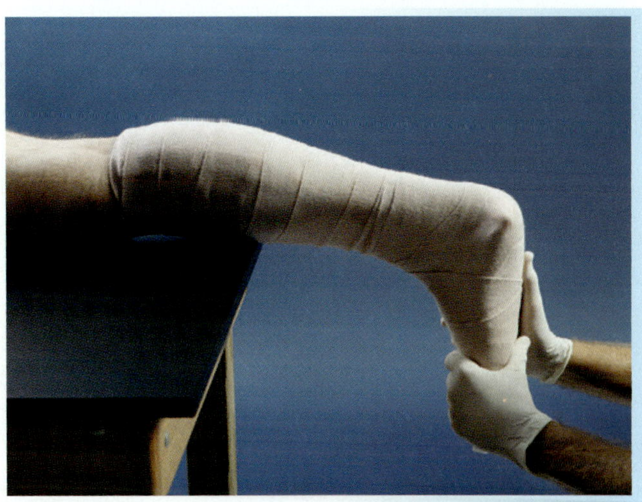

**Fig. 4–10 C**

**STEP 5:** Using another 4 inch width by 10 yard length elastic wrap, attach the splint with moderate roll tension to the posterior lower leg, ankle, and foot in a spiral, distal-to-proximal pattern ◀▬▬▶ (Fig. 4–10D). Anchor the wrap with metal clips or loosely applied 1½ inch non-elastic tape or 2 inch self-adherent wrap. The patient will require crutches for non–weight-bearing ambulation.

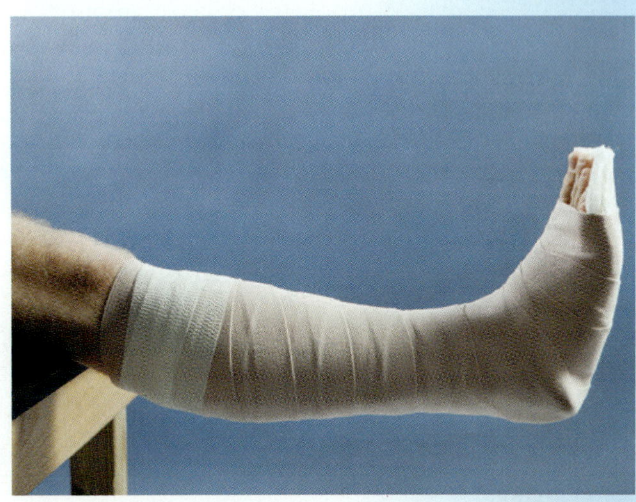

**Fig. 4–10 D**

### Clinical Application Question 2

Through the outpatient orthopedic clinic, you perform outreach services with an amateur rugby team. A flanker on the team suffers a syndesmosis sprain of his left ankle. Following rehabilitation, a physician allows the flanker to return to practice and competition with appropriate ankle support.

➡ **Question: What taping techniques can be used in this situation?**

# Wrapping Techniques

Wrapping techniques are used to provide compression to control swelling and effusion, to provide support, and to reduce range of motion.

## FOOT AND ANKLE COMPRESSION WRAP   Figure 4–11

➡ **Purpose:** The foot and ankle compression wrap technique is used in the acute treatment of inversion, eversion, and syndesmosis sprains to control mild, moderate, or severe swelling and effusion (Fig. 4–11).

➥ **Materials:**
- 2 inch, 3 inch, or 4 inch width by 5 yard length elastic wrap, metal clips, 1½ inch non-elastic or 2 inch elastic tape, taping scissors

*Options:*
- ¼ inch or ½ inch foam or felt
- 2 inch, 3 inch, or 4 inch self-adherent wrap or elastic tape, pre-wrap, thin foam pads

➥ **Position of the patient:** Sitting on a taping table or bench with the leg extended off the edge and the foot in pain-free dorsiflexion.

➥ **Preparation:** Apply the technique directly to the skin.

*Option:* Cut a ¼ inch or ½ inch foam or felt horseshoe pad (see Fig. 4–19A–D). With the use of elastic tape, apply one layer of pre-wrap directly to the skin and use thin foam pads over the heel and lace areas.

➥ **Application:**

**STEP 1:** The wrap technique for the ankle is identical to the compression technique for the foot illustrated in Chapter 3, Figure 3–17. Apply the greatest amount of roll tension distally and lessen tension as the wrap continues proximally.

*Option:*   *Apply the ¼ inch or ½ inch foam or felt horseshoe pad to the medial and/or lateral aspect of the ankle to provide additional compression to assist in the control of swelling and effusion (Fig. 4–11). If an elastic wrap is not available, 2 inch, 3 inch, or 4 inch self-adherent wrap or elastic tape may be used.*

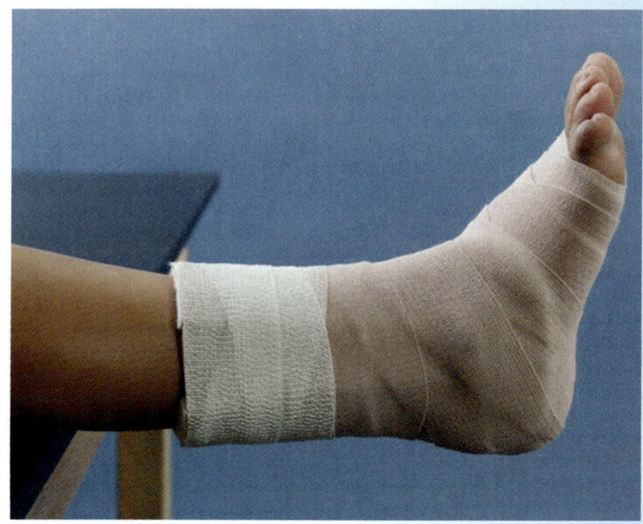

**Fig. 4–11**

---

**...IF/THEN...**

**IF** the elastic compression wrap migrates or slides over or off the calcaneus during ambulation and movement of footwear, **THEN** loosely apply a 1½ inch non-elastic or 2 inch elastic tape or self-adherent wrap circular strip from the lace area, across the plantar calcaneus, and finish over the lace area to anchor the elastic wrap ◂▥▸.

---

## FOOT AND ANKLE COMPRESSION SLEEVE    Figure 4–12

➥ **Purpose:** Use the foot and ankle compression sleeve technique to provide compression when controlling mild, moderate, or severe swelling and effusion when treating sprains (Fig. 4–12). Unlike elastic wraps, this compression technique, with proper instruction, can be applied and removed by the patient without assistance.

➥ **Materials:**
- 2½ inch, 3 inch, or 3½ inch elastic sleeve, taping scissors

*Option:*
- ¼ inch or ½ inch foam or felt

➥ **Position of the patient:** Sitting on a taping table or bench with the leg extended off the edge or sitting in a chair.

➥ **Preparation:** Cut a sleeve from a roll to extend from the proximal toes to the distal lower leg. Cut and use a double-length sleeve to provide additional compression.

➥ **Application:**

**STEP 1:**   Pull the sleeve onto the foot and ankle directly to the skin in a distal-to-proximal direction (Fig. 4–12). If using a double-length sleeve, pull the distal end over the first layer to provide an additional layer. No anchors are required; the sleeve can be cleaned and reused.

*Option:*   *Apply the ¼ inch or ½ inch foam or felt horseshoe pad to the medial and/or lateral aspect of the ankle to provide additional compression.*

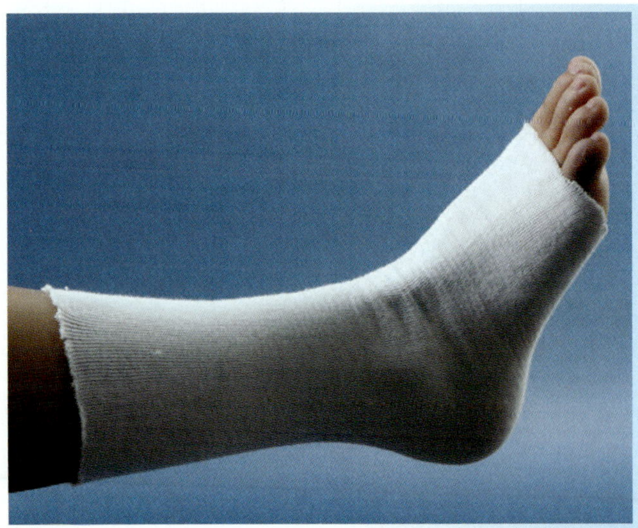

**Fig. 4–12**

## SOFT CAST   Figure 4–13

➠ **Purpose:** Compression and mild support can be provided with the soft cast technique in the acute treatment of sprains (Fig. 4–13). Because of the materials used, this technique is perhaps the most comfortable for the patient with moderate or severe swelling and can be left in place for several days.

➠ **Materials:**
  • 2 inch, 3 inch, or 4 inch width cast padding, 2 inch, 3 inch, or 4 inch width by 5 yard length elastic or self-adherent wrap

➠ **Position of the patient:** Sitting on a taping table or bench with the leg extended off the edge and the foot in pain-free dorsiflexion.

➠ **Preparation:** Apply the soft cast directly to the skin.

➠ **Application:**

**STEP 1:**   Apply 2 inch, 3 inch, or 4 inch width cast padding from the proximal toes to the distal lower leg in a spiral, distal-to-proximal pattern with moderate roll tension ◀▬▬▶ (Fig. 4–13A). Applying three layers of the material should provide adequate compression around the ankle.

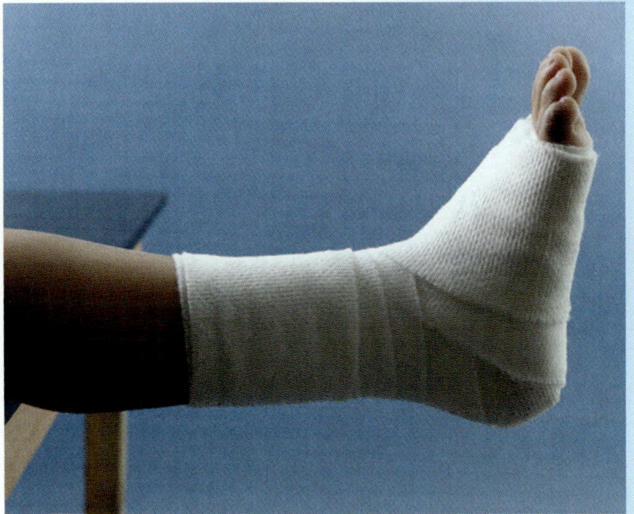

**Fig. 4–13 A**

*Steps Cont.*

**STEP 2:** Next, apply the foot and ankle compression wrap technique over the cast padding with a 2 inch, 3 inch, or 4 inch width by 5 yard length elastic wrap or self-adherent wrap (Fig. 4–13B).

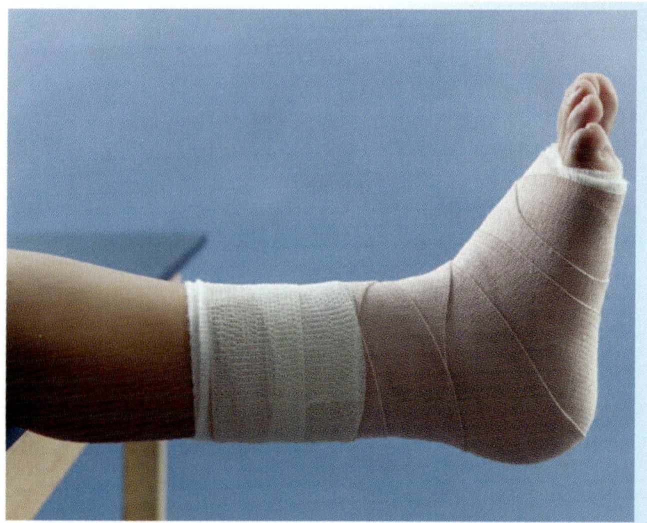

**Fig. 4–13 B**

## CLOTH WRAP    Figure 4–14

➡ **Purpose:** Use the cloth wrap technique to provide mild support in preventing inversion and eversion sprains during athletic activities (Fig. 4–14).
➡ **Materials:**
  • 2 inch width by 72–96 inch length cloth wrap, thin foam pads, 1½ inch or 2 inch non-elastic tape
➡ **Position of the patient:** Sitting on a taping table or bench with the leg extended off the edge with the foot in 90 degrees of dorsiflexion.
➡ **Preparation:** Apply over a sock and use thin foam pads over the heel and lace areas to lessen irritation.
➡ **Application:**

**STEP 1:** Place the end of a 72–96 inch length cloth wrap on the distal lateral lower leg superior to the lateral malleolus and anchor around the leg in a lateral-to-medial direction (Fig. 4–14A).

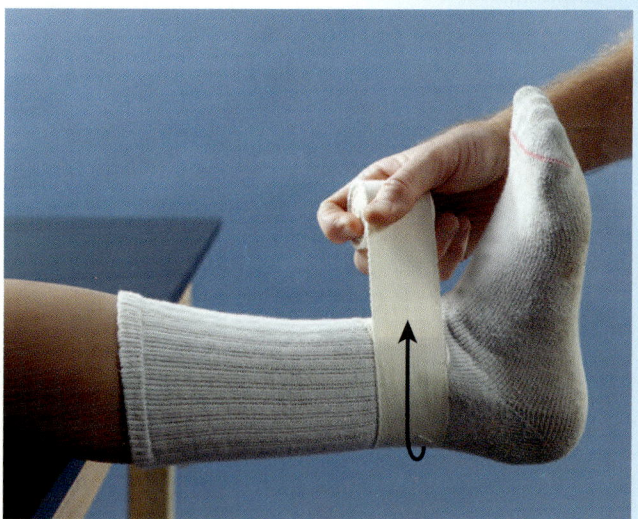

**Fig. 4–14 A**

**STEP 2:** Continue applying the wrap with the continuous heel lock technique with moderate roll tension (Fig. 4–14B). The length of the cloth wrap should allow for the application of at least two sets of heel locks.

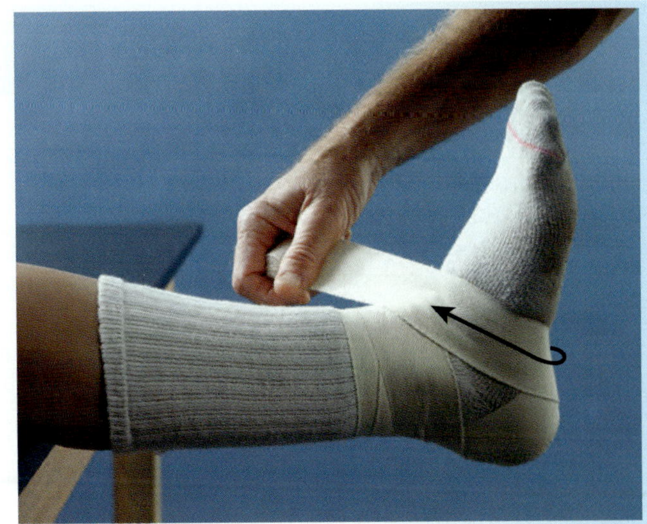

**Fig. 4–14 B**

**STEP 3:** Finish the wrap around the distal lower leg and anchor with 1½ inch or 2 inch non-elastic tape ◀▬▬▶ (Fig. 4–14C).

**STEP 4:** Heel locks may be applied with 1½ inch or 2 inch non-elastic tape with moderate roll tension over the cloth wrap for additional support.

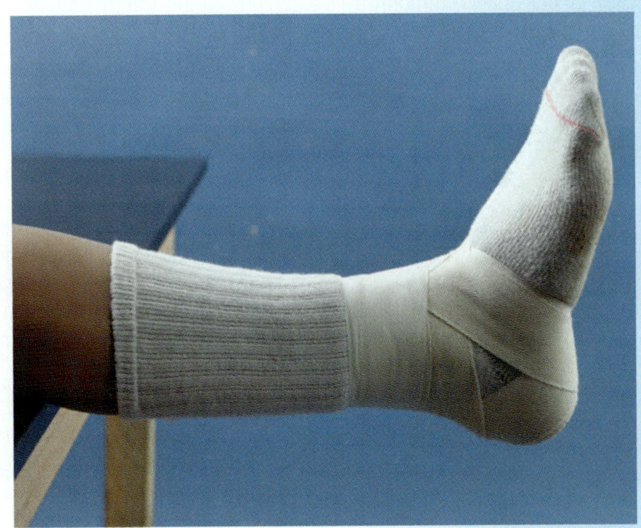

**Fig. 4–14 C**

## Clinical Application Question 3

While working on a job site, an electrician steps off the unfinished stairs that lead to an outside door. His right foot lands on several pieces of scrap wood, causing a moderate inversion ankle sprain. A physician applies an air/gel bladder brace on the ankle for support and compression. The electrician is also placed on crutches for ambulation.

➡ **Question: What type of compression wrap technique can you use with the brace?**

## ...IF/THEN...

**IF** a patient has swelling following an ankle sprain but will not be seen for treatment for an extended period of time because of work commitments, **THEN** consider using an elastic sleeve to provide compression; after receiving application instruction, the patient can apply and remove the sleeve herself or himself.

# Bracing Techniques

Bracing techniques for preventing and treating ankle sprains generally can be classified into four categories: lace-up, semirigid, air/gel bladder, and wrap. Bracing offers several advantages over taping in preventing and treating injuries. With fitting instructions, a patient can apply and remove the braces, and they can be reused. During activity, straps and/or laces can be adjusted to maintain proper fit, comfort, and support. Several braces are designed to assist in venous return in the treatment of swelling and effusion. Using braces also has been proved cost-effective for reducing the incidence of ankle sprains.[12–14]

## LACE-UP    Figure 4–15

➡ **Purpose:** Lace-up braces are designed to provide moderate support and limit inversion, eversion, plantar flexion, and dorsiflexion in preventing and treating inversion and eversion ankle sprains (Fig. 4–15).

### DETAILS

Lace-up braces are commonly used when preventing and treating inversion and eversion sprains of athletes in a variety of sports. The braces can also be used with work and casual footwear. Lace-up ankle braces may be used in combination with the closed basketweave, elastic, Spartan Slipper, and subtalar sling taping techniques to provide maximal support during activities.

➡ **Design:**
- The braces are available off-the-shelf in predetermined sizes, corresponding either to ankle circumference or to shoe size.
- Some designs are universal and can be used on either ankle, while others are purchased in a right or left style.
- The brace is applied directly over a sock and is constructed of a variety of strong, breathable materials, such as ballistic nylon, neoprene, nylon/polyester fabric, vinyl laminate, or mesh fabric. Some designs can be worn directly on the skin.
- Eyelets for lacing are located on the anterior aspect of the brace in a longitudinal pattern. The tongue, located beneath the laces, is constructed of a durable, padded material to lessen irritation. This padded material is also found over the posterior heel area.
- To provide additional support, outer straps or flaps are incorporated into the designs. Nylon straps with Velcro closures are applied in a figure-of-eight and/or heel lock pattern over the brace. Flaps are used to secure the laces and prevent loosening.
- Many of the designs that have straps contain an elastic Velcro closure strip to anchor the strap and lace ends at the proximal end of the brace on the distal lower leg.
- From the basic lace-up design, many braces include various plastic or steel materials or use additional straps to provide support.
- Insert plastic stays to serve as stirrups with some designs. Others are manufactured with an internal thermoplastic shell that forms to the contour of the ankle during use.
- Some designs have forefoot and calcaneal straps to restrict range of motion in those areas.
- Several other design features found in lace-up braces include buttress pads, which prevent migration and lessen swelling; tabs, which speed lacing and assist with application; elastic, neoprene, or gel materials, which prevent irritation; and contoured arches, which provide support.

➡ **Position of the patient:** Sitting on a taping table or bench or chair.

➡ **Preparation:** Apply a sock over the foot and ankle. Loosen the laces and straps of the brace.

Specific instructions for fitting and applying the brace are included with each design. For proper fit and support, carefully follow the step-by-step procedures from the manufacturer. The following application guidelines pertain to most braces.

➡ **Application:**

**STEP 1:**   Over a sock, hold each side of the brace and pull it over the foot until the heel is firmly positioned in the brace (Fig. 4–15A).

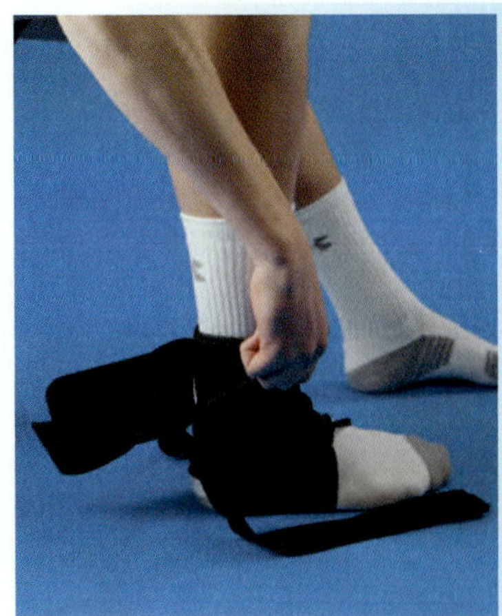

**Fig. 4–15 A**

**STEP 2:**   Put the laces through the eyelets in a distal-to-proximal pattern and tie at the proximal end (Fig. 4–15B). With many designs, the distance between the left and right eyelets should be less than 2 inches. If greater, use the next larger brace size. If the brace does not utilize straps, application is complete.

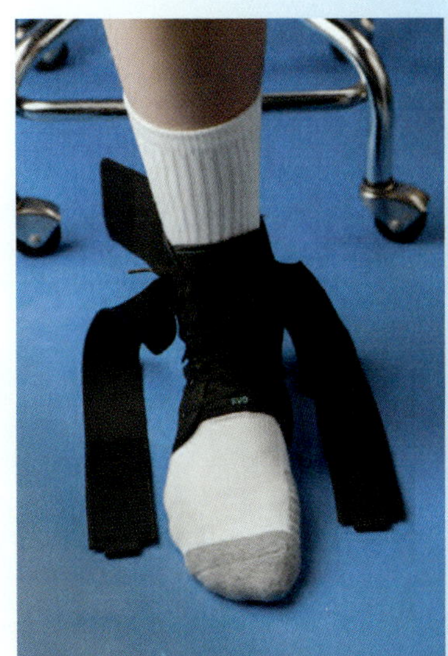

**Fig. 4–15 B**

**STEP 3:**   Applying straps will depend on the specific brace design. Figure-of-eight and heel lock straps commonly begin with application over the dorsum of the foot, continuing under the longitudinal arch, around the heel, and anchoring on the lateral or medial lower leg (Fig. 4–15C).

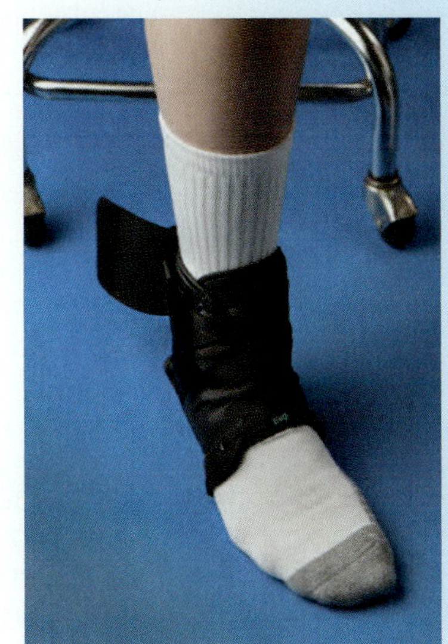

**Fig. 4–15 C**

*Steps Cont.*

**STEP 4:**    Pull these straps tight and secure to the brace with Velcro. Anchor the strap and lace ends with the elastic closure strip (Fig. 4–15D).

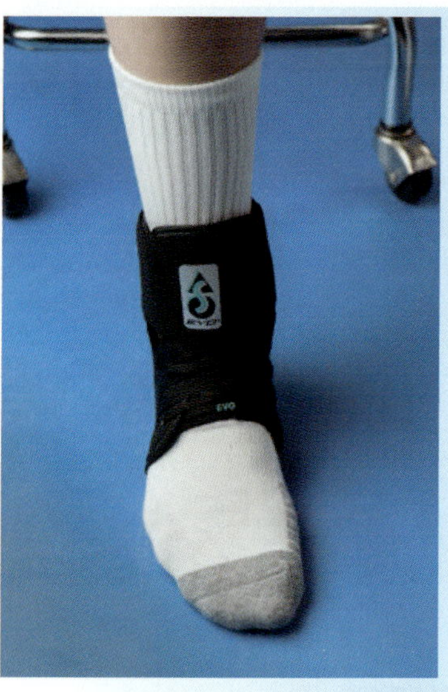

**Fig. 4–15 D**

## ... IF/THEN ...

**IF** lace-up braces gradually stretch after days or weeks of use, **THEN** wash and air-dry the braces and laces to shrink the materials to near original size to achieve proper fit.

## SEMIRIGID    Figure 4–16

➡ **Purpose:** Semirigid braces provide moderate support and are used when preventing and treating inversion, eversion, and syndesmosis ankle sprains. These braces limit inversion, eversion, and rotation, allowing normal plantar flexion and dorsiflexion (Fig. 4–16).

### DETAILS

Semirigid designs are very popular with basketball and volleyball players because these designs do not restrict plantar flexion and dorsiflexion range of motion. However, athletes in a variety of sports can also wear the braces. The braces can also be used with casual and work footwear. Use semirigid designs in combination with the closed basketweave, elastic, Spartan Slipper, and subtalar sling taping techniques to provide maximal support during activities.

➡ **Design:**
- The braces are manufactured in universal or individual fit designs in predetermined sizes.
- Most semirigid designs consist of a medial and lateral stirrup attached through a hinge to either a heel or foot plate. The stirrups and plates are constructed from semirigid plastics and carbon composites.
- Several designs allow for custom molding and fitting.
- Semirigid braces are lined with EVA, neoprene, or air cell padding to provide compression, support, and comfort during activity.
- Various nylon straps with Velcro attachments incorporated into the stirrups anchor the brace to the distal lower leg.
- Many of the semirigid braces are available with extra design features to assist with support and comfort.
- Some designs have a nylon foam liner that wraps around the lower leg and calcaneus with anterior laces to provide additional support.
- The medial and lateral stirrups of other designs contain a reinforced shell to further limit range of motion.

- The foot plates of some designs are molded similarly to an orthotic to support the longitudinal arch. Other foot plates have small cleats on the plantar surface to prevent migration during activity.
- In several designs, the lining of the stirrups can be changed to accommodate abnormal body contours and to vary the amount of compression.
- In several designs, the anchor strap can be adjusted according to the size and shape of the leg and the type of footwear worn, such as low or high top athletic styles.

➠ **Position of the patient:** Sitting on a taping table or bench or chair.

➠ **Preparation:** Apply a sock over the foot and ankle.

Application of semirigid designs should follow manufacturers' instructions, which are included with the braces when purchased. The following general application guidelines apply to most semirigid designs.

➠ **Application:**

**STEP 1:** Begin by loosening the straps and positioning the foot onto the heel or foot plate. Align the stirrups over the lateral and medial malleoli. Bring the stirrups snugly together and anchor the distal lower leg strap (Fig. 4–16A).

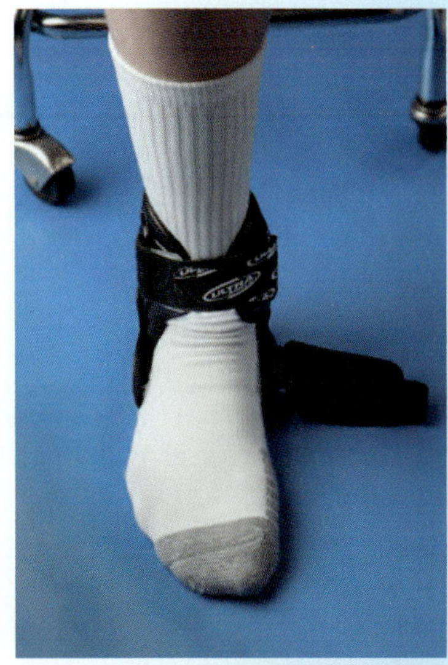

**Fig. 4–16 A**

**STEP 2:** Position the pad and straps over the midfoot and anchor (Fig. 4–16B).

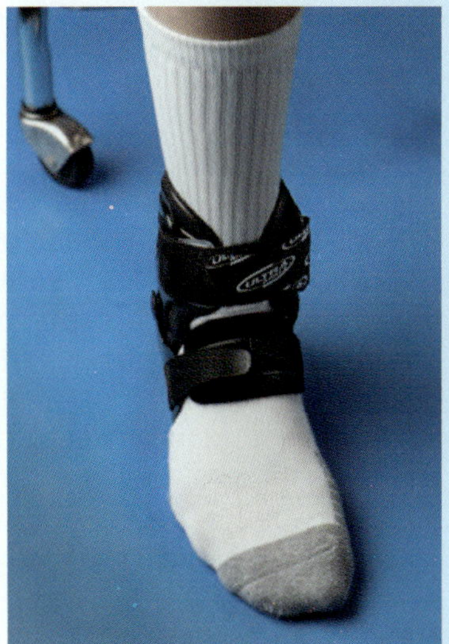

**Fig. 4–16 B**

*Steps Cont.*

**STEP 3:**    Loosen the shoe laces and place the foot inside the shoe, sliding the heel against the heel box. Finish by tying the shoe laces (Fig. 4–16C).

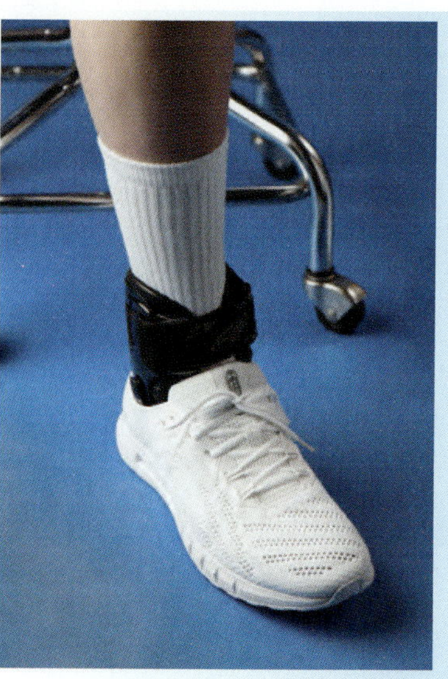

**Fig. 4–16 C**

## AIR/GEL BLADDER        Figure 4–17

➠ **Purpose:** Air/gel bladder braces are designed only to limit inversion and eversion in preventing and treating inversion and eversion ankle sprains (Fig. 4–17). The braces are used most often during the acute phase of treatment to provide compression and moderate support.

### DETAILS

The braces are used to prevent and treat sprains for athletes participating in a variety of sports. While somewhat larger than lace-up, semirigid, and wrap designs, air/gel bladder braces can be used with work and casual footwear. Air/gel bladder braces may be used in combination with the closed basketweave, elastic, Spartan Slipper, and subtalar sling taping techniques to provide maximal support during activities and with the compression, sleeve, and soft cast wrapping techniques to provide moderate support during the acute phase of treatment.

➠ **Design:**
  • The braces are available in universal or individual fit designs of various widths and lengths in predetermined sizes.
  • Air/gel bladder designs consist of medial and lateral thermoplastic stirrups or shells, pre-molded to the contours of the lower leg and ankle.
  • The stirrups/shells are lined with various combinations of air and/or gel bladders. Many pre-inflated air bladder liners contain a proximal valve that allows for adjustments in compression. Some of the air/gel and gel liners may be removed and placed in a freezer to cool. After the liners are cooled, reattach the liners to the stirrups/shells to provide compression and cryotherapy. Several liner designs are covered with soft foam material for additional comfort.
  • The stirrups/shells are connected with an adjustable nylon strap that is worn across the plantar calcaneus.
  • Some designs have a nylon foam lower leg and midfoot wrap to provide additional compression and support.
  • The braces are anchored to the lower leg and ankle with two vinyl straps with Velcro closures.
➠ **Position of the patient:** Sitting on a taping table or bench or chair.
➠ **Preparation:** Apply a sock over the foot and ankle.
Instructions for application are included with each brace. The following guidelines pertain to most designs.
➠ **Application:**

**STEP 1:**  Begin by loosening the lower leg straps and distal air/gel bladders from the stirrups/shells to expose the plantar calcaneus strap (Fig. 4–17A). Adjust the calcaneus strap to allow the stirrups/shells to fit snugly around the lower leg and ankle.

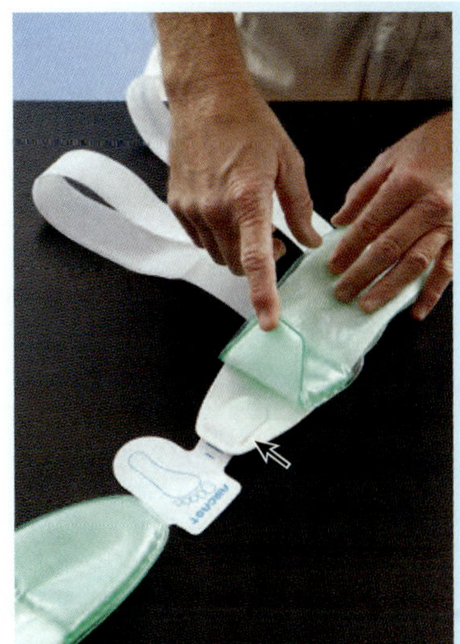

**Fig. 4–17 A** *Plantar calcaneus strap.*

**STEP 2:**  Over a sock, place the heel onto the calcaneus strap and position the stirrups/shells over the ankle and lower leg (Fig. 4–17B).

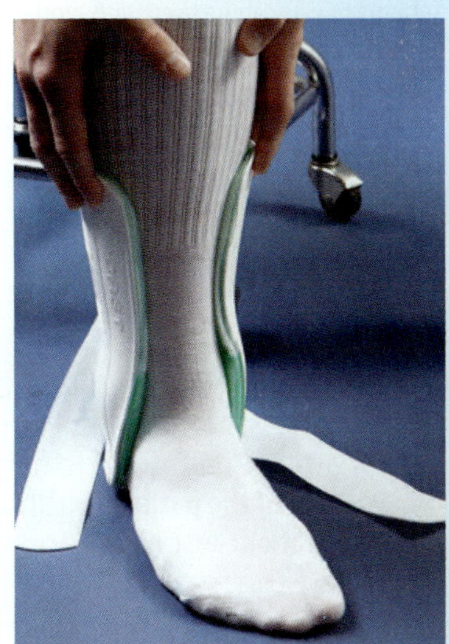

**Fig. 4–17 B**

**STEP 3:**  Anchor the brace with the lower leg straps.

**STEP 4:**  Place the foot and brace into the shoe and adjust the straps if needed to achieve a snug fit (Fig. 4–17C).

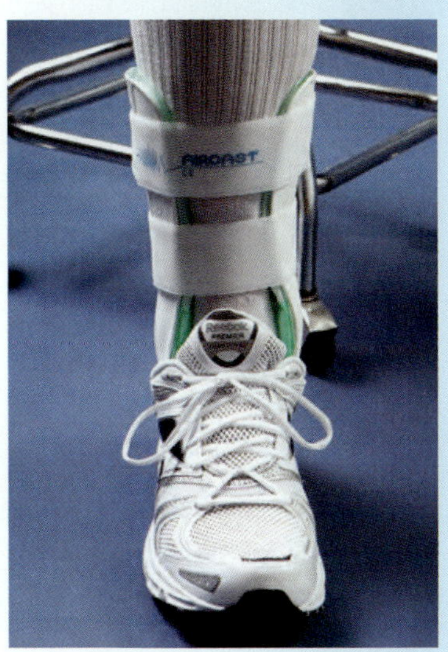

**Fig. 4–17 C**

## Clinical Application Question 4

Near the conclusion of the spring semester, an intercollegiate soccer midfielder who sustained a right ankle syndesmosis sprain during spring practice comes into the athletic training facility. She plans to participate in a summer league at home and asks about what type of protection she can use for her right ankle during practices and competitions. The Spartan Slipper and subtalar sling taping techniques were applied when she returned to practice in the spring. These techniques allowed a return but limited her ability to dribble and shoot the ball on goal.

➡ **Question: What technique(s) can you use in this situation?**

## WRAP     Figure 4–18

➡ **Purpose:** Wrap braces are used in the prevention and treatment of inversion and eversion ankle sprains and provide mild support (Fig. 4–18). These off-the-shelf braces can be categorized into two basic designs based on their function: support or treatment.

### DETAILS

Support braces can be used with work and casual footwear and for athletes participating in a variety of sports. The support design may be used in combination with the closed basketweave, elastic, Spartan Slipper, and subtalar sling taping techniques to provide moderate support. The treatment brace, on the other hand, is designed to be used for non–weight-bearing therapeutic activities to provide compression.

➡ **Design:**
- Support designs are available in universal or individual fit in predetermined sizes. The braces are constructed of ballistic nylon, nylon/Lycra, elastic/Lycra, or neoprene. Support to the ankle is provided through various nylon straps with Velcro closures that are applied in figure-of-eight and/or heel lock patterns.
- Treatment designs are available in universal fit and are made of neoprene with removable gel packs attached in the inner liner of the brace. Many packs can be removed and heated and/or cooled, then reattached to provide treatment to the ankle. Anchor the treatment designs with Velcro closures.

➡ **Position of the patient:** Sitting on a taping table or bench or chair.

➡ **Preparation:** Apply support designs over a sock. Apply treatment designs over a sock or directly to the skin. Follow the manufacturer's instructions when applying the braces.

➡ **Application:**

**STEP 1:** Apply some of the support designs by loosening the closures, positioning the foot onto the brace, wrapping the brace around the foot and ankle, and anchoring with Velcro closures (Fig. 4–18A).

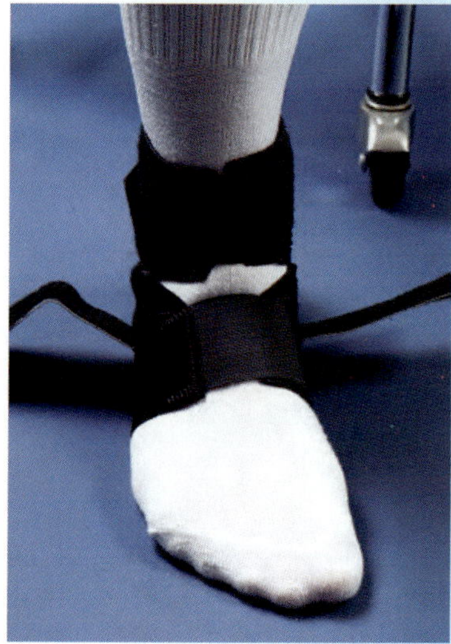

**Fig. 4–18 A**

**STEP 2:** Apply the nylon straps in a figure-of-eight, heel lock, and/or stirrup pattern as indicated by the manufacturer (Fig. 4–18B). Pull other designs onto the foot and ankle in a distal-to-proximal pattern.

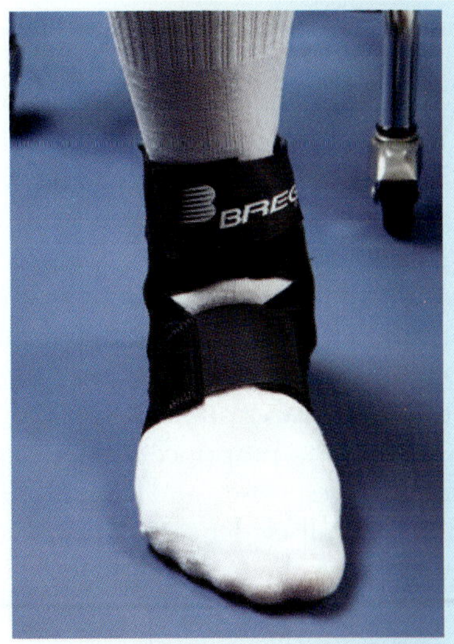

**Fig. 4–18 B**

**STEP 3:** Apply the treatment designs by positioning the foot onto the brace, wrapping around the foot and ankle, and anchoring with the Velcro closures (Fig. 4–18C).

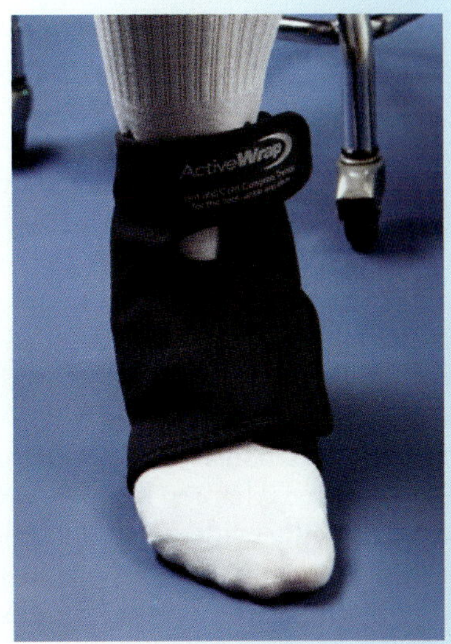

**Fig. 4–18 C**

## Clinical Application Question 5

This season, you decide to purchase and use lace-up ankle braces in place of taping techniques to prevent ankle sprains in the basketball athletes. During the first few practices, several athletes complain about the fit of the braces and the lack of support provided.

➡ **Question: What can you do to accommodate the basketball athletes?**

### . . . IF/THEN . . .

**IF** choosing a brace design for an athlete returning to practice following a syndesmosis ankle sprain, **THEN** consider a semirigid design, which will limit external rotation. Also consider using the brace in combination with several taping techniques to provide maximal support.

### . . . IF/THEN . . .

**IF** support is needed in the acute treatment of a first-degree eversion sprain with mild to moderate swelling, **THEN** consider the use of an air/gel bladder brace design, which limits inversion and eversion and can be applied over a compression wrap technique in the control of swelling.

## EVIDENCE SUMMARY

Health care professionals use a variety of taping and lace-up, semirigid, air/gel bladder, and wrap bracing techniques in preventing and treating ankle sprains. The high incidence of ankle sprains[15] has led to the development of these multiple tape techniques and brace designs. Investigations of taping and bracing techniques are numerous in the literature. The majority of the research has examined the influence of ankle taping and bracing on ankle range of motion, proprioception, balance, postural control, muscle response, and overall functional performance. The overall evidence from these clinical studies appears to support the use of taping and bracing to reduce range of motion and provide mechanical stability and improve neuromuscular control with a minimal negative effect on functional performance. Despite these clinical findings, a limited amount of research has investigated the effectiveness of taping and bracing in preventing the rate of ankle sprains among active populations.

A 2013 National Athletic Trainers' Association (NATA) position statement[16] presented recommendations for the conservative management and prevention of ankle sprains in athletes. The recommendations in the statement are supported by relevant, patient-oriented evidence available in articles and reviews. The evidence was graded based on the Strength of Recommendation Taxonomy developed by the American Academy of Family Physicians.[17] (For more complete information on the scale, see Chapter 1, Further Reading). The authors[16] examined the evidence to determine the efficacy of tape and brace techniques/designs in the prevention of first-time and recurrent ankle sprains. Studies[18–25] included in the statement demonstrated that tape and lace-up and semirigid braces reduced the incidence of ankle sprains among athletes in various sports. Some researchers[23] found no differences between tape and braces in lessening rates of injury, while others[12,24,25] reported that braces were more effective than tape in preventing ankle sprains. An additional and important finding was that tape and brace designs were more effective in the prevention of ankle sprains among athletes with a history of sprains compared with those who had no history of ankle injury.[12,18,20,21,26] Based on the evidence, the position statement[16] recommends athletes with a history of previous ankle sprains should use prophylactic ankle bracing and taping for all practices and games. Lace-up and semirigid braces and traditional taping are recommended to reduce the rate of recurrent ankle sprains in athletes. A 2018 clinical practice guideline[27] provided recommendations for the diagnosis, treatment, and prevention of lateral ankle sprains. Examining injury prevention, the authors[27] concluded that the use of tape and brace techniques lessened the risk of first-time and recurrent ankle sprains. Tape and braces were more effective in the prevention of recurrent sprains compared to first-time injuries. The recommendations demonstrated no differences between tape and braces in the prevention of recurrent sprains.

Recommendations from the NATA position statement[16] and clinical practice guideline[27] and findings from clinical research support the use of ankle taping and bracing, but guidance for the most effective prophylactic technique/design is unclear. Determining the most appropriate technique/design to utilize should be based on the patient as well as available resources such as budget, availability, and skill of the health care professional. Many[12,18,20,21,26] have shown that taping and bracing are more effective in preventing ankle sprains in athletes with a history of ankle injury. This finding should be considered in clinical decisions of whether to prophylactically tape or brace an entire team or only those with a history of ankle injury.[16] Researchers[12] have conducted a numbers-needed-to-treat (NNT) and cost-benefit analysis examining the effectiveness of ankle taping and bracing. The NNT analysis was performed to determine how many athletes must be taped or braced to prevent one ankle sprain. The cost-benefit analysis determined implications of the interventions on facility budgets.[12] Findings from three studies in the analysis[12] showed fewer athletes with a history of ankle injury needed to be taped or braced to prevent one sprain compared to taped or braced athletes without a history of ankle injury. The cost of taping an athlete one time is less than bracing the athlete one time, but braces were found to be cost-effective over a competitive season.[12] Additionally, following instruction, bracing requires less time from the athlete and health care professional for application than taping over a season.

Numerous taping and bracing techniques and designs are available to implement in the prevention and treatment of ankle sprains. Health care professionals can integrate the existing evidence, clinical expertise with the interventions, and patient preferences and needs to guide clinical decisions. Future randomized controlled trials and long-term prospective studies examining the efficacy of different methods of taping and designs of bracing can produce additional evidence in determining the most effective intervention for preventing ankle sprains among patients with a history of ankle injury and those without a history of injury.

## WALKING BOOT

➡ **Purpose:** Walking boots or walkers (see Fig. 3–22) are used in treating inversion, eversion, and syndesmosis ankle sprains, as well as with stable acute and stress fractures.
  • Use the boots in the postacute treatment and rehabilitation period when limited range of motion and weight-bearing are allowed to provide support.
  • The ability to remove the boot for treatment, adjust the range of motion, and proceed with gait training provides an effective bracing technique at a lower cost than traditional casting.

# Padding Techniques

Use padding techniques to lessen shear forces and provide compression with various injuries and conditions of the ankle. Applying taping, wrapping, and bracing techniques can cause trauma to the skin and result in irritation, blisters, and lacerations. Several padding techniques can be used to prevent and treat these injuries and conditions.

## HORSESHOE PAD    Figure 4–19

➡ **Purpose:** Use the horseshoe pad technique in the acute treatment of ankle sprains to provide additional compression to assist with reducing swelling and effusion (Fig. 4–19).
➡ **Materials:**
  • ¼ inch or ½ inch foam or felt, taping scissors
➡ **Position of the patient:** Sitting on a taping table or bench with the leg extended off the edge and the foot in pain-free dorsiflexion.
➡ **Preparation:** Cut the horseshoe pad from ¼ inch or ½ inch foam or felt to fit over the medial and/or lateral aspect of the ankle. Off-the-shelf pre-cut designs are also available.
➡ **Application:**

**STEP 1:**   Cut a piece of foam or felt approximately 4–5 inches in width and 6–8 inches in length.

**STEP 2:**   Cut a narrow "U"-shaped pattern 5–7 inches lengthwise into the foam or felt (Fig. 4–19A). Another horseshoe technique is to cut a hole in the middle of the foam or felt 5–7 inches from the proximal end (Fig. 4–19B).

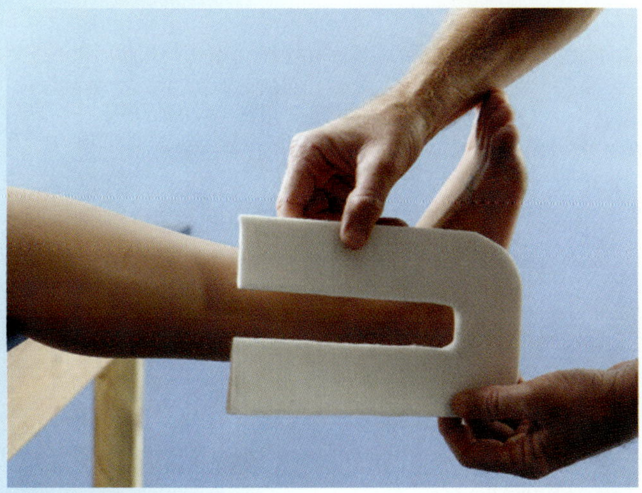

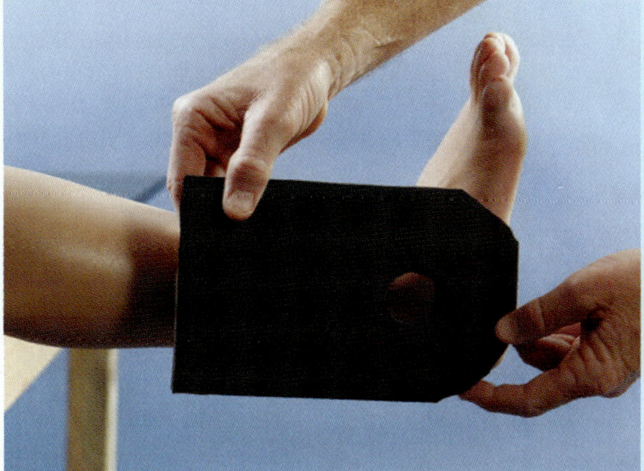

**Fig. 4–19 A**

**Fig. 4–19 B**

*Steps Cont.*

**STEP 3:** Position the horseshoe pad over the medial and/or lateral ankle with the malleoli placed at the bottom of the "U" or in the hole of the pad (Fig. 4–19C).

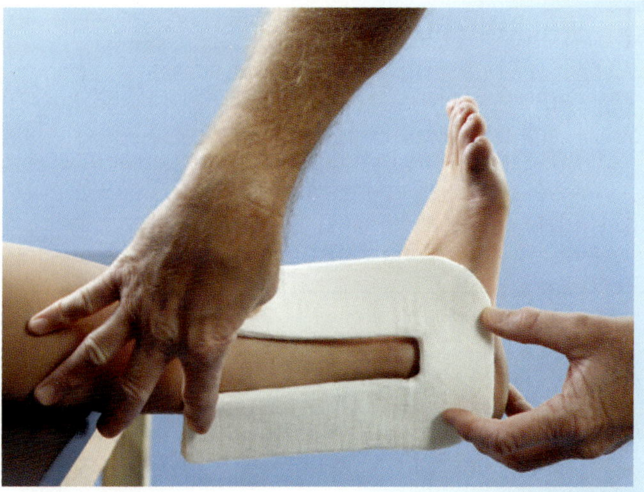

**Fig. 4–19 C**

**STEP 4:** Apply the foot and ankle compression or sleeve wrapping techniques over the horseshoe pad to anchor (Fig. 4–19D).

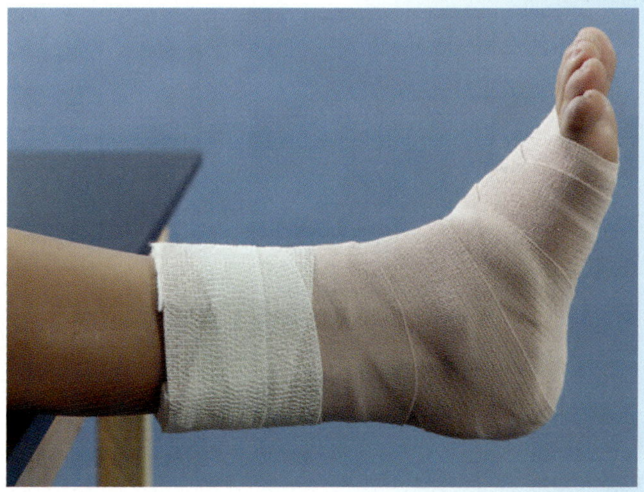

**Fig. 4–19 D**

## DONUT PADS

**Purpose:** Donut pads can be used to reduce shearing forces on the ankle in the treatment of skin irritations (see Fig. 3–26). Blisters are common over the heel, lace, and medial and lateral malleoli and are caused by footwear and the application of tapes, wraps, and braces.
- Cut pads from ⅛ inch or ¼ inch foam or felt and place them over the medial and/or lateral malleoli.
- The pad may be used under taping, wrapping, and bracing techniques.
- With taping techniques, attach the pad directly to the skin with adhesive gauze material (see Fig. 3–15) prior to tape application or with pre-wrap (see Fig. 4–4A) during the taping technique.
- When applying wrapping techniques, anchor the pad within the technique.
- With bracing techniques, attach the pad with adhesive gauze material (see Fig. 3–15) or pre-wrap and 1½ inch or 2 inch elastic tape using the heel lock technique (see Fig. 4–5).

## ACHILLES TENDON STRIPS

**Purpose:** The Achilles tendon strip technique also reduces shearing forces that may occur when using taping and bracing techniques. This technique and steps of application can be found on FADavis.com.

## DETAILS

Applying taping and bracing techniques daily to prevent and treat ankle sprains often causes irritation of the skin. Taping technique closure strips and/or brace straps can cause irritation, especially over the Achilles tendon. Abnormal body contours, such as malalignment of the Achilles tendon, may also lead to irritation.

## Clinical Application Question 6

After several weeks of treatment and rehabilitation for an ankle sprain/fracture, a salesperson for an automobile dealership returns to work. The physician recommends that all work activities be performed with a semirigid brace on the ankle. Soon, the brace begins to cause skin irritation over the lateral malleolus.

➡ **Question: How can you manage this situation?**

## . . . IF/THEN . . .

**IF** using foam or felt materials for padding in combination with an ankle taping, wrapping, or bracing technique, **THEN** choose the appropriate thickness of the material; the material should reduce shear forces but not affect the fit and support provided by the technique, which can occur with an excessively thick pad.

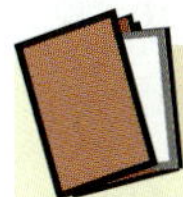

## EVIDENCE-BASED PRACTICE

Meghan Johnson is a two-sport athlete at G. Wilson College, participating on the volleyball team in the fall and the softball team in the spring. During the first competitive volleyball match of the season, Meghan jumped to block a spike at the net. When she landed, her right foot struck a teammate's shoe, causing a moderate inversion and plantar flexion force. Meghan has no history of ankle injury and was not wearing a prophylactic tape, brace, or wrap technique. Meghan was taken to the athletic training facility for evaluation by Dean Fish, AT, and by the team physician. Following an evaluation and subsequent radiographs, Meghan was diagnosed by the physician with a moderate right ankle inversion sprain. The team physician ordered Meghan to be immobilized at 90 degrees of ankle dorsiflexion, non–weight-bearing, for 5–10 days. During this time, Meghan could receive treatment to her ankle. Dean and the team physician discussed various taping and bracing techniques that could be used to immobilize Meghan's right ankle. Dean decided to check several types of immobilization techniques before speaking again with the team physician and selecting one for Meghan.

Meghan progressed well within the therapeutic exercise program Dean and the team physician designed. Meghan was ready to begin sport-specific drills during volleyball practice. The team physician requested that Meghan's ankle be supported during these drills and for the remainder of the season. Dean used EBP and selected an appropriate technique to support Meghan's ankle during volleyball activities.

Meghan finished the volleyball season without further injury and began practice with the softball team. Meghan asked Dean if she could continue with some type of ankle support during softball practices. Dean agreed and continued applying the technique used for volleyball practices and competitions. During softball practice, a base running drill required Meghan to sprint from home plate to second base. As she stepped on first base, her right ankle was forced into dorsiflexion, and she experienced pain. Meghan finished practice and returned to the athletic training facility to talk to Dean about a different technique for support. Dean began to think about a technique that will provide support and limit dorsiflexion to allow Meghan to participate pain-free.

1.  Develop two clinically relevant questions from the case in the PICO format to generate answers for the selection of a (1) technique for immobilization for 5–10 days and (2) technique for softball activities for Meghan. The questions should include the population or problem, the intervention, a comparison intervention (if relevant), and the clinical outcome of interest.

2.  Design a search strategy and search to find the best evidence to answer the clinical questions. The strategies should include relevant search terms, electronic databases, online journals, and print journals to use for the search. Discussions with your clinical preceptor and other health care professionals can provide evidence from expert opinion.

*Continued*

3. Choose two to three full text studies or reviews from each of your searches or the chapter references. Evaluate and appraise each article to determine its value and usefulness to the case. Ask these questions for each study: (1) Are the results of the study valid? (2) What are the actual results? and (3) Are the findings clinically relevant to my patients? Prepare a summary of the evaluation with answers to the questions and rank the articles based on the evidence hierarchy in Chapter 1.

4. Integrate findings from the evidence, your clinical experience, and Meghan's goals and preferences into the case. Consider which techniques may be appropriate for each situation.

5. Evaluate the EBP process and your experience within the case. Consider these questions in the evaluation.

Were the clinical questions answered?
Did the searches generate quality evidence?
Was the evidence evaluated appropriately?
Was the evidence, your clinical experience, and Meghan's goals and values integrated to make the clinical decisions?
Did the interventions produce successful clinical outcomes for Meghan?
Was the EBP experience positive for Dean and Meghan?

## WRAP-UP

- Ankle sprains are caused by excessive range of motion and are common in athletic activities. Fractures can occur in combination with sprains.
- Blisters can result from repetitive shearing forces caused by footwear and the application of taping, wrapping, and bracing techniques.
- The closed basketweave, heel lock, elastic, Spartan Slipper, subtalar sling, and spatting techniques provide support and reduce range of motion of the subtalar and talocrural joints.
- Cast tape and off-the-shelf fiberglass splints provide immobilization in treating sprains and fractures.
- Elastic wraps, tapes, and sleeves, as well as soft cast compression techniques, control swelling and effusion following injury.
- Cloth wraps provide mild support when preventing ankle sprains.
- Lace-up, semirigid, air/gel bladder, and wrap braces provide support and compression and limit range of motion when preventing and treating ankle sprains and fractures.
- Walking boots and posterior splints can be used to provide support and immobilization.
- Donut and Achilles tendon strip pad techniques reduce shearing forces.
- The horseshoe pad technique provides compression to reduce swelling and effusion.

## FADAVIS ONLINE RESOURCES

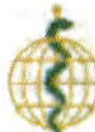
Go to the online resource center at http://Fadavis.com/ to view these additional techniques for the ankle.

- Spatting taping technique
- Posterior splint technique two
- Achilles tendon strip padding technique

## WEB REFERENCES

**National Athletic Trainers' Association**
**National Athletic Trainers' Association Position Statement: Conservative Management and Prevention of Ankle Sprains in Athletes**
http://natajournals.org/doi/pdf/10.4085/1062-6050-48.4.02?code=nata-site
- This site allows access to recommendations on the management and prevention of ankle sprains among athletes.

**American Academy of Orthopaedic Surgeons**
https://www.aaos.org
- This website allows you to search for information about the mechanism, treatment, and rehabilitation of ankle injuries, including the American Academy of Orthopaedic Surgeons Clinical Practice Guidelines.

**The American College of Foot & Ankle Orthopedics & Medicine**
https://www.acfaom.org
- This site provides general information on common injuries and conditions.

## REFERENCES


1. Doherty, C, Delahunt, E, Caulfield, B, Hertel, J, Ryan, J, and Bleakley, C: The incidence and prevalence of ankle sprain injury: A systematic review and meta-analysis of prospective epidemiological studies. Sports Med 44:123–140, 2014.

2. Gibney, VP: Sprained ankle: A treatment that involves no loss of time, requires no crutches, and is not attended with an ultimate impairment of function. NY Med J 61:193–197, 1985.

3. Purcell, SB, Schuckman, BE, Docherty, CL, Schrader, J, and Poppy, W: Differences in ankle range of motion

before and after exercise in 2 tape conditions. Am J Sports Med 37:383–389, 2009.

4. Wilkerson, GB: Biomechanical and neuromuscular effects of ankle taping and bracing. J Athl Train 37:436–445, 2002.

5. Wilkerson, GB: Comparative biomechanical effects of the standard method of ankle taping and a taping method designed to enhance subtalar stability. Am J Sports Med 19:588–595, 1991.

6. Wilkerson, GB, Kovaleski, JE, Meyer, M, and Stawiz, C: Effects of the subtalar sling ankle taping technique on combined talocrural-subtalar joint motions. Foot Ankle Int 26:239–246, 2005.

7. Pederson, TS, Ricard, MD, Merrill, G, Schulthies, SS, and Allsen, PE: The effects of spatting and ankle taping on inversion before and after exercise. J Athl Train 32:29–33, 1997.

8. Trower, B, Buxton, BP, German, TL, Joyner, AB, McMillan, JL, and Tsang, KKW: The effects of prophylactic taping on ankle joint motion and performance. J Athl Train 32:S14, 1997.

9. Udermann, BE, Miller, KC, Doberstein, ST, Reineke, DM, Murray, SR, and Pettitt, RW: Spatting restricts ankle motion more effectively than taping during exercise. Int J Exerc Sci 2:72–82, 2009.

10. Bernitt, CJ, Powers, ME, and Gildard, M: A comparison of ankle strapping and spatting on range of motion and performance. J Athl Train 51:S59, 2016.

11. Reuter, GD, Dahl, AR, and Senchina, DS: Ankle spatting compared to bracing or taping during maximal-effort sprint drills. Int J Exerc Sci 4:49–64, 2011.

12. Olmsted, LC, Vela, LI, Denegar, CR, and Hertel, J: Prophylactic ankle taping and bracing: A numbers-needed-to-treat and cost-benefit analysis. J Athl Train 39:95–100, 2004.

13. Cordova, ML, Ingersoll, CD, and LeBlanc, MJ: Influence of ankle support on joint range of motion before and after exercise: A meta-analysis. J Orthop Sports Phys Ther 30:170–182, 2000.

14. Cordova, ML, Ingersoll, CD, and Palmieri, RM: Efficacy of prophylactic ankle support: An experimental perspective. J Athl Train 37:446–457, 2002.

15. Fong, DT, Hong, Y, Chan, LK, Yung, PS, and Chan, KM: A systematic review on ankle injury and ankle sprain in sports. Sports Med 37:73–94, 2007.

16. Kaminski, TW, Hertel, J, Amendola, N, Docherty, CL, Dolan, MG, Hopkins, JT, Nussbaum, E, Poppy, W, and Richie, D: National Athletic Trainers' Association position statement: Conservative management and prevention of ankle sprains in athletes. J Athl Train 48:528–545, 2013.

17. Ebell, MH, Siwek, J, Weiss, BD, Woolf, SH, Susman, J, Ewigman, B, and Bowman, M: Strength of recommendation taxonomy (SORT): A patient-centered approach to grading evidence in the medical literature. Am Fam Physician 69:548–556, 2004.

18. Garrick, JG, and Requa, RK: Role of external support in the prevention of ankle sprains. Med Sci Sports 5:200–203, 1973.

19. Sitler, M, Ryan, J, Wheeler, B, McBride, J, Arciero, R, Anderson, J, and Horodyski, M: The efficacy of a semirigid ankle stabilizer to reduce acute ankle injuries in basketball. A randomized clinical study at West Point. Am J Sports Med 22:454–461, 1994.

20. Tropp, H, Askling, C, and Gillquist, J: Prevention of ankle sprains. Am J Sports Med 13:259–262, 1985.

21. Surve, I, Schwellnus, MP, Noakes, T, and Lombard, C: A fivefold reduction in the incidence of recurrent ankle sprains in soccer players using the Sport-Stirrup orthosis. Am J Sports Med 22:601–606, 1994.

22. McGuine, TA, Brooks, A, and Hetzel, S: The effect of lace-up ankle braces on injury rates in high school basketball players. Am J Sports Med 39:1840–1848, 2011.

23. Mickel, TJ, Bottoni, CR, Tsuji, G, Chang, K, Baum, L, and Tokushige, KA: Prophylactic bracing versus taping for the prevention of ankle sprains in high school athletes: A prospective, randomized trial. J Foot Ankle Surg 45:360–365, 2006.

24. Rovere, GD, Clarke, TJ, Yates, CS, and Burley, K: Retrospective comparison of taping and ankle stabilizers in preventing ankle injuries. Am J Sports Med 16:228–233, 1988.

25. Sharpe, SR, Knapik, J, and Jones, B: Ankle braces effectively reduce recurrence of ankle sprains in female soccer players. J Athl Train 32:21–24, 1997.

26. Dizon, JM, and Reves, JJ: A systematic review on the effectiveness of external ankle supports in the prevention of inversion ankle sprains among elite and recreational players. J Sci Med Sport 13:309–317, 2010.

27. Vuurberg, G, Hoorntje, A, Wink, LM, van der Doelen, BFW, van den Bekerom, MP, Dekker, R, van Dijk, CN, Krips, R, Loogman, MCM, Ridderikhof, ML, Smithuis, FF, Stufkens, SAS, Verhagen, EALM, de Bie, RA, and Kerkhoffs, GMMJ: Diagnosis, treatment and prevention of ankle sprains: Update of an evidence-based clinical guideline. Br J Sports Med 52:956. doi: 10.1136/bjsports-2017-098106, 2018.

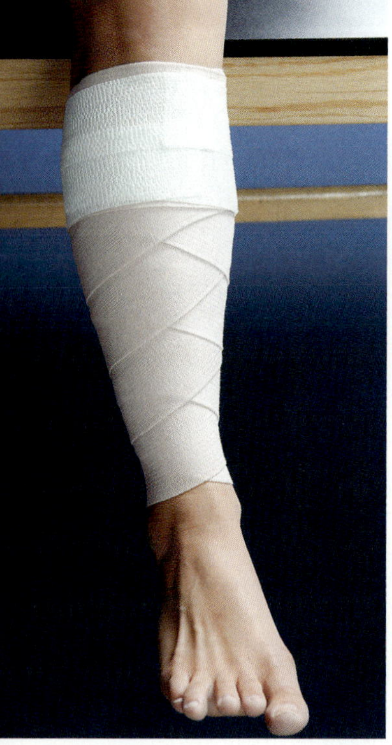

# 5

# Lower Leg



## INJURIES AND CONDITIONS

Acute and chronic injuries and conditions of the lower leg can result from direct force, excessive range of motion, rapid acceleration and/or deceleration, and repetitive stress. Sudden acceleration, such as that experienced by a sprinter pushing off from the blocks or a softball outfielder chasing a fly ball, can cause excessive plantar flexion and/or dorsiflexion of the ankle and can result in a strain or rupture of the lower leg musculature. Moreover, repetitive running and jumping can cause inflammation of, and injury to, the soft tissues. Common injuries to the lower leg include:

- Contusions
- Strains
- Ruptures
- Overuse injuries and conditions

## Contusions

Contusions to the lower leg are caused by direct forces and typically involve the tibia and/or posterior musculature. The tibia is susceptible to injury because overlying soft tissue does not provide a lot of protection. Direct forces to the tibia often affect the **periosteum** and cause irritation. Contusions to the posterior musculature frequently involve the gastrocnemius (Fig. 5–1). These injuries are common in many athletic activities as a result of being kicked or struck with equipment.

## Strains

Strains to the lower leg musculature are caused by a variety of mechanisms during athletic and work activities. Achilles tendon strains are caused by excessive dorsiflexion of the ankle[1] (see Fig. 5–1). For example, a strain can occur as a soccer player suddenly decelerates, changes direction, and accelerates in the opposite direction off the right foot, causing excessive dorsiflexion of the right ankle. An inversion force to the ankle, excessive dorsiflexion, or a direct force to the posterior lateral malleolus can cause a peroneal tendon strain (Fig. 5–2). With a violent eversion and dorsiflexion or inversion and plantar flexion force, the **peroneal retinaculum** can tear, causing a peroneal tendon **subluxation** and/or **dislocation** (see Fig. 5–2). A subluxation and/or dislocation can result, for example, when a wrestler's left foot is caught on the

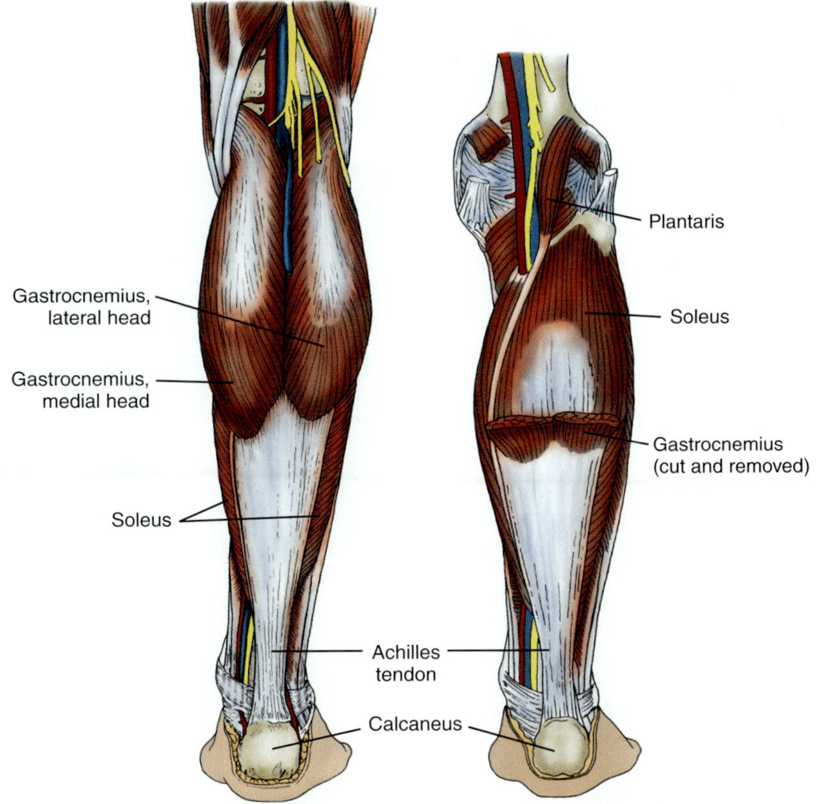



**Fig. 5–1** *Superficial muscles of the posterior lower leg.*

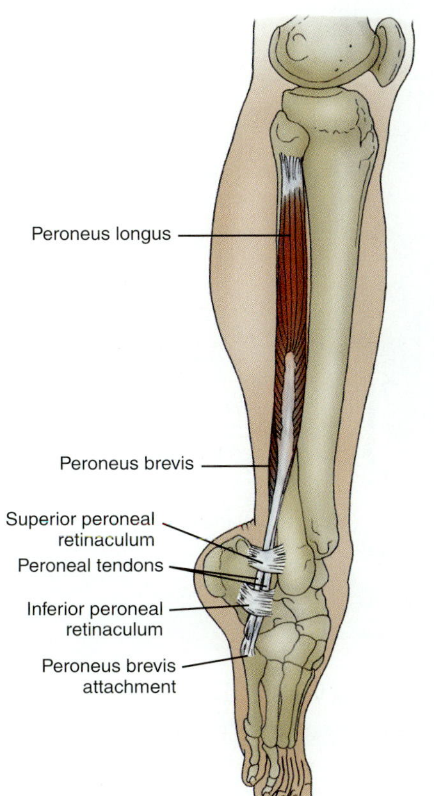



**Fig. 5–2** *Peroneal muscles of the lateral lower leg.*

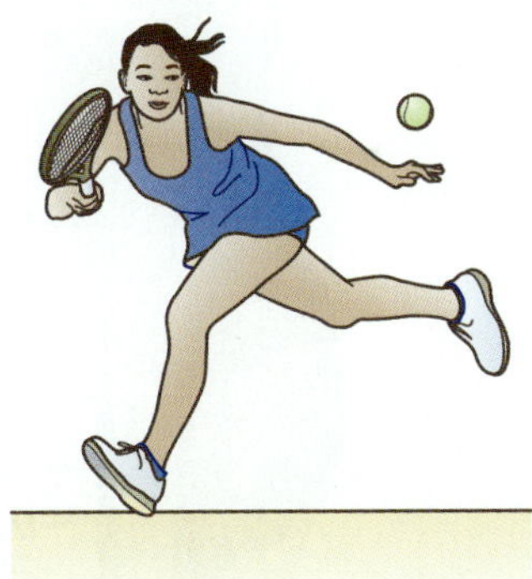

**Fig. 5–3** *Gastrocnemius strain in tennis. Note dorsiflexion of the left foot with forced knee extension.*

mat while the trunk is forced forward by an opponent during a takedown, causing eversion and dorsiflexion of the left ankle. Injury to the gastrocnemius, commonly the medial head, can result from activities involving rapid acceleration, deceleration, and jumping. Two common causes of gastrocnemius injury include dorsiflexion of the foot with forced knee extension (Fig. 5–3) and extension of the knee with forced foot dorsiflexion.

## Ruptures

Complete rupture of the Achilles tendon is caused by the sudden acceleration that is common with many athletic activities (Fig. 5–4). During the toe-off phase of the running gait, the foot is placed in plantar flexion while the knee moves toward full extension. While more common in males 30 years of age or older, perhaps because of chronic inflammation and degeneration, ruptures can be associated with patients of all sex and age groups.[2]

## Overuse

Overload and repetitive stress from weight-bearing activities and structural abnormalities can cause lower leg overuse injuries and conditions. Repetitive tensile stress caused by excessive weight-bearing can result in **Achilles tendinitis**. Repetitive running on a

downhill grade may lead to **anterior tibialis tendinitis** (Fig. 5–5). **Posterior tibialis tendinitis** can be associated with foot pronation. Supination and pronation of the foot (Fig. 5–6) can result in **peroneal**

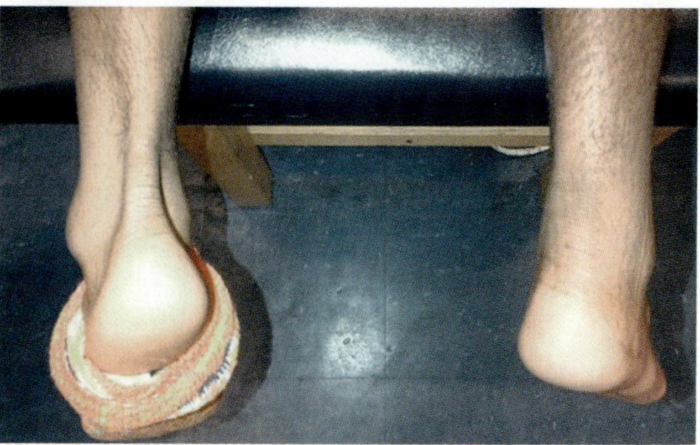

**Fig. 5–4** *Ruptured Achilles tendon. The patient's right Achilles tendon has been ruptured. Note the depression proximal to the calcaneus and the involved swelling. (Courtesy of Starkey, C and Brown, SD. Examination of Orthopedic & Athletic Injuries. 4th ed. Philadelphia, PA: F.A. Davis Company: 2015.)*

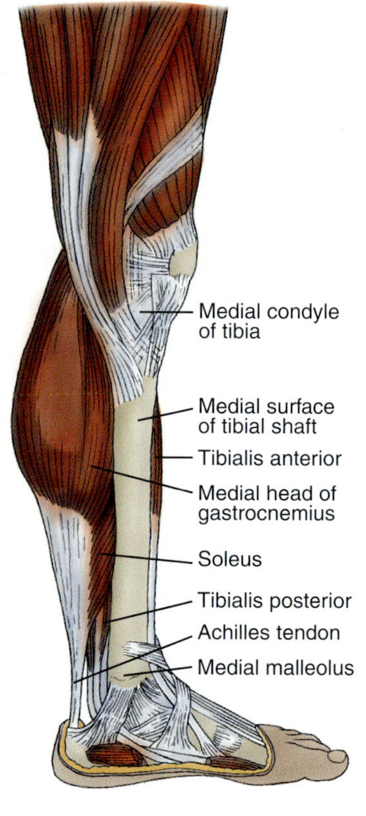



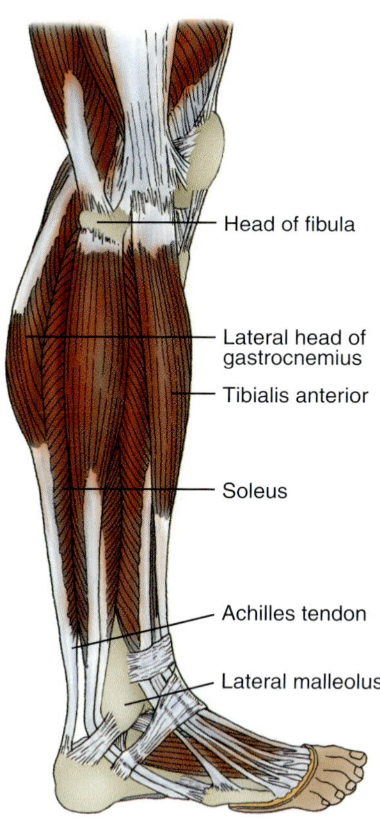



**Fig. 5–5** *Superficial muscles of the lower leg.*

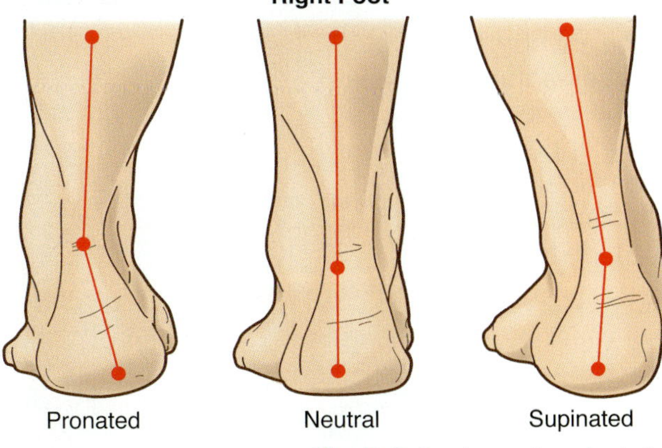


**Fig. 5–6** *Excessive pronation and supination.*

**tendinitis**. Repetitive stress, supination or pronation of the foot, inflexibility and/or weakness of the musculature, and training errors can cause **medial tibial stress syndrome (MTSS)**. Excessive running on hard surfaces such as asphalt or concrete in shoes without appropriate support or shock absorption can lead to the development of MTSS. Furthermore, **stress fractures** of the tibia or fibula may result from overload, foot pronation, pes cavus, training errors, **amenorrhea, oligomenorrhea**, and disordered eating and associated nutritional deficiencies. Overload and repetitive stress may also lead to **exertional compartment syndrome**.

# Taping Techniques

Use several taping techniques to treat lower leg injuries and conditions, to limit excessive range of motion, to support the musculature and soft tissue, and to immobilize the foot, ankle, and lower leg.

## ACHILLES TENDON — Figures 5–7 and 5–8

➡ **Purpose:** Use the Achilles tendon technique to treat strains and tendinitis, to limit excessive dorsiflexion and stretch on the tendon. Two interchangeable methods are illustrated in the application of the technique. Choose according to patient preferences (Fig. 5–7).

### Achilles Tendon Technique One

➡ **Materials:**
- 1½ inch non-elastic tape or 2 inch self-adherent wrap, 2 inch and 3 inch elastic tape, 3 inch heavyweight elastic tape, adherent tape spray, thin foam pads, taping scissors

*Option:*
- Pre-wrap

➡ **Position of the patient:** Prone, sitting, or kneeling on a taping table or bench, with the lower leg extended off the edge. Determine the range of dorsiflexion that produces pain by stabilizing the mid-to-distal lower leg. Place a hand on the plantar surface of the distal foot and slowly move the foot into dorsiflexion until pain occurs. Once painful range of motion is determined, place the involved foot in a pain-free range and maintain this position during application.

➡ **Preparation:** Apply adherent tape spray to the distal lower leg and distal plantar surface of the foot. Place a thin foam pad over the heel area to prevent irritation. Apply Technique One directly to the skin.

*Option:*
Apply pre-wrap over the area to lessen irritation.

➡ **Application:**

**STEP 1:** Apply two anchors around the distal lower leg, with 1½ inch non-elastic tape or 2 inch self-adherent wrap, and one anchor around the ball of the foot, with 2 inch elastic tape or self-adherent wrap with moderate roll tension ◄▬▬► (Fig. 5–7A). The lower leg anchor may be placed inferior to the knee, around the upper portion of the gastrocnemius belly. Using this anchor will allow for additional tensile strength of the heavyweight elastic tape in limiting range of motion. Use 2 inch or 3 inch elastic tape for the anchor to prevent constriction.

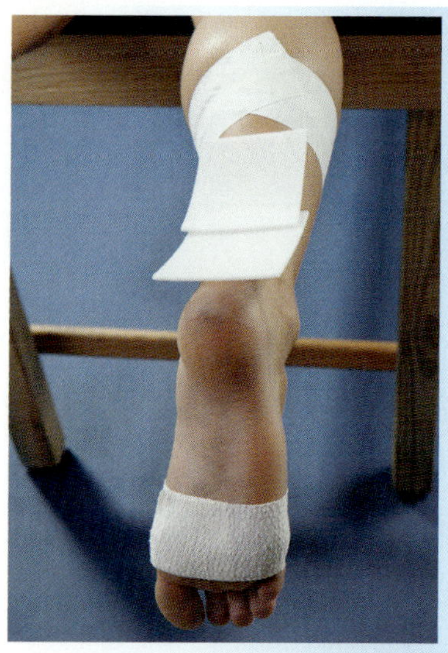

**Fig. 5-7 A**

**STEP 2:** Using 3 inch heavyweight elastic tape, anchor a strip on the mid-to-distal plantar foot and pull up toward the calcaneus (Fig. 5–7B).

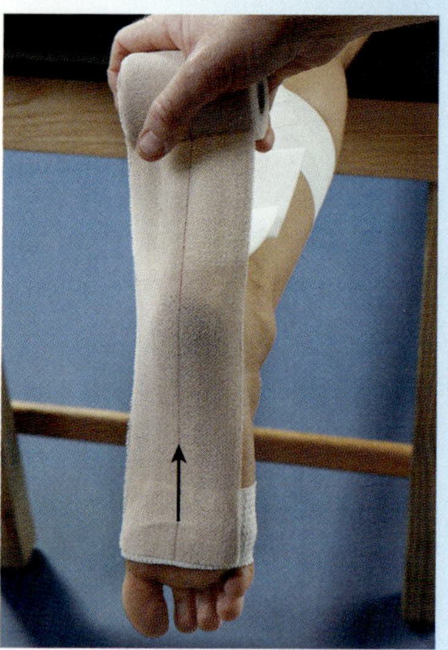

**Fig. 5-7 B**

**STEP 3:** Continue across the middle calcaneus, over the posterior lower leg, and finish on the posterior distal lower leg anchor (Fig. 5–7C). Apply moderate roll tension with the tape and monitor the pain-free position of the foot.

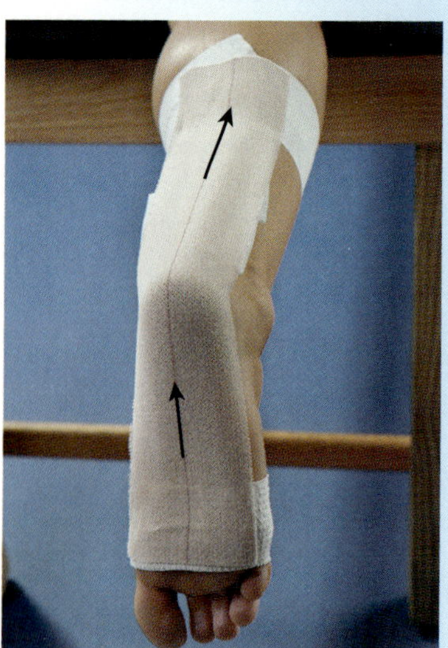

**Fig. 5-7 C**

**STEP 4:**  Anchor an additional 3 inch heavyweight elastic tape strip on the plantar foot over the first strip and pull the additional strip toward the distal lower leg anchor (Fig. 5–7D). Cut or tear this strip approximately 3 to 4 inches beyond the distal lower leg anchor.

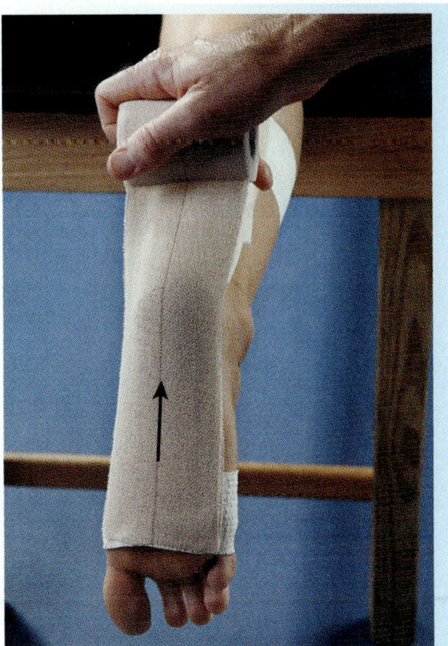

**Fig. 5–7 D**

**STEP 5:**  Tear or cut the proximal end of this strip lengthwise down the middle to an area just superior to the insertion of the Achilles tendon on the calcaneus (Fig. 5–7E).

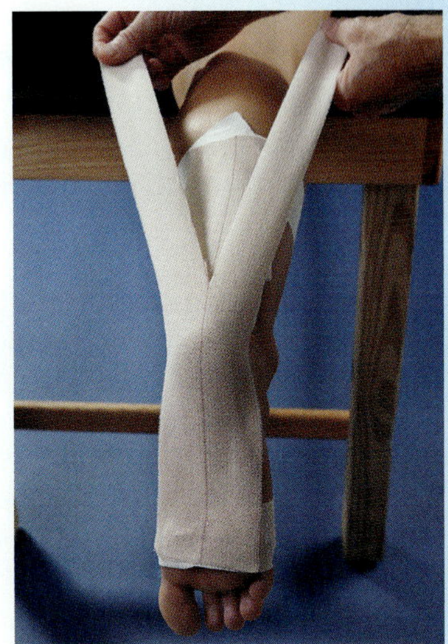

**Fig. 5–7 E**

**STEP 6:**  Apply moderate tension on the tape ends and wrap each, in opposite directions, around the lower leg in a spiral pattern. Finish the pattern on the distal lower leg anchor (Fig. 5–7F).

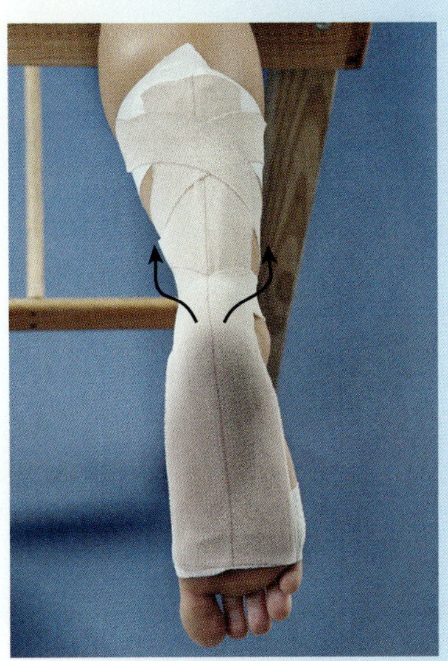

**Fig. 5–7 F**

*Steps Cont.*

**STEP 7:** Apply two to four circular strips of 2 inch elastic tape around the midfoot and distal foot and four to six circular strips of 2 inch elastic tape around the lower leg with mild to moderate roll tension ◄▦► (Fig. 5–7G). Additional strips of non-elastic tape are not required.

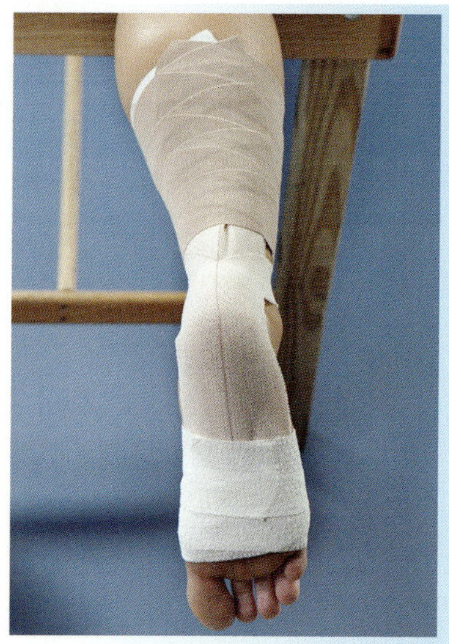

**Fig. 5–7 G**

### Achilles Tendon Technique Two

▦ **Materials:**
- 1½ inch non-elastic tape or 2 inch self-adherent wrap, 2 inch and 3 inch elastic tape, 2 inch heavyweight elastic tape, adherent tape spray, thin foam pads, taping scissors
  
  **Option:**
  - Pre-wrap

▦ **Position of the patient:** Prone, sitting, or kneeling on a taping table or bench, with the lower leg extended off the edge. Determine the range of dorsiflexion that produces pain, as explained above. After the painful range of motion has been determined, place the involved foot in a pain-free range and maintain this position during application.

▦ **Preparation:** Apply adherent tape spray to the distal lower leg and distal plantar surface of the foot. Place a thin foam pad over the heel area to prevent irritation. Apply Technique Two directly to the skin.

  **Option:** Apply pre-wrap over the area to lessen irritation.

▦ **Application:**

**STEP 1:** Apply anchors as illustrated in Figure 5–7A.

**STEP 2:** Anchor a strip of 2 inch heavyweight elastic tape on the mid-to-distal plantar foot. Proceed over the middle calcaneus, and finish on the distal lower leg anchor (Fig. 5–8A). Apply moderate roll tension during strip application and monitor the pain-free position of the foot.

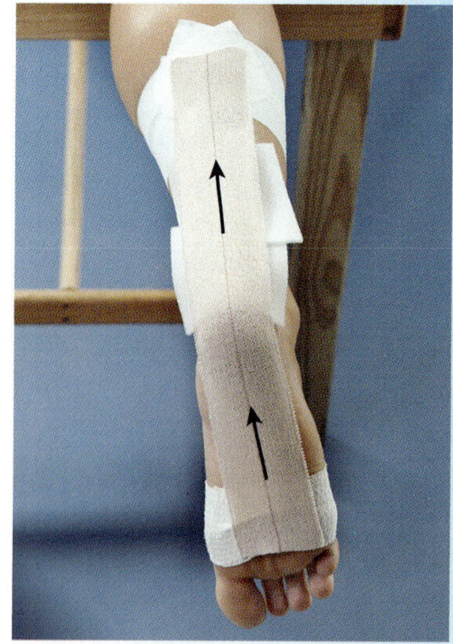

**Fig. 5–8 A**

**STEP 3:** Anchor the next 2 inch heavyweight elastic tape strip at an angle over the head of the fifth metatarsal. Continue over the medial calcaneus, and anchor on the medial lower leg (Fig. 5–8B).

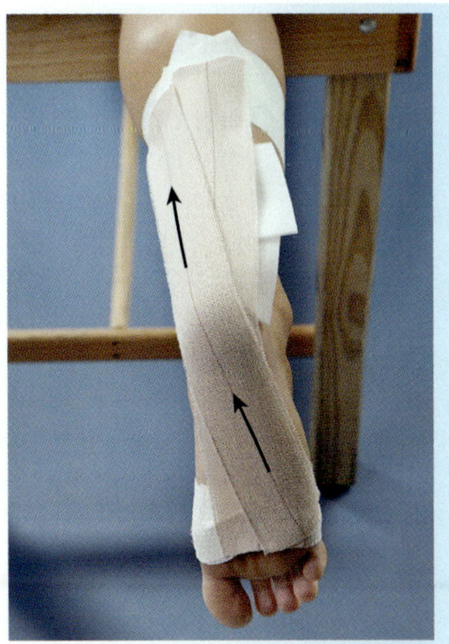

**Fig. 5–8 B**

**STEP 4:** Place the last 2 inch heavyweight elastic tape strip at an angle over the head of the first metatarsal, proceed over the lateral calcaneus, and anchor on the lateral lower leg (Fig. 5–8C).

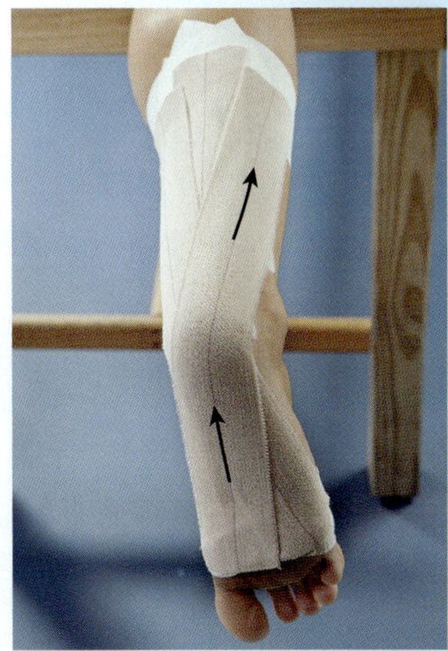

**Fig. 5–8 C**

**STEP 5:** Apply circular strips around the foot and lower leg with 2 inch elastic tape ◄▬▬► (Fig. 5–8D).

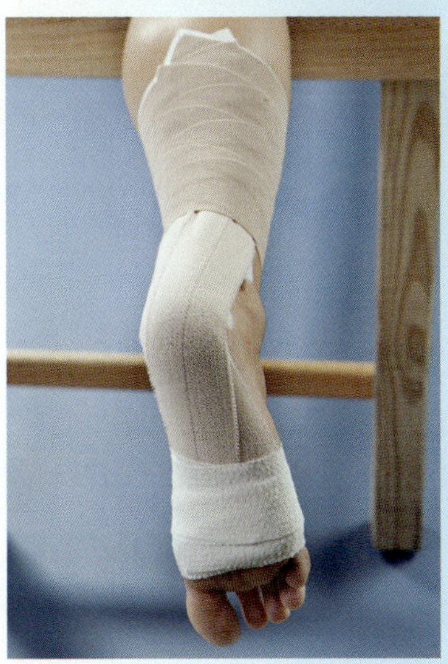

**Fig. 5–8 D**

## DORSAL BRIDGE    Figure 5–9

➡ **Purpose:** The dorsal bridge technique limits excessive plantar flexion and stretch on the tendon when treating anterior tibialis tendinitis (Fig. 5–9). This technique also can be used with ankle sprains to limit plantar flexion, which is often temporarily lost following injury. When treating sprains, the dorsal bridge may be used in combination with the closed basketweave (see Fig. 4–4), elastic (see Fig. 4–7), Spartan Slipper (see Fig. 4–8), or subtalar sling (see Fig. 4–9) taping techniques to limit excessive plantar flexion further and lessen additional stress on bony and ligamentous structures.

➡ **Materials:**
  • 1½ inch non-elastic tape or 2 inch self-adherent wrap, 2 inch elastic tape, 3 inch heavyweight elastic tape, adherent tape spray, thin foam pads, taping scissors
  ***Option:***
  • Pre-wrap

➡ **Position of the patient:** Sitting on a taping table or bench with the lower leg extended off the edge. Determine the range of plantar flexion that produces pain by stabilizing the mid-to-distal lower leg. Place a hand on the dorsal surface of the distal foot. Slowly move the foot into plantar flexion until pain occurs. After painful range of motion has been determined, place the involved foot in a pain-free range and maintain this position during application.

➡ **Preparation:** Apply adherent tape spray to the distal lower leg and foot. Place a thin foam pad over the lace area to prevent irritation. Apply the dorsal bridge directly to the skin.
  ***Option:*** Apply pre-wrap over the area to lessen irritation.

➡ **Application:**

**STEP 1:**   Place two anchor strips around the distal lower leg, with 1½ inch non-elastic tape or 2 inch self-adherent wrap, and place one anchor around the ball of the foot, with 2 inch elastic tape or self-adherent wrap ◄———►.

**STEP 2:**   Anchor a strip of 3 inch heavyweight elastic tape on the mid-to-distal dorsal foot and pull with moderate tension toward the lower leg. Anchor the strip on the middle anterior lower leg (Fig. 5–9A). An additional bridge may be applied over the first strip.

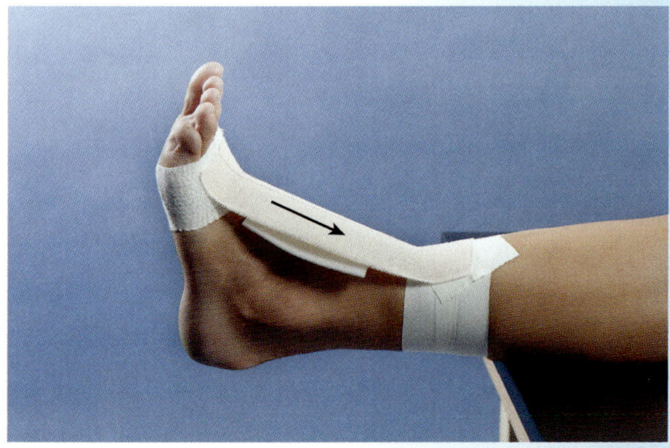

**Fig. 5–9 A**

**STEP 3:**   To prevent migration or slippage of the strip(s) during activity, tear or cut the ends lengthwise down the middle and anchor on the distal foot and lower leg in a spiral pattern (Fig. 5–9B).

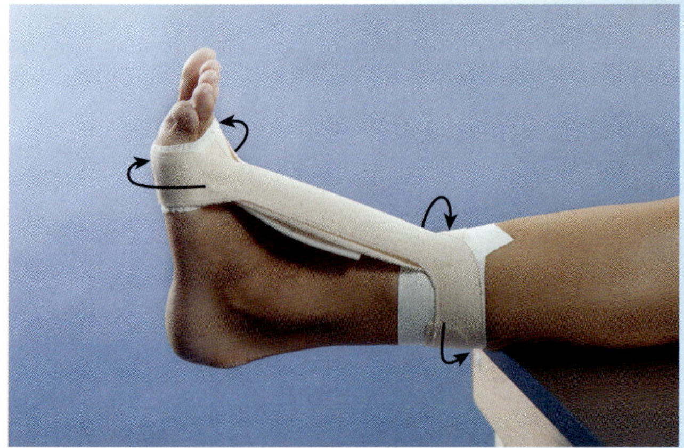

**Fig. 5–9 B**

**Helpful Hint |**
If migration of the heavyweight elastic tape strips used with the Achilles tendon or dorsal bridge taping techniques continues, use longer strips and anchor in a spiral pattern as before. The longer strips will allow for additional anchoring on the foot and lower leg, and should lessen migration.

**STEP 4:** Apply two to four circular strips of 2 inch elastic tape around the lower leg and two to three strips of 2 inch elastic tape around the distal foot with mild to moderate roll tension ◄▦▶ (Fig. 5–9C). Additional strips of non-elastic tape are not required.

**STEP 5:** Following application of the ankle taping technique, place pre-wrap or self-adherent wrap from the midfoot closure strips to the ball of the foot ◄▦▶.

**STEP 6:** Place an anchor around the ball of the foot ◄▦▶ and proceed with the application of the dorsal bridge.

**STEP 7:** Finish with the application of circular strips with 1½ inch non-elastic or 2 inch elastic tape on the lower leg and 2 inch elastic tape around the foot ◄▦▶ (Fig. 5–9D). A strip of 1½ inch non-elastic tape may be placed over the bridge from the lateral malleolus to the medial malleolus. Do not encircle the ankle with this strip.

**Helpful Hint |**
To prevent skin irritation from gaps, check to be sure the circular strips on the foot overlap with the midfoot closure strips of the ankle taping technique.

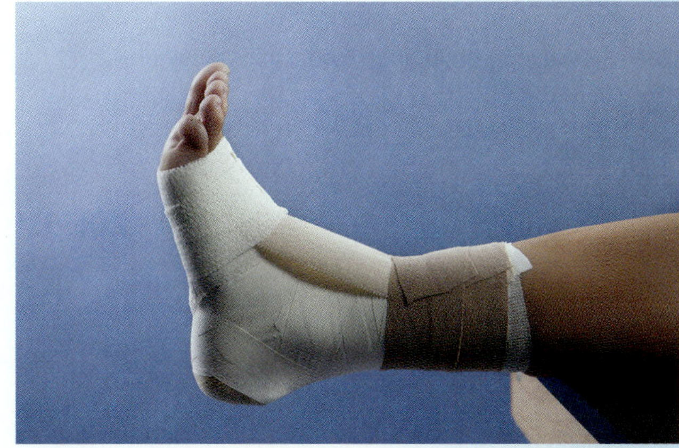

**Fig. 5–9 C**

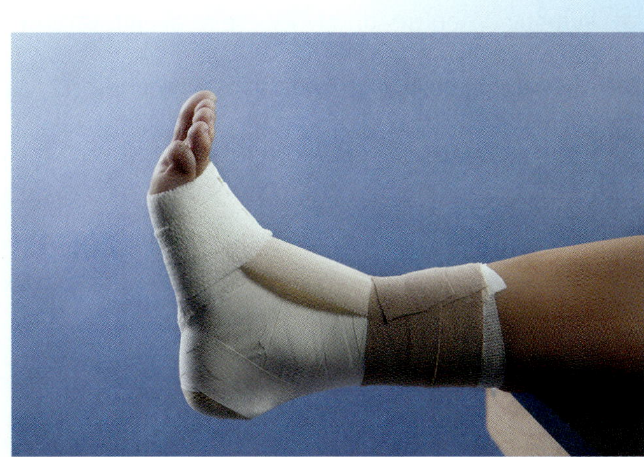

**Fig. 5–9 D**

## ✿ PERONEAL TENDON

▦▶ **Purpose:** The peroneal tendon technique can be used to treat strains when a patient is returning to activity. This technique is effective because it limits excessive inversion and eversion at the subtalar joint and provides moderate support and stability to the tendon as it passes posterior to the lateral malleolus. This technique and steps of application can be found on FADavis.com.

## POSTERIOR SPLINT

➡ **Purpose:** Use the posterior splint technique to immobilize the foot and ankle when treating an Achilles tendon rupture and peroneal tendon subluxation and/or dislocation (see Fig. 4–10 and FADavis.com 💲). The techniques are commonly used in the acute treatment stages as temporary immobilization but can also be used for extended periods of immobilization.
  • Rigid, padded splints are available off-the-shelf in pre-cut widths and lengths and can be molded quickly to the patient.
  • Use rigid cast tape over stockinet to immobilize the area.
  • Off-the-shelf and cast tape splints require an elastic wrap to attach the splint to the lower leg, ankle, and foot.
  • The patient will require crutches for non–weight-bearing ambulation.

## CAST TAPE

➡ **Purpose:** Orthopedic technicians or physicians commonly apply rigid cast tape to immobilize the foot, ankle, and lower leg completely when treating peroneal tendon subluxations and/or dislocations, Achilles tendon ruptures, gastrocnemius strains, posterior tibialis tendinitis, MTSS, and stress fractures.
  • Periods of immobilization are typically determined by a physician.
  • The majority of the rigid casts applied for these injuries are referred to as short-leg, extending from the inferior knee to the toes.
  • Cast tape is applied over stockinet and soft cast or Gore-Tex padding.

## CIRCULAR, "X," LOOP, AND WEAVE ARCH

➡ **Purpose:** When treating MTSS, several arch taping techniques provide support to the foot and correct structural abnormalities.
  • Use the circular arch (see Fig. 3–6) technique to provide mild support to the longitudinal arch.
  • Use the "X" (see Fig. 3–7), loop (see Fig. 3–8), and weave (see Fig. 3–9) arch techniques to provide mild to moderate support to both the longitudinal arch and forefoot.

## LOW-DYE

➡ **Purpose:** Use the Low-Dye technique to provide moderate support of the foot/forefoot and limit excessive pronation when treating peroneal and posterior tibialis tendinitis and MTSS. The two methods are illustrated (see Fig. 3–10 and FADavis.com 💲), in the context of arch strains and plantar fasciitis treatment.

### Clinical Application Question 1

The personnel manager at the local textile manufacturing plant suffers a mild left Achilles tendon strain when playing basketball at the high school gym. You apply the Achilles tendon technique to limit excessive dorsiflexion prior to his athletic activities. Shortly after he begins to play, the taping technique migrates distally, allowing full dorsiflexion.

➡ **Question: How can you manage this problem?**

### ...IF/THEN...

**IF** using the circular, "X," loop, or weave arch taping techniques to support the longitudinal arch and/or forefoot when treating MTSS and pain is not lessened, **THEN** consider applying the Low-Dye taping technique or using a soft, semirigid, or rigid orthotic design; these techniques provide support to the longitudinal arch and/or forefoot and correct structural abnormalities, such as excessive pronation in the treatment of MTSS. These techniques also may lessen pain.

# Wrapping Techniques

Use compression wrap techniques to control swelling in the acute treatment of Achilles tendon strains and ruptures, peroneal tendon and gastrocnemius strains, and muscle and/or bone contusions. There are three wrapping techniques, using elastic wraps and sleeves, that provide mechanical pressure over the lower leg or lower leg, ankle, and foot following injury to control and lessen distal migration of swelling.

## FOOT, ANKLE, AND LOWER LEG COMPRESSION WRAP — Figure 5–10

➠ **Purpose:** The wrap technique for many lower leg strains, ruptures, and distal contusions should include the foot, ankle, and lower leg to assist in controlling swelling and lessening distal migration. The foot, ankle, and lower leg compression wrap technique controls mild, moderate, or severe swelling (Fig. 5–10).

➠ **Materials:**
- 3 inch, 4 inch, or 6 inch width by 5 or 10 yard length elastic wrap, or 3 inch, 4 inch, or 6 inch width self-adherent wrap, metal clips, 1½ inch non-elastic or 2 inch elastic tape, taping scissors

*Option:*
- ¼ inch or ½ inch foam or felt

➠ **Position of the patient:** Sitting on a taping table or bench with the leg extended off the edge and the foot in pain-free dorsiflexion.

➠ **Preparation:** Apply the compression wrap directly to the skin.

➠ **Application:**

**STEP 1:** Anchor the end of the wrap on the distal plantar foot and apply the foot and ankle compression wrap (see Fig. 3–17).

**STEP 2:** At the distal lower leg, continue the spiral wrap proximally to the inferior knee ◄█████► (Fig. 5–10). Apply the greatest amount of roll tension distally and over the injured area. Lessen the roll tension as the wrap continues proximally from the injured area. The technique may require using multiple elastic wraps or rolls of self-adherent wrap. Anchor the wrap with Velcro, metal clips, or loosely applied 1½ inch non-elastic or 2 inch elastic tape ◄█████►.

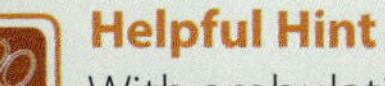

**Helpful Hint |**
With ambulation, monitor the proximal gastrocnemius and popliteal space for irritation from the wrap, which may occur with repetitive knee flexion.

*Option:*  *The horseshoe pad technique (see Fig. 4–19), along with the compression wrap, may be used when treating peroneal tendon subluxations and/or dislocations to provide additional compression over the area and assist in venous return. Place the pad directly on the skin over the lateral malleolus and cover it with the foot, ankle, and lower leg compression wrap.*

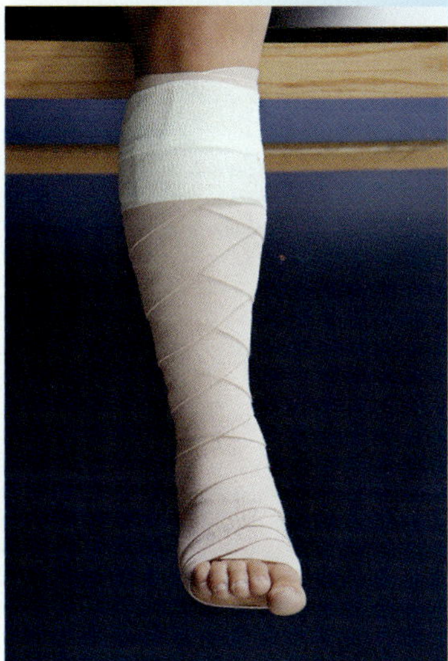

**Fig. 5–10**

## LOWER LEG COMPRESSION WRAP — Figure 5–11

➠ **Purpose:** Use the lower leg compression wrap technique to assist in reducing mild or moderate swelling in the acute treatment of muscle and/or bone contusions to the mid and proximal lower leg (Fig. 5–11).

➡ **Materials:**
- 3 inch or 4 inch width by 5 yard length elastic wrap or 3 inch or 4 inch width self-adherent wrap, metal clips, 1½ inch non-elastic or 2 inch elastic tape, taping scissors
  
  ***Option:***
- ⅛ inch or ¼ inch foam or felt

➡ **Position of the patient:** Sitting on a taping table or bench with the leg extended off the edge.

➡ **Preparation:** Apply the compression wrap directly to the skin.

  ***Option:*** Cut a ⅛ inch or ¼ inch foam or felt pad and place it over the inflamed area directly to the skin to provide additional compression and assist in venous return.

➡ **Application:**

**STEP 1:** Anchor the wrap around the distal lower leg and continue in a distal-to-proximal spiral pattern toward the inferior knee ◄▦► (Fig. 5–11A). Apply the greatest amount of roll tension distally and lessen as the wrap continues proximally.

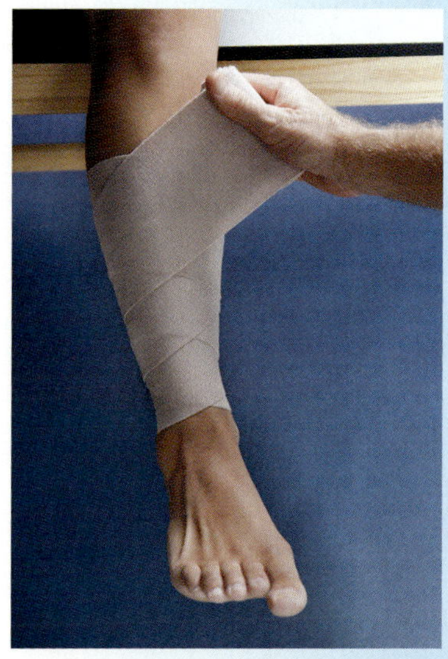

**Fig. 5–11 A**

**STEP 2:** Anchor with Velcro, metal clips, or loosely applied 1½ inch non-elastic or 2 inch elastic tape ◄▦► (Fig. 5–11B).

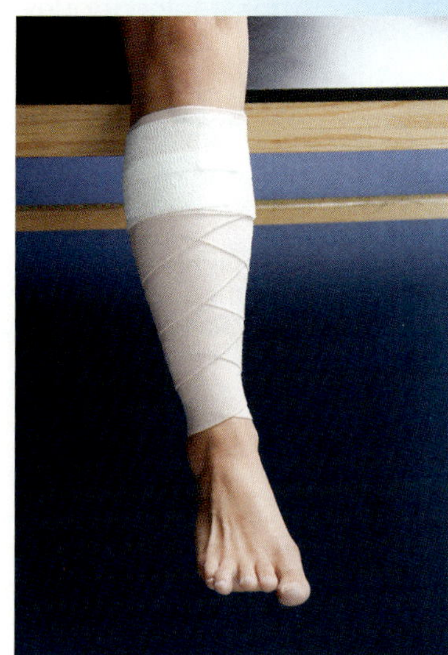

**Fig. 5–11 B**

## LOWER LEG COMPRESSION SLEEVE   Figure 5–12

➡ **Purpose:** Using the lower leg compression sleeve technique will also control mild, moderate, or severe swelling (Fig. 5–12). After receiving instructions on application, the patient can apply and remove this compression technique without assistance.

➡ **Materials:**
- 3 inch, 3½ inch, or 4 inch elastic sleeve, taping scissors
  *Option:*
- ⅛ inch or ¼ inch foam or felt

➡ **Position of the patient:** Sitting on a taping table or bench with the leg extended off the edge.

➡ **Preparation:** Apply the elastic sleeve directly to the skin.
  *Option:* Cut a ⅛ inch or ¼ inch foam or felt pad and place it over the inflamed area directly to the skin to assist in the control of swelling.

➡ **Application:**

**STEP 1:** Cut a sleeve from a roll to extend from the inferior knee to the distal lower leg. A double-length sleeve may also be cut and used to provide additional compression.

**STEP 2:** Pull the sleeve onto the lower leg in a distal-to-proximal direction (Fig. 5–12). If using a double-length sleeve, pull the distal end over the first layer to provide an additional layer. No anchors are required. Clean and reuse the sleeve.

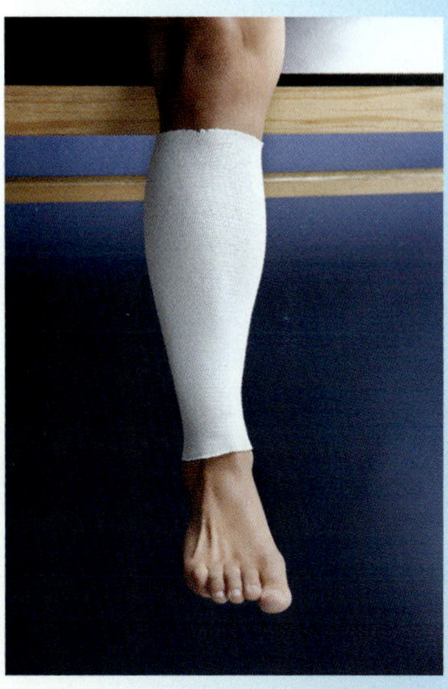

**Fig. 5–12**

---

### Clinical Application Question 2

Two days ago, a warehouse worker was struck in the proximal right lower leg with a metal cart. He was sent to a physician for evaluation and was diagnosed with a moderate proximal tibial contusion. An elastic wrap was applied over the proximal lower leg to control swelling. Today, he returns with ecchymosis and swelling in the distal lower leg and foot.

➡ **Question: What wrapping techniques can be used in this situation?**

---

### . . . IF/THEN . . .

**IF** an athlete is recovering from a mid tibial contusion and the physician allows a return to practice even though mild swelling remains in the area, **THEN** consider using an elastic sleeve under the protective pad to control the swelling; the sleeve may be more comfortable than an elastic wrap during practice.

# Bracing Techniques

Many of these bracing techniques have been discussed previously and can be used to treat a variety of lower leg injuries and conditions. Walking boots and orthotics, discussed in greater detail in Chapter 3, are used to prevent and treat lower leg strains, ruptures, and overuse injuries and conditions. Ankle braces, illustrated in Chapter 4, can be used to treat strains and overuse injuries and conditions.

## WALKING BOOT

➡ **Purpose:** Use walking boots (see Fig. 3–22) to provide complete support and immobilization when treating peroneal tendon subluxations and/or dislocations, gastrocnemius strains, Achilles tendon ruptures, posterior tibialis tendinitis, MTSS, and stress fractures.
• Use the boots to provide lower leg, ankle, and foot support during non–weight-bearing and full weight-bearing rehabilitation periods.

> **Helpful Hint |**
> When using walking boots in warm, humid environments, place a sock over the involved foot, ankle, and lower leg before applying the boot to absorb perspiration and reduce soiling of the inner lining.

• The boots are commonly used in place of rigid casts. The boot allows for removal and treatment, range of motion adjustments, and gait training.

## ORTHOTICS

➡ **Purpose:** Soft, semirigid, and rigid orthotic designs provide support, absorb shock, and correct structural abnormalities, while preventing and treating lower leg injuries and conditions.
• Use soft orthotic designs (see Fig. 3–18), such as heel cups and full-length neoprene, silicone, thermoplastic rubber, polyurethane foam, and viscoelastic polymer insoles, to provide shock absorption when treating MTSS and stress fractures. These designs assist in lessening repetitive stress to the lower leg.
• Use semirigid (see Fig. 3–19) and rigid (see Fig. 3–20) orthotics to provide support and correct structural abnormalities, such as excessive foot pronation or supination, when treating Achilles, posterior tibialis, and peroneal tendinitis, stress fractures, MTSS, and exertional compartment syndrome.

## NEOPRENE SLEEVE     Figure 5–13

➡ **Purpose:** Neoprene sleeves provide compression and mild support when treating gastrocnemius strains, muscle and bone contusions, and MTSS (Fig. 5–13). Anecdotal information indicates that compression over inflamed areas may lessen pain levels. However, with some patients, this technique may increase pain. Following application, monitor for an increase in pain levels during activity.
➡ **Design:**
• Neoprene sleeves come in off-the-shelf designs in predetermined sizes that correspond to lower leg circumference measurements.
• Some designs are constructed with protective padding incorporated into the sleeve.
• Several designs use a strap with a Velcro closure to provide additional support and compression.
• Extended wear and cleaning of neoprene sleeves may cause them to shrink, resulting in difficulties during daily application.

**Helpful Hint |**
Lessen neoprene sleeve application problems by first turning the sleeve inside-out
(Fig. 5–13A). Next, place the smaller end over the foot
(Fig. 5–13B). Pull the sleeve proximally onto the lower leg,
and stop when the smaller end approaches its normal
distal location on the lower leg (Fig. 5–13C). Last, pull the
larger end proximally and over the sleeve to its normal
location (Fig. 5–13D). Talcum powder may also be
applied on the inside of the sleeve to lessen problems.

➡ **Position of the patient:** Sitting on a taping table or bench with the leg
extended off the edge or in a chair.
➡ **Preparation:** Apply neoprene sleeves directly to the skin; no anchors are
required.
➡ **Application:**

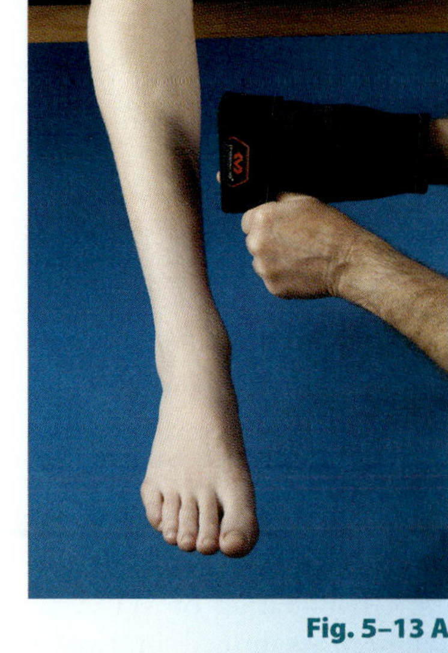

**Fig. 5–13 A**

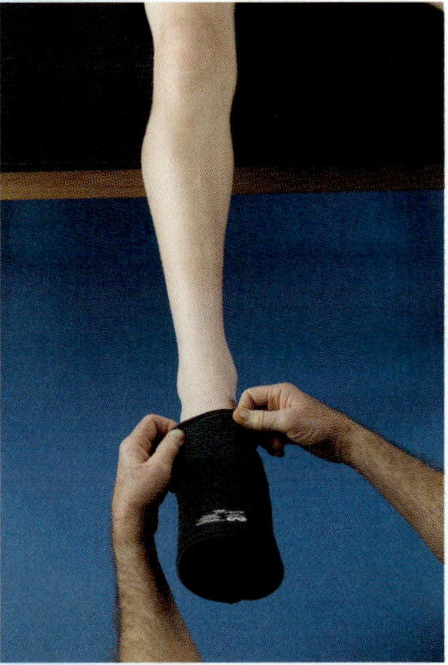

**Fig. 5–13 B**

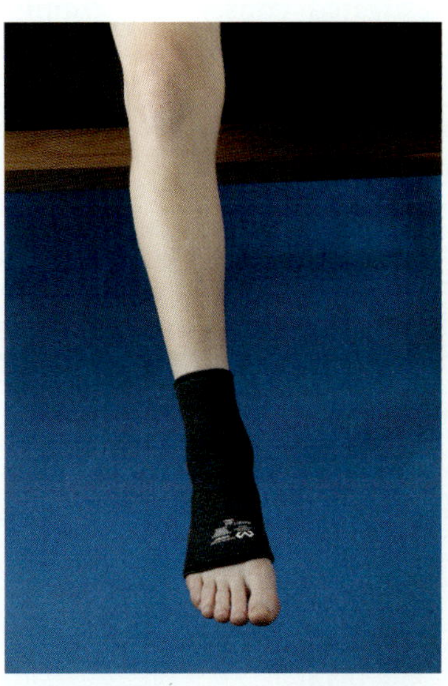

**Fig. 5–13 C**

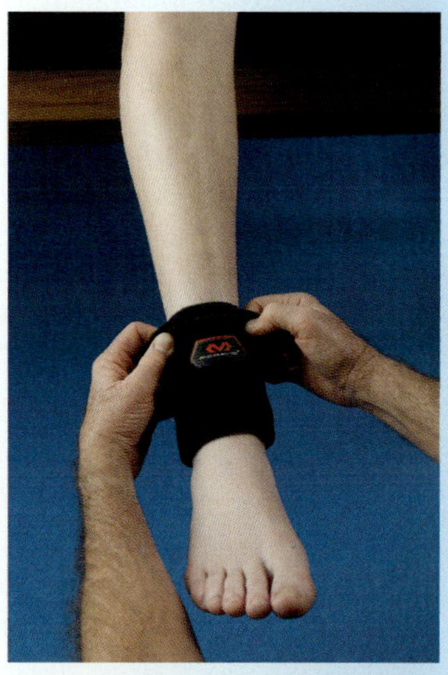

**Fig. 5–13 D**

**STEP 1:** To apply, hold each side of the sleeve and place the larger end over
the foot. Continue to pull proximally until the sleeve is positioned
on the lower leg (Fig. 5–13E).

### Clinical Application Question 3

A cross-country runner was diagnosed by the team
physician with MTSS several weeks ago. Treatment and
rehabilitation, which included therapeutic modalities,
stretching and strengthening exercises, and off-the-
shelf soft orthotics, allowed a full return to practice.
Recently, the runner asks if some type of support can
be applied to the lower leg during practice.

➡ **Question: What are the alternative techniques
you can use?**

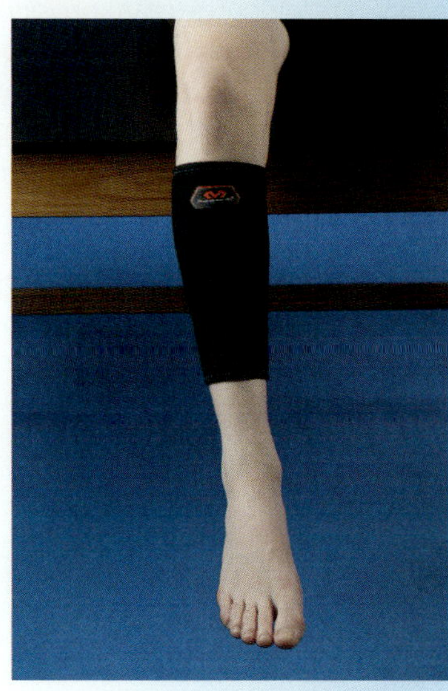

**Fig. 5–13 E**

## ANKLE BRACES

➠ **Purpose:** Several ankle brace designs can be used to treat peroneal tendon and stress fracture injuries. The braces provide compression and/or moderate support when treating these injuries and can be applied by the patient, following proper instruction.
- Use air/gel bladder braces (see Fig. 4–17) to provide additional compression to control swelling in the acute treatment of subluxations and/or dislocations. These braces may be used in combination with the compression wrap techniques (see Figs. 3–17 and 5–10) to assist in venous return.
- Air/gel bladder braces are also used when treating stress fractures of the tibia and/or fibula. Lower leg designs are constructed with longer medial and lateral stirrups or shells to provide support to the proximal, mid, and distal lower leg.

## EVIDENCE SUMMARY

The efficacy of various interventions for the treatment and rehabilitation of MTSS and tibial stress fractures has been examined in two separate evidence-based reviews. A 2013 meta-analysis[3] investigated conservative interventions among active duty military subjects with MTSS. Three randomized controlled trials (RCTs) compared the use of air/gel bladder braces or a neoprene sleeve with an incorporated aluminum bar and no brace or sleeve during rehabilitation following diagnosis. The researchers found no differences in the time to complete a progressive rehabilitation and running program and a measured run without pain among the subjects. Based on this review,[3] the evidence is insufficient to support the use of braces/sleeves to accelerate a return to full activity. A separate 2005 meta-analysis[4] examined interventions for the treatment and rehabilitation of tibial stress fractures. The findings from three small RCTs among military personnel and recreational athletes demonstrated that the use of air/gel bladder braces resulted in a faster rehabilitation period and return to activity following diagnosis. While this review provided some evidence for the benefit of air/gel bladder braces, further investigations are needed to determine their effectiveness with tibial stress fractures.

- Use lace-up (see Fig. 4–15) and semirigid (see Fig. 4–16) designs during a return to athletic or work activities to limit inversion, eversion, plantar flexion, dorsiflexion, and rotation with peroneal tendon strains.
- Air/gel, lace-up, and semirigid braces are available off-the-shelf in predetermined sizes.

### Clinical Application Question 4

During the second half of the women's basketball game, an official sprints down the court in advance of a fast break. The team misses the layup, and the opponents start a fast break toward their goal. The official quickly stops, turns, and sprints toward the other end of the court. He feels a pop in his left lower leg and immediately stops, suffering a ruptured Achilles tendon. The team physician refers the official to a local orthopedic surgeon for further evaluation.

➠ **Question: What immobilization options are available in this situation and under what circumstances would you choose one option over another?**

### . . . IF/THEN . . .

**IF** applying the peroneal tendon taping technique and adequate compression and support is not provided to the tendon in the fibular groove, **THEN** consider using a lace-up or semirigid ankle brace in combination with the taping technique to provide additional compression over the tendon and further limit excessive inversion and eversion at the subtalar joint.

# Padding Techniques

Use foam, felt, and thermoplastic materials to offer support, absorb shock, and provide protection when preventing and treating lower leg injuries and conditions. Foam and felt materials can be used to provide support and absorb shock when treating strains, ruptures, and overuse injuries and conditions. Foam and thermoplastic materials are used to prevent and treat contusions. Several high school and intercollegiate sports require mandatory padding of the lower leg. These padding techniques will be discussed in Chapter 13.

## OFF-THE-SHELF    Figure 5–14

➡ **Purpose:** Padding materials may be molded and attached to off-the-shelf pad designs to provide additional protection following a contusion (Fig. 5–14). Off-the-shelf designs can be found in Chapter 13.
➡ **Materials:**
  • ⅛ inch, ¼ inch, or ½ inch open-cell foam, rubber cement, 2 inch elastic tape, thermoplastic material, taping scissors
➡ **Position of the patient:** Sitting on a taping table or bench with the lower leg extended off the edge in a functional position.
➡ **Preparation:** Cut the appropriate size of foam to overlap the shin guard.
➡ **Application:**

**STEP 1:** Cut a piece of open-cell foam ¼ inch or ½ inch larger than the shin guard and attach the foam to the inside surface with rubber cement or 2 inch elastic tape (Fig. 5–14A). Cut a hole or donut in the foam over the contusion to disperse the impact force.

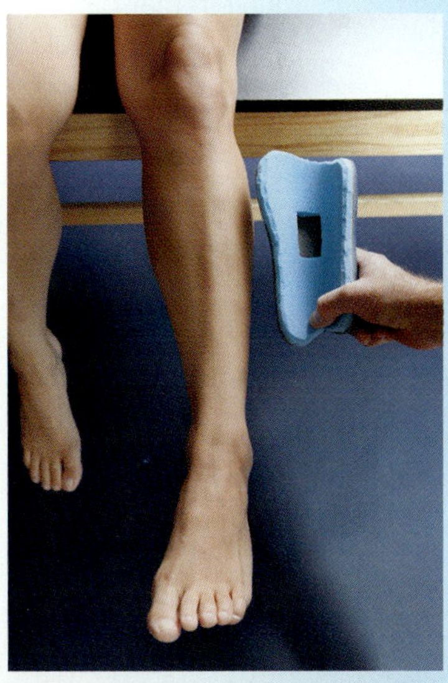

**Fig. 5–14 A**

**STEP 2:** Consider molding and attaching a piece of thermoplastic material with rubber cement or 2 inch elastic tape to a shin guard to protect a medial or lateral contusion (Fig. 5–14B).

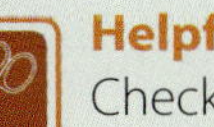

**Helpful Hint |**
Check to make sure normal range of motion is allowed at the knee, talocrural, and/or subtalar joints when using off-the-shelf or thermoplastic pads over the proximal or distal lower leg.

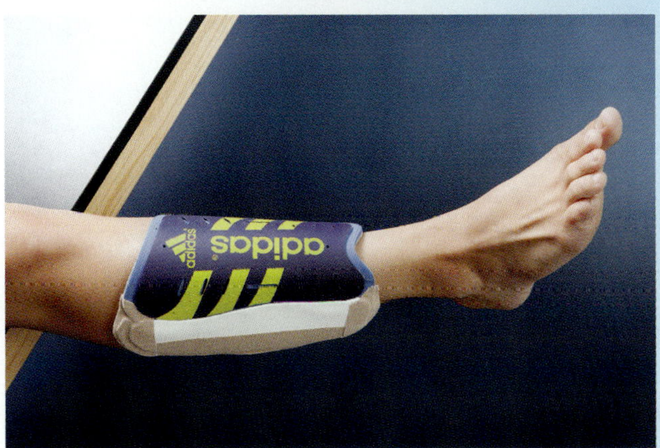


**Fig. 5–14 B**

## | **CUSTOM-MADE**   Figure 5–15

➡ **Purpose:** Use thermoplastic material to construct custom-made pads to provide protection when preventing and treating lower leg muscle and bone contusions (Fig. 5–15). Many construct these pads when off-the-shelf designs are not available or a comfortable fit cannot be achieved.

➡ **Materials:**
- Paper, felt tip pen, thermoplastic material, ⅛ inch or ¼ inch foam or felt, taping scissors, a heating source, 2 inch or 3 inch elastic tape or self-adherent wrap, pre-wrap, an elastic wrap, soft, low-density foam, rubber cement

*Option:*
- 1 inch or 1½ inch non-elastic or 1 inch or 2 inch elastic tape

➡ **Position of the patient:** Sitting on a taping table or bench with the lower leg extended off the edge in a functional position.

➡ **Preparation:** Design the pad with a paper pattern (see Fig. 1–10). Cut, mold, and shape the thermoplastic material on the lower leg over the injured area. Attach soft, low-density foam to the inside surface of the material (see Fig. 1–11).

➡ **Application:**

**STEP 1:**   Attach the pad to the lower leg with 2 inch or 3 inch elastic tape, or self-adherent wrap over pre-wrap, or directly to the skin. Use strips or a circular pattern with moderate roll tension ◀▬▶ (Fig. 5–15A). One to two circular strips of 1½ inch non-elastic tape may be applied loosely around the pad for additional anchors. Monitor roll tension over the gastrocnemius to prevent constriction.

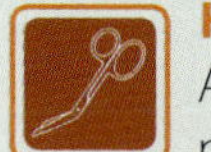

**Helpful Hint |**
Anchor the elastic tape directly on the thermo-plastic material and continue with application. The tape adhesive bond on the thermoplastic material will lessen migration of the pad during activity.

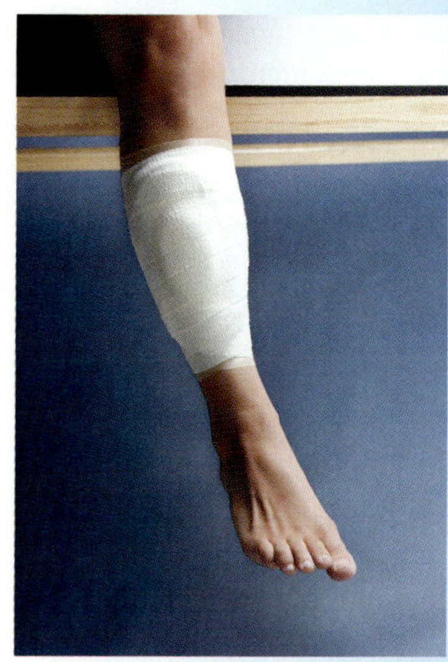

**Fig. 5–15 A**

*Option:*   *Attach the pad to the lower leg by placing the pad underneath a knee-high sock. Apply strips of 1 inch or 1½ inch non-elastic or 1 inch or 2 inch elastic tape over the sock to provide additional anchors ◀▬▶ (Fig. 5–15B).*

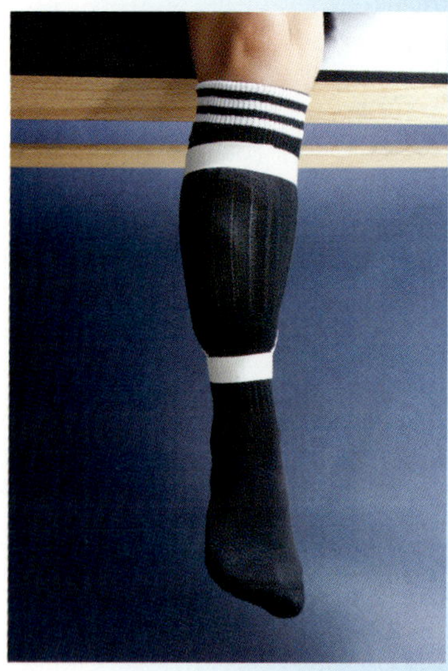

**Fig. 5–15 B**

## HEEL LIFT　　Figure 5–16

➡ **Purpose:** Use this heel lift pad technique to absorb shock, elevate the hindfoot, and lessen the stress and stretch on the tendon and muscle during activity, when treating strains, tendinitis, ruptures of the Achilles tendon, and strains of the gastrocnemius (Fig. 5–16). The heel pad technique, constructed of foam, illustrated in Chapter 3 (see Fig. 3–27), also provides shock absorption when treating MTSS. When soft heel cups are not available, foam heel pads may be used to lessen repetitive stress to the lower leg.

➡ **Materials:**
- ⅛ inch, ¼ inch, or ½ inch felt, taping scissors

➡ **Position of the patient:** Sitting on a taping table or bench with the leg extended off the edge and the foot in a dorsiflexed position.

➡ **Preparation:** Construct the pads from ⅛ inch, ¼ inch, or ½ inch felt or purchase in pre-cut designs with adhesive backing. The pads should cover the entire heel or shoe liner heel area. To prevent adaptive changes with the use of one pad, such as changes in walking and/or running gaits, place a heel lift on each heel or in each shoe.

➡ **Application:**

**STEP 1:** Taper the distal end of the pad and attach it to the heel with adhesive gauze material (see Fig. 3–27) or with 2 inch elastic tape or self-adherent wrap (see Fig. 4–5) or cement the pad to the shoe liner (Fig. 5–16).

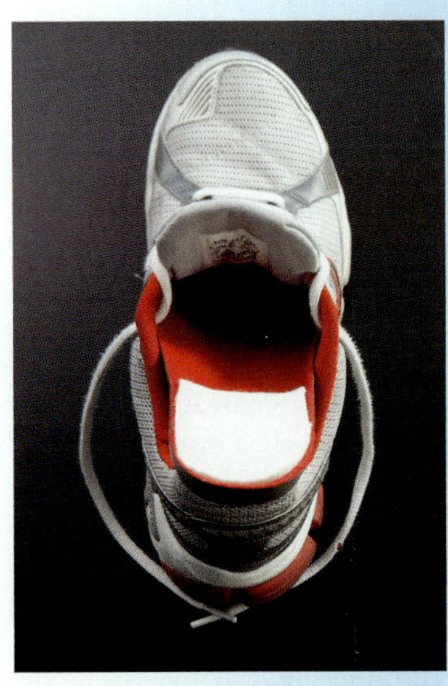

**Fig. 5–16**

### DETAILS
Using certain types of footwear can also elevate the hindfoot and lessen the stress and stretch on the Achilles tendon and gastrocnemius. Shoes with medium heels of 1–2 inches can elevate the hindfoot and lessen stress and stretch on these structures. Cowboy boots are a common shoe design that can be used.

## LONGITUDINAL ARCH

➡ **Purpose:** Use the longitudinal arch pad technique to provide mild to moderate support of the arch when treating MTSS and stress fractures (see Fig. 3–25). The pads are available off-the-shelf or cut from foam or felt. These pads may be used when orthotics are not available. Attach the pad with the circular arch technique (see Fig. 3–6).

## MANDATORY PADDING

The NCAA[5] and the NFHS[6] require the use of mandatory protective equipment for the lower leg in several sports. Baseball, field hockey, ice hockey, girls' lacrosse (goalkeeper), soccer, and softball athletes are required to wear protective padding on the lower leg during all practices and competitions. The majority of these pads come in off-the-shelf designs. An in-depth discussion of these pads can be found in Chapter 13.

### Clinical Application Question 5

While batting in the fourth inning, the right fielder on the baseball team fouls a ball off his right lateral lower leg. After several days of treatment, the physician allows him to return to activity if protected with padding.

➥ **Question: What padding techniques are appropriate in this situation?**

### . . . IF/THEN . . .

**IF** felt heel lifts are effective in lessening the stress and stretch of the Achilles tendon when treating tendinitis, **THEN** consider using custom-made orthotics with heel lifts, which will eliminate the need for daily construction and application of the felt pad.

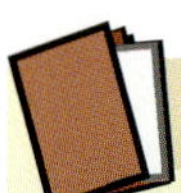

## EVIDENCE-BASED PRACTICE

Melissa Hoover is an investment banker at Kozack Financial Services in town. She is currently in week 6 of a 20 week training schedule for the local marathon. Melissa has been running for the past 3 years, averaging approximately 12–15 miles per week. During the past 3 years, she has experienced occasional lower leg pain, which she always relieved by purchasing new shoes. Melissa's training schedule was designed by a local running club, specifically for first-time marathoners. Week 1 began with a total of 16 miles and progressed to 21 miles at week 6. The scheduled mileage peaks at week 18 with a total of 36 miles, then decreases as the marathon approaches. Monday and Friday are rest days, and a long run is scheduled for each Sunday.

During week 3, Melissa began to experience a periodic dull ache in her distal right lower leg. She continued training as scheduled. Melissa noticed that the dull ache progressed to constant pain in the area during week 4, especially at night following her morning run. Again, she continued the scheduled training. As week 5 progressed, she began to experience the pain prior to, during, and after each run. The pain was centered in her distal right posteromedial tibia. She also noticed that the medium/high-heeled shoes she wore to work increased the intensity of the pain. Melissa believed that some amount of pain was normal for this type of training and attempted to continue with the training. She decided to take an extra rest day in week 6 and resume training the following day. But Melissa was unable to run the scheduled mileage because of the intense pain in her right lower leg. After obtaining a physician's referral, she contacts a friend, Jennifer Duke, who is a PT/AT at Tolsma Orthopedic Clinic, and schedules an appointment.

Following a static and dynamic evaluation, Jennifer discovers excessive right foot pronation during walking and running gaits. The wear pattern on Melissa's running and work shoes demonstrates the pronation. Jennifer finds point tenderness with palpation, along the distal posteromedial border of the tibia. Bilateral range of motion and strength are normal, but pain is produced with resisted plantar flexion in the right foot. Active weight-bearing movements on the distal right toes also produce pain. Jennifer notes inflexibility of the right heel cord. Jennifer refers Melissa to a physician for further evaluation of suspected medial tibial stress syndrome. The physician finds point tenderness in the distal right tibia with no crepitus, deformity, or neurological symptoms. Radiographs and bone scan reveal no bony pathology. The physician's recommendation is to begin treatment of medial tibial stress syndrome.

Jennifer designs a therapeutic exercise program for Melissa that includes rest, flexibility and strengthening exercises, and modalities for symptomatic treatment. Melissa asks Jennifer for her advice on including taping and/or bracing techniques in the program. Jennifer has used several techniques with previous patients with medial tibial stress syndrome to provide support, shock absorption, and correction of structural abnormalities, but the outcomes have been mixed. Jennifer tells Melissa that she will explore the options and choose the most effective technique(s) to return her to running.

1. Develop a clinically relevant question from the case in the PICO format to generate answers for the selection of taping and/or bracing techniques for Melissa. The question should include the population or problem, the intervention, a comparison intervention (if relevant), and the clinical outcome of interest.

2. Design a search strategy and search to find the best evidence to answer the clinical question. The strategy should include relevant search terms, electronic databases, online journals, and print journals to use for the search. Discussions with your faculty, preceptor, and other health care professionals can provide evidence from expert opinion.
3. Choose three to five full text studies or reviews from your search or the chapter references. Evaluate and appraise each article to determine its value and usefulness to the case. Ask these questions for each study: (1) Are the results of the study valid? (2) What are the actual results? and (3) Are the findings clinically relevant to my patients? Prepare a summary of the evaluation with answers to the questions and rank the articles based on the evidence hierarchy in Chapter 1.

4. Integrate findings from the evidence, your clinical experience, and Melissa's goals and preferences into the therapeutic exercise program for Melissa. Consider which taping and/or bracing techniques may be appropriate for Melissa.
5. Evaluate the EBP process and your experience within the case. Consider these questions in the evaluation.

Was the clinical question answered?
Did the search generate quality evidence?
Was the evidence evaluated appropriately?
Was the evidence, your clinical experience, and Melissa's goals and values integrated to make the clinical decision?
Did the intervention produce successful clinical outcomes for Melissa?
Was the EBP experience positive for Jennifer and Melissa?

## WRAP-UP

- Lower leg contusions, strains, ruptures, and overuse injuries and conditions can be caused by excessive range of motion and acute and chronic stresses.
- The Achilles tendon, dorsal bridge, and peroneal tendon taping techniques limit excessive dorsiflexion, plantar flexion, and inversion/eversion of the foot, respectively.
- The Low-Dye and arch taping techniques provide support to the foot and correct structural abnormalities.
- The posterior splint and cast tape techniques provide immobilization of the foot, ankle, and lower leg.
- Elastic wraps and sleeves and self-adherent wraps provide mechanical pressure to the lower leg in the acute treatment of swelling.
- Walking boots and ankle braces provide support and limit range of motion.
- Orthotics can be used when treating acute and chronic lower leg injuries.
- A neoprene sleeve provides support and compression to the lower leg.
- The heel lift and longitudinal arch padding techniques provide shock absorption, support, and correction of structural abnormalities.
- Thermoplastic materials provide protection when preventing and treating lower leg contusions.
- The NCAA and NFHS require the use of mandatory protective equipment for the lower leg in several sports.

## FADAVIS ONLINE RESOURCES

- Peroneal tendon taping technique

## WEB REFERENCES

**Wheeless' Textbook of Orthopaedics**
http://www.wheelessonline.com/
- This website allows access to anatomy, diagnostic imaging, and management information on a variety of injuries.

**American Orthopaedic Foot & Ankle Society**
http://www.aofas.org/Pages/Home.aspx
- This site provides access to lower leg information on injuries and conditions as well as treatment methods.

**SportsInjuryClinic.net**
https://www.sportsinjuryclinic.net/
- This site allows you to search an injury index for the treatment and rehabilitation of a variety of lower leg injuries and conditions.

## REFERENCES

1. Prentice, WE: Principles of Athletic Training: A Guide to Evidence-Based Clinical Practice, ed 16. McGraw-Hill, New York, 2017.
2. Claessen, FM, de Vos, RJ, Reijman, M, and Meuffels, DE: Predictors of primary Achilles tendon ruptures. Sports Med 44:1241–1259, 2014.
3. Winters, M, Eskes, M, Weir, A, Moen, MH, Backx, FJG, and Bakker, EWP: Treatment of medial tibial stress

syndrome: A systematic review. Sports Med 43:1315–1333, 2013.

4. Rome, K, Handoll, HHG, and Ashford, RL: Interventions for preventing and treating stress fractures and stress reactions of bone of the lower limbs in young adults. Cochrane Database Syst Rev (2);CD000450, 2005.

5. National Collegiate Athletic Association: 2014–15 Sports Medicine Handbook, ed 25. NCAA, Indianapolis, 2014. http://www.ncaapublications.com/productdownloads/MD15.pdf.

6. National Federation of State High School Associations: 2018–2019 Soccer Rules Book. National Federation of State High School Associations, Indianapolis, 2019.

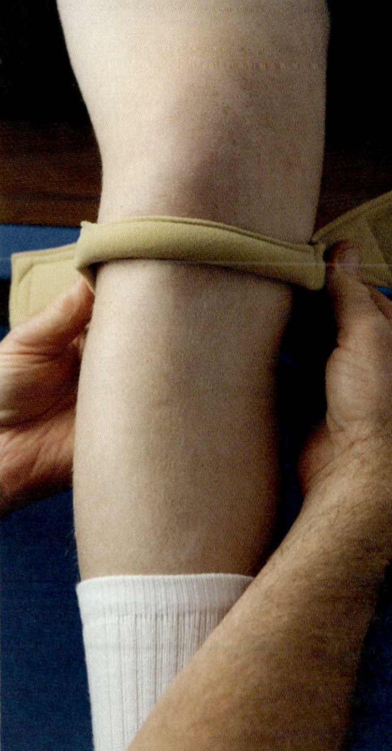

# Knee





1. Discuss common injuries that occur to the knee.
2. Demonstrate the application of taping, wrapping, bracing, and padding techniques when preventing, treating, and rehabilitating knee injuries.
3. Explain and demonstrate evidence-based practice for the implementation of taping, wrapping, bracing, and padding techniques for the knee within a clinical case.

## INJURIES AND CONDITIONS

Injury to the knee can occur from acute and chronic forces during contact and/or non-contact athletic and work activities. During athletic and work activities, extreme forces are placed on the knee. Because soft tissue structures act as the main stabilizers of the knee joint, injuries occur more frequently to ligaments, menisci, bursae, and tendons as a result of compression, friction, repetitive movements, and rotary and shearing forces. Common injuries to the knee include the following:

- Contusions
- Sprains
- Meniscal tears
- Plica syndrome
- Anterior knee pain
- Nerve contusion
- Fractures
- Dislocations/subluxations
- Bursitis
- Overuse injuries and conditions

## Contusions

Contusions to the soft tissue and bone of the knee can be caused by compressive forces. Falling on the knee and being struck by a direct force may result in pain, swelling, and loss of range of motion. A direct blow, chronic compression from kneeling, and being pinched between the tibia, patella, and femur can cause an **infrapatellar fat pad** contusion (Fig. 6–1).

## Sprains

Knee sprains are caused by **unidirectional, multidirectional,** and/or **rotary forces** during contact or non-contact activities. Depending on the force, a sprain of the knee can result in damage to single or multiple ligamentous structures. A valgus force on the lateral aspect of the knee can result in a **medial collateral ligament (MCL)** sprain (Figs. 6–2 and 6–3). Adduction and internal rotation of the knee is a common mechanism of MCL injury.[1] For example, a sprain can occur as a football offensive linemen pass blocks and another player is pushed or falls against the lateral aspect of the linemen's right knee, causing a valgus force. The **lateral collateral ligament (LCL)** is injured by a varus force on the medial aspect of the knee, commonly with internal rotation of the tibia. Medial or lateral lower leg rotation on a planted foot, direct force causing hyperextension, and external tibia rotation with the knee in a valgus position can cause injury to the **anterior cruciate ligament (ACL)** (Fig. 6–4). ACL injuries typically occur with quick deceleration, cutting, twisting, and landing

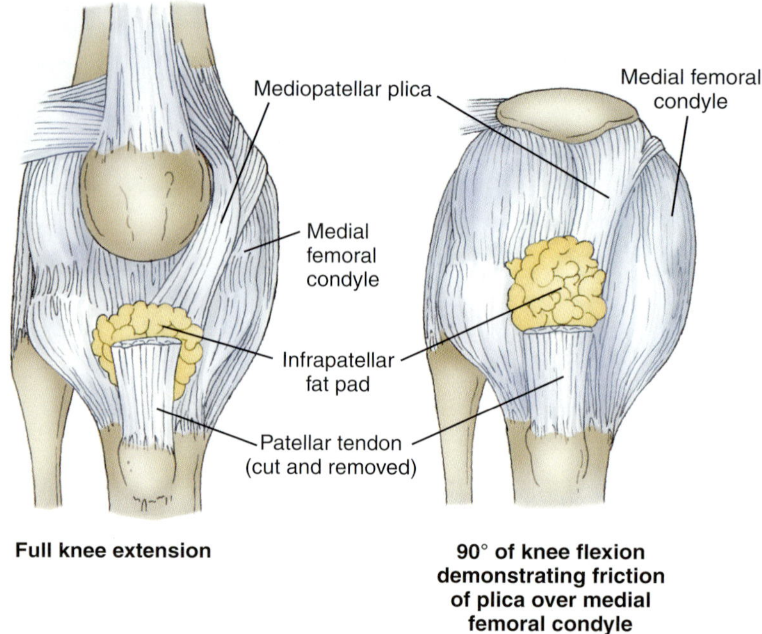



**Fig. 6–1** *Anterior view of the knee.*

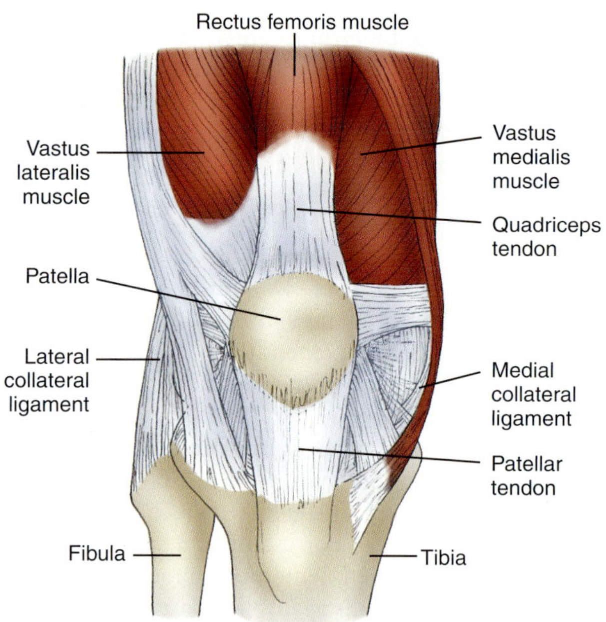



**Fig. 6–2** *Anterior view of the ligaments and muscles of the knee.*

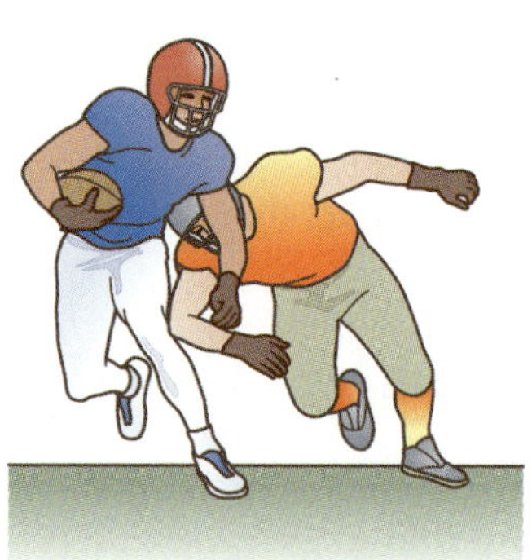

**Fig. 6–3** *Valgus force causing medial collateral ligament (MCL) sprain.*

movements (Fig. 6–5). An ACL sprain can result as a lacrosse midfielder sprints down the field and suddenly stops, then pivots on the left foot and quickly turns to the right, causing external rotation of the left tibia and valgus stress at the knee (Fig. 6–6). The **posterior cruciate ligament (PCL)** can be injured by a fall on the anterior knee while in a flexed position with foot plantar flexion, a direct force to the proximal lower leg, hyperextension, or a rotational force (see Fig. 6–4).

With multidirectional and rotary forces, injury commonly occurs to more than one structure.

## Meniscal Tears

Tears to the **medial** and **lateral menisci** are caused by compression and shearing forces (see Fig. 6–4). Injury to the medial meniscus is more common because of its connection to the joint capsule surrounding the knee and the deep fibers of the MCL. Tears can occur from twisting or cutting movements on a planted foot during flexion or extension of the knee.[2] Medial meniscal tears are also associated with multiple sprains of the MCL, caused by the loss of medial stability and their structural connection.

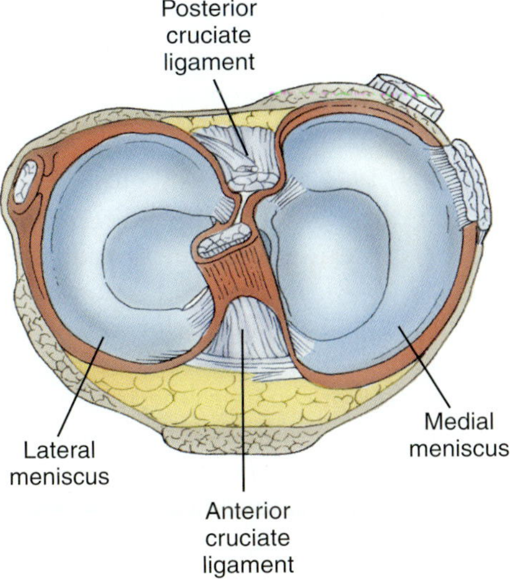



**Fig. 6–4** *Superior view of the cruciate ligaments and menisci.*

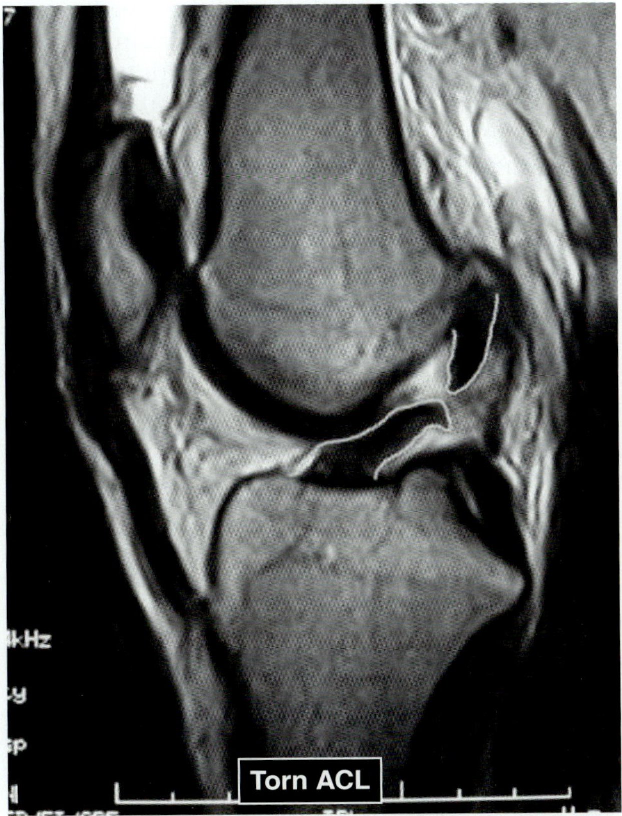



**Fig. 6–5** *Sagittal MRI demonstrating disruption in linear continuity of ACL (outlined). (Courtesy of McKinnis, LN. Fundamentals of Musculoskeletal Imaging, 4th ed. Philadelphia, PA: F.A. Davis Company: 2014.)*

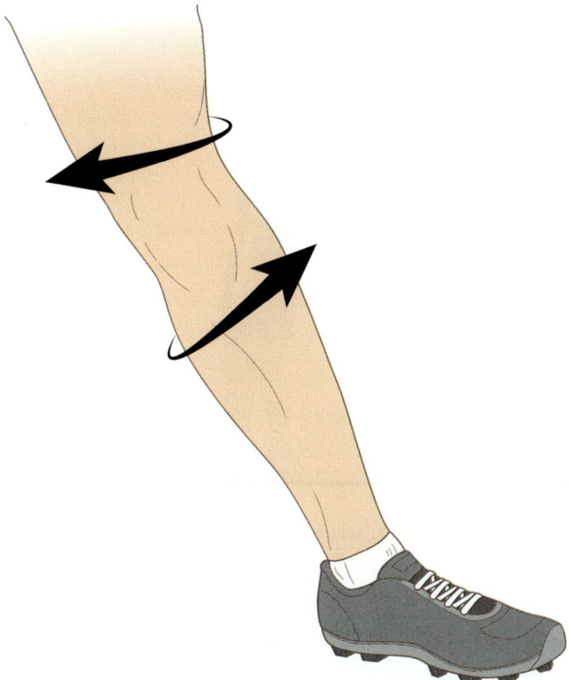

**Fig. 6–6** *Anterior cruciate ligament (ACL) sprain.*

## Medial Plica Syndrome

The most commonly injured **plica** is the mediopatellar, which originates on the medial knee and crosses the medial femoral condyle (see Fig. 6–1). A direct blow to the medial knee as a result of being kicked or repetitive friction of the plica over the medial femoral condyle during knee flexion and extension can cause inflammation and additional thickening.

## Anterior Knee Pain

Anterior knee pain is commonly associated with injury or structural abnormalities involving the extensor mechanism, consisting of the distal quadriceps, quadriceps tendon, patella, and patellar tendon (see Fig. 6–2). **Patellofemoral pain (PFP)** is caused by inflexibility of the posterior leg musculature and lateral retinaculum, pronation of the foot, and weakness of the medial quadriceps and hip adductors resulting in abnormal tracking of the patella within the femoral groove. Compressive and shear forces and abnormal tracking of the patella caused by pronation of the foot, external torsion of the tibia, **patella alta,** and degeneration can result in **chondromalacia patella. Patellar tendinitis (jumper's knee)** or patellar tendinopathy is caused by repetitive jumping, running, or kicking (Fig. 6–7). These movements can also result in tendinitis of the quadriceps tendon. Repetitive tension on the patellar tendon in the adolescent can lead to **Osgood-Schlatter disease (OSD)** or **Sinding-Larsen Johansson disease (SLJ).** Ruptures of the patellar or quadriceps tendon can occur with violent eccentric quadriceps contractions and often follow injuries and conditions that have caused degenerative changes in these structures.

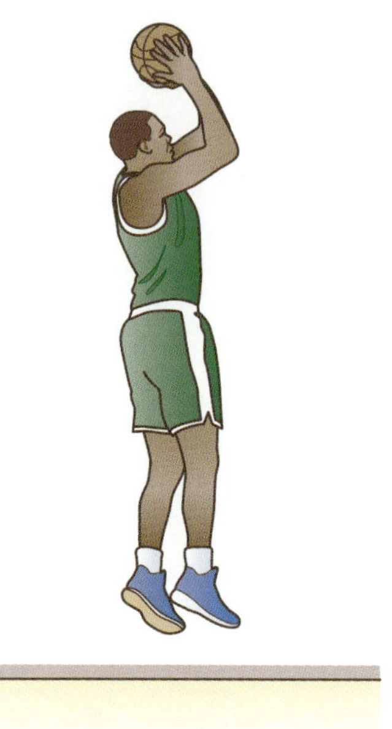

**Fig. 6–7** *Patellar tendinitis (jumper's knee) or patellar tendinopathy is common in basketball.*

# Nerve Contusion

A direct blow or excessive compression to the inferior aspect of the fibular head can cause a peroneal nerve contusion. The force is commonly a result of being kicked or excessive compression from a wrap or brace.

# Fractures

Fractures of the patella can be caused by a direct blow occurring with a fall or a blow to the anterior knee or an eccentric contraction of the quadriceps occurring with jumping or running movements.[3] **Osteochondral** and **chondral fractures** can occur from a direct blow or violent twisting, cutting, or rotational movement. Overuse, direct trauma, or a violent muscular contraction can result in an avulsion fracture. A fracture of the tibial tubercle can be caused by active contraction of the quadriceps with forced flexion of the knee and may follow the development of OSD.[3]

# Dislocations/Subluxations

Dislocations of the knee are caused by multidirectional and/or rotary forces and are associated with injury to other structures in and around the knee. Acute patellar subluxations or dislocations can be caused by sudden deceleration with an associated cutting movement, as is experienced by football wide receivers while running pass routes. Individuals with flat lateral femoral condyles, pronated feet, **genu valgum,** externally rotated patellas, and/or medial knee laxity and lateral knee tightness are predisposed to lateral subluxations or dislocations.[1]

# Bursitis

**Bursitis** of the knee can be caused by direct force or overuse. Compressive force from a direct blow or excessive kneeling can cause inflammation of the **prepatellar bursa** (Fig. 6–8). Repetitive friction of the patellar tendon can result in inflammation of the **deep infrapatellar bursa.** Compressive force from a direct blow, genu valgum, quadriceps weakness, or inflexibility of the hamstrings can result in inflammation of the **pes anserinus bursa**. Ligamentous or meniscal injuries of the knee can cause inflammation of the **semimembranosus bursa (Baker's cyst).**

# Overuse

Overuse injuries and conditions of the knee are caused by repetitive stress and structural abnormalities. **Iliotibial band syndrome** is caused by repetitive stress and friction as the iliotibial band passes over the lateral femoral condyle (see Figs. 6–9 and 7–4). The syndrome is often associated with excessive foot pronation, leg-length discrepancy, **genu varus,** and training errors. Genu valgum, quadriceps weakness, and overuse can cause **pes anserinus tendinitis** (see Fig. 6–8). Stress fractures of the tibial tubercle, tibial plateau, and femoral condyles can be the result of repetitive jumping or running movements and training errors.

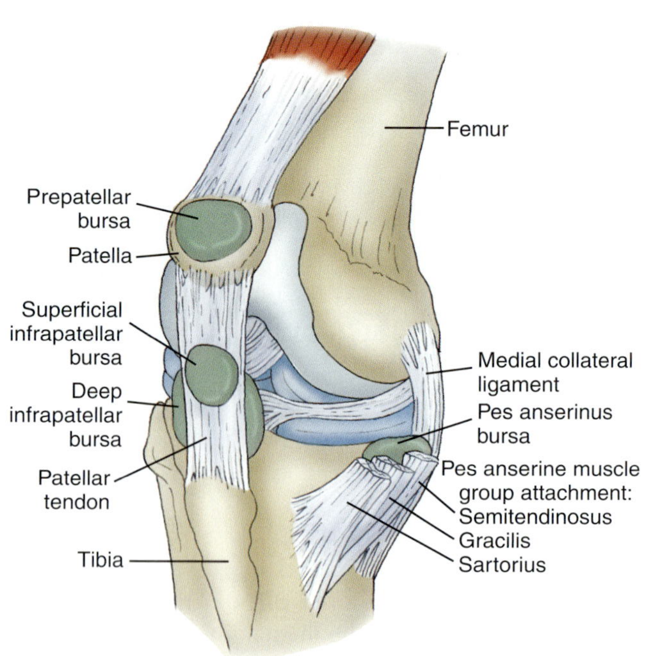


**Fig. 6–8** *Bursae of the anterior and medial knee.*

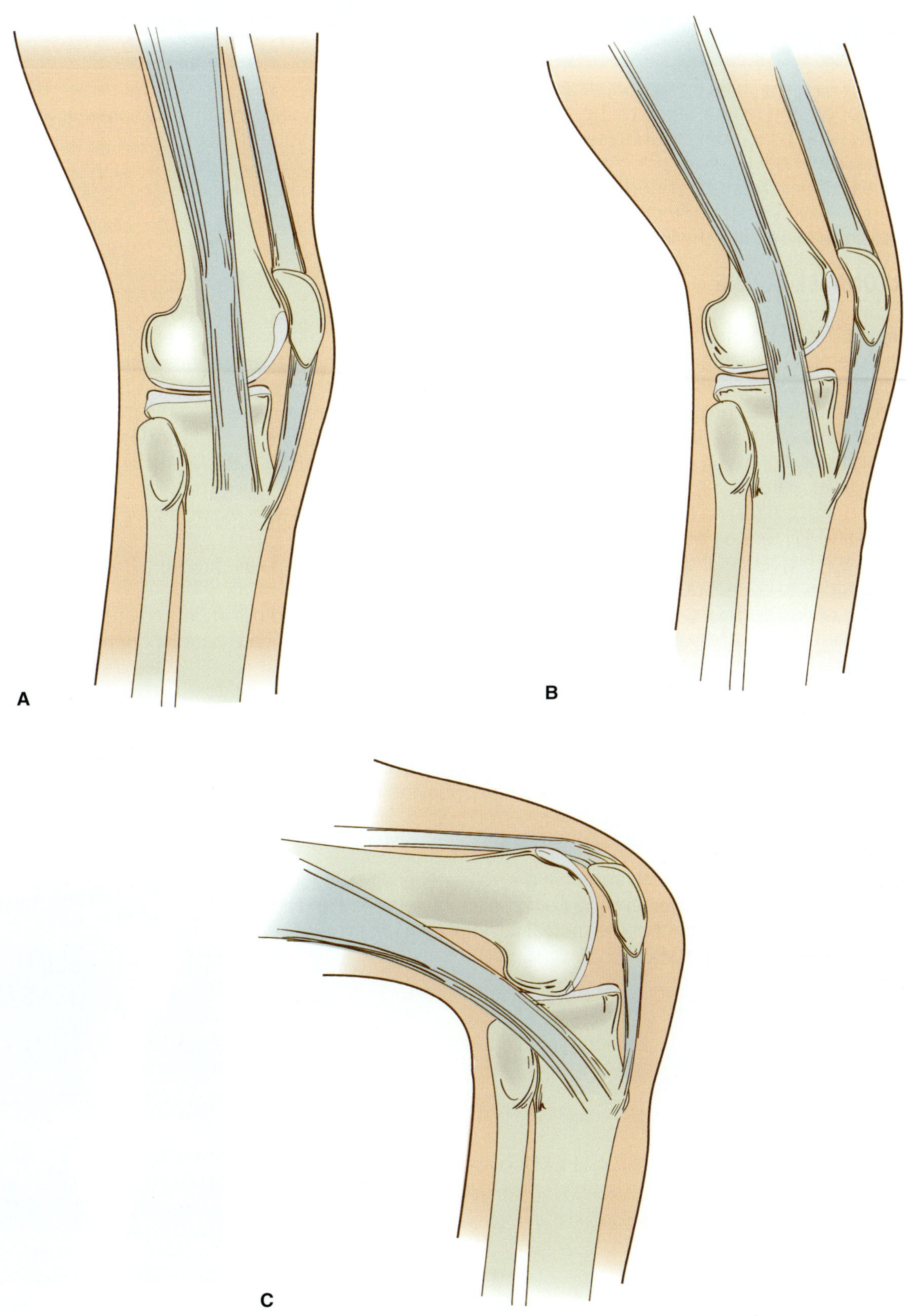



**Fig. 6–9** *Iliotibial band syndrome.* **A** *Full knee extension,* **B** *Iliotibial band moving posteriorly over lateral femoral condyle with knee flexion,* **C** *90° of knee flexion with iliotibial band positioned posterior to lateral femoral condyle.*

**Knee**

# Taping Techniques

Provide support and reduce stress to the soft tissue, limit excessive range of motion, and prevent and treat knee injuries and conditions by using several taping techniques. Techniques that are applied after a sprain protect against knee hyperextension and valgus and varus forces. For overuse injuries and conditions, several techniques correct structural abnormalities and lessen tension of the patellar tendon on the tibial tubercle. A technique may be effective for one patient but ineffective for another. Prior to application, consider the purpose of the technique, the injury, the patient, and the activity.

## McCONNELL TAPING        Figure 6–10

➠ **Purpose:** The McConnell taping technique[4] is used to treat PFP and to provide relief of pain and correct patellofemoral malalignment (Fig. 6–10). Use the technique within a therapeutic exercise program that consists of stretching tight lateral structures, retraining and strengthening the vastus medialis oblique muscle, mobilizing the patella, and correcting structural foot abnormalities.[4–6]
  • Rigid non-elastic tape in 1½ inch width is placed over adhesive gauze material and is used to correct patellar malalignment. Many manufacturers offer the tape; it is also available in kits containing the adhesive gauze material.
  • Design the application of the technique specifically for the patient with regard to the sequence of tape strips and roll tension or how tightly the tape is applied.
  • Begin the sequence of strips with correction of the most excessive malalignment component. Use additional strips to correct other components if necessary.
  • After applying each strip, reevaluate the painful activity. There should be an immediate decrease in pain. If the pain does not lessen or if it worsens, reapply the strips or reevaluate patellar orientation.
➠ **Materials:**
  • 1½ inch rigid non-elastic tape, 2 inch adhesive gauze material, taping scissors
➠ **Position of the patient:** Sitting on a taping table or bench with the knee in extension and the quadriceps relaxed.
➠ **Preparation:** Perform a static and dynamic evaluation of the patient to determine patellar glide, rotation, tilt, and anteroposterior orientation components. Shaving may be necessary for effective application.
➠ **Application:**

**STEP 1:**  Apply two strips of 2 inch adhesive gauze material directly to the skin over the patella, extending from the lateral femoral condyle to the posterior aspect of the medial femoral condyle to serve as a base ◄▦▦► (Fig. 6–10A).

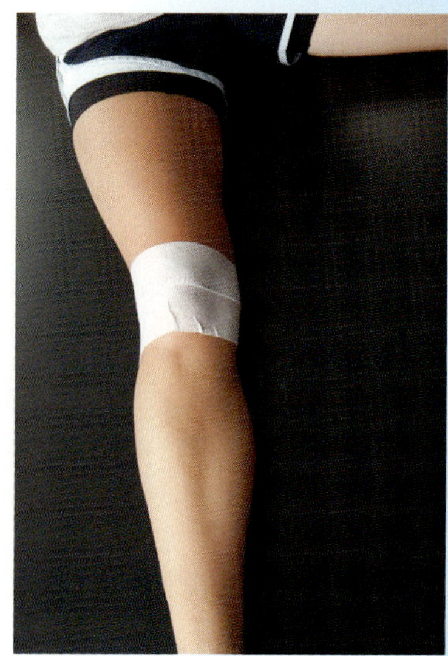

**Fig. 6–10 A**

**STEP 2:**   To correct the glide component (typically a positive lateral glide), anchor a strip of rigid non-elastic tape on the lateral border of the patella (Fig. 6–10B). Pull the strip in a medial direction and push the soft tissue on the medial aspect of the knee toward the patella, and anchor on the adhesive gauze material over the medial femoral condyle (Fig. 6–10C).

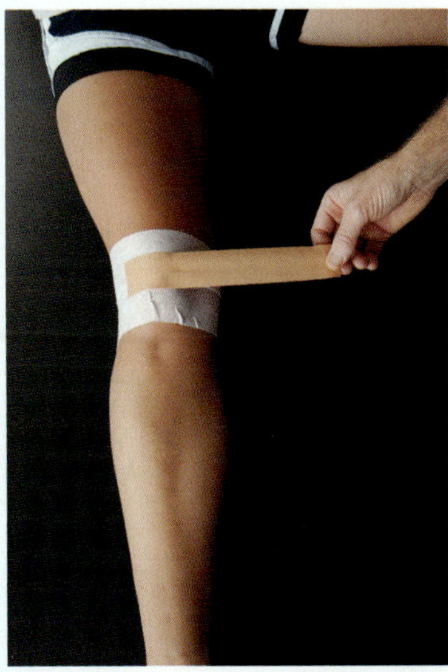

**Fig. 6–10 B**

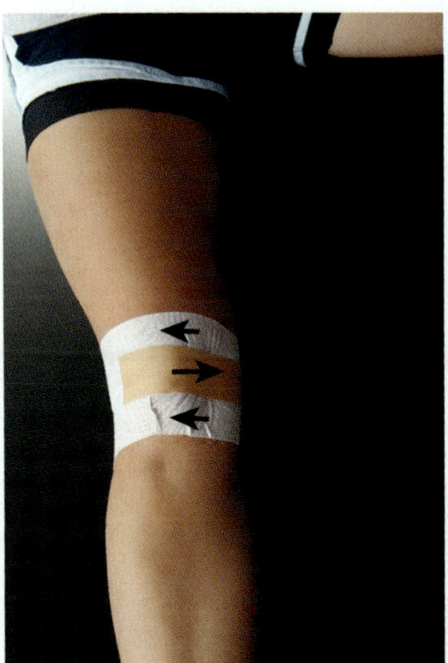

**Fig. 6–10 C**

**STEP 3:**   To correct the rotation component (commonly positive external rotation of the inferior pole), place a strip of rigid tape on the middle of the inferior pole of the patella at an angle (Fig. 6–10D). Pull the strip upward and medially and anchor on the medial aspect of the knee (Fig. 6–10E). The superior pole of the patella should rotate laterally.

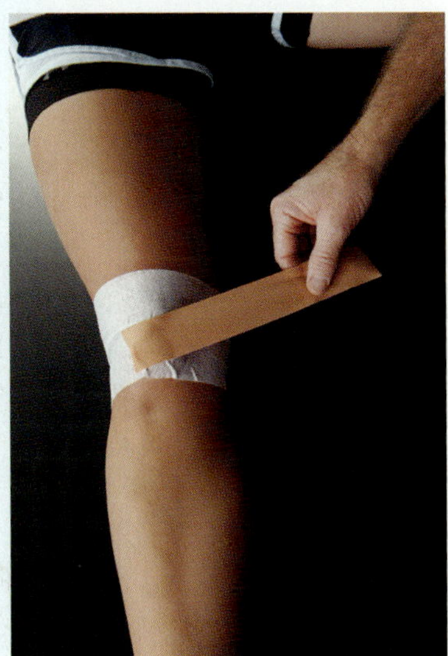

**Fig. 6–10 D**

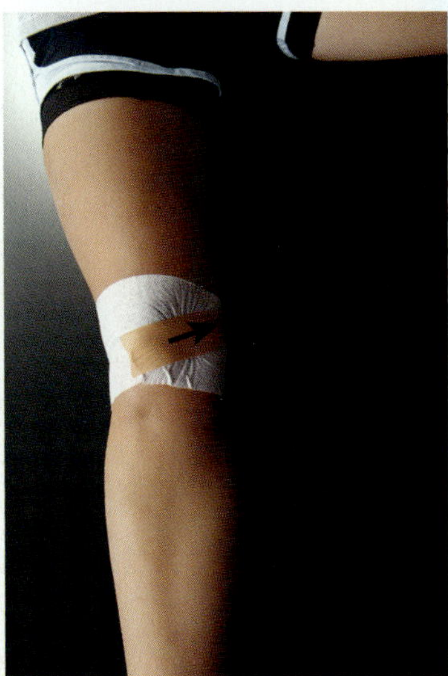

**Fig. 6–10 E**

*Steps Cont.*

**Knee**

**STEP 4:** To correct the tilt component (often a positive lateral tilt), anchor a strip of rigid tape on the middle of the patella (Fig. 6–10F). Pull the strip medially, push the medial knee soft tissue toward the patella, and anchor on the medial femoral condyle (Fig. 6–10G).

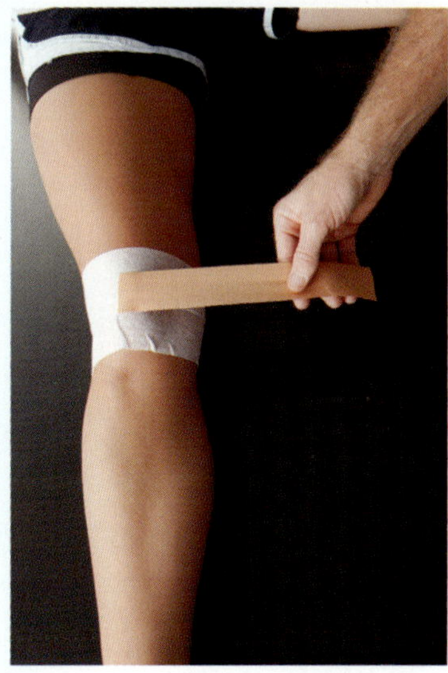

**Fig. 6–10 F**                    **Fig. 6–10 G**

**STEP 5:** To correct the anteroposterior component (commonly a positive inferior tilt), place a strip of rigid tape across the upper half of the patella and anchor the strip on the lateral and medial femoral condyles (Fig. 6–10H).

> **Helpful Hint |**
> A positive anteroposterior inferior tilt may require correction first in the taping sequence to lift the inferior pole of the patella away from the infra-patellar fat pad to prevent irritation and pain.[5]

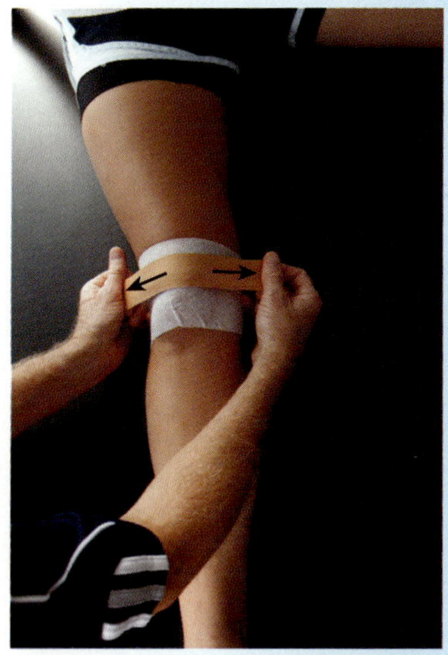

**Fig. 6–10 H**

# EVIDENCE SUMMARY

The McConnell taping technique is used by many health care professionals when treating PFP. Although positive outcomes have been demonstrated when the technique has been used in the clinical setting, many questions remain unanswered. Several evidence-based reviews have examined patellar taping to determine the efficacy in the treatment of PFP.

A 2012 meta-analysis[7] investigated the effects of patellar taping on knee pain, function, and activity scores among adults with PFP. Three randomized controlled trials (RCTs) examined pain levels with two comparisons: (1) taping and a placebo taping or no-tape situation and (2) taping within therapeutic exercise (lower extremity strengthening and flexibility exercises) and placebo taping or no-tape situation with therapeutic exercise. The researchers found no significant differences in visual analogue scales of pain perception with taping after 1 week to 3 months. The findings from individual trials in the review[7] demonstrated conflicting results for knee function and activity scores. Two trials showed taping and therapeutic exercise resulted in significantly higher patient-reported scores at 3 and 4 weeks compared with placebo taping or no-tape with therapeutic exercise. In contrast, one trial reported no significant differences in patient-reported scores at 3 and 12 month periods between taping and a placebo and no-tape situation and taping within a therapeutic exercise program and a placebo or no-tape situation with therapeutic exercise. Although this review provided some support for the use of patellar taping, the overall evidence is of low-quality and insufficient to determine the efficacy of patellar taping when used alone or within a therapeutic exercise program in the treatment of PFP.[7]

In a 2015 review, researchers[8] examined the effects of patellar taping on knee biomechanics and muscle activation patterns during functional weight-bearing activities (single leg squat, stepping activities, stair climbing). The findings from three trials in the review demonstrated no significant differences between taping and placebo tape or no-tape situation in average knee extensor moments during loading response among patients with PFP. Three trials investigated the average vastus medialis oblique and vastus lateralis activation ratio in patients with PFP and found no differences between taping and placebo tape or no-tape situation.

The timing of vastus medialis oblique and vastus lateralis activation during functional activity was examined in three trials, and no differences were revealed between taping and placebo tape or no-tape situation. Individual trials in the review[8] examining kinematics produced conflicting findings, perhaps from the lack of standardization among outcome measures. Based on the review findings, there is insufficient evidence to establish the effectiveness of patellar taping in the treatment of PFP.[8]

A 2017 systematic review[9] of five RCTs investigated the efficacy of patellar taping on visual analogue scales of pain perception among patients with PFP. Comparisons among patellar and placebo taping, therapeutic exercise, taping and exercise alone, and combinations of taping and exercise were examined in the review. The results from four trials showed greater improvements in pain scores with placebo taping within therapeutic exercise compared with patellar taping with therapeutic exercise. Three trials demonstrated placebo taping with therapeutic exercise produced lower pain scores when compared to therapeutic exercise alone. Among five trials, the researchers[9] found greater reductions in pain scores with patellar taping within therapeutic exercise compared to patellar taping alone. The findings from this review appear to support the use of patellar and placebo taping within therapeutic exercise programs to lessen pain in the treatment of PFP.

A 2018 International Patellofemoral Pain Research Retreat consensus statement[10] presented recommendations for therapeutic exercise and physical interventions for the management of PFP. While acknowledging that patellar taping may be beneficial, the authors[10] found insufficient evidence to recommend taping in the treatment of PFP.

The effect and role of patellar taping in the treatment of PFP is unclear based on insufficient evidence produced from evidence-based reviews and statements.[7–10] Further research is needed to support or refute the current clinical practice of patellar taping in the treatment of PFP. RCTs should investigate the long-term effects of taping, used alone or in combination with therapeutic exercise, on standardized outcome measures during work, athletic, or casual weight-bearing activities among patients with PFP.

## | HYPEREXTENSION    Figure 6–11

**➠ Purpose:** The hyperextension technique is used to limit hyperextension of the knee and stretch on the soft tissues when treating sprains. Two methods are interchangeable in applying the hyperextension technique; the first is illustrated here (Fig. 6–11) and the second is online at FADavis.com.  Use the different methods to accommodate patient preferences and available supplies.

**Knee**

### Hyperextension Technique One

➡ **Materials:**
- Pre-wrap, thin foam pads, 3 inch heavyweight elastic tape, adherent tape spray, skin lubricant, taping scissors

***Option:***
- 6 inch width by 5 yard length elastic wrap

➡ **Position of the patient:** Standing on a taping table or bench with the majority of the weight on the non-involved leg. Determine the range of extension that produces pain by having the patient actively contract the quadriceps and slowly extend the knee until pain occurs. Once painful range of motion is determined, place the involved knee in a pain-free range and, using a heel lift, maintain this position during application.

> **Helpful Hint |**
> You can construct a quick and inexpensive heel lift from paper or plastic tape cores of 1½ inch or 2 inch width tape. Place 5 to 7 of these cores together and apply non-elastic or elastic tape around them, completely covering all sides. You can store the lift in a taping table or bench between uses.

➡ **Preparation:** Shave the leg from the mid thigh to mid lower leg. The technique is applied directly to the skin or over one layer of pre-wrap. Cover the popliteal space with thin foam pads to prevent irritation. A skin lubricant can also be used. Apply adherent tape spray from the mid thigh to the mid lower leg area.

> **Helpful Hint |**
> Closely monitor the skin of the thigh and lower leg for irritation from heavyweight elastic tape and/or adherent tape spray with daily application of the hyperextension and/or collateral "X" taping techniques. If irritation occurs, apply the tape over pre-wrap or replace the taping technique with a bracing technique.

➡ **Application:**

**STEP 1:** Apply two anchors of 3 inch heavyweight elastic tape around the mid thigh and mid lower leg with mild roll tension ◄▬▬► (Fig. 6–11A).

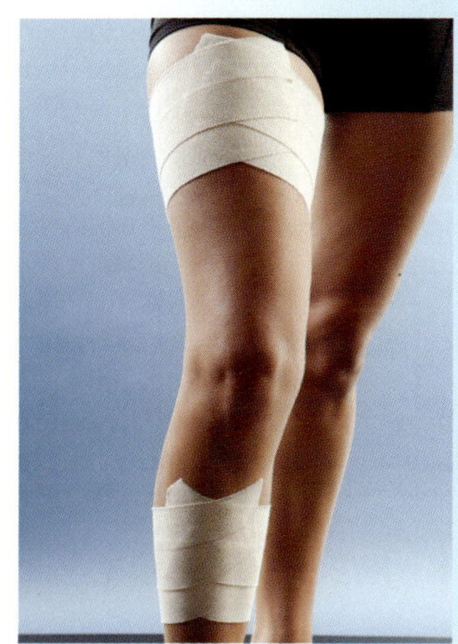

**Fig. 6–11 A**

**STEP 2:** Using 3 inch heavyweight elastic tape, apply a strip from the middle posterior lower leg to the posterior middle thigh (Fig. 6–11B). Apply moderate roll tension with the tape and monitor the pain-free position of the knee.

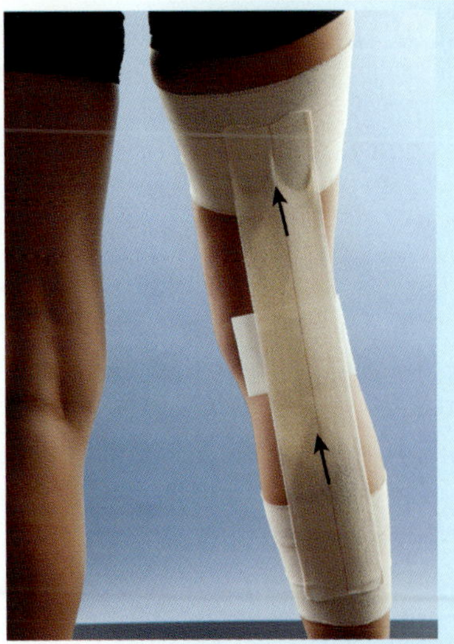

**Fig. 6–11 B**

**STEP 3:** Place another strip of 3 inch heavyweight elastic tape on the anterior lateral lower leg, continue across the popliteal area, and anchor on the anterior medial thigh (Fig. 6–11C).

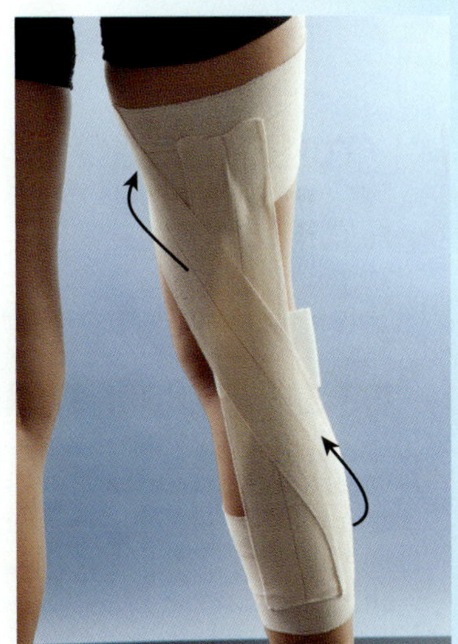

**Fig. 6–11 C**

**STEP 4:** Begin the next strip on the anterior medial lower leg, across the popliteal area, and anchor on the anterior lateral thigh (Fig. 6–11D). These strips should form an "X" over the posterior knee. These strips (see Figs. 6–11C and D) can be repeated with moderate tension, overlapping by ⅓ of the tape width.

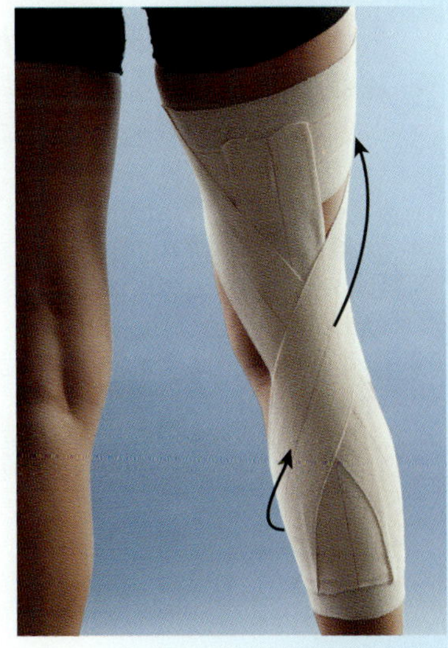

**Fig. 6–11 D**

*Steps Cont.*

**STEP 5:** Apply three to four circular closure patterns around the thigh and lower leg with mild roll tension, overlapping each ◄▬▬► (Fig. 6–11E). Non-elastic tape anchors are not necessary.

*Option:* *Consider applying a 6 inch width by 5 yard length elastic wrap in a circular pattern over the technique with moderate roll tension in a distal-to-proximal direction to lessen migration and unraveling of the tape* ◄▬▬►. *Anchor with elastic tape* ◄▬▬►.

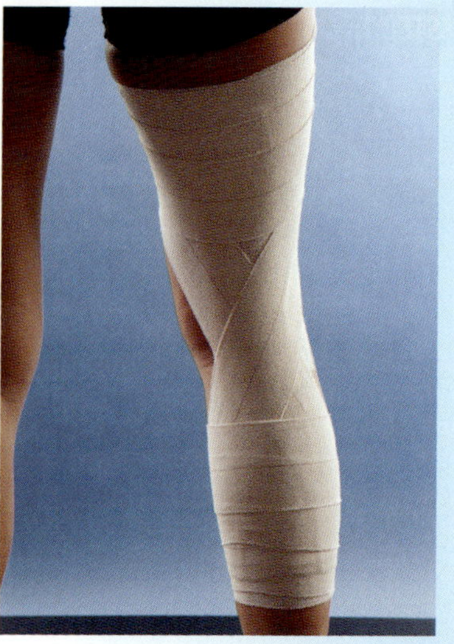

**Fig. 6–11 E**

## COLLATERAL "X"

► **Purpose:** The collateral "X" technique is used in the treatment of medial and lateral collateral ligament sprains to provide mild to moderate support and protection against valgus and varus forces at the knee. This technique and steps of application can be found on FADavis.com.

## PATELLAR TENDON STRAP        Figures 6–12 and 6–13

► **Purpose:** Use the strap technique to treat patellar tendinitis, OSD, PFP, and chondromalacia and to reduce the tension or pull of the tendon on the inferior pole of the patella and/or tibial tubercle. The straps can be made from taping materials or purchased off-the-shelf. The off-the-shelf designs are illustrated in the Bracing section. Three methods are interchangeable in applying the patellar tendon strap technique: The first and second are illustrated here (Figs. 6–12 and 6–13), and the third is online at FADavis.com. ⊕ Choose according to patient preferences and available supplies.

### Patellar Tendon Strap Technique One

► **Materials:**
• 2 inch heavyweight elastic tape, ½ inch non-elastic tape, taping scissors
**Option:**
• 2 inch self-adherent wrap
► **Position of the patient:** Sitting on a taping table or bench, or in a chair, with the knee in a flexed position.
► **Preparation:** Cut a piece of 2 inch heavyweight elastic tape in a 25–30 inch length strip.
**Option:**
Cut a piece of 2 inch self-adherent wrap in a 25–30 inch length strip.
► **Application:**

**STEP 1:** Fold the 2 inch heavyweight elastic tape strip over into one piece lengthwise, adhering both sides together. Grasp the ends of this 1 inch strip and rub over a table edge to enhance adhesion (Fig. 6–12A).

*Option:* *2 inch self-adherent wrap may be used if 2 inch heavyweight elastic tape is not available.*

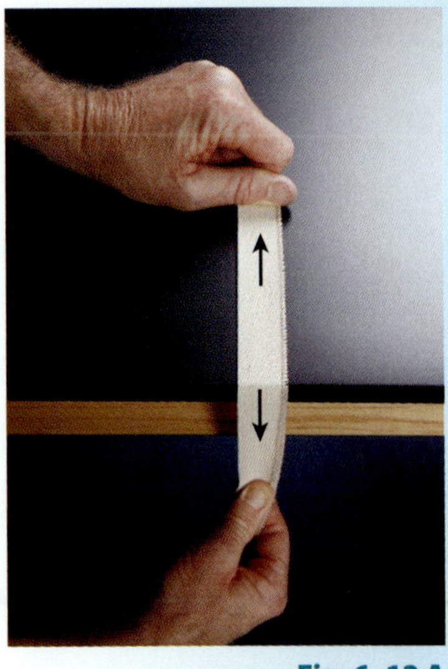

**Fig. 6–12 A**

**STEP 2:** Locate the mid portion of the tendon between the inferior pole of the patella and the tibial tubercle. Anchor the strip directly to the skin on the medial proximal lower leg, continue laterally across the mid portion of the patellar tendon, around the posterior knee, and return to the anchor position (Fig. 6–12B).

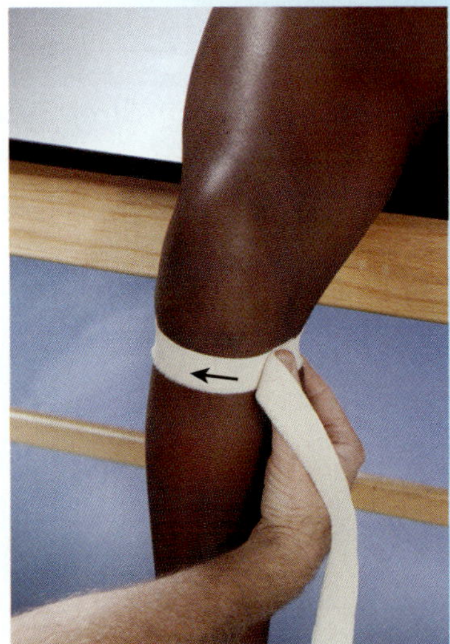

**Fig. 6–12 B**

**STEP 3:** Without overlapping, continue to apply the strip around the knee and finish on the medial lower leg, cutting any excess of the strip (Fig. 6–12C). The elastic tape strip should be applied with moderate tension.

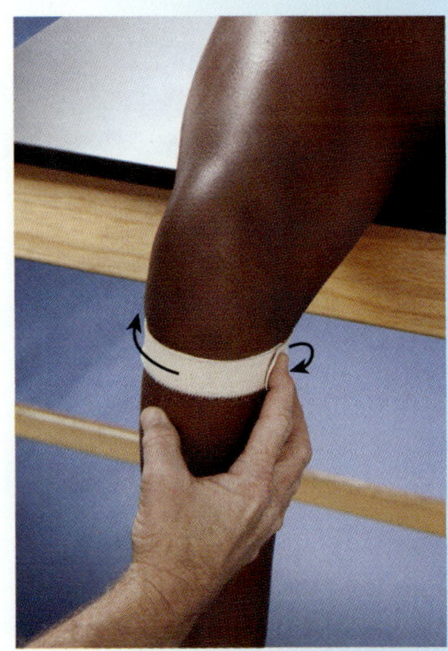

**Fig. 6–12 C**

*Steps Cont.*

**STEP 4:** Anchor ½ inch non-elastic tape on the anterior knee and apply two to four continuous strips over the elastic tape in a medial-to-lateral direction (Fig. 6–12D).

**Helpful Hint |**
To achieve proper tension and pain relief, the roll tension of the non-elastic tape will vary among patients. Check the tension of the strips by allowing the patient to perform a previously painful activity. Readjust the tension of the non-elastic strips if necessary. The elastic strip can be reused several times.

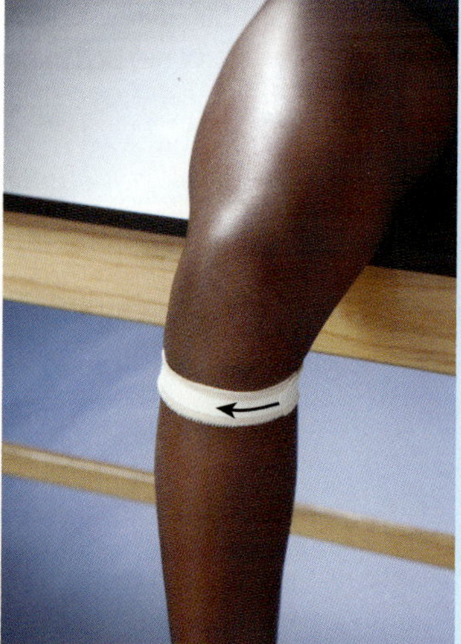

Fig. 6–12 D

### Patellar Tendon Strap Technique Two

➠ **Materials:**
• Pre-wrap, 2 inch lightweight elastic tape, taping scissors
➠ **Position of the patient:** Sitting on a taping table or bench, or in a chair, with the knee in a flexed position.
➠ **Preparation:** Apply the strap directly to the skin.
➠ **Application:**

**STEP 1:** Using pre-wrap, roll the wrap onto itself and continue until a sausage-sized roll is produced (Fig. 6–13A). Apply 2 inch lightweight elastic tape around the roll.

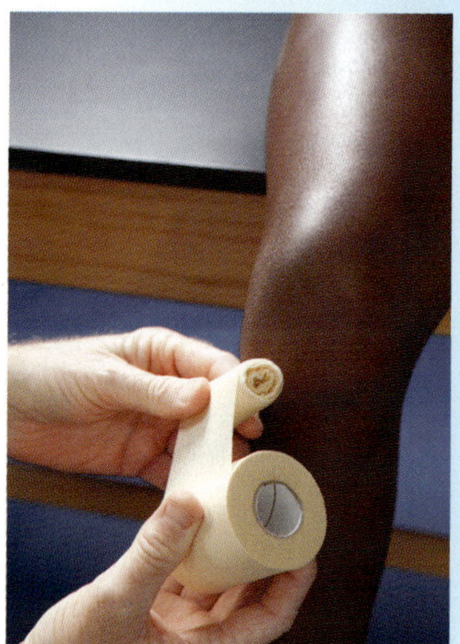

Fig. 6–13 A

**STEP 2:** Palpate the anterior knee and place the roll over the mid portion of the patellar tendon directly to the skin. Attach the roll to the knee by applying pre-wrap in a circular pattern around the proximal lower leg ⬅️▬▬➡️ (Fig. 6–13B).

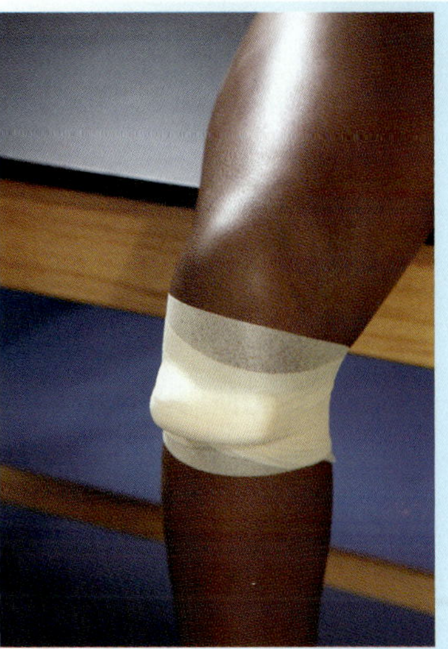

**Fig. 6–13 B**

**STEP 3:** With 2 inch lightweight elastic tape, anchor on the medial lower leg and apply two to four continuous strips over the pre-wrap and roll in a medial-to-lateral direction (Fig. 6–13C). Roll tension will vary among patients. Additional non-elastic tape strips are not necessary. The pre-wrap roll can be reused.

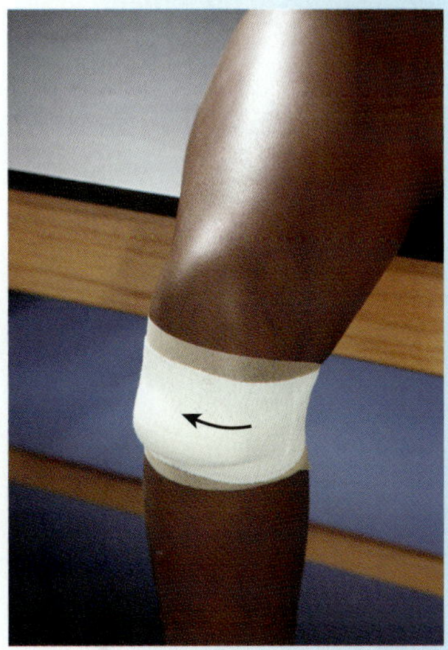

**Fig. 6–13 C**

## Clinical Application Question 1

Over the past 6 months, a competitive weightlifter has experienced periodic pain in his left patellar tendon during intense workouts. He has been evaluated by a physician and has undergone treatment for patellar tendinitis that included an off-the-shelf patellar tendon strap. When he initially applies the strap with maximal tension, his pain lessens. However, during workouts, the strap loosens when perspiration collects on the neoprene strap and Velcro closure, lessening tension over the patellar tendon.

➡️ **Question: What techniques can you use to maintain maximal tension during workouts?**

## ...IF/THEN...

**IF** limits in hyperextension are required over several weeks during a return to activity, **THEN** consider the use of a neoprene sleeve with hinged bars brace, which will allow for range of motion control. Most designs will be cost-effective.

# Wrapping Techniques

Use compression wrap techniques to control swelling and effusion when treating contusions, sprains, meniscal tears, bursitis, iliotibial band friction syndrome, and patellar fractures, dislocations, and subluxations. Three wrapping methods can provide compression over the knee following injury. Choose a technique based on the amount of swelling and effusion.

## KNEE COMPRESSION WRAP    Figure 6–14

➡ **Purpose:** Apply the knee compression wrap technique for injuries and conditions of the knee that cause mild to moderate swelling and effusion (Fig. 6–14).

➡ **Materials:**
• 4 inch or 6 inch width by 5 yard length elastic wrap, metal clips, 1½ inch non-elastic or 1½ inch or 2 inch elastic tape, taping scissors
*Option:*
• ¼ inch or ½ inch open-cell foam

➡ **Position of the patient:** Standing on a taping table or bench with the majority of the weight on the non-involved leg and the involved knee placed in a pain-free, slightly flexed position. Also, sitting on a taping table or bench with the leg extended off the edge.

➡ **Preparation:** To lessen migration, apply adherent tape spray, tape strips, or anchors directly to the skin (see Fig. 1–7).

➡ **Application:**

**STEP 1:**   Anchor the extended end of the wrap directly to the skin around the proximal lower leg and encircle the anchor ⬅➡ (Fig. 6–14A).

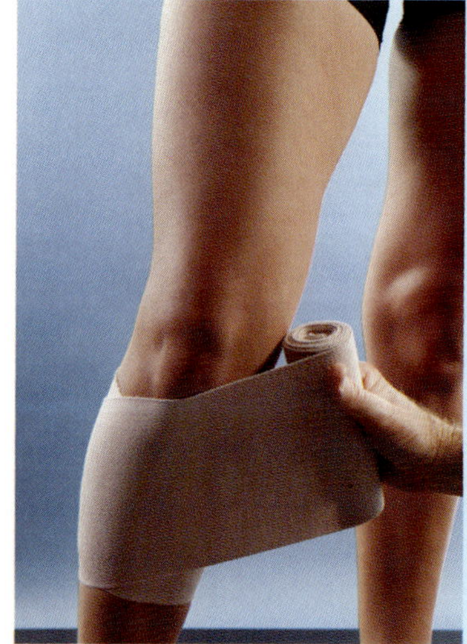

**Fig. 6–14 A**

**STEP 2:** Continue to apply the wrap in a spiral pattern, overlapping by ½ of the wrap width, in a distal-to-proximal direction (Fig. 6–14B). Apply the greatest roll tension distally and lessen tension as the wrap continues proximally.

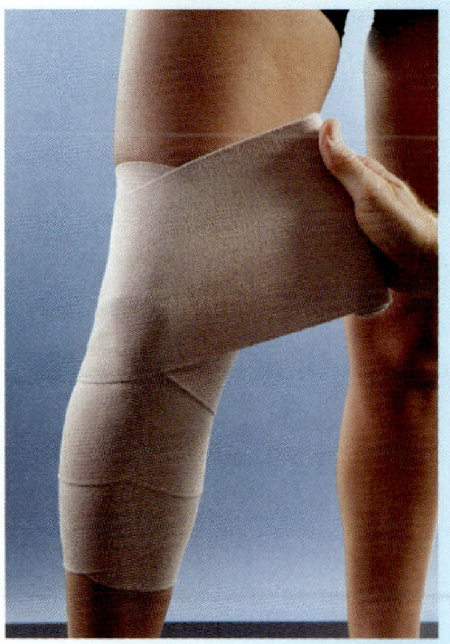

**Fig. 6–14 B**

**STEP 3:** Finish the wrap over the mid thigh area. Anchor the wrap with Velcro, metal clips, or loosely applied 1½ inch non-elastic or 1½ inch or 2 inch elastic tape (Fig. 6–14C).

*Option:* *It is possible to place a ¼ inch or ½ inch open-cell foam pad over the anterior knee, extending from the lateral femoral condyle to the medial femoral condyle, for additional compression around the patella to assist in venous return (see Fig. 6–28A). Place the pad directly on the skin and cover it with the compression wrap.*

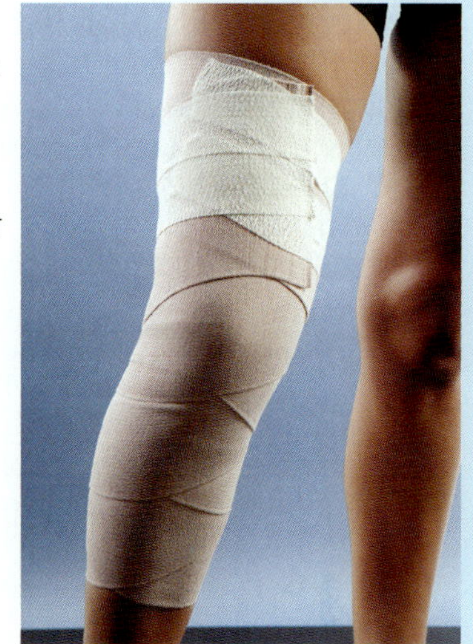

**Fig. 6–14 C**

## FOOT, ANKLE, LOWER LEG, AND KNEE COMPRESSION WRAP　　Figure 6–15

➠ **Purpose:** With some knee injuries, such as third-degree sprains of the ACL, swelling and effusion can be immediate and severe. To lessen the deleterious effects of moderate to severe swelling/effusion and distal migration, use the foot, ankle, lower leg, and knee compression wrap technique (Fig. 6–15).

➠ **Materials:**
 • 4 inch or 6 inch width by 10 yard length elastic wrap, metal clips, 1½ inch non-elastic or 1½ inch or 2 inch elastic tape, taping scissors
 **Option:**
 • ¼ inch or ½ inch open-cell foam

➠ **Position of the patient:** Sitting on a taping table or bench with the leg extended off the edge, knee in a pain-free, slightly flexed position, and the ankle placed in 90 degrees of dorsiflexion.

➠ **Preparation:** To lessen migration, apply adherent tape spray, tape strips, or anchors directly to the skin (see Fig. 1–7).

➠ **Application:**

Knee

**STEP 1:** Anchor the end of the wrap on the distal plantar foot and apply the foot, ankle, and lower leg compression wrap directly to the skin (see Fig. 5–10).

**STEP 2:** At the inferior knee, continue the spiral wrap proximally to the mid thigh area ◀━━━━. Apply the greatest amount of roll tension distally and lessen as the wrap continues proximally.

**STEP 3:** Anchor the wrap with Velcro, metal clips, or loosely applied 1½ inch non-elastic or 1½ inch or 2 inch elastic tape ◀━━━▶ (Fig. 6–15).

*Option:* *Consider using a ¼ inch or ½ inch open-cell foam pad over the anterior knee for additional compression to control swelling and effusion.*

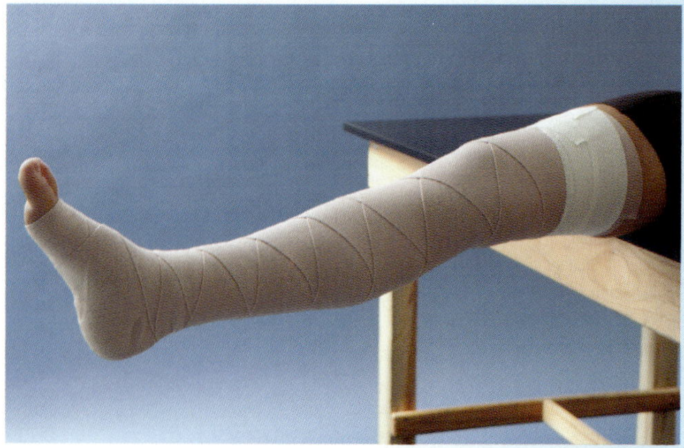

**Fig. 6–15**

## ▌KNEE COMPRESSION SLEEVE    Figure 6–16

▶ **Purpose:** The knee compression sleeve technique may also be used to control mild to moderate swelling and effusion (Fig. 6–16). Following proper instruction, this compression technique can be applied and removed by the patient without assistance.

▶ **Materials:**
- 3 inch, 4 inch, or 5 inch width elastic sleeve determined by the size of the lower leg and thigh, taping scissors

  ***Option:***
- ¼ inch or ½ inch open-cell foam

▶ **Position of the patient:** Sitting on a taping table or bench with the leg extended off the edge.

▶ **Preparation:** Cut a sleeve from a roll to extend from the proximal lower leg to the mid thigh area or from the distal lower leg to the mid thigh area. Cut and use a double-length sleeve to provide additional compression.

▶ **Application:**

**STEP 1:** Pull the sleeve onto the knee in a distal-to-proximal direction. If using a double-length sleeve, pull the distal end over the first layer to provide an additional layer (Fig. 6–16). No anchors are required. The elastic sleeve can be cleaned and reused.

*Option:* *An open-cell foam pad may be cut and placed over the anterior knee to assist in controlling swelling and effusion.*

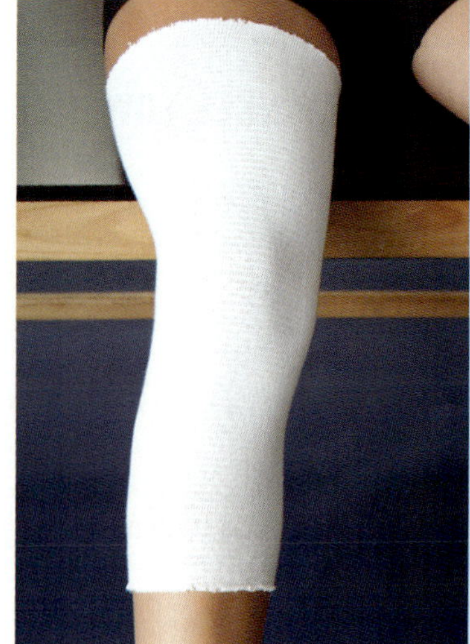

**Fig. 6–16**

**Clinical Application Question 2**

Several members of a high school wrestling team practice daily without any type of anterior knee padding. One particular athlete in the 103 lb weight class complains of pain over the prepatellar region with direct compression and passive knee flexion. Swelling has developed over the prepatellar area. Treatment consisting of ice, a compression wrap, and protective pad returns him to pain-free activity. Two weeks later, swelling returns to the prepatellar region and remains despite the use of a compression wrap. He is able to continue practice pain-free.

➡ **Question: What techniques are available to lessen the swelling?**

**. . . IF/THEN . . .**

**IF** considering when to use a compression wrap technique safely and effectively, **THEN** remember that an elastic wrap or sleeve can be used immediately following most injuries and/or surgeries to control swelling and effusion.

# Bracing Techniques

Bracing techniques for the knee provide immobilization, support, and compression, and they correct structural abnormalities when preventing and treating injuries and conditions. Generally, knee braces can be classified into three categories: prophylactic, rehabilitative, and functional. Other bracing techniques—also often used interchangeably within these categories—include neoprene sleeves, neoprene sleeves with hinged bars or buttress pads, and patellar tendon straps. Knee braces are available in off-the-shelf and custom-made designs and can be used for a variety of injuries and conditions.

## PROPHYLACTIC        Figure 6–17

➡ **Purpose:** Prophylactic braces are designed to prevent or reduce the severity of knee injuries (Fig. 6–17). The braces provide moderate support and are primarily used to protect the knee from valgus forces and injury to the MCL.

### DETAILS
Prophylactic knee braces are commonly used for preventing MCL sprains of athletes in collision and contact sports, such as football and ice hockey. The nonpliable brace materials are covered with padding that meets NCAA[11] and NFHS[12] rules.

➡ **Design:**
- The braces are available off-the-shelf in predetermined sizes, corresponding either to circumference measurements of the thigh and lower leg or the height of the patient.
- The braces are manufactured in a universal fit design and can be used on either knee.
- Most prophylactic designs consist of a stainless steel, polycarbonate, or aircraft aluminum bar with single, dual, or polycentric hinges.
- The braces contain a hyperextension block to prevent excessive range of motion.
- Several designs have additional nylon straps to limit migration.
- To provide additional stability, some designs contain a pressure pad that fits under the hinged bar over the lateral joint line of the knee.

**Knee**

➠ **Materials:**
 • 2 inch or 3 inch heavyweight elastic tape, pre-wrap, self-adherent wrap, adherent tape spray, taping scissors

➠ **Position of the patient:** Standing on a taping table or bench with the majority of the weight on the non-involved leg and the involved knee placed in slight flexion. Maintain this position by placing a 1½ inch lift under the heel.

➠ **Preparation:** Some prophylactic designs are attached directly to the skin over the lateral aspect of the thigh and lower leg with neoprene wraps, cuffs, or sleeves. Other designs are attached directly to the skin with elastic tape or over one layer of pre-wrap or self-adherent wrap. Apply adherent tape spray underneath neoprene, pre-wrap, or self-adherent wrap to lessen brace migration.

   Application of prophylactic designs should follow manufacturers' instructions, which are included with the braces when purchased. The following application guidelines pertain to most braces.

➠ **Application:**

**STEP 1:**   If using designs with neoprene attachments, begin by loosening the wraps, cuffs, or sleeves. Center the brace hinge over the lateral joint line of the knee with the bars extending proximally over the lateral thigh and distally over the lateral lower leg (Fig. 6–17A).

> **Helpful Hint |**
> Accommodate for migration during the initial positioning of the brace. After centering the hinge, reposition the hinge slightly superior to the lateral joint line. During activity, the hinge will migrate distally into the correct position over the lateral joint line.

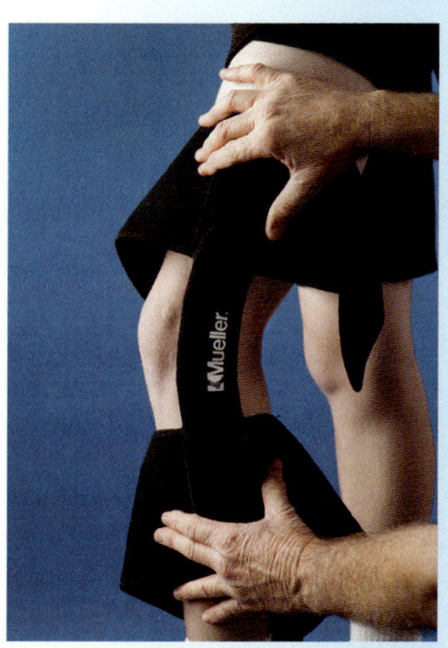

**Fig. 6–17 A**

**STEP 2:**   The application of neoprene wraps, cuffs, or sleeves will depend on the specific brace design. Apply most of these designs by wrapping the neoprene around the lower leg and thigh and anchoring with Velcro (Fig. 6–17B). With some designs, anchor additional straps over the neoprene.

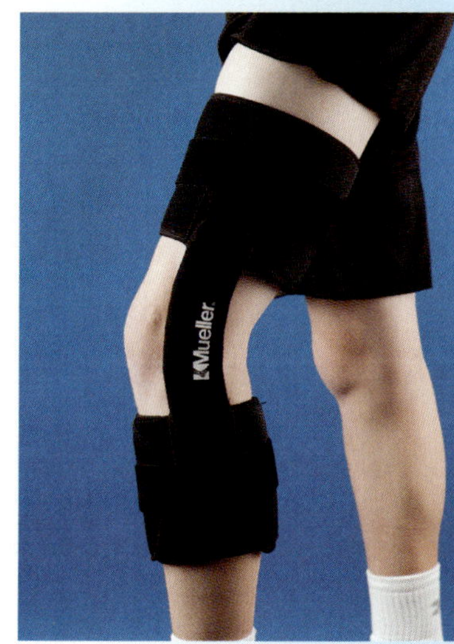

**Fig. 6–17 B**

**STEP 3:** With other designs, apply one layer of pre-wrap or self-adherent wrap directly over the distal thigh and proximal lower leg ◀▦▶. Anchor 2 inch or 3 inch heavyweight elastic tape directly on the proximal end of the brace bar and proceed around the thigh in a circular pattern with mild to moderate roll tension, overlapping the tape by ½ of its width with each pass ◀▦▶. Cover the entire end of the bar and anchor on the anterior thigh (Fig. 6–17C). Avoid gaps, wrinkles, and inconsistent roll tension. The tape may also be applied directly to the skin.

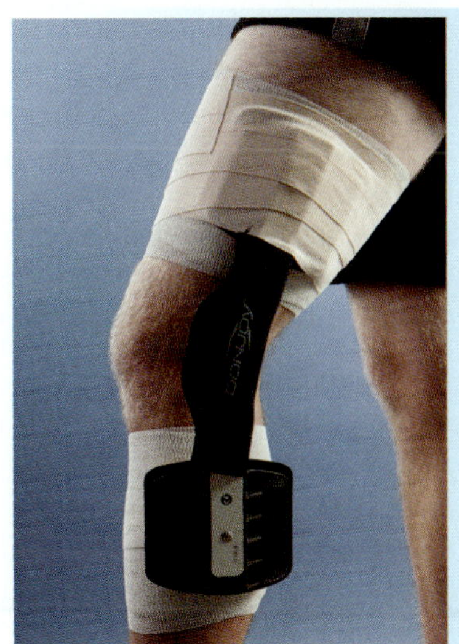

**Fig. 6–17 C**

**STEP 4:** Anchor 2 inch or 3 inch heavyweight elastic tape on the distal brace bar and proceed around the lower leg in a circular pattern with mild to moderate roll tension ◀▦▶ (Fig. 6–17D). Cover the entire end of the bar and anchor on the anterior lower leg. No additional anchors are required.

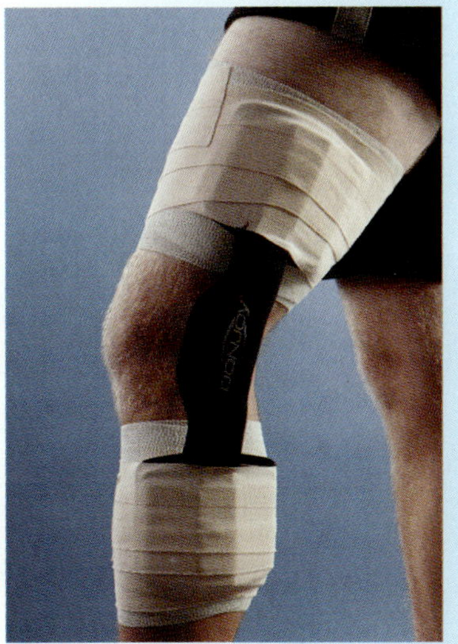

**Fig. 6–17 D**

## EVIDENCE SUMMARY

Prophylactic braces are designed and worn in an attempt to prevent injury to the structures of the knee. Health care professionals have a variety of brace designs from which to choose based on athlete needs, preferences, and comfort, facility financial resources, and available evidence supporting their effectiveness. Past investigations have examined the effects of prophylactic designs on the amount of protection they can provide against injurious forces and on functional performance outcomes. While some researchers found braces decreased injurious loads on the MCL and ACL in the laboratory using mechanical limb models or cadaver specimens, others found no protective benefit. Investigations focusing on the effects of brace wear on forward and backward sprint times, agility drills, and lower extremity muscle activity have produced conflicting findings.

Several evidence-based reviews have examined the effectiveness of prophylactic braces in the prevention of ligamentous knee injuries. A 2008 systematic review[13] included seven studies among intramural and intercollegiate tackle football athletes. The findings revealed that the use of prophylactic braces decreased the incidence of injury in three studies but increased injury incidence in four studies. These conflicting findings from studies conducted in the 1980s and 1990s among multiple prophylactic designs produced inconclusive evidence for the efficacy of prophylactic braces among American football athletes. A separate 2010 systematic review[14] that included six studies examined prophylactic braces among intramural, high school, and intercollegiate tackle football athletes. The findings from this review also produced inconclusive results. One study in the review[14] demonstrated a significant reduction in the incidence of knee injury with brace use and a separate investigation revealed a nonsignificant trend in lower injury incidence with braces. However, two studies showed no differences in injury incidence and two investigations reported an increased incidence of injury with the use of braces. Based on the limited evidence in the literature, the American Academy of Orthopaedic Surgeons[15] evidence-based clinical practice guidelines for the management of ACL injuries does not recommend the use of prophylactic braces to prevent injury to the ACL.

Preventing knee injuries is a concern for both the patient and health care professional. For the patient, issues such as lost time from athletic and work activities, quality of life, and cost of medical services must be considered. The health care professional must examine the personnel required for the application of preventive techniques and subsequent treatment and rehabilitation of injury and the cost-effectiveness of prophylactic brace use.

The limited, inconclusive evidence neither supports nor refutes the efficacy of prophylactic braces in preventing knee injuries. Future research with randomized controlled trials using current prophylactic designs among sports and activities with a high risk of knee injury are needed to determine the exact role and effectiveness of the braces in preventing injury.

## | REHABILITATIVE     Figures 6–18 and 6–19

➠ **Purpose:** Rehabilitative braces are designed to support, immobilize, and allow protected range of motion of the knee following injury and surgery. The braces can be used to treat knee sprains, meniscal tears, tendon ruptures, OSD, SLJ, fractures, dislocations, and subluxations. Two rehabilitative designs are illustrated below.

### *Rehabilitative: Immobilizer/Splint*

➠ **Purpose:** The immobilizer/splint brace provides mild to moderate support and complete immobilization of the knee (Fig. 6–18).

### DETAILS

The braces are commonly used (following acute injury or surgery) with crutches for non–weight-bearing ambulation. The braces may be removed for treatment and rehabilitation.

Consider using the braces in combination with the knee compression wrapping techniques to control swelling and effusion (see Figs. 6–14, 6–15, and 6–16).

➠ **Design:**
- These universal fit designed braces are available in predetermined sizes based on thigh and lower leg circumference measurements.
- The braces are available in various lengths, measured from the proximal/mid thigh to the mid/distal lower leg, to accommodate the height of the patient.
- The braces are constructed of foam and nylon/fiber laminate panels with Velcro strap closures.
- The designs have removable plastic or aluminum stays incorporated into the panels on the medial, lateral, and posterior surfaces.
- Some designs have popliteal pads to provide additional support and to lessen brace migration.
- Another design uses a rigid posterior splint incorporated into padded straps to provide immobilization.

➠ **Position of the patient:** Sitting on a taping table or bench with the knee in full extension.
➠ **Preparation:** Apply the braces directly to the skin or over tight-fitting pants.
   Specific instructions for applying the braces are included with each design. The following general application guidelines apply to most designs.
➠ **Application:**

**STEP 1:**    Begin by loosening the straps and unfolding the brace.

**STEP 2:**    With assistance, position the brace under the involved leg of the patient. Ensure proper alignment of the medial, lateral, and posterior stays as well as the patellar opening (Fig. 6–18A). Reposition the brace if necessary.

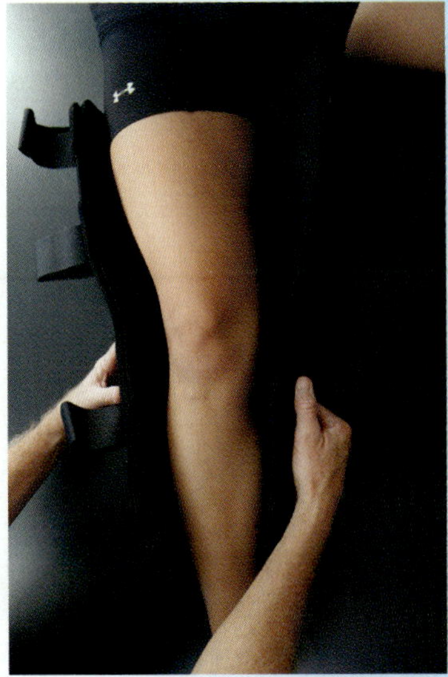

**Fig. 6–18 A**

**STEP 3:**    Bring the panels together over the anterior thigh, knee, and lower leg. Beginning at the superior patella, pull the strap tight and secure to the brace with Velcro (Fig. 6–18B). Next, pull the inferior patellar strap and anchor (Fig. 6–18C).

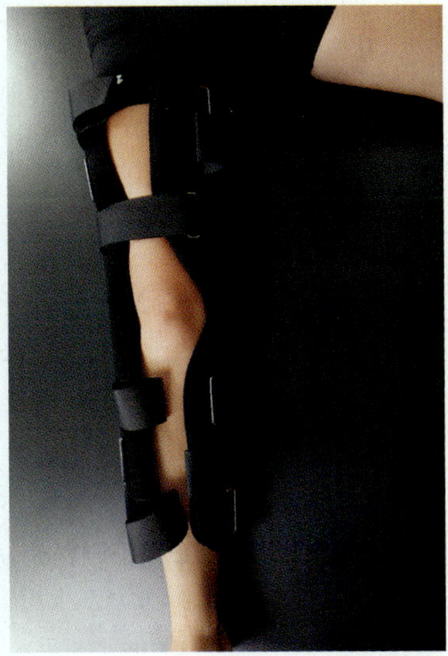

**Fig. 6–18 B**

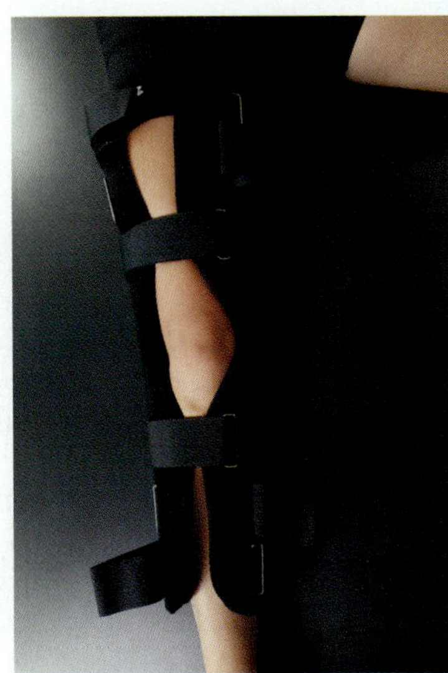

**Fig. 6–18 C**

*Steps Cont.*

**STEP 4:**  Continue to anchor the straps in this alternating pattern until all straps are anchored (Fig. 6–18D).

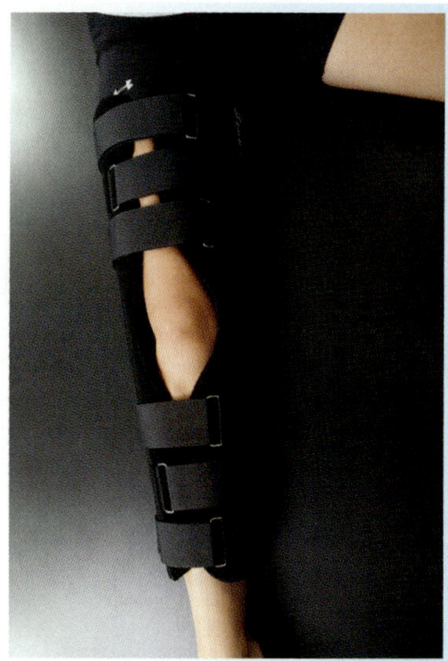

**Fig. 6–18 D**

### *Rehabilitative: Postsurgical*

➟ **Purpose:** Use the postsurgical brace to provide mild to moderate support, immobilization, and protected range of motion (Fig. 6–19). These braces can replace a plaster or fiberglass cast or a splint. The advantages of the braces include the following: they are removable, which allows for treatment and rehabilitation; they have adjustable range of motion; they are of lightweight design; and they support and control early weight-bearing.

---

**DETAILS**

The braces can be used following acute injury or surgery, with or without the use of crutches. This design may be used in combination with the compression wrapping techniques to control swelling and effusion (see Figs. 6–14, 6–15, 6–16).

---

➟ **Design:**
- The braces are manufactured in universal fit designs in predetermined sizes, corresponding either to circumference measurements of the thigh or the height of the patient.
- The designs are available in various lengths depending on the objective of the technique.
- Most designs consist of foam or polyethylene thigh and lower leg wraps or cuffs with medial and lateral hinged aluminum bars, attached with Velcro. The wraps or cuffs may be cut to achieve proper fit.
- Some designs have telescoping hinge bars to assist with comfort and size adjustments.
- The polycentric hinges on most designs allow for control and locking of range of motion. Some designs have easy-to-use dials for quick range of motion settings.
- Some designs have soft condyle pads to assist with repositioning of the knee joint angle.
- The designs have adjustable straps incorporated into the bars to anchor the brace to the thigh and lower leg with Velcro or buckles.

➟ **Position of the patient:** Sitting on a taping table or bench with the involved knee in a pain-free range of motion.

➟ **Preparation:** Set the brace range of motion at the desired settings of flexion and extension as indicated by a physician and/or therapeutic exercise program. Apply the brace directly to the skin or over tight-fitting pants.

Again, instructions for application are included with each brace. The following guidelines pertain to most designs.

> **Helpful Hint |**
> Following application of the brace, check the
> actual range of flexion and extension with a
> goniometer to ensure the correct settings.

**➡ Application:**

**STEP 1:**   Begin the application by loosening the straps and unfolding
the brace.

**STEP 2:**   Position the brace under the involved leg. Center the hinges with
the joint line and the bars along the medial and lateral thigh and
lower leg (Fig. 6–19A). Reposition the bars on the wraps or cuffs
with the Velcro attachments if necessary.

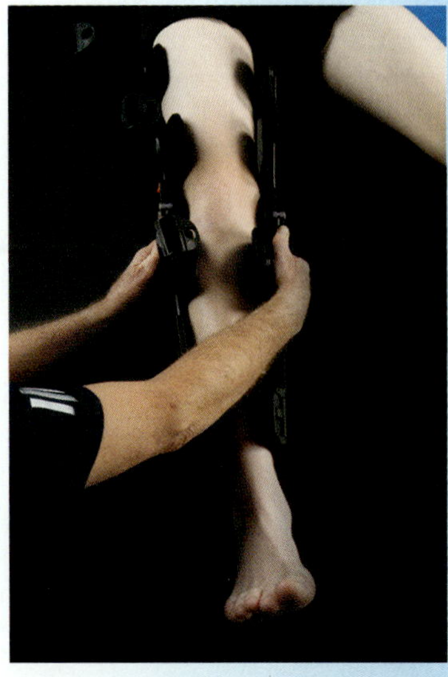

**Fig. 6–19 A**

**STEP 3:**   Anchor the wraps or cuffs around the thigh and lower leg. At the
superior patella, pull the strap tight and anchor. Next, anchor the
inferior patellar strap. Continue to anchor the remaining straps in
this alternating pattern (Fig. 6–19B).

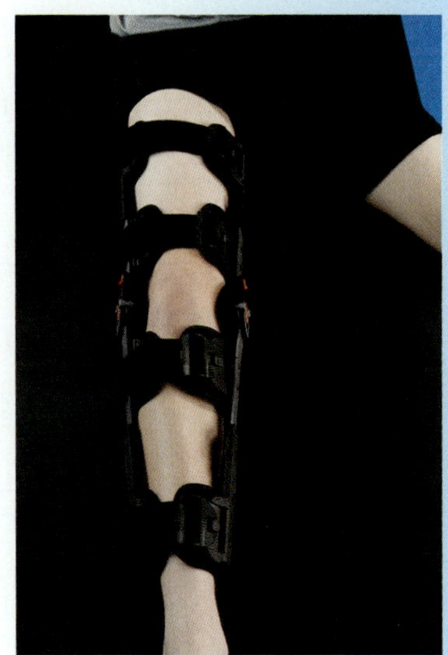

**Fig. 6–19 B**

**. . . IF/THEN . . .**

**IF** budget constraints allow for the purchase of only one type of rehabilitative brace, **THEN** consider the postsurgical
design, which allows for range of motion adjustments, from complete immobilization (the purpose of the immobilizer/
splint design) to full protected range of motion.

# EVIDENCE SUMMARY

Rehabilitative brace designs are used following injury and/or surgery to control flexion and extension and prevent valgus and varus stresses to provide protection for healing structures. The effectiveness of these brace designs on clinical and functional outcomes following ACL reconstruction has been investigated in three separate systematic reviews.[16–18] A 2008 review[16] included seven randomized controlled trials (RCTs) with brace wear during the early rehabilitative period (3 weeks to 3 months) following bone–patellar tendon–bone surgical techniques within an accelerated therapeutic exercise program. The findings demonstrated minimal long-term differences in knee laxity, swelling, pain, and range of motion, isokinetic peak torque of the quadriceps and hamstrings, functional tests, and complications when rehabilitative braces were compared to no braces. A 2012 review[17] included six RCTs examining brace wear during the early postoperative period (3 days to 6 weeks) following bone–patellar tendon–bone or hamstring autograft techniques within varied therapeutic exercise programs. The results showed no clinically significant differences between the use of braces and no braces at 14 days to 2-year periods in the outcomes of knee pain, laxity, joint position sense, isokinetic quadriceps and hamstring strength, and quadriceps and hamstring atrophy. In a 2016 review,[18] 20 studies among post-ACL reconstruction patients revealed insufficient evidence that brace wear within varied rehabilitation programs improved pain, stability, rehabilitation, and functional outcomes compared with no brace. Evidence-based clinical practice guidelines for the management of ACL injuries were developed in 2014 by the American Academy of Orthopaedic Surgeons[15] and do not recommend the use of postoperative functional bracing following isolated ACL reconstruction. Although using rehabilitative braces following isolated ACL reconstruction techniques is widely practiced by health care professionals, the evidence does not demonstrate their efficacy on long-term clinical and functional outcomes compared with no brace. Additionally, implementing this evidence into clinical practice may decrease the overall cost of rehabilitation[15] for the patient and health care facility.

## FUNCTIONAL       Figure 6–20

➡ **Purpose:** Functional braces are designed to provide moderate stability to the unstable knee following injury and surgery (Fig. 6–20). The braces are commonly used when treating ACL, PCL, MCL, and LCL sprains to control anterior tibial translation and rotary stress. Some health care professionals use functional braces prophylactically with athletes in collision and contact sports to provide optimal protection against unidirectional and multidirectional forces.

### DETAILS

Functional braces are commonly used to provide knee stability for athletes in a variety of sports. The braces can also be useful with work and casual activities.

The nonpliable materials of the brace must be padded to meet NCAA and NFHS rules. Off-the-shelf brace covers are available from some manufacturers to meet the standards.

➡ **Design:**
- Functional braces are available in three designs: bilateral hinge-post-shell, bilateral hinge-post-strap, and unilateral hinge-post-shell.[19]
- Bilateral hinge-post-shell designs consist of a rigid frame or shell, medial and lateral hinges, and soft straps. Bilateral hinge-post-strap designs are manufactured with medial and lateral hinges and soft straps. Unilateral hinge-post-shell designs are constructed of a rigid frame or shell, a medial or lateral hinge, and soft straps.
- These braces are available in off-the-shelf and custom-made designs in a right or left style.

- Off-the-shelf designs are manufactured in predetermined sizes corresponding to knee joint, distal thigh, and/or lower leg circumference measurements. The designs allow for small size adjustments during wear.
- Custom-made designs are manufactured for a specific patient following fitting by a manufacturer representative or orthopedic technician. The size cannot be adjusted after a custom-made brace is constructed.
- Most braces are available in short and standard length designs to accommodate different heights of patients and activities such as motocross, horseback riding, and skiing.
- Functional brace designs consist of a frame or shell, condyle pads, liners, and straps. With most designs, the liners and straps may be cut to achieve proper fit.
- The frames are constructed of tempered aluminum, carbon composite, metallic plastic composite, carbon fiber titanium, or carbon/graphite laminate materials with monocentric or polycentric hinges.
- The hinges allow control over the range of motion; most designs contain a hyperextension block.
- Most designs have suede and chamois condyle pads and liners and nylon straps with Velcro closures.
- Some designs have pneumatic condyle pads and liners to enhance fit and comfort.

➠ **Position of the patient:** Sitting in a chair with the knee in approximately 30 to 45 degrees of flexion.

➠ **Preparation:** Apply functional braces directly to the skin or over a Lycra or neoprene sleeve. Set the brace range of motion at the desired settings of flexion and extension. Loosen all straps.

Specific instructions for application of functional braces are included with each design. For proper application and use, follow the step-by-step procedure. The following general application guidelines apply to most functional designs.

➠ **Application:**

| **STEP 1:** | Hold each hinge and guide the patient to place the leg into the brace. Position the condyle pads just superior to the patella. Push the lower leg cuff in a posterior direction on the lower leg (Fig. 6–20A). |

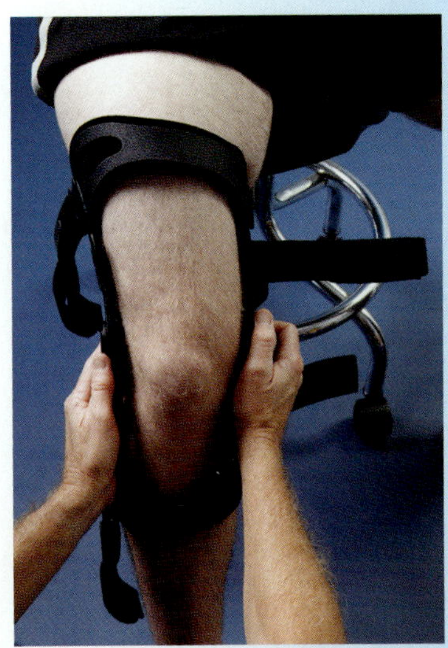

**Fig. 6–20 A**

*Steps Cont.*

**Knee**

**STEP 2:** Applying straps will depend on the specific brace design. Begin application of some designs by anchoring the distal posterior lower leg strap (Fig. 6–20B). Next, anchor the distal posterior thigh strap (Fig. 6–20C).

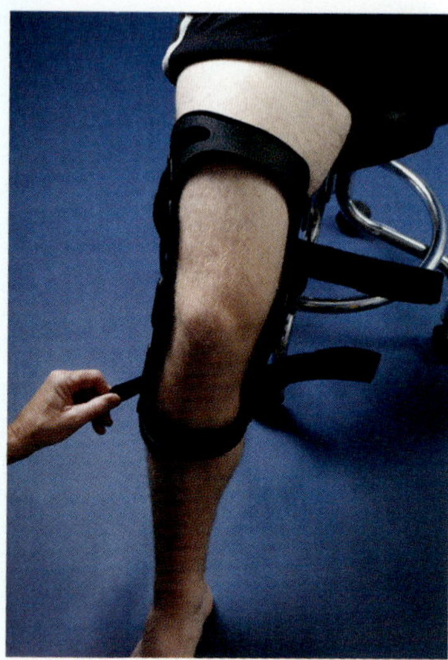

**Fig. 6–20 B**

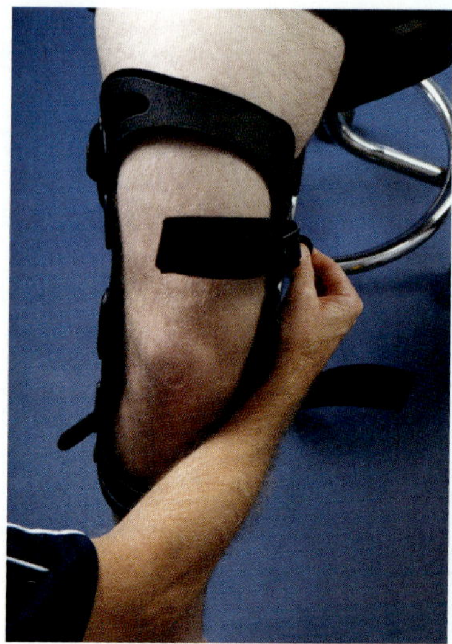

**Fig. 6–20 C**

**STEP 3:** With the thigh cuff firmly on the thigh, anchor the proximal posterior thigh strap (Fig. 6–20D).

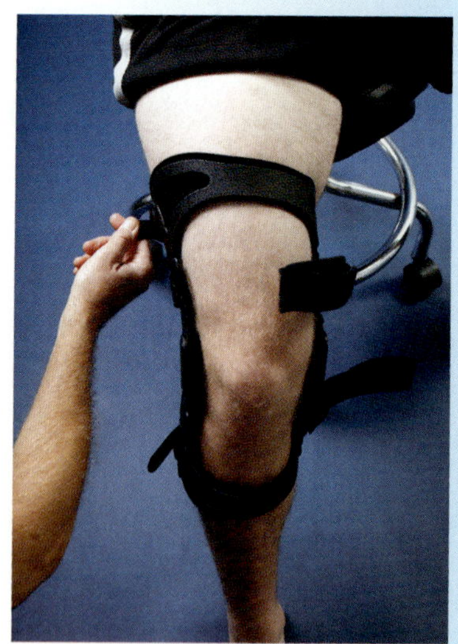

**Fig. 6–20 D**

**STEP 4:** Continue and anchor the distal anterior lower leg strap (Fig. 6–20E). Next, anchor the proximal posterior lower leg strap (Fig. 6–20F).

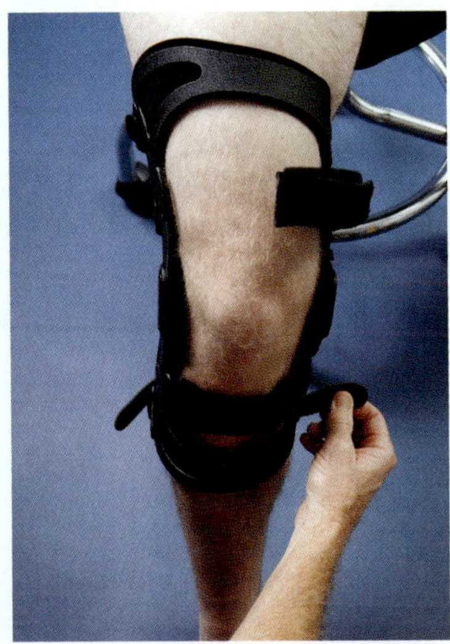

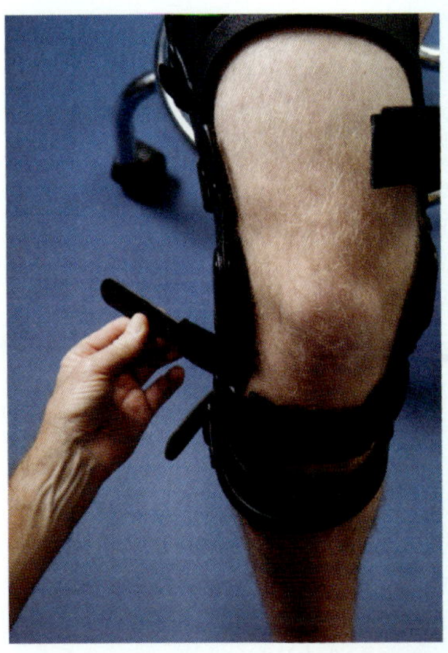

**Fig. 6–20 E**    **Fig. 6–20 F**

**STEP 5:** Allow the patient to stand and anchor the proximal anterior thigh strap (Fig. 6–20G). Allow the patient to walk to ensure proper fit. Retighten the straps and/or reposition the brace if necessary.

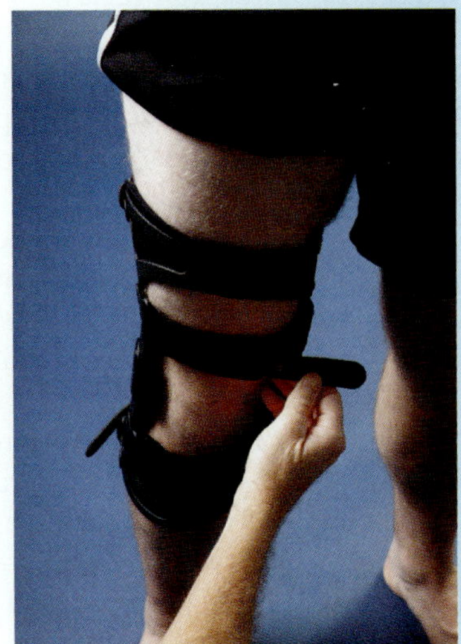

**Fig. 6–20 G**

# EVIDENCE SUMMARY

Functional braces are used to protect the unstable knee following injury and/or surgery. These braces have been used for many years by health care professionals during various phases of the treatment and rehabilitation process, and manufacturers continue to develop new designs. However, most functional braces are designed for the ACL-deficient or postreconstruction knee, with limited designs for PCL injuries. Research conducted to examine the effectiveness of functional bracing techniques has been inconsistent, and many questions remain unanswered. Two evidence-based reviews have investigated the effects of functional braces among post-ACL reconstruction patients.

A 2016 critically appraised topic[20] examined the effects of functional knee braces on knee joint position sense. The findings from three studies in the review were inconsistent that brace use produced improvements in active knee joint angle reproduction (active reproduction of a joint position) and threshold to detection of passive motion values (active detection of a change in joint position). Additionally, knee joint position sense in the included studies was evaluated in an open kinetic chain position. The researchers[20] suggested additional studies are needed to evaluate joint position sense in closed kinetic chain positions to determine the efficacy of functional braces on functional outcomes.

A 2017 systematic review[21] that included 15 studies investigated the effects of functional braces on knee kinematics, proprioception, muscle response, functional performance, and patient-reported outcomes among post-ACL reconstruction patients. Examining knee kinematics, six studies demonstrated that functional braces reduced anterior tibial translation force and tibial rotation and increased knee flexion angle and peak knee abduction moment. One study showed improvements in valgus/varus symmetry with brace wear. In contrast, two studies in the review reported no differences in valgus/varus symmetry between a brace and no-brace situation. The effects of functional braces on lower extremity proprioception was investigated in three studies. Functional braces were shown to increase joint angle replication and accuracy scores. Other studies in the review revealed no improvements in threshold to detection of passive motion values and balance test scores. Focusing on muscle response, three studies revealed functional braces decreased isokinetic peak torque of the quadriceps and hamstrings. Brace wear of 1 to 2 years was shown to decrease quadriceps muscle strength at 60 degrees of flexion, and brace wear of 3 months significantly increased quadriceps atrophy. However, there was no significant difference in quadriceps atrophy at 6 months between braces and non-braced subjects. Twelve studies in the review examined the effect of functional braces on functional performance and outcomes. The overall data showed no differences in knee joint laxity and range of motion and performance of single-leg hop, agility, jumping, landing accuracy, and running tests with brace wear compared to no brace. Several studies demonstrated no significant differences among brace and no-brace subjects for isokinetic quadriceps and hamstrings strength outcomes. Among post-ACL reconstruction skiers, one study demonstrated the use of functional braces reduced the risk of reinjury. Patient-reported function, quality of life, and pain outcomes were examined in three studies. The researchers[21] reported no significant differences in scores among braced and unbraced subjects. The results of this review[21] suggest that functional braces may protect the patient from tibial translation and rotation stresses, reducing the risk of reinjury without negative effects on functional performance. However, the investigators[21] cautioned that further research is needed to determine the efficacy of the designs in the prevention of injury.

Functional knee braces are widely used with ACL-deficient and post-ACL reconstruction patients to provide stability and lessen the risk of reinjury. Among members of the American Academy of Orthopaedic Surgeons, 62.9% recommended the use of functional braces for sports participation following ACL reconstruction.[22] Health care professionals can choose from a variety of off-the-shelf and custom-made functional brace designs when treating and rehabilitating knee injuries. Overall, the research to support the use of functional brace designs for ACL-deficient and post-ACL reconstruction patients and athletes is limited. Currently, there is no one best brace design available. Based on the vast use of functional braces for the prevention and treatment of ACL, PCL, MCL, and LCL injuries, additional research is needed to provide evidence to guide brace use and the development of future designs. Quality research examining the effects of functional braces on unidirectional, multidirectional, and rotary forces on the knee, injury incidence, long-term functional outcomes, and patient comfort and compliance can assist health care professionals in the selection of the most appropriate brace design.

## ...IF/THEN...

**IF** protection from valgus and varus forces is needed following a sprain, **THEN** use a functional brace design; remember that most prophylactic braces are constructed with a single hinged bar designed to prevent or lessen injury only from valgus forces.

## Clinical Application Question 3

A rookie defensive end on a professional football team sustains a first-degree MCL sprain of the left knee during training camp. His history includes two previous first-degree MCL sprains of the same knee that occurred during his 4 year intercollegiate career. After completing a rehabilitation program, he is allowed to return to practice. The team physician is concerned about laxity of the MCL and the risk of trauma to other structures in the left knee.

➡ **Question: What techniques can be used in this situation?**

## NEOPRENE SLEEVE    Figure 6–21

➡ **Purpose:** Neoprene sleeves provide compression and mild support when treating contusions, sprains, meniscal tears, PFP, quadriceps tendinitis, chondromalacia, plica, bursitis, and overuse injuries and conditions (Fig. 6–21).

### DETAILS

The sleeves may be used during rehabilitative, athletic, work, and casual activities.

➡ **Design:**
- The off-the-shelf sleeves are manufactured in universal fit designs in predetermined sizes corresponding to thigh and knee circumference measurements.
- Some designs cover the patella (closed patella), while others are cut-out (open patella) over the area.
- Several designs also have a cut-out area over the popliteal space (open popliteal).
- Another design uses a strap that wraps around the knee and waist to control excessive internal rotation of the hip.

➡ **Position of the patient:** Sitting on a taping table or bench with the leg extended off the edge, or in a chair, with the knee in approximately 45 degrees of flexion.

➡ **Preparation:** Apply neoprene sleeves directly to the skin; no anchors are required.

➡ **Application:**

**STEP 1:**   Hold each side of the sleeve and place the larger end over the foot. Pull in a proximal direction until the sleeve is positioned on the knee (Fig. 6–21).

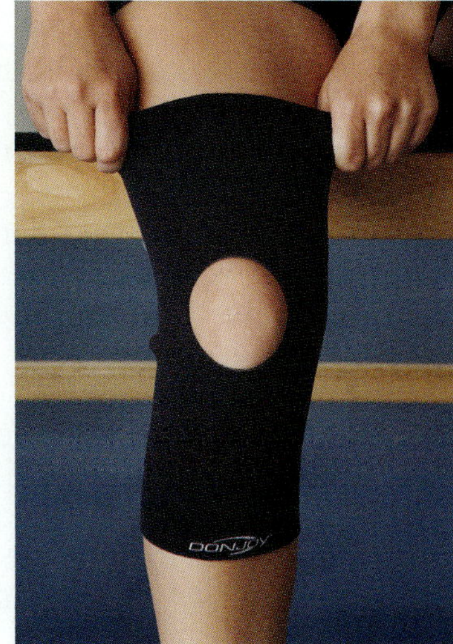

**Fig. 6–21**

## EVIDENCE SUMMARY

Neoprene knee sleeves are typically used to provide warmth, compression, and mild support following injury. Despite their frequent use, there is a limited amount of research examining the efficacy of neoprene sleeves. A 2017 systematic review[23] investigated the effects of various knee sleeves on gait, balance, proprioception, and functional performance. Among osteoarthritic patients, the review demonstrated that knee sleeves significantly improved knee flexion angle and reduced knee adduction angle during walking. Other researchers found knee sleeves produced no significant changes in tibial rotation during walking among healthy subjects. Two studies in the review[23] found significant improvements in anterior/posterior, static, and dynamic balance scores with sleeves among healthy and osteoarthritic subjects. A separate study among osteoarthritic subjects demonstrated no significant differences in center of pressure sway with brace wear. Examining joint position sense, knee sleeves were shown to improve accuracy and awareness among healthy and post-ACL reconstruction subjects. Knee sleeves did not change threshold to detection of passive motion among healthy subjects. One study in the review[23] demonstrated improvements in acuity among healthy subjects with poor baseline acuity during non-fatigued and isokinetic knee extensor and flexor fatigued conditions. The effects of knee sleeves on functional performance parameters among healthy, post-ACL reconstruction, and osteoarthritic subjects revealed improved scores in mobility, balance, and muscular power tests. Other studies in the review found no differences among knee sleeves in vertical jump and single-leg hop measures. Based on the various neoprene brace designs examined in the studies, the authors[23] suggested that different designs could influence outcome measures; sleeves with hinged bars may provide additional lateral knee stability and designs with an open patella greater patella stability.

The limited results appear to indicate that neoprene sleeves influence gait, balance, proprioception, and specific functional performance measures among various populations. Health care professionals should consider the construction and materials of neoprene sleeves to guide the selection of the most appropriate design based on the patient's injury or condition. Additional research is needed with well-designed randomized controlled trials with longer intervention durations to determine the efficacy of neoprene knee sleeves to guide prevention and rehabilitation interventions.

## NEOPRENE SLEEVE WITH HINGED BARS    Figure 6–22

➡ **Purpose:** Neoprene sleeves with hinged bars provide compression and mild to moderate support to the knee following injury (Fig. 6–22). These braces are commonly used when treating mild and moderate MCL and LCL and mild ACL and PCL sprains to control valgus, varus, and rotary stresses.

### DETAILS

Use the sleeves during rehabilitation, athletic, work, and casual activities. The nonpliable materials, commonly the hinges, must be padded to meet NCAA[11] and NFHS[12] rules.

➡ **Design:**
- The universal fit sleeves are available off-the-shelf in predetermined sizes corresponding to thigh, knee, and/or lower leg circumference measurements.
- The sleeves are manufactured in standard and short length designs to accommodate patient height differences.
- Most designs consist of a one-piece neoprene sleeve with medial and lateral hinged aluminum bars and two or four nylon strap closures. Other sleeves are constructed of breathable materials such as latex-free nylon and polyester Lycra.
- Some designs use a contoured sleeve that wraps around the knee to accommodate hard-to-fit leg shapes. These designs are anchored on the anterior thigh and lower leg with Velcro.
- The sleeves are constructed with an open patella front; some sleeves also have an open popliteal space cut-out.

- Most designs have a polycentric hinge that allows for range of motion control. A hyperextension block is also available.
- Most designs are constructed with proximal and distal pockets or pouches that anchor the medial and lateral bars to the sleeve. Outer nylon straps provide further support to the bars.
- To provide additional support, some designs have condyle pads located under the hinges at the joint line, attached to the sleeve with Velcro.
- Some designs are available with a fixed and/or adjustable buttress incorporated into the sleeve.

➡ **Position of the patient:** Sitting on a taping table or bench with the leg extended off the edge, or in a chair, with the knee in approximately 45 degrees of flexion.

➡ **Preparation:** Apply neoprene sleeves with hinged bars directly to the skin; no anchors are required. Set the brace range of motion at the desired settings of flexion and extension.

Follow the instructions of the manufacturer when applying the sleeves. The following application guidelines pertain to most sleeves.

➡ **Application:**

**STEP 1:**    Begin by loosening the thigh and lower leg straps.

**STEP 2:**    Grasp the loops above the proximal ends of the bars and pull the brace in a proximal direction over the knee. Center the hinges over the joint line with the cut-out positioned over the patella (Fig. 6–22A).

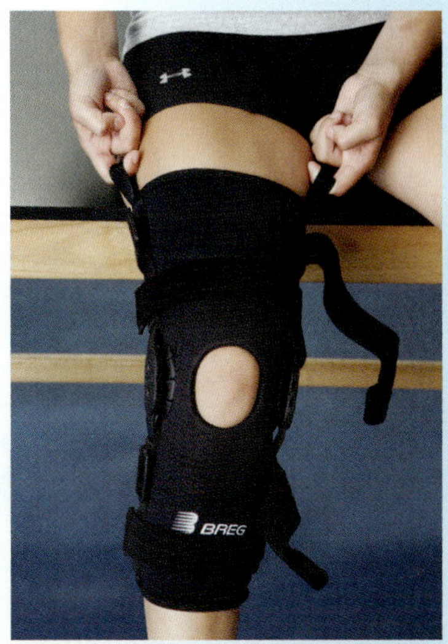

**Fig. 6–22 A**

**STEP 3:**    With the contoured or wraparound design, position the brace on the posterior thigh and lower leg. Wrap the sleeve around and anchor on the anterior thigh and lower leg with Velcro closures (Fig. 6–22B). Center the hinges over the joint line.

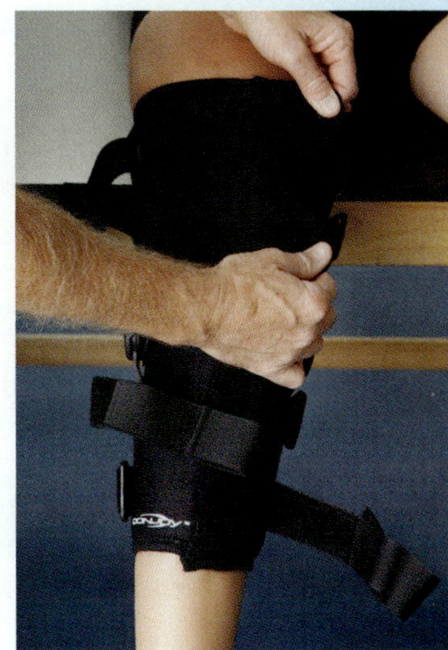

**Fig. 6–22 B**

*Steps Cont.*

**Knee**

**STEP 4:**   The application of straps will depend on the specific sleeve design. Apply most by pulling the straps tight and anchoring with Velcro (Fig. 6–22C).

**Helpful Hint |**
Elastic wrap, clothing fibers, and debris from playing surfaces often adhere to the male ends of the Velcro closures and lessen adherence. To increase adherence, clean the male ends of fibers and debris with small, pointed scissors or tweezers.

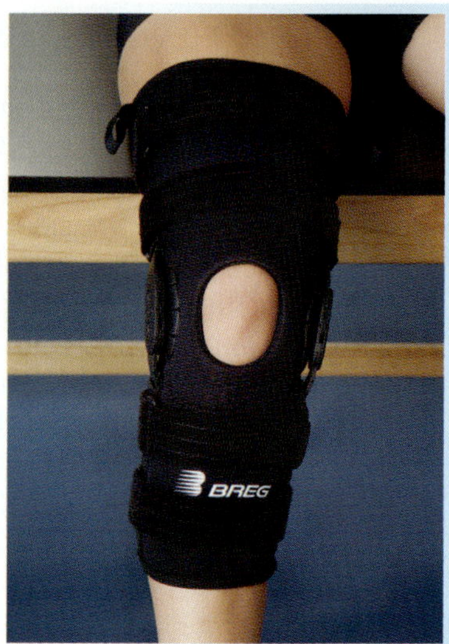

**Fig. 6–22 C**

**. . . IF/THEN . . .**

**IF** support and protection are needed following a MCL sprain and taping is not an option, **THEN** consider using a prophylactic or neoprene sleeve with hinged bars brace design, which will protect against valgus forces and further injury.

**Clinical Application Question 4**

A forward on an intercollegiate ice hockey team suffers a first-degree LCL sprain of the right knee. Following a short period of rehabilitation, the athlete is allowed to return to activity. The team physician requests that the knee be supported and protected from further injury for a period of 2 weeks during all practices and competitions. During this 2 week period, 10 practices and two competitions will occur.

➡ **Question: Which taping or bracing technique can you use? Which technique would be cost-effective?**

## NEOPRENE SLEEVE WITH BUTTRESS     Figures 6–23 and 6–24

➡ **Purpose:** Neoprene sleeves with buttresses provide compression, reduce friction and stress, provide mild to moderate support, and correct structural abnormalities. Use these sleeves when treating PFP, chondromalacia, patellar dislocations and subluxations, patellar tendinitis, and OSD. A variety of buttress sleeve designs are available to treat these injuries and conditions.

### DETAILS
Fixed and adjustable sleeves can be used with athletic, work, and casual activities.

- These sleeves may be purchased off-the-shelf in right and left styles, with predetermined sizes corresponding to thigh and knee circumference measurements.
- The designs consist of a neoprene or breathable material sleeve with a fixed or adjustable buttress with various straps.

### *Fixed Buttress*

➠ **Design:**
- Fixed buttresses are incorporated into the brace and do not allow for adjustments during application or activity (Fig. 6–23).
- Fixed buttress sleeves are constructed with an open patella front, surrounded by a felt, silicone, rubber, foam, or pneumatic buttress in the shape of an uppercase "C," "H," "J," or "U," or circular pattern.
- The "C"- and "J"-shaped buttresses are designed to limit lateral movement of the patella.
- The "H"-shaped buttress is designed to limit inferior and superior patellar movement, while the "U"-shaped buttress limits inferior movement.
- Circular buttresses are designed to stabilize the patella in multidirectional ranges of motion.
- Many designs are available with an open popliteal space.
- Some designs have proximal and distal straps with Velcro closures to support and stabilize the buttress and anchor the brace to the thigh and lower leg.
- Several designs are constructed with medial and lateral hinged aluminum bars with polycentric hinges.

➠ **Position of the patient:** Sitting on a taping table or bench with the leg extended off the edge, or in a chair, with the knee in approximately 45 degrees of flexion.

➠ **Preparation:** Apply fixed buttress sleeves directly to the skin; no anchors are required.

➠ **Application:**

**STEP 1:** Place the larger end of the sleeve over the foot and pull in a proximal direction. Position the cut-out over the patella and the buttress against the patella. Following the manufacturer's instructions, pull the straps tight and secure to the sleeve with Velcro (Fig. 6–23).

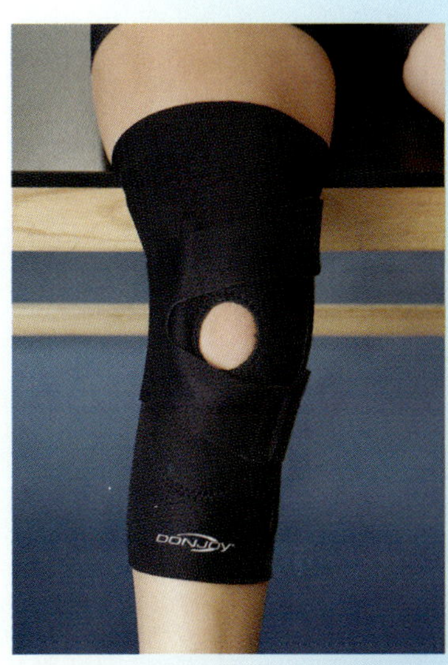

**Fig. 6–23**

### *Adjustable Buttress*

➠ **Design:**
- These designs allow adjustment of the buttress that is incorporated into the sleeve and/or adjustment of various straps to provide additional support to the patella (Fig. 6–24).
- The sleeves are manufactured with an open patella front; some sleeves also have an open popliteal space.
- Many adjustable designs contain a "C," "H," "J," "U," or circular buttress that one can reposition and/or trim to achieve the desired compression and support.
- Some designs use various straps with Velcro attachments incorporated into the sleeve to limit excessive patellar range of motion.

- Several other sleeves are manufactured with a fixed buttress and adjustable straps.
- Most strap designs are attached on the lateral aspect of the sleeve. The straps are normally pulled in a medial direction to limit lateral movement of the patella.
- Some adjustable designs use both a buttress incorporated into the sleeve and an external buttress to limit excessive patellar range of motion.
- Another design uses an external buttress plate attached to a tension hinge to adjust support to the patella throughout knee range of motion.
- Some designs use an elastomeric web or strap to adjust support and compression to the patella.
- Several designs are available with medial and lateral hinged aluminum bars with polycentric hinges.

➠ **Position of the patient:** Sitting on a taping table or bench with the leg extended off the edge, or in a chair, with the knee in approximately 45 degrees of flexion.

➠ **Preparation:** Apply adjustable buttress sleeves directly to the skin; no anchors are required.

   The manufacturer includes specific instructions for fitting and application. For proper fit and support, follow the step-by-step procedures. The following application guidelines apply to most sleeves.

➠ **Application:**

**STEP 1:**   To apply, pull the sleeve over the foot and onto the knee. Adjust the cut-out and buttress over and around the patella (Fig. 6–24A).

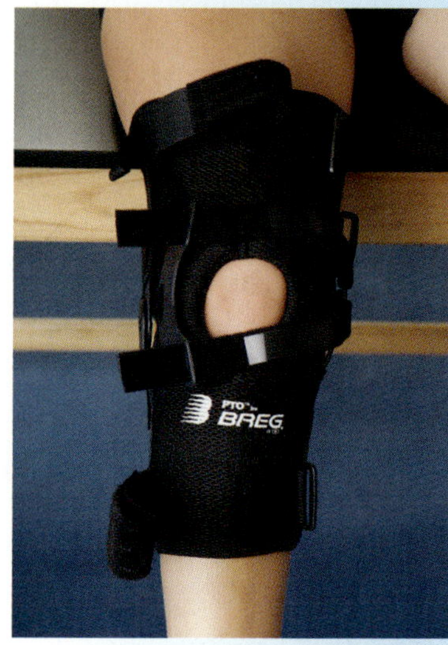

**Fig. 6–24 A**

**STEP 2:**   Applying straps will depend on the specific brace design. Generally, pull these straps tightly in a medial direction over the thigh and lower leg and anchor on the medial or lateral sleeve with Velcro (Fig. 6–24B).

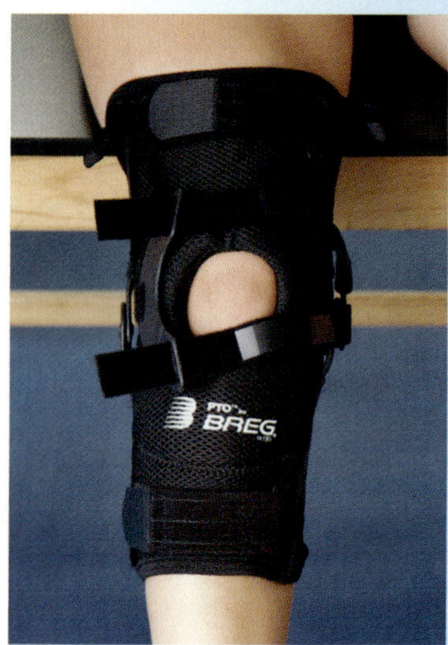

**Fig. 6–24 B**

**STEP 3:** Position the external buttresses just next to the lateral patella and pull the straps across the superior and inferior patella; anchor on the medial or lateral sleeve (Fig. 6–24C).

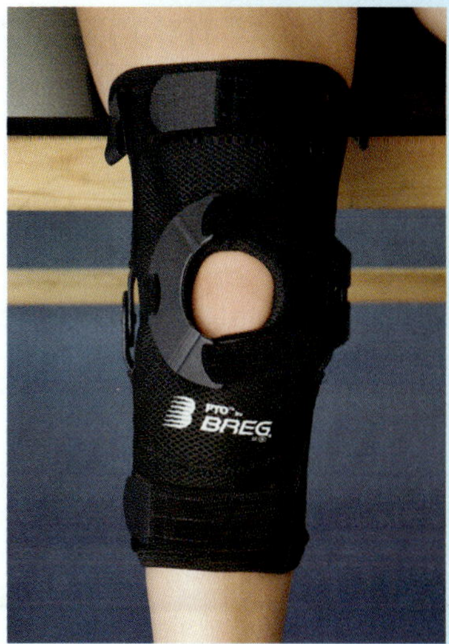

**Fig. 6–24 C**

**...IF/THEN...**

**IF** an athlete requires support of the patella in the treatment of PFP or patellar subluxation, **THEN** use a neoprene sleeve with buttress brace; although a neoprene sleeve does provide support, a fixed or adjustable buttress brace provides greater support and stabilization of the patella and surrounding soft tissues, lessening excessive movement.

## EVIDENCE SUMMARY

Neoprene sleeves with buttresses are designed to influence the position of the patella in the trochlear groove and correct abnormal patellar tracking in the treatment of many anterior knee injuries and conditions.[24] In a 2015 evidence-based review,[25] researchers demonstrated a lack of evidence to determine the efficacy of various knee brace designs in the treatment of patellofemoral pain (PFP) among adults in outpatient orthopedic and military settings. Examining patient-reported knee pain and function scores, the review[25] found no clinically significant differences between neoprene sleeve, neoprene sleeve with buttress, and patellar tendon strap designs worn within a therapeutic exercise program and therapeutic exercise alone after 6 to 12 weeks. Therapeutic exercise programs varied among the five trials in the review and included isometric and isotonic hip and lower extremity strengthening and flexibility exercises and/or military training. Other results showed no differences in pain and function scores between neoprene sleeves with therapeutic exercise and neoprene sleeves with buttress and patellar tendon strap braces with therapeutic exercise at 8 to 12 week periods. No significant differences were found in the review[25] for pain and function scores between the use of neoprene sleeves and neoprene sleeves with buttresses within a therapeutic exercise program after 12 weeks. Based on the limited findings from the low-quality trials in the review,[25] neoprene sleeve, neoprene sleeve with buttress, and patellar tendon strap braces used in combination with therapeutic exercise appear to be ineffective in reducing knee pain and improving knee function after 12 weeks[25] among adults with PFP. The 2018 International Patellofemoral Pain Research Retreat consensus statement[10] found insufficient evidence to recommend patellar bracing in the management of PFP. Further research is needed with high-quality randomized controlled trials among various populations to determine the long-term effects of knee braces used alone or within a comprehensive therapeutic exercise program. This evidence can be integrated with clinician expertise with bracing designs and specific patient needs to guide clinical decisions for the treatment of anterior knee injuries and conditions.

Knee

## PATELLAR TENDON STRAP    Figure 6–25

➠ **Purpose:** Several patellar tendon strap brace designs exist to lessen tension on the tendon at the inferior pole of the patella and/or at the tibial tubercle to treat patellar tendinitis, OSD, PFP, and chondromalacia (Fig. 6–25).

### DETAILS
Use the straps with athletic, work, or casual activities. Patellar tendon straps may be used in combination with neoprene sleeves to provide compression and support.

➠ **Design:**
- The straps are available off-the-shelf in universal styles and predetermined sizes that correspond to inferior knee circumference measurements. Some designs are available in universal sizes.
- The straps are constructed of neoprene or foam composite materials with Velcro closures.
- Most designs contain a semitubular or tubular foam, viscoelastic, foam/air cell, or padded plastic buttress incorporated into the strap. Some designs allow for custom molding and fitting.

➠ **Position of the patient:** Sitting on a taping table or bench, or in a chair, with the knee placed in slight flexion.

➠ **Preparation:** Apply patellar tendon straps directly to the skin; no anchors are required.

➠ **Application:**

**STEP 1:**   To apply, place the semitubular/tubular buttress over the patellar tendon, between the inferior pole of the patella and tibial tubercle (Fig. 6–25A).

**STEP 2:**   Pull the ends snugly together and anchor on the posterior knee with the Velcro closures (Fig. 6–25B). Allow the patient to perform a previously painful activity. Readjust the strap if necessary.

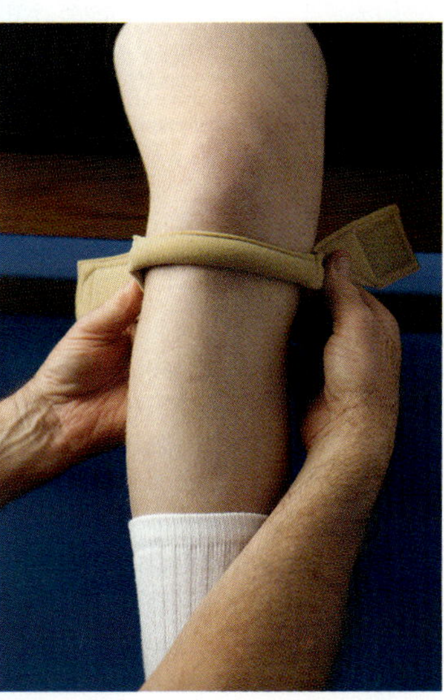

**Fig. 6–25 A**

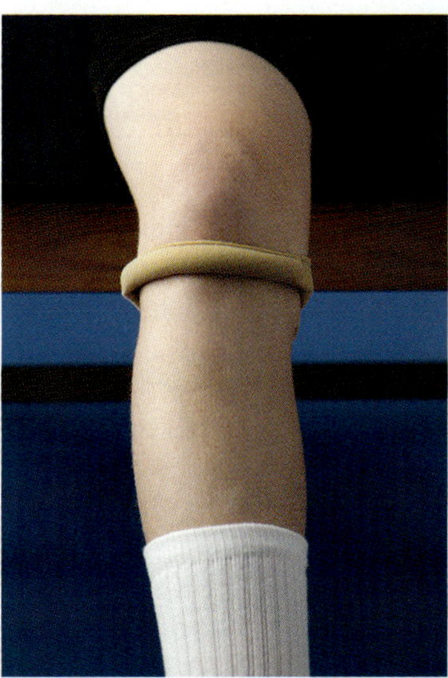

**Fig. 6–25 B**

## EVIDENCE SUMMARY

A brace technique for the patellar tendon was first introduced in 1978,[26] and many designs are currently available and used by patients to lessen pain associated with patellar tendinitis or tendinopathy. However, limited investigations have examined the clinical and biomechanical effects of patellar tendon braces among patients with patellar tendinitis.

The effects of patellar tendon strap braces and patellar taping on pain associated with patellar tendinopathy have resulted in positive outcomes. Researchers[27] found significant reductions in visual analogue scales of pain perception with the use of patellar tendon strap braces and patellar taping during performance of a single-leg decline squat compared with a no-brace and no-tape situation. However, during vertical jump and triple-hop tests, no significant differences in pain scores were demonstrated among patellar braces and taping, placebo taping, and a control. Patellar tendon strap braces, patellar taping, and placebo taping resulted in significant reductions in pain 2 hours after completion of sport activity compared to no-brace and no-tape situations.[27] Following 1 week of sports participation with these interventions, patellar and placebo taping produced significant reductions in pain scores. Other researchers demonstrated significant reductions in visual analogue scales of pain perception with patellar tendon strap braces during drop jump,[28] single-leg jump,[28] and single-leg landing[29] tests compared to no-brace controls. However, no significant differences in pain scores were revealed during squat jump and double-leg continuous jump tests and overall jumping performance among brace and no-brace situations.[28]

Other researchers[30] have examined the effects of patellar tendon strap braces on proprioception among subjects with and without patellar tendinopathy. The findings demonstrated a significant improvement in threshold to detection of passive motion in both groups of subjects compared to no-strap. The strap brace was also shown to significantly improve threshold to detection of passive motion in both groups of subjects categorized with low proprioceptive acuity. Other researchers[31–33] have demonstrated improvements in

knee extensor mechanism (distal quadriceps, quadriceps tendon, patella, and patellar tendon) function and decreased muscular reaction time with patellar tendon braces. Examining subjects with and without patellar tendinopathy, researchers[34] demonstrated significantly lower electromyographic activity of the vastus lateralis among the strap brace group than among the no-brace group during pre-landing of a double-leg drop activity. During the performance of a single-leg landing test, researchers[29] revealed significant decreases in hip internal rotation, knee adduction, ankle inversion, and peak vertical ground reaction force with patellar strap braces compared to no-brace. The researchers[29] suggested the influence of strap braces on jump landing may indicate a more neutral landing alignment, lessening tension on the patellar tendon. Few studies have examined the mechanical effects of these braces to determine the specific mechanism of action. Using knee cadaver specimens, several investigators found patellar tendon braces decreased patellar contact area and pressure and infrapatellar tissue pressure.[35]

Based on the available evidence in the literature, additional studies are necessary to investigate patellar tendon braces. Future research should examine the long-term effects of these braces on the patellar tendon, patella, and surrounding musculature to understand the mechanism of development and progression to effectively guide prevention and treatment interventions.

## | ORTHOTICS

- ➡ **Purpose:** Orthotics provide support, absorb shock, and correct structural abnormalities when treating knee injuries and conditions.
  - Use soft orthotic designs (see Fig. 3–18) to absorb shock and lessen stress on the patellar tendon to treat OSD and SLJ. The soft designs can also be used to absorb shock when preventing and treating stress fractures of the tibial tubercle, tibial plateau, and femoral condyles. Heel cups and full-length neoprene, silicone, and viscoelastic polymer insoles are available in off-the-shelf designs.
  - Use semirigid (see Fig. 3–19) and rigid (see Fig. 3–20) orthotics to provide support and correct structural abnormalities like excessive foot pronation, leg-length discrepancy, genu varus or valgum, or external tibial torsion. Semirigid and rigid orthotics can be used to treat iliotibial band friction syndrome, chondromalacia, PFP, and pes anserinus bursitis and tendinitis. The designs can be purchased off-the-shelf or custom-made.

## EVIDENCE SUMMARY

A 2011 meta-analysis[36] investigated the efficacy of orthotics among adults with patellofemoral pain. Two randomized controlled trials (RCTs) compared the use of off-the-shelf EVA orthotics with a therapeutic exercise program consisting of hip and thigh stretching and strengthening. One RCT included patellar mobilization and taping in the program. The researchers found no differences in patient-reported knee pain and function scores between orthotics used in combination with therapeutic exercise and therapeutic exercise alone after 6, 8, and 52 weeks. Other findings showed the use of orthotics improved knee function scores after 6 and 52 weeks when compared to therapeutic exercise, but no differences were found in knee pain scores during the reporting periods. One RCT in the review[36] examined orthotics and insoles and found insoles reduced knee pain scores after 6 weeks, but there were no differences in pain scores at 52 weeks and in knee function scores at 6 and 52 weeks. This review[36] provides limited evidence to support the use of orthotics in the management of patellofemoral pain in adults. A consensus statement[10] from the International Patellofemoral Research Retreat recommends the use of therapeutic exercise with off-the-shelf orthotics, patellar taping, or manual therapy for the reduction of short- and medium-term patellofemoral pain. Recommendations also support the use of off-the-shelf orthotics to reduce short-term knee pain. The authors[10] found no evidence to recommended therapeutic exercise, off-the-shelf orthotics, patellar taping, and manual therapy in the management of long-term patellofemoral pain in adolescents and adults. Additionally, no evidence was demonstrated for the use of custom-made orthotics to lessen knee pain. While these findings provided some evidence for the use of orthotics, further research is needed to determine their role and efficacy among various populations for the development of evidence-based management protocols.

### Clinical Application Question 5

The first mate on a charter fishing boat sustains a torn ACL of the left knee. After imaging studies and a clinical examination by a surgeon, the surgeon schedules ACL reconstruction. The surgeon schedules the procedure 2 weeks post-injury to allow for a reduction in effusion and an increase in range of motion. The first mate will receive daily therapy at a local out-patient orthopedic clinic and can ambulate as tolerated.

➡ **Question: What wrapping and bracing techniques can you use during the 2 week period?**

# Padding Techniques

A variety of off-the-shelf padding techniques can prevent and treat injuries and conditions of the knee. Another option is using foam and felt to provide compression, reduce stress, and absorb shock. The use of padding for the knee is mandatory with several interscholastic and intercollegiate sports. These mandatory techniques will be discussed further in Chapter 13.

## OFF-THE-SHELF   Figures 6–26 and 6–27

➡ **Purpose:** Off-the-shelf padding techniques are available from manufacturers in a variety of designs. These techniques provide shock absorption and protection when preventing and treating bursitis, OSD, SLJ, and contusions of the soft tissue and bone of the knee. Following is a description of two basic designs.

### Soft, Low-Density

**DETAILS**

Soft, low-density pads are commonly used to provide shock absorption to the knees of athletes in sports such as baseball, basketball, football, ice hockey, lacrosse, softball, volleyball, and wrestling. Use the pads with work and casual activities.

➡ **Design:**
- The pads are manufactured in a universal fit design in predetermined sizes, corresponding either to circumference measurements of the thigh or the weight of the patient (Fig. 6–26A).
- Most pads are constructed of varying thicknesses of high-impact open- and closed-cell foams, covered with polyester/spandex or woven fabric materials.
- Several designs consist of a neoprene sleeve with additional foam incorporated on the anterior aspect.
- Some designs have an open popliteal space, while others have a closed space.

➠ **Position of the patient:** Sitting on a taping table or bench with the leg extended off the edge, or in a chair, with the knee in approximately 45 degrees of flexion.
➠ **Preparation:** Apply the soft, low-density designs directly to the skin or over tight-fitting clothing.
➠ **Application:**

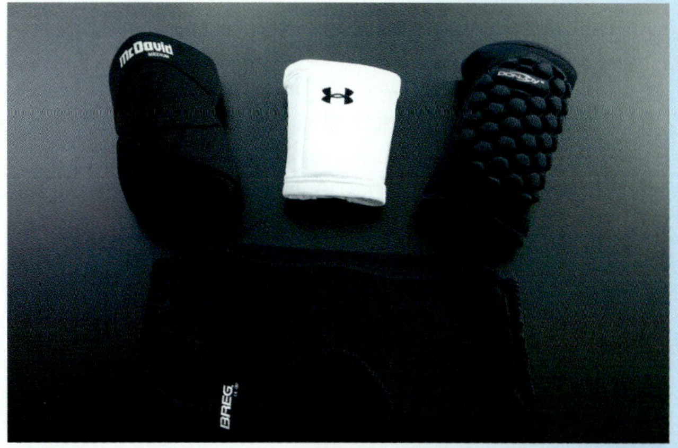

**Fig. 6–26 A** *Variety of soft, low-density pads. (Bottom) Padded cover for a functional ACL knee brace.*

**STEP 1:**  To apply the pad, place the larger end over the foot and pull in a proximal direction onto the knee (Fig. 6–26B).

**Helpful Hint |**
Off-the-shelf soft, low-density pads can cause irritation in the popliteal space. To lessen the chance of irritation, apply a skin lubricant and/or thin foam pads over the area or purchase pad designs with an open popliteal space.

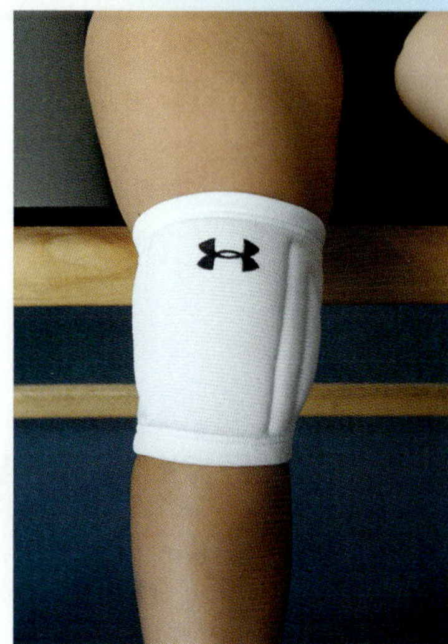

**Fig. 6–26 B**

### Hard, High-Density

**DETAILS**
Hard, high-density pads are commonly used to provide shock absorption to the knees of athletes in sports such as baseball, ice hockey, and softball. Use the pads in work and casual activities, such as kneeling, which may result in chronic or prolonged compression.

➠ **Design:**
  • The universal fit designs are available in predetermined sizes based on lower leg circumference measurements or age of the patient (Fig. 6–27A).
  • Most designs are constructed of a polycarbonate or plastic material outer shell pre-molded to the contours of the knee.
  • The outer shell is lined with open- and closed-cell foams and is incorporated into a vinyl pad that extends in all directions to provide shock absorption.
  • Another design uses a polycarbonate cup lined with foam that attaches to the hinges of functional knee braces to protect the patella.

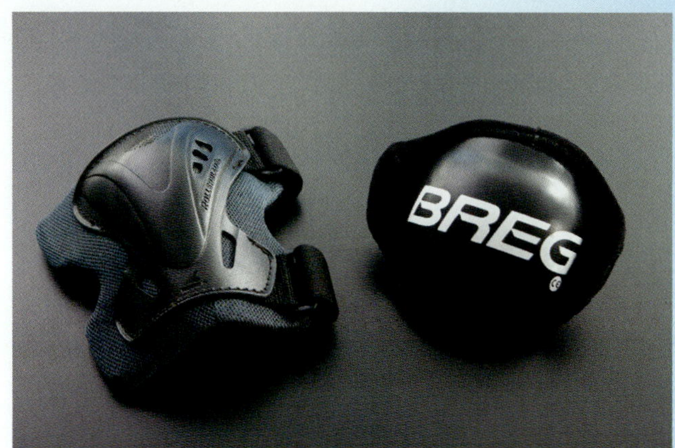

**Fig. 6–27 A** *Variety of hard, high-density pads. (Right) Pad that can be attached to a functional ACL knee brace to protect the anterior knee.*

- The pads are available in various lengths depending on the technique objective.
- Hard, high-density pads are attached to the knee with various adjustable nylon straps with Velcro or buckle closures.

➡ **Position of the patient:** Sitting on a taping table or bench with the leg extended off the edge, or in a chair, with the knee in approximately 45 degrees of flexion.

➡ **Preparation:** Apply the hard, high-density designs directly to the skin or over tight-fitting clothing.

➡ **Application:**

**STEP 1:**  Place the pad over the anterior knee. Applying straps will depend on the specific design. Normally, pull the straps across the posterior knee and anchor on the pad with Velcro or buckle closures (Fig. 6–27B). Readjust the straps if necessary for proper fit. Pad all nonpliable materials to meet NCAA and NFHS rules.

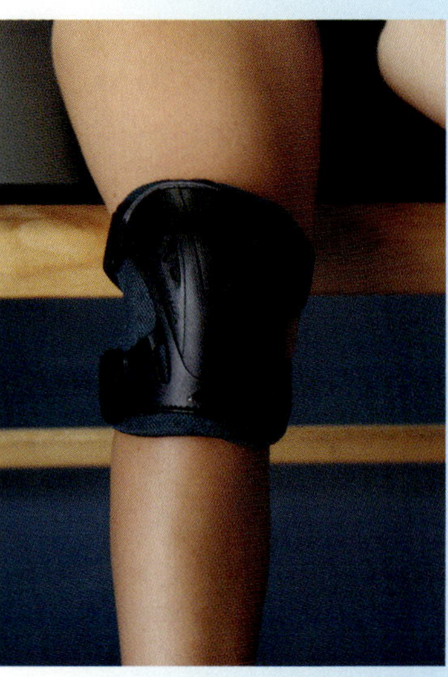

**Fig. 6–27 B**

## COMPRESSION WRAP PAD          Figure 6–28

➡ **Purpose:** The compression wrap pad technique helps to reduce mild, moderate, or severe swelling and effusion in the acute treatment of knee contusions, sprains, meniscal tears, fractures, dislocations/subluxations, bursitis, and overuse conditions (Fig. 6–28).

➡ **Materials:**
- ¼ inch or ½ inch open-cell foam, taping scissors

➡ **Position of the patient:** Sitting on a taping table or bench with the leg extended off the edge.

➡ **Preparation:** Apply the pad directly to the skin.

➡ **Application:**

**STEP 1:**  Extend the pad across the anterior knee, from the medial-to-lateral joint line and from the suprapatellar pouch to the tibial tubercle (Fig. 6–28A).

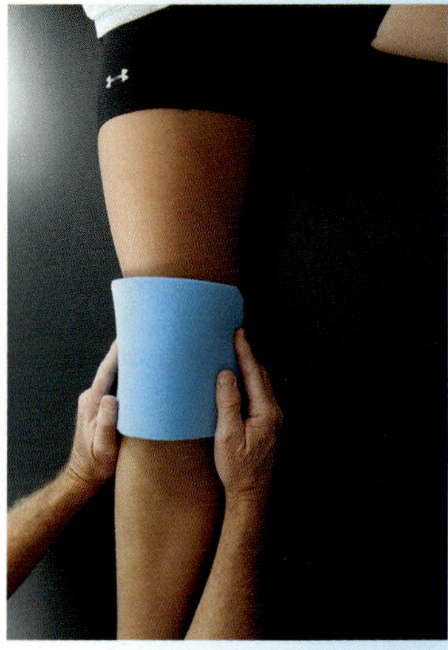

**Fig. 6–28 A**

**STEP 2:** Position the pad over the anterior knee and apply the compression wrap technique to anchor (see Figs. 6–14, 6–15, 6–16, and 6–28B).

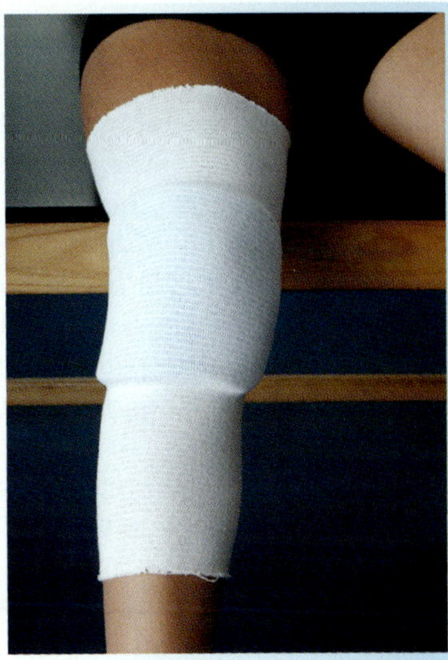

**Fig. 6–28 B**

## HEEL LIFT

→ **Purpose:** The heel lift pad technique (see Fig. 5–16) reduces stress in the treatment of an infrapatellar fat pad contusion. The heel lift elevates the hindfoot and lessens stress on the fat pad that may occur during knee extension.
- Construct the heel lift pads from ½ inch or 1 inch felt, or purchase heel lift pads with an adhesive backing.
- Cut the pad to cover the heel or shoe liner area.
- Use a pad on each heel or in each shoe to prevent adaptive changes.
- Apply the pad to the heel or shoe liner (see Fig. 5–16).

## DONUT PADS

→ **Purpose:** Use the donut pad technique (see Fig. 3–26) to lessen the amount of stress over an inflamed area when treating contusions and bursitis.
- Make the pads from ⅛ inch or ¼ inch foam or felt or purchase them pre-cut with adhesive backing.
- Attach the pad directly to the skin over the prepatellar, infrapatellar, pes anserinus, or semimembranosus bursa, the infrapatellar fat pad, or the peroneal nerve using adhesive gauze material (see Fig. 3–15) or attach in a circular pattern with loosely applied 1½ inch or 2 inch elastic tape.
- Consider anchoring the pad with the compression wrapping techniques (see Figs. 6–14, 6–15, and 6–16).

## MANDATORY PADDING

Mandatory protective equipment for the knee is required by the NCAA[11] and the NFHS[12] in several sports. Athletes participating in baseball, field hockey, football, ice hockey, and softball must wear protective padding during all practices and competitions. These padding techniques are available in a variety of off-the-shelf designs. Chapter 13 provides a full discussion of these padding techniques.

### Clinical Application Question 6
Over the past week, a tile layer has noticed tingling and numbness along the lateral aspect of his lower leg that radiates in a distal direction toward his foot. The pain is worse at the end of the work day. Recently, his company issued new hard, high-density knee pads to all employees that fit snugly around the proximal lower leg.
→ **Question: How can you manage this situation?**

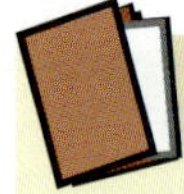

# EVIDENCE-BASED PRACTICE

Over the past several weeks, Ron Daubenmire has experienced a progressively worsening dull, aching pain in the right anterior knee. Ron is a science teacher at Helmick High School and rides with a local cycling club on Saturdays. He first noticed the pain at school when descending stairs and rising from a prolonged sitting position. The pain has progressed and is now present during walking, running, and squatting movements. During most weeks, he runs 5–6 miles and cycles 20–35 miles in preparation for a 30–50 mile Saturday club ride. However, his schedule has not allowed him to visit a fitness center or gym for strengthening and flexibility exercises. Ron enjoys cycling with the club and does not want to take any time off to treat his right anterior knee pain. Last Saturday during a club ride, he noticed that he was unable to perform to the level of the other members because of muscular fatigue and pain in the right knee.

Ron decides to walk down to the football stadium after school the next week to seek assistance from the sports medicine staff. He enters the athletic training facility and speaks with Angela Waybright, the AT at the high school. After gathering a history from Ron, Angela tells him to return later that afternoon for an evaluation. During the evaluation, Angela finds point tenderness along the lateral facet of the right patella, tightness of the lateral retinaculum, and lateral tracking of the patella. Compression of the patella into the patellofemoral groove also produces pain. Angela discovers inflexibility of the right posterior leg musculature with bilateral range of motion testing. Manual muscle testing reveals weaknesses in the right medial quadriceps and hip adductors. Ron is placed on a treadmill for a dynamic evaluation, and Angela finds excessive pronation of the right foot during walking and running gaits. Angela begins to discuss her findings with Ron as the team physician arrives in the athletic training facility for the afternoon injury clinic. Angela continues talking with Ron; when she is finished, the team physician examines Ron. The evaluation produces the same positive findings, and the team physician and Angela agree that Ron is suffering from PFP. The team physician recommends that Ron be placed into a comprehensive treatment program for the condition.

Angela and the team physician decide to place Ron into a therapeutic exercise protocol that uses rest, avoidance of painful activities, flexibility exercises for tight structures, retraining and strengthening of weak musculature, correction of structural abnormalities, and modalities for symptomatic treatment. Ron tells Angela about a friend in the cycling club who had similar knee pain last year. Ron remembers the friend wore a bracing technique for his knee and was told the technique lessened the pain, but was uncomfortable to wear while cycling. Angela is not certain of the specific bracing technique used by Ron's friend. Angela decides to research taping and bracing techniques that would support and correct the structural abnormalities and lessen stress and pain to allow Ron to continue to comfortably ride with the cycling club.

1. Develop a clinically relevant question from the case in the PICO format to generate answers for the integration of taping and bracing techniques for Ron. The question should include the population or problem, the intervention, a comparison intervention (if relevant), and the clinical outcome of interest.
2. Design a search strategy and search to find the best evidence to answer the clinical question. The strategy should include relevant search terms, electronic databases, online journals, and print journals to use for the search. Discussions with your faculty, preceptor, and other health care professionals can provide evidence from expert opinion.
3. Choose three to five full text studies or reviews from your search or the chapter references. Evaluate and appraise each article to determine its value and usefulness to the case. Ask these questions for each study: (1) Are the results of the study valid? (2) What are the actual results? and (3) Are the findings clinically relevant to my patients? Prepare a summary of the evaluation with answers to the questions and rank the articles based on the evidence hierarchy in Chapter 1.
4. Integrate findings from the evidence, your clinical experience, and Ron's goals and preferences into the therapeutic exercise program for Ron. Consider which taping and bracing techniques may be appropriate.
5. Evaluate the EBP process and your experience within the case. Consider these questions in the evaluation.

Was the clinical question answered?
Did the search generate quality evidence?
Was the evidence evaluated appropriately?
Was the evidence, your clinical experience, and Ron's goals and values integrated to make the clinical decision?
Did the intervention produce successful clinical outcomes for Ron?
Was the EBP experience positive for Angela and Ron?

## WRAP-UP

- Unidirectional, multidirectional, rotary, and compression forces; structural abnormalities; inflexibility and weakness of soft tissue; and repetitive stress can cause injury to the knee.
- The McConnell taping technique provides support when correcting patellofemoral malalignment.
- The hyperextension and collateral "X" taping techniques can be used to reduce range of motion and provide support when treating sprains.
- The patellar tendon strap taping and bracing techniques lessen the tension of the tendon on the inferior pole of the patella and/or the tibial tubercle.
- Elastic wraps and sleeves control swelling and effusion following injury.
- Prophylactic knee braces provide protection and reduce severity of injury, rehabilitative braces provide support and protected range of motion following injury/surgery, and functional braces provide stability following injury/surgery.
- The neoprene sleeve and sleeve with hinged bars bracing techniques provide compression and support to the knee.
- Neoprene sleeves with buttress braces provide compression, reduce stress, and correct structural abnormalities when treating acute and chronic injuries.
- Orthotics and the heel lift padding technique can be used to provide support, absorb shock, and correct structural abnormalities.
- Soft, low-density; hard, high-density; and donut padding techniques provide shock absorption, protection, and compression, and reduce stress.
- Mandatory protective equipment is required for the knee in several sports by the NCAA and NFHS.

## ⓢ FADAVIS ONLINE RESOURCES

- Collateral "X" taping technique
- Hyperextension taping technique two
- Patellar tendon strap technique three

## WEB REFERENCES

**American Academy of Orthopaedic Surgeons**
  https://www.aaos.org/
  - This website allows you to search for information on the mechanism, treatment, and rehabilitation of knee injuries, including the American Academy of Orthopaedic Surgeons Clinical Practice Guidelines.

**United States National Library of Medicine**
  https://www.nlm.nih.gov/
  - This website provides access to knee injury prevention, treatment, and rehabilitation information among a variety of populations.

**Arthritis Foundation**
  https://www.arthritis.org/
  - This site allows you to search for information about the causes and treatment of knee pain associated with arthritis.

**International Patellofemoral Research Network**
  https://ipfrn.org/
  - This site allows access to the research group for information on the causes and recommendations for the treatment and rehabilitation of patellofemoral pain.

## REFERENCES


1. Prentice, WE: Principles of Athletic Training: A Guide to Evidence-Based Clinical Practice, ed 16. McGraw-Hill, New York, 2017.
2. Bernstein, J: Meniscal tears of the knee: Diagnosis and individualized treatment. Phys Sportsmed 28:83, 2000.
3. Anderson, MK: Foundations of Athletic Training: Prevention, Assessment, and Management, ed 6. Wolters Kluwer, Philadelphia, 2017.
4. McConnell, JS: The management of chondromalacia patellae: A long term solution. Austr J Physiother 32:215–233, 1986.
5. Crossley, K, Cowan, SM, Bennell, KL, and McConnell, J: Patellar taping: Is clinical success supported by scientific evidence? Manual Ther 5:142–150, 2000.
6. McConnell, J: A novel approach to pain relief pretherapeutic exercise. J Sci Med Sport 3:325, 2000.
7. Callaghan, MJ, and Selfe, J: Patellar taping for patellofemoral pain syndrome in adults. Cochrane Database Syst Rev (4):CD006717, 2012.
8. Leibbrandt, DC, and Louw, QA: The use of McConnell taping to correct abnormal biomechanics and muscle activation patterns in subjects with anterior knee pain: A systematic review. J Phys Ther Sci 27:2395–2404, 2015.
9. Logan, CA, Bhashyam, AR, Tisosky, AJ, Haber, DB, Jorgensen, A, Roy, A, and Provencher, MT: Systematic review of the effect of taping techniques on patellofemoral pain syndrome. Sports Health 9:456–461, 2017.
10. Collins, NJ, Barton, CJ, van Middelkoop, M, Callaghan, MJ, Rathleff, MS, Vicenzino, BT, Davis, IS, Powers, CM, Macri, EM, Hart, HF, de Oliveira Silva, D, and Crossley, KM: 2018 consensus statement on exercise therapy and physical interventions (orthoses, taping and manual therapy) to treat patellofemoral pain: Recommendations from the 5th International Patellofemoral Pain Research Retreat, Gold Coast, Australia, 2017. Br J Sports Med 52:1170–1178, 2018.
11. National Collegiate Athletic Association: 2014–15 Sports Medicine Handbook, ed 25. NCAA, Indianapolis, 2014. http://www.ncaapublications.com/productdownloads/MD15.pdf.

12. National Federation of State High School Associations: 2018 Football Rules Book. National Federation of State High School Associations, Indianapolis, 2019.

13. Pietrosimone, BG, Grindstaff, TL, Linens, SW, Uczekaj, E, and Hertel, J: A systematic review of prophylactic braces in the prevention of knee ligament injuries in collegiate football players. J Athl Train 43:409–415, 2008.

14. Salata, MJ, Gibbs, AE, and Sekiya, JK: The effectiveness of prophylactic knee bracing in American football: A systematic review. Sports Health 2:375–379, 2010.

15. American Academy of Orthopaedic Surgeons. Management of Anterior Cruciate Ligament Injuries: Evidence-based Clinical Practice Guideline. https://www.aaos.org/globalassets/quality-and-practice-resources/anterior-cruciate-ligament-injuries/anterior-cruciate-ligament-injuries-clinical-practice-guideline-4-24-19.pdf, 2019.

16. Smith, TO, and Davies, L: A systematic review of bracing following reconstruction of the anterior cruciate ligament. Physiotherapy 94:1–10, 2008.

17. Kruse, LM, Gray, B, and Wright, RW: Rehabilitation after anterior cruciate ligament reconstruction. J Bone Joint Surg Am 94:1737–1748, 2012.

18. Rodríguez-Merchán, EC: Knee bracing after anterior cruciate ligament reconstruction. Orthopedics 39:e602–e609, 2016.

19. Liu, SH, and Mirzayan, R: Current review: Functional knee bracing. Clin Orthop Relat Res 317:273–281, 1995.

20. Sugimoto, D, LeBlanc, JC, Wooley, SE, Micheli, LJ, and Kramer, DE: The effectiveness of functional knee brace on joint position sense in anterior cruciate ligament reconstructed individuals. J Sport Rehabil 25:190–194, 2016.

21. Lowe, WR, Warth, RJ, Davis, EP, and Bailey, L: Functional bracing after anterior cruciate ligament reconstruction: A systematic review. J Am Acad Orthop Surg 25:239–249, 2017.

22. Marx, RG, Jones, EC, Angel, M, Wickiewicz, TL, and Warren, RF: Beliefs and attitudes of members of the American Academy of Orthopaedic Surgeons regarding the treatment of anterior cruciate ligament injury. Arthroscopy 19:762–770, 2003.

23. Mohd Sharif, NA, Goh, SL, Usman, J, and Wan Safwani, WKZ: Biomechanical and functional efficacy of knee sleeves: A literature review. Phys Ther Sport 28:44–52, 2017.

24. Bizzini, M, Childs, JD, Piva, SR, and Delitto, A: Systematic review of the quality of randomized controlled trials for patellofemoral pain syndrome. J Orthop Sports Phys Ther 33:4–20, 2003.

25. Smith, TO, Drew, BT, Meek, TH, and Clark, AB: Knee orthoses for treating patellofemoral pain syndrome. Cochrane Database Syst Rev (12):CD010513, 2015.

26. Levine, I: A new brace for chondromalacia patellae and kindred conditions. Am J Sports Med 3:137–140, 1978.

27. de Vries, A, Zwerver, J, Diercks, R, Tak, I, van Berkel, S, van Cingel, R, van der Worp, H, and van den Akker-Scheek, I: Effect of patellar strap and sports tape on pain in patellar tendinopathy: A randomized controlled trial. Scan J Med Sci Sports 26:1217–1224, 2016.

28. Dar, G, and Mei-Dan, E: Immediate effect of infrapatellar strap on pain and jump height in patellar tendinopathy among young athletes. Prosthet Orthot Int 43:21–27, 2019.

29. Rosen, AB, Ko, J, and N Brown, C: Single-limb landing biomechanics are altered and patellar tendinopathy related pain is reduced with acute infrapatellar strap application. Knee 24:761–767, 2017.

30. de Vries, AJ, van den Akker-Scheek, I, Diercks, RL, Zwerver, J, and van der Worp, H: The effect of a patellar strap on knee joint proprioception in healthy participants and athletes with patellar tendinopathy. J Sci Med Sport 19:278–282, 2016.

31. Cowan, SM, Bennell, KL, and Hodges, PW: Therapeutic patellar taping changes the timing of vastus muscle activation in people with patellofemoral pain syndrome. Clin J Sport Med 12:339–347, 2002.

32. Gilleard, W, McConnell, J, and Parsons, D: The effect of patellar taping on the onset of vastus medialis obliquus and vastus lateralis muscle activity in persons with patellofemoral pain. Phys Ther 78:25–32, 1998.

33. Ng, GY: Patellar taping does not affect the onset of activities of vastus medialis obliquus and vastus lateralis before and after muscle fatigue. Am J Phys Med Rehabil 84:106–111, 2005.

34. Rosen, AB, Ko, J, Simpson, KJ, and Brown, CN: Patellar tendon straps decrease pre-landing quadriceps activation in males with patellar tendinopathy. Phys Ther Sport 24:13–19, 2017.

35. Bohnsack, M, Halcour, A, Klages, P, Wilharm, A, Ostermeier, S, Rühmann, O, and Hurschler, C: The influence of patellar bracing on patellar and knee load-distribution and kinematics: An experimental cadaver study. Knee Surg Sports Traumatol Arthrosc 16:135–141, 2008.

36. Hossain, M, Alexander, P, Burls, A, and Jobanputra, P: Foot orthoses for patellofemoral pain in adults. Cochrane Database Syst Rev (1):CD008402, 2011.

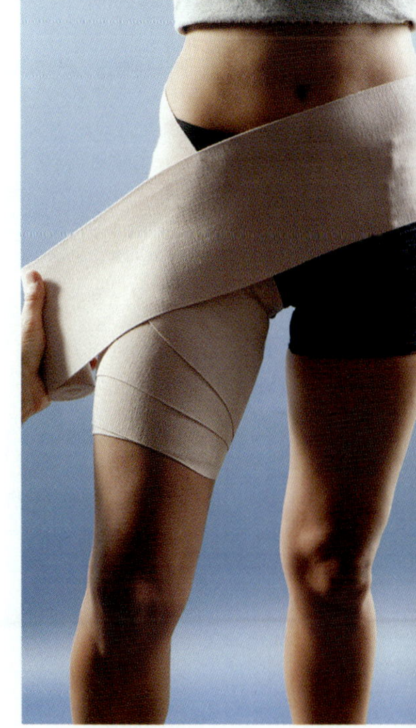

**7**

# Thigh, Hip, and Pelvis



## INJURIES AND CONDITIONS

Acute and chronic injuries can occur to the thigh, hip, and pelvis in athletic and work activities. Thigh and hip contusions are common in athletic activities but vary in severity. Many athletes are able to return to activity following a mild contusion with additional padding, while a severe contusion may require hospitalization. Strains of the thigh and hip musculature can occur in athletic and work activities and are typically caused by rapid movements. Repetitive stress to the thigh, hip, and pelvis can result in chronic inflammation and/or stress fractures. Common injuries to the thigh, hip, and pelvis include:

• Contusions
• Strains
• Overuse injuries and conditions

## Contusions

Contusions to the thigh, hip, and pelvis are caused by direct forces. These areas are susceptible to injury in many sports that do not require protective padding. Thigh contusions **(charley horse)** typically involve the anterior and/or lateral aspect (Fig. 7–1). A contusion can result, for instance, when a soccer sweeper is struck in the anterior/lateral right thigh by an opponent's knee while attempting to stop a breakaway (Fig. 7–2). **Heterotopic ossification** (sometimes referred to as **myositis ossificans**) may result from a single, violent direct force or repeated direct forces to the anterior or lateral thigh[1,2] (Fig. 7–3). A delay in treatment, forceful manipulation, or a quick return to activity following a quadriceps contusion can also lead to the development of heterotopic ossification.[3,4] A direct force or fall on the hip can cause an iliac crest contusion **(hip pointer)** with associated injury to the abdominal soft tissue (Figs. 7–4 and 12–2). These contusions are common in collision and contact sport activities (Fig. 7–5).

## Strains

Strains to the thigh, hip, and pelvis are caused by a variety of mechanisms during athletic and work activities. A rapid stretch, contraction, or change in direction, eccentric overload, fatigue, and muscular weakness and imbalance can result in a quadriceps, hamstrings, adductor, gluteal, and iliopsoas strain (see Figs. 7–1,

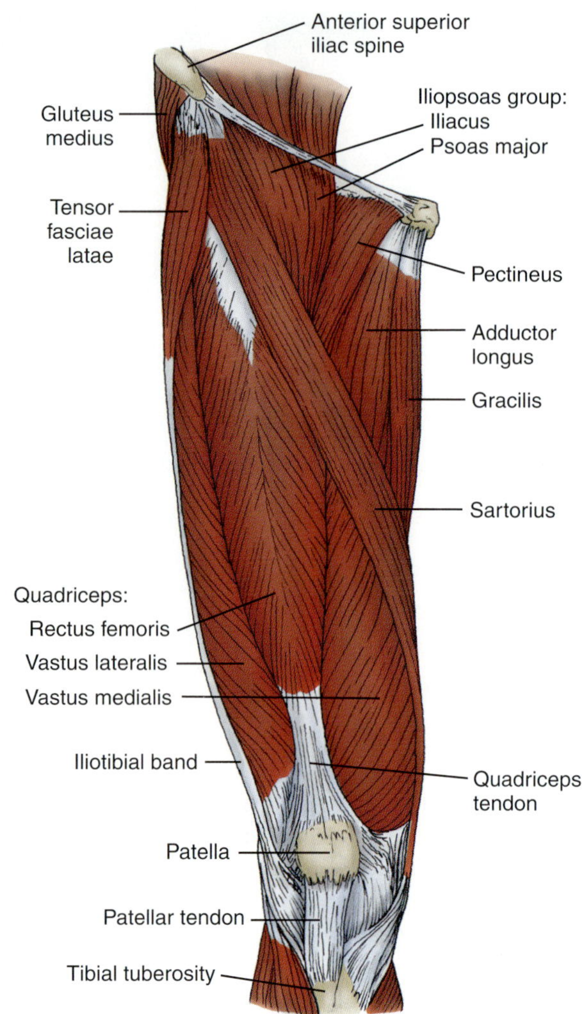



**Fig. 7–1** *Superficial muscles of the anterior thigh.*

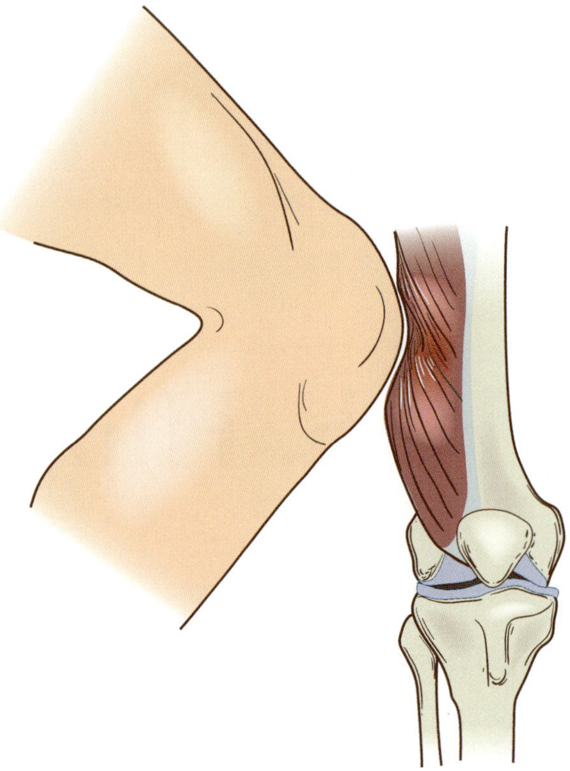

**Fig. 7–2** *Quadriceps contusion.*

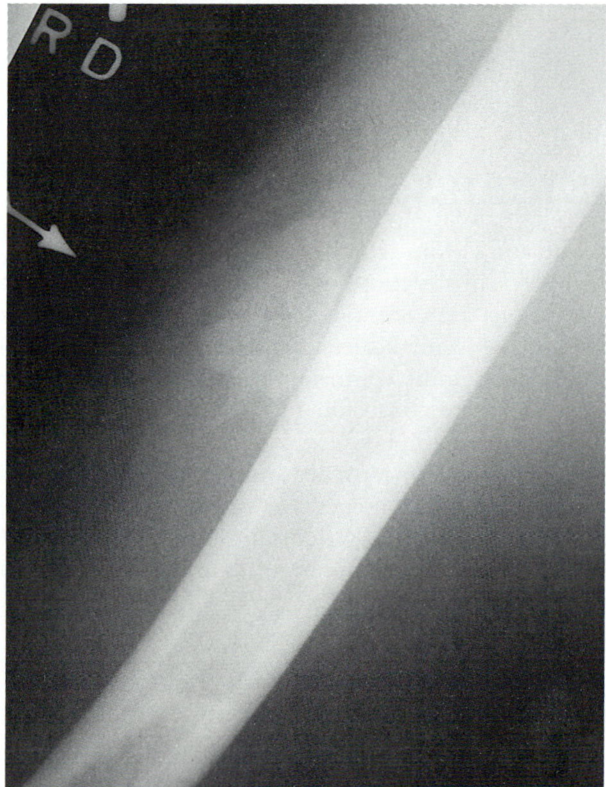



**Fig 7–3** *Femoral heterotopic ossification resulting from a quadriceps contusion. (Courtesy of Starkey, C. and Brown, SD. Examination of Orthopedic & Athletic Injuries. 4th ed. Philadelphia, PA: F.A. Davis Company: 2015.)*

7–4, 7–6). Abnormal posture and leg-length discrepancy may contribute to a hamstring strain. Strains occur more frequently to the hamstrings; these injuries often have a chronic history and reinjuries are commonly more severe than the initial injury.[5,6] For example, a quadriceps strain can occur as a volleyball player jumps to spike the ball at the net, causing an explosive contraction of the quadriceps. A hamstring strain can result when a sprinter increases the stride length at the finish line, causing a violent stretch of the musculature.

## Overuse

Structural abnormalities and repetitive stress can cause overuse injuries to the hip, thigh, and pelvis. Repetitive running on banked surfaces, training errors, leg-length discrepancy, and an increased **Q angle** can result in **greater trochanteric bursitis**.[7] A single direct force

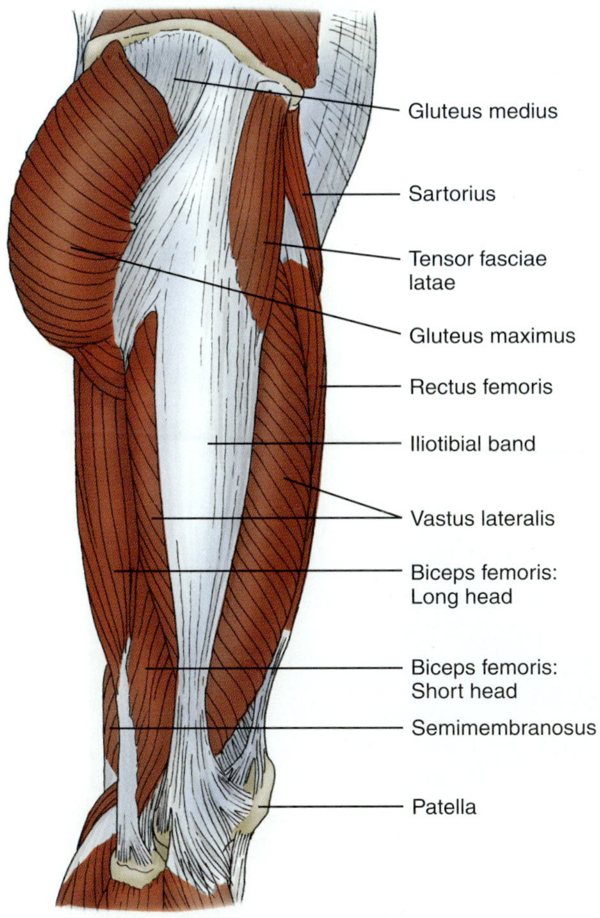


**Fig. 7–4** *Superficial muscles of the lateral thigh and hip.*

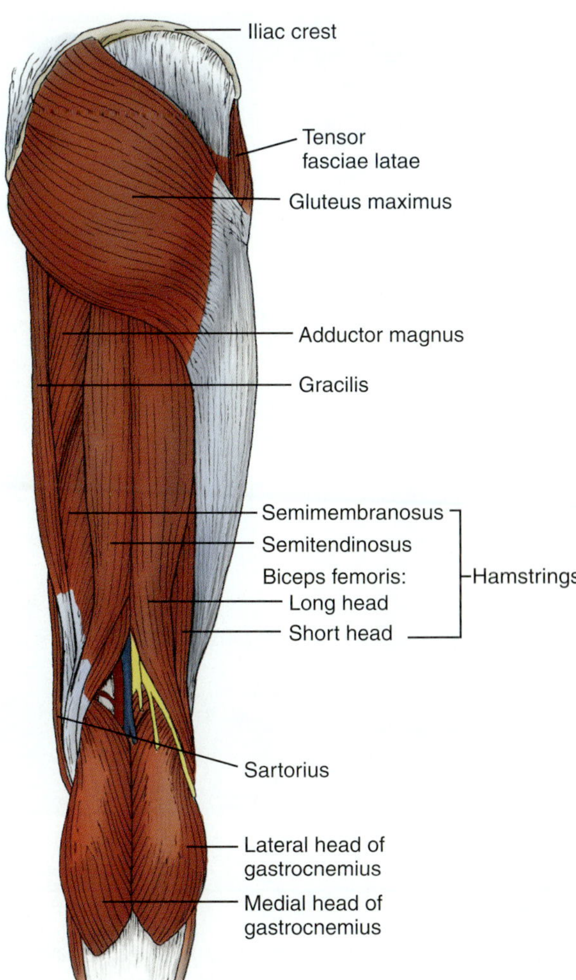


**Fig. 7–6** *Superficial muscles of the posterior thigh and hip.*

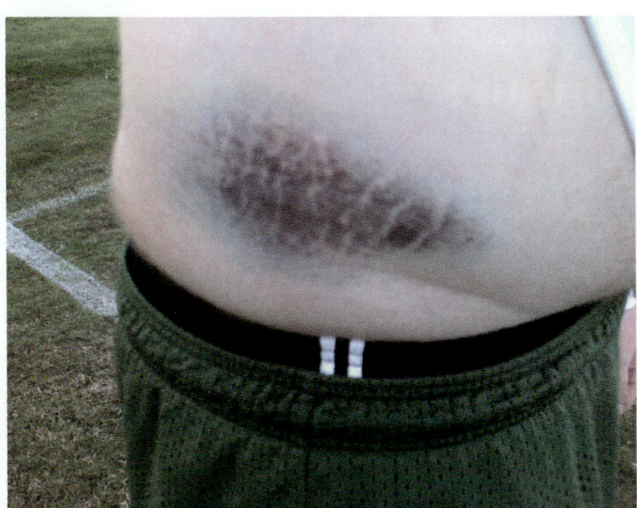

**Fig. 7–5** *Contusion to the iliac crest. This injury, the so-called "hip pointer," results in gross discoloration, swelling, pain, and loss of function. (Courtesy of Starkey, C. and Brown, SD. Examination of Orthopedic & Athletic Injuries. 4th ed. Philadelphia, PA: F.A. Davis Company: 2015.)*

to the trochanteric bursa causing chronic inflammation can also lead to bursitis.[8] **Osteitis pubis** is caused by repetitive tension from the adductor musculature on the pubic symphysis,[9–11] which occurs with repeated twisting and change in direction activities (Fig. 7–7). A reduction in internal rotation of the hip may also cause shearing stress at the pubic symphysis.[12] The repetitive kicking and pivoting on one leg experienced by rugby players may lead to the development of osteitis pubis. Stress fractures of the femur, hip, and pelvis may arise from overload, training errors, amenorrhea, oligomenorrhea, and disordered eating. For example, repetitive distance running without appropriate footwear, recovery, and caloric and nutrient intake could cause a stress fracture.

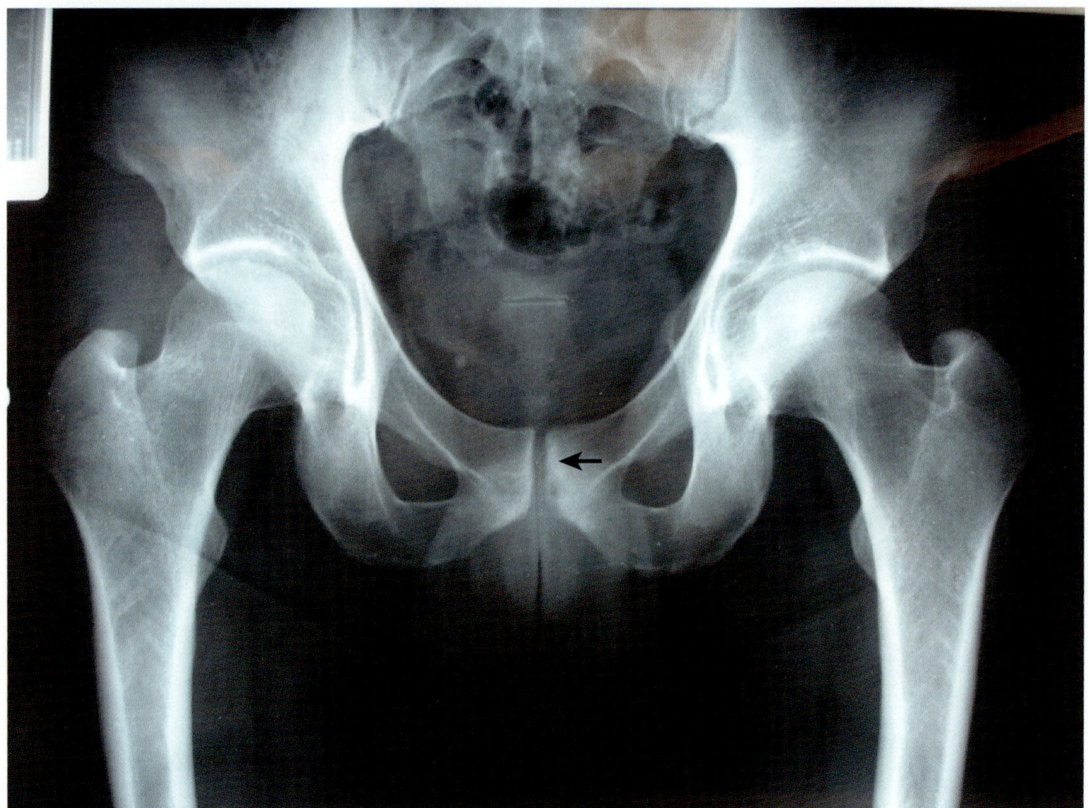

**Fig. 7–7** *Osteitis pubis. Pelvic radiograph of a 40-year-old recreational runner presenting with chronic hip pain demonstrating cystic changes and sclerosis.*

## DETAILS

The name "charley horse" was created by major league baseball players in the early 20th century when horses were used to pull lawn mowers, including a horse known as Charley at Ebbets Field in New York. Charley suffered from a chronic limp; when a player sustained a thigh contusion that caused a limp, others reportedly said the player was limping like Charley the horse.[13]

# Taping Techniques

Taping techniques are used to anchor protective padding to the thigh, hip, and pelvis following a quadriceps contusion or hip pointer. Protective padding techniques are illustrated in the Padding section.

## CIRCULAR THIGH    Figure 7–8

➡ **Purpose:** The circular thigh technique provides mild support and anchors protective padding to the thigh (Fig. 7–8). Use this technique with off-the-shelf and custom-made pads upon a return to activity to absorb shock and prevent further injury for a quadriceps contusion or heterotopic ossification.

➡ **Materials:**
• Pre-wrap or self-adherent wrap, 3 inch or 4 inch elastic tape, adherent tape spray, taping scissors
*Option:*
• 1½ inch non-elastic tape

➠ **Position of the patient:** Standing on a taping table or bench with the majority of the weight on the non-involved leg and the involved leg placed in a neutral position with slight knee flexion. Maintain this position during application with the use of a heel lift.

➠ **Preparation:** Apply adherent tape spray to the thigh, then pre-wrap or self-adherent wrap.

➠ **Application:**

**STEP 1:**    Place the pad over the injured area. Anchor 3 inch or 4 inch elastic tape directly on the distal pad (Fig. 7–8A).

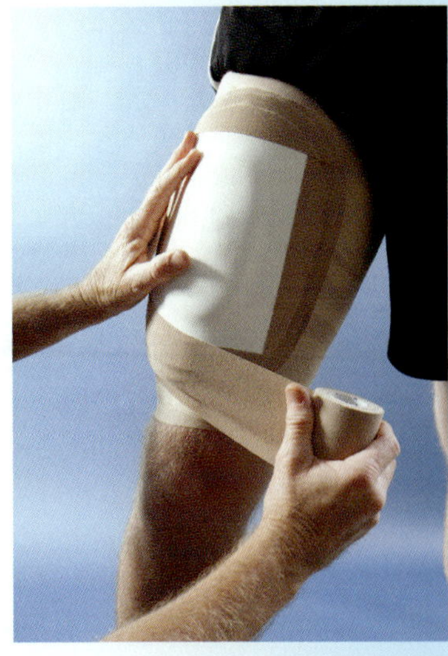

**Fig. 7–8 A**

**STEP 2:**    Continue around the thigh with moderate roll tension in a circular, distal-to-proximal pattern, overlapping the tape by ½ of its width ◀▥▥▥▶ (Fig. 7–8B). Cover the entire pad and anchor on the top of the pad to prevent irritation. Avoid gaps, wrinkles, and inconsistent roll tension.

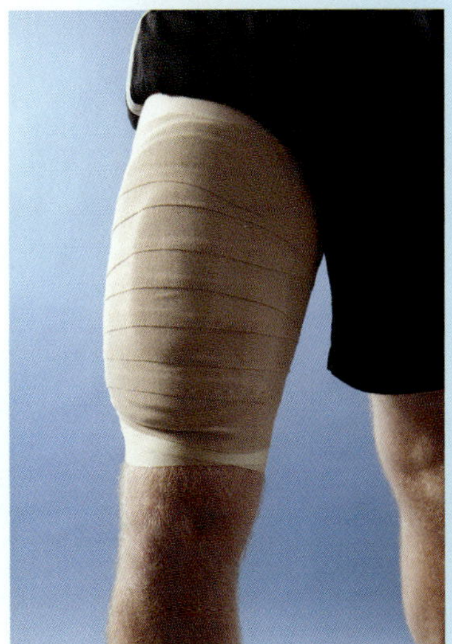

**Fig. 7–8 B**

*Steps Cont.*

**STEP 3:**   To prevent migration, a distal circular strip of elastic tape may be applied with distal-to-proximal tension, or the proximal portion of the elastic tape may be applied partially on the skin (Fig. 7–8C).

*Option:*   *Apply one to two circular strips of 1½ inch non-elastic tape loosely around the pad for additional anchors* ◀▥▥▥▶.

**Helpful Hint |**
Near the completion of the technique, angle a strip distally, across the distal portion of the pad with moderate roll tension. Then continue sharply in a proximal direction, and finish the circular pattern (Fig. 7–8D).

This strip provides additional tension and support to lessen distal migration of the pad.

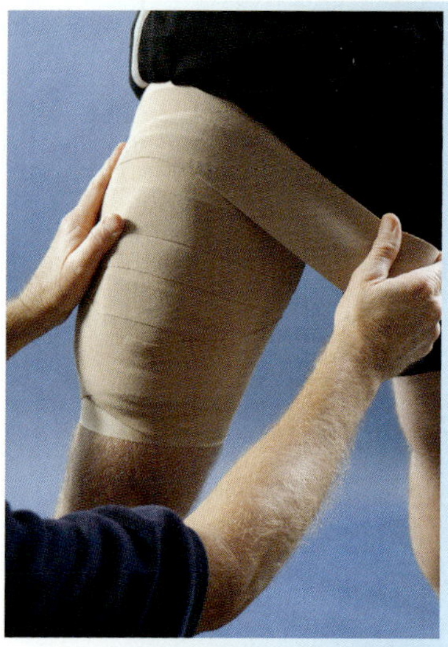

**Fig. 7–8 C**

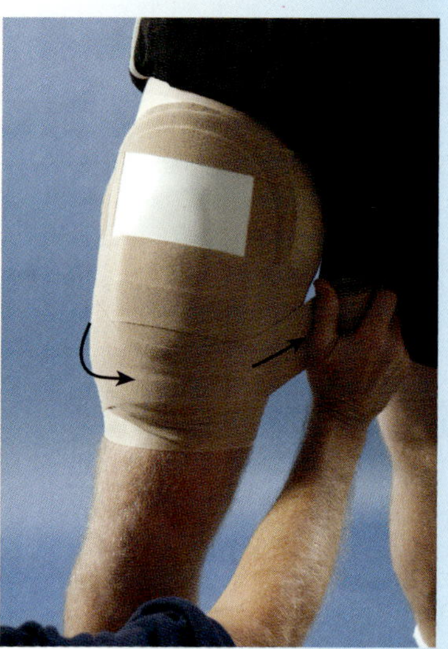

**Fig. 7–8 D**

## HIP POINTER TAPE      Figure 7–9

▥▶ **Purpose:** Use the hip pointer technique to absorb shock when preventing and treating contusions and to anchor off-the-shelf and custom-made pads to the iliac crest (Fig. 7–9).

▥▶ **Materials:**
  • 2 inch or 3 inch heavyweight elastic tape, adherent tape spray, taping scissors

▥▶ **Position of the patient:** Standing on a taping table, bench, or floor with the majority of the weight on the non-involved leg and the involved leg placed in a neutral position with slight knee flexion. Maintain this position during application with the use of a heel lift.

▥▶ **Preparation:** Apply the hip pointer technique directly to the skin.

▥▶ **Application:**

**STEP 1:**   Apply adherent tape spray over the pad area and 4–6 inches beyond, over the hip and low back. Allow the spray to dry.

**STEP 2:**   Cut several strips of 2 inch or 3 inch heavyweight elastic tape in lengths that will cover the pad and extend 4–6 inches beyond the pad on the two sides. Place the pad over the injured area.

**STEP 3:**  Anchor the first tape strip on the abdomen or anterior hip 4–6 inches from the edge of the pad and pat down (Fig. 7–9A). Do not stretch the tape as the anchor is applied.

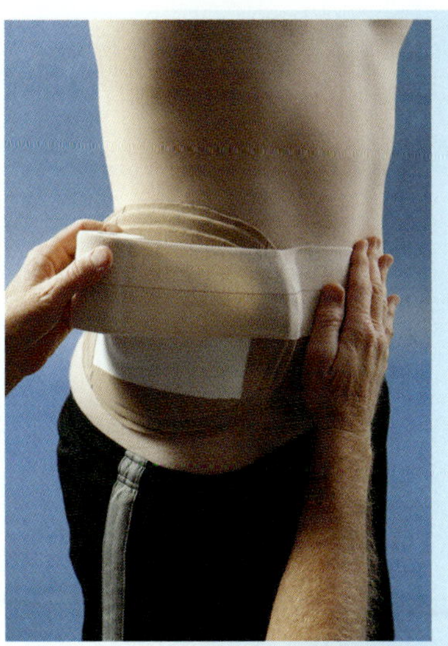

**Fig. 7–9 A**

**STEP 4:**  Continue to apply the strip to the edge of the pad. At the edge, hold the strip on the abdomen/anterior hip and pad with one hand and pull the strip over the pad with tension on the tape (Fig. 7–9B).

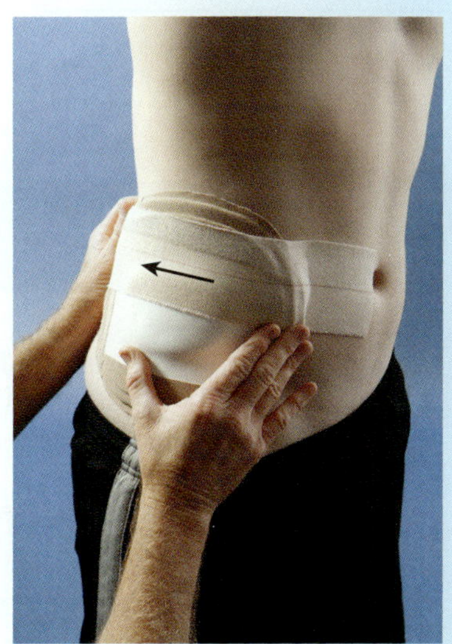

**Fig. 7–9 B**

**STEP 5:**  When the strip completely covers the pad, release the tension in the tape and anchor to the low back and pat down (Fig. 7–9C). This technique is the release-stretch-release sequence illustrated in Figure 8–10A to D.

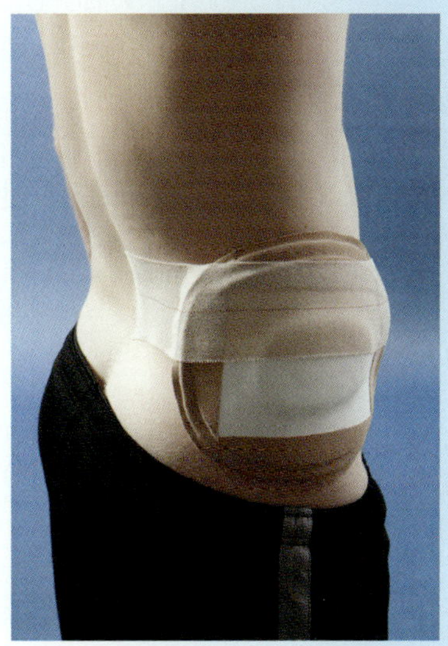

**Fig. 7–9 C**

*Steps Cont.*

**STEP 6:**   Continue with additional strips in the same manner, overlapping each by ½ the width of the tape (Fig. 7–9D).

**STEP 7:**   Apply enough strips to cover the majority of the pad.

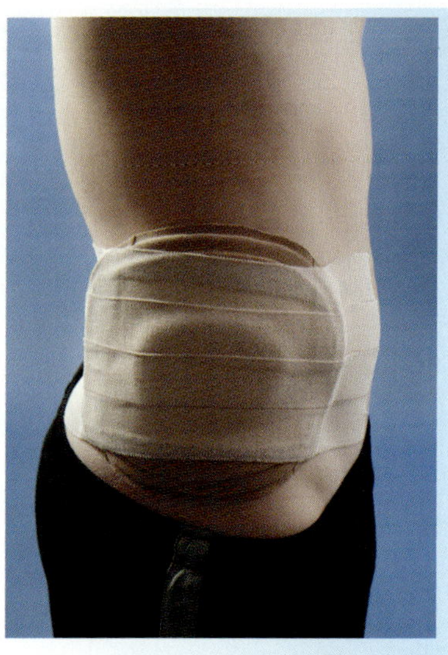

**Fig. 7–9 D**

# Wrapping Techniques

Use wrapping techniques to provide compression and support and to attach protective pads to the thigh, hip, and pelvis. The techniques can be used to prevent and treat quadriceps contusions and strains; hamstrings, adductor, and hip flexor strains; iliac crest contusions; and heterotopic ossification.

## THIGH COMPRESSION WRAP    Figure 7–10

➠ **Purpose:** Apply the thigh compression wrap technique to control mild to moderate swelling with mild thigh contusions and strains (Fig. 7–10).

➠ **Materials:**
• 4 inch or 6 inch width by 5 yard length elastic wrap determined by the size of the thigh, metal clips, 1½ inch non-elastic or 2 inch or 3 inch elastic tape, taping scissors
*Options:*
• ¼ inch or ½ inch foam or felt
• 4 inch or 6 inch width self-adherent wrap

➠ **Position of the patient:** Standing on a taping table or bench with the majority of the weight on the non-involved leg and the involved leg placed in a pain-free, slightly flexed position. Maintain this position during application with the use of a heel lift.

➠ **Preparation:** To lessen migration, apply adherent tape spray, tape strips, or anchors directly to the skin (see Fig. 1–7).
*Option:*
Cut a ¼ inch or ½ inch foam or felt pad and place it over the inflamed area directly to the skin to provide additional compression and assist in venous return.

➠ **Application:**

**STEP 1:**  Anchor the wrap around the distal thigh directly to the skin and encircle the anchor ◀▦▦▶ (Fig. 7–10A).

*Option:*  *If an elastic wrap is not available, 4 inch or 6 inch self-adherent wrap may be used.*

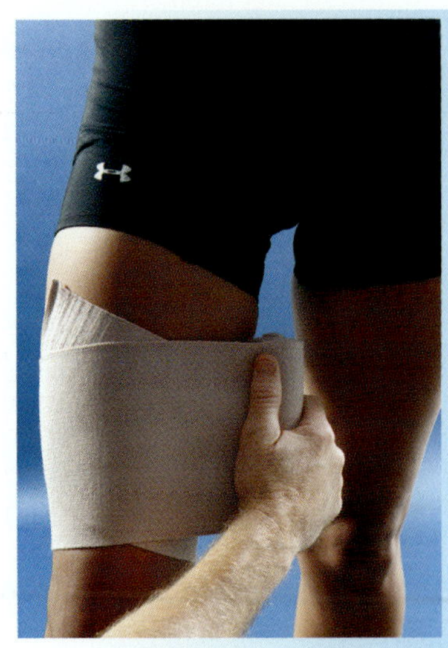

**Fig. 7–10 A**

**STEP 2:**  Continue to apply the wrap in a spiral pattern in a distal-to-proximal direction, overlapping the wrap by ½ of its width (Fig. 7–10B). Apply the greatest amount of roll tension distally and over the inflamed area. Lessen the roll tension as the wrap continues proximally from the injured area.

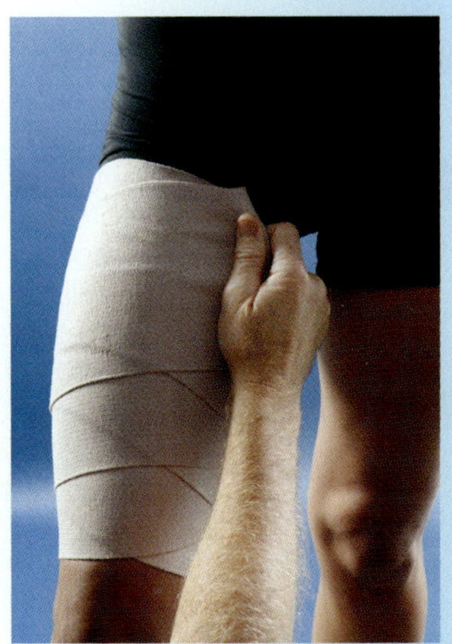

**Fig. 7–10 B**

**STEP 3:**  Finish the wrap over the proximal thigh and anchor with Velcro, metal clips, or loosely applied 1½ inch non-elastic or 2 inch or 3 inch elastic tape ◀▦▦▶ (Fig. 7–10C).

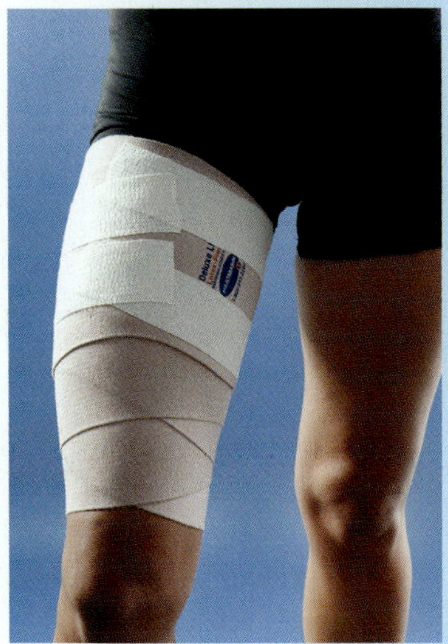

**Fig. 7–10 C**

## FOOT, ANKLE, LOWER LEG, KNEE, AND THIGH COMPRESSION WRAP    Figure 7–11

➡ **Purpose:** With second- and third-degree thigh contusions and strains, swelling can be severe. Use the foot, ankle, lower leg, knee, and thigh compression wrap technique to control moderate to severe swelling and prevent distal migration of post-injury swelling (Fig. 7–11).

➡ **Materials:**
- 4 inch or 6 inch width by 10 yard length elastic wrap, metal clips, 1½ inch non-elastic or 2 inch or 3 inch elastic tape, taping scissors

*Option:*
- ¼ inch or ½ inch foam or felt

➡ **Position of the patient:** Sitting on a taping table or bench with the leg extended off the edge, knee in a pain-free, slightly flexed position, and the ankle placed in 90 degrees of dorsiflexion.

➡ **Preparation:** To lessen migration, apply adherent tape spray, tape strips, or anchors directly to the skin.

*Option:*
Cut a ¼ inch or ½ inch foam or felt pad and place it over the inflamed area directly to the skin to assist in controlling swelling.

➡ **Application:**

**STEP 1:**    Anchor the elastic wrap on the distal plantar foot and apply the foot, ankle, lower leg, and knee compression wrap directly to the skin (see Fig. 6–15).

**STEP 2:**    At the mid thigh, continue the spiral wrap to the proximal thigh ◄▥▥► (Fig. 7–11). Apply the greatest amount of roll tension distally and lessen tension as the wrap continues proximally.

**STEP 3:**    Anchor the wrap with Velcro, metal clips, or loosely applied 1½ inch non-elastic or 2 inch or 3 inch elastic tape.

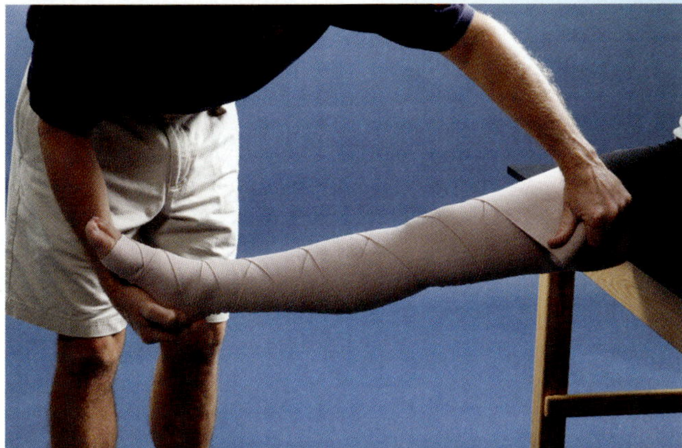

**Fig. 7–11**

**Helpful Hint |**
When treating a quadriceps contusion, place the knee in maximal pain-free flexion to stretch the quadriceps. Use a 4 inch or 6 inch width by 10 yard length elastic wrap to provide compression, anchor an ice bag, and maintain knee flexion by encircling the thigh and proximal lower leg (Fig. 7–12).

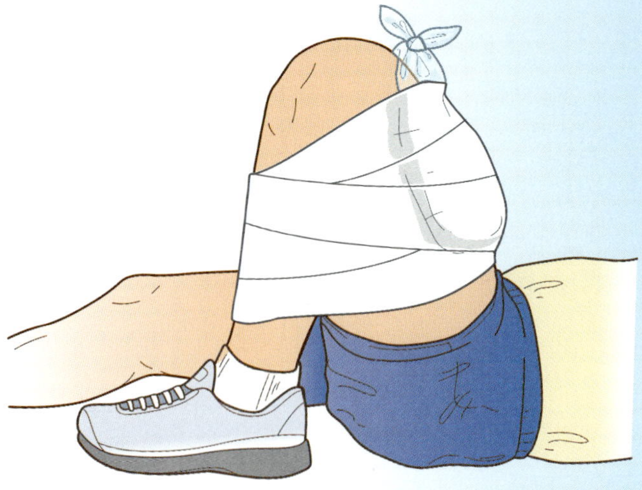

**Fig. 7–12** *Treatment of a quadriceps contusion.*

## THIGH COMPRESSION SLEEVE     Figure 7–13

➠ **Purpose:** Use the thigh compression sleeve technique to control mild to moderate swelling (Fig. 7–13). The benefit of this technique is that the patient can apply the sleeve without assistance following application instruction.

➠ **Materials:**
- 4 inch, 5 inch, or 6 inch width elastic sleeve determined by the size of the thigh, taping scissors
*Option:*
- ¼ inch or ½ inch foam or felt

➠ **Position of the patient:** Sitting on a taping table or bench with the leg extended off the edge.

➠ **Preparation:** Cut an elastic sleeve from a roll to extend from the superior knee to the proximal thigh area. Cut and use a double-length sleeve to provide additional compression.
*Option:*
Cut a ¼ inch or ½ inch foam or felt pad and place it over the inflamed area directly to the skin to assist in venous return.

➠ **Application:**

**STEP 1:**   Pull the sleeve onto the thigh in a distal-to-proximal pattern. If using a double-length sleeve, pull the distal end over the first layer (Fig. 7–13). No anchors are required; the sleeve can be cleaned and reused.

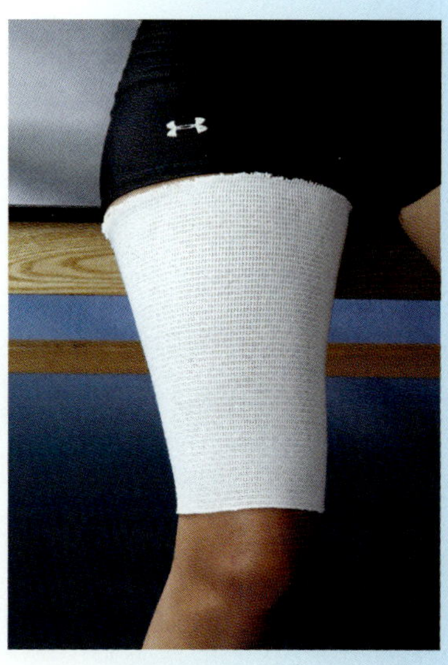

**Fig. 7–13**

## QUADRICEPS STRAIN WRAP     Figure 7–14

➠ **Purpose:** The quadriceps strain technique is used to provide compression and mild to moderate circular support when treating strains. This technique may be used to anchor protective padding for a quadriceps contusion or heterotopic ossification. Two methods of the technique are available to accommodate patient preferences and available supplies. The first is illustrated here (Fig. 7–14), and the second is online at FADavis.com. ✦ Protective padding techniques are illustrated in the Padding section (see Fig. 7–22).

### Quadriceps Strain Technique One

➠ **Materials:**
- 4 inch or 6 inch width by 5 yard length elastic wrap, metal clips, 1½ inch non-elastic tape, 2 inch, 3 inch, or 4 inch elastic tape, taping scissors

➠ **Position of the patient:** Standing on a taping table or bench with the majority of the weight on the non-involved leg and the involved leg placed in a neutral position with slight knee flexion. Maintain this position during application with the use of a heel lift.

➠ **Preparation:** To lessen migration, apply adherent tape spray, tape strips, or anchors directly to the skin. To anchor a pad, place the pad over the injured area.

➠ **Application:**

**STEP 1:** Anchor the extended end of the elastic wrap on the lateral distal thigh directly to the skin and proceed around the thigh in a medial direction to encircle the anchor (Fig. 7–14A).

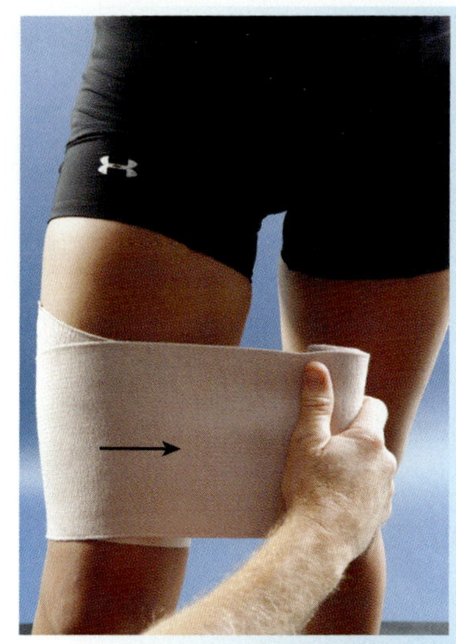

**Fig. 7–14 A**

**STEP 2:** Continue to apply the wrap in a lateral-to-medial circular pattern with moderate roll tension, overlapping by ½ of the wrap width, moving in a distal-to-proximal direction (Fig. 7–14B). Avoid gaps, wrinkles, and inconsistent roll tension.

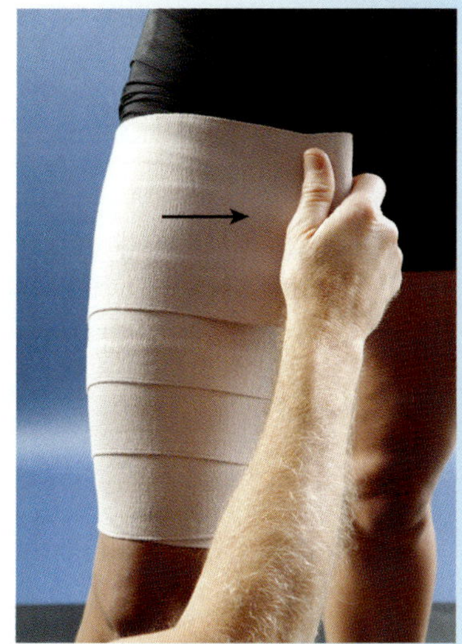

**Fig. 7–14 B**

**STEP 3:** Finish the wrap over the proximal thigh. The wrap should extend above and below the injured area. During non-athletic or non-work activities, anchor the wrap with Velcro, metal clips, or loosely applied 1½ inch non-elastic tape in a lateral-to-medial circular pattern (Fig. 7–14C).

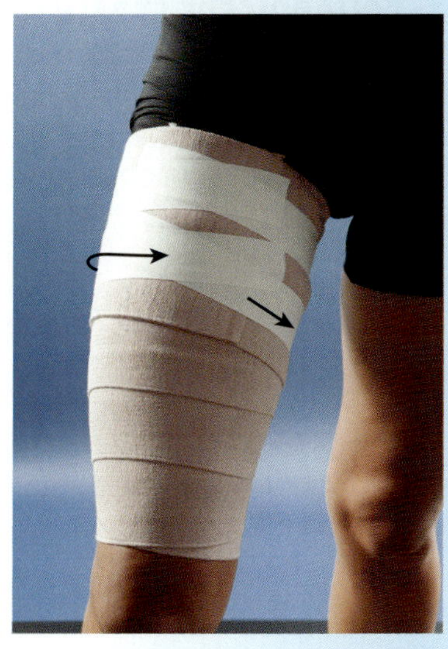

**Fig. 7–14 C**

**STEP 4:**  With athletic or work activities, anchor 2 inch, 3 inch, or 4 inch elastic tape on the lateral distal thigh and apply two to four continuous lateral-to-medial circular patterns with moderate roll tension, finishing on the proximal thigh (Fig. 7–14D). To ensure adherence, anchor the loose end of the elastic tape on the circular tape pattern rather than on the wrap. Additional anchors are not required.

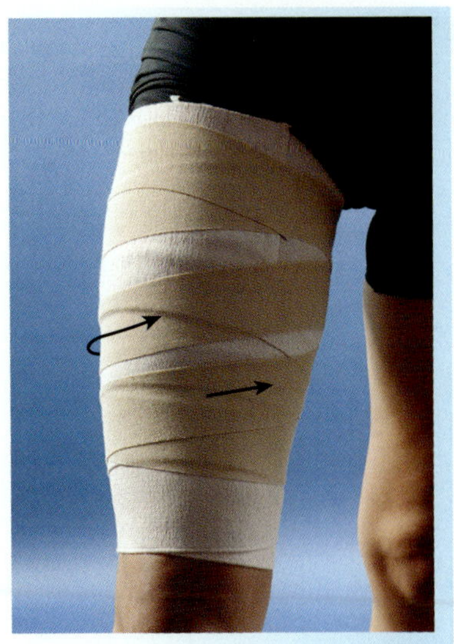

**Fig. 7–14 D**

## HAMSTRINGS STRAIN WRAP        Figure 7–15

➡ **Purpose:** Use the hamstrings strain technique to provide compression and mild to moderate circular support when treating strains. Two methods are available to accommodate patient preferences and available supplies. The first is illustrated here (Fig. 7–15) and the second is online at FADavis.com ✥.

### Hamstrings Strain Technique One

➡ **Materials:**
   • 4 inch or 6 inch width by 5 yard length elastic wrap, metal clips, 1½ inch non-elastic tape, 2 inch, 3 inch, or 4 inch elastic tape, taping scissors
➡ **Position of the patient:** Standing on a taping table or bench with the majority of the weight on the non-involved leg and the involved leg placed in a neutral position with slight knee flexion. Maintain this position during application with the use of a heel lift.
➡ **Preparation:** To lessen migration, apply adherent tape spray, tape strips, or anchors directly to the skin.
➡ **Application:**

**STEP 1:**  When treating a medial hamstrings strain, anchor the extended end of the wrap on the distal, posterior medial thigh directly to the skin and proceed in a lateral direction around the thigh to encircle the anchor (Fig. 7–15A).

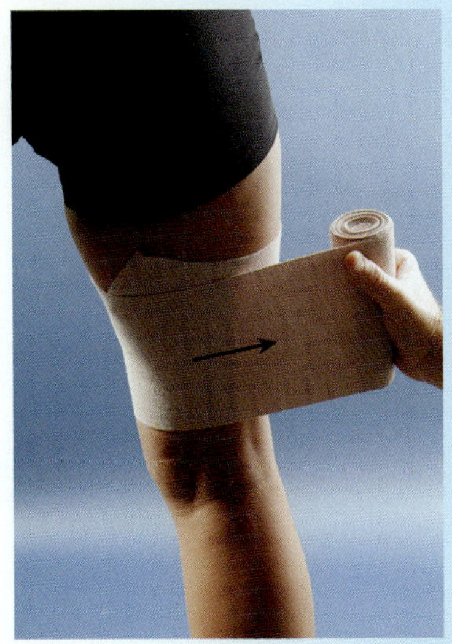

**Fig. 7–15 A**

*Steps Cont.*

**STEP 2:** Continue to apply the wrap with moderate roll tension in a medial-to-lateral circular pattern. Overlap the wrap by ½ of the width and apply it in a distal-to-proximal direction (Fig. 7–15B). Avoid gaps, wrinkles, and inconsistent roll tension.

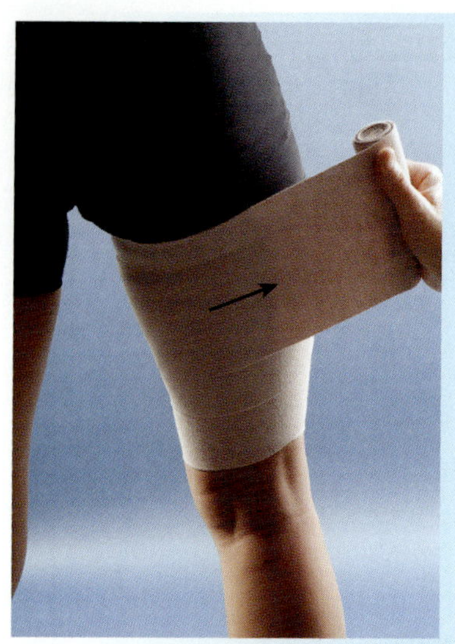

**Fig. 7–15 B**

**STEP 3:** Finish the wrap over the proximal thigh, extending above and below the injured area. Anchor the wrap as illustrated in Figures 7–14C or 7–14D, but apply the 1½ inch non-elastic or 2 inch, 3 inch, or 4 inch elastic tape in a medial-to-lateral circular pattern (Fig. 7–15C). Additional anchors are not necessary.

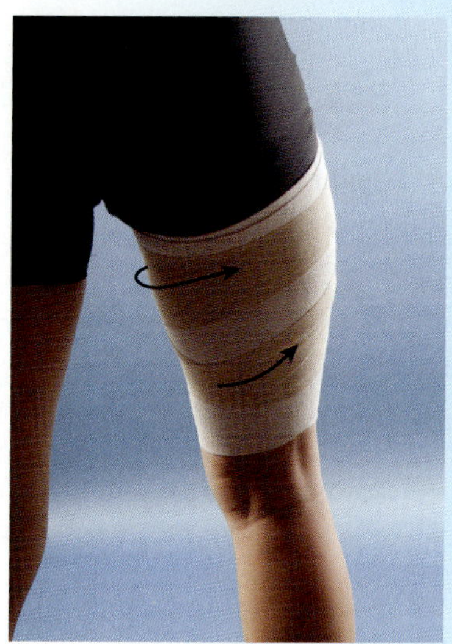

**Fig. 7–15 C**

**STEP 4:** When treating a lateral hamstrings strain, anchor the extended end of the wrap on the distal, posterior lateral thigh directly to the skin and proceed around the thigh in a medial direction to encircle the anchor (Fig. 7–15D).

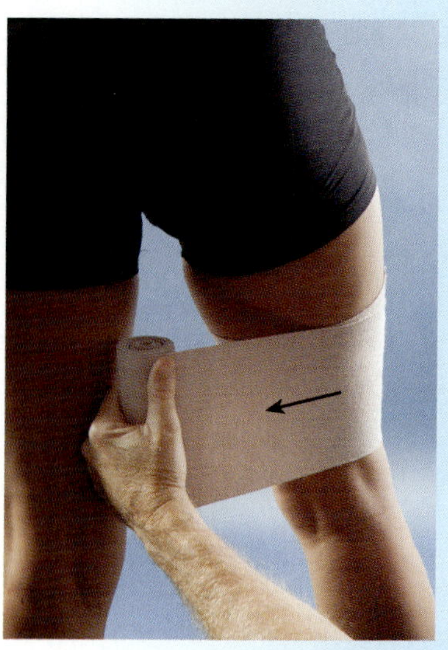

**Fig. 7–15 D**

**STEP 5:**  Continue to apply the wrap in a lateral-to-medial circular pattern, overlapping the wrap by ½ of the width, moving in a distal-to-proximal direction with moderate roll tension (Fig. 7–15E).

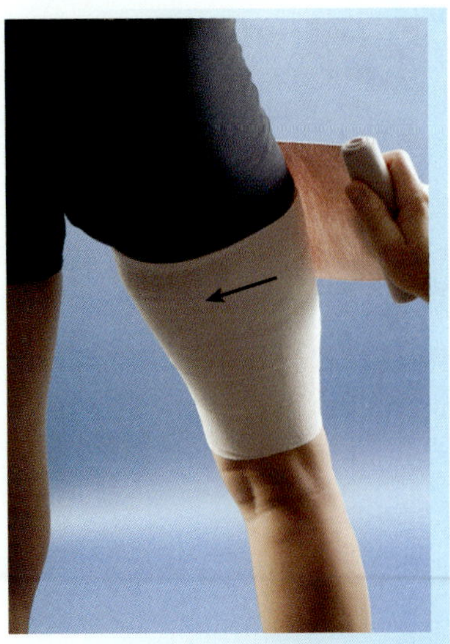

**Fig. 7–15 E**

**STEP 6:**  Finish over the proximal thigh and anchor as shown in Figures 7–14C or 7–14D, applying the 1½ inch non-elastic or 2 inch, 3 inch, or 4 inch elastic tape in a lateral-to-medial circular pattern (Fig. 7–15F).

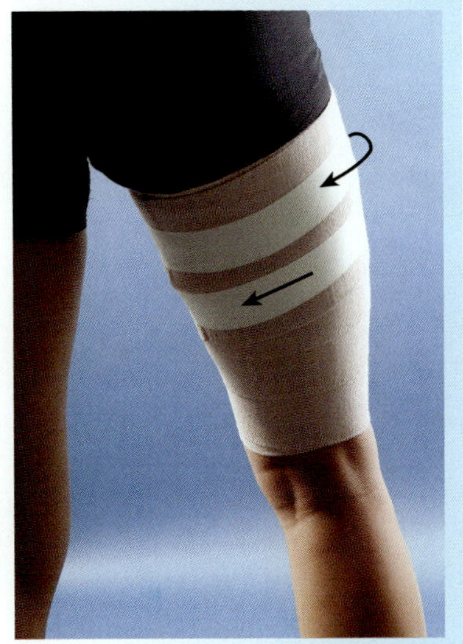

**Fig. 7–15 F**

**. . . IF/THEN . . .**

**IF** the quadriceps and/or hamstrings strain wrapping technique one migrates distally during activity, **THEN** consider applying technique two (FADavis.com), incorporating the waist, to lessen migration.

## ADDUCTOR STRAIN WRAP     Figure 7–16

➡ **Purpose:** The adductor strain technique is used to provide compression and mild to moderate support of hip adduction when treating strains (Fig. 7–16).

➡ **Materials:**
- 4 inch or 6 inch width by 10 yard length elastic wrap, metal clips, 1½ inch non-elastic tape, 2 inch, 3 inch, or 4 inch elastic tape, taping scissors

➠ **Position of the patient:** Standing on a taping table, bench, or floor with the majority of the weight on the non-involved leg and the involved leg in an internally rotated position with slight knee flexion. Maintain this position during application.

➠ **Preparation:** To lessen migration, apply adherent tape spray, tape strips, or anchors directly to the skin.

➠ **Application:**

**STEP 1:**  Anchor the extended end of the elastic wrap on the lateral distal thigh directly to the skin and continue in a medial direction to encircle the anchor (Fig. 7–16A).

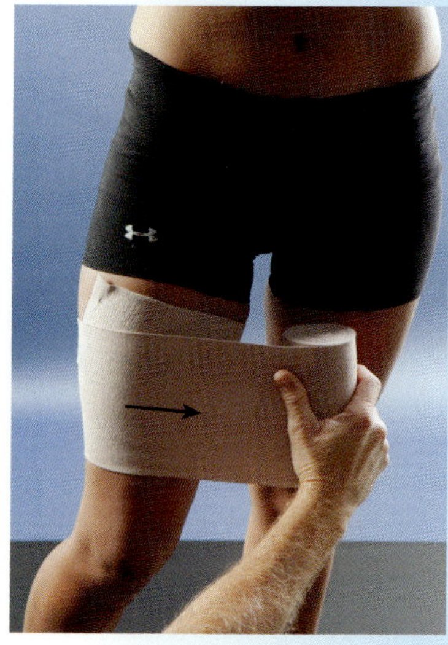

**Fig. 7–16 A**

**STEP 2:**  Continue to apply the wrap in a lateral-to-medial circular pattern with moderate roll tension, supporting internal rotation of the leg (Fig. 7–16B). Move in a distal-to-proximal direction and overlap the wrap by ½ of the width. Avoid gaps, wrinkles, and inconsistent roll tension.

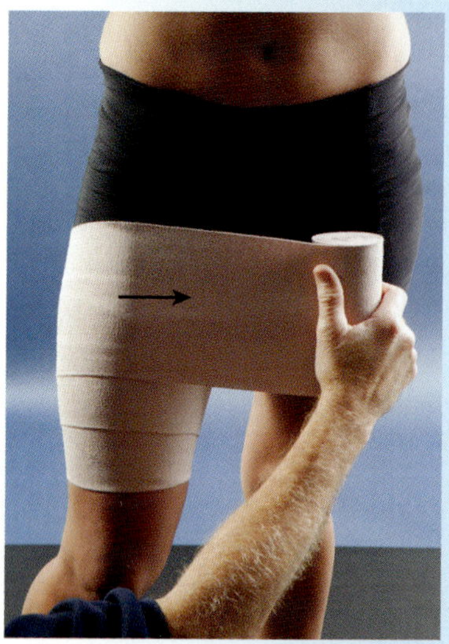

**Fig. 7–16 B**

**STEP 3:**  At the proximal thigh, continue in a lateral-to-medial direction across the lateral hip, abdomen, and waist with mild roll tension (Fig. 7–16C). Next, continue to apply the wrap distally across the medial proximal thigh with a moderate downward pull, supporting internal rotation of the leg, then continue around the proximal thigh (Fig. 7–16D). Monitor roll tension to prevent constriction and irritation of the lower abdominal and back and medial thigh soft tissue.

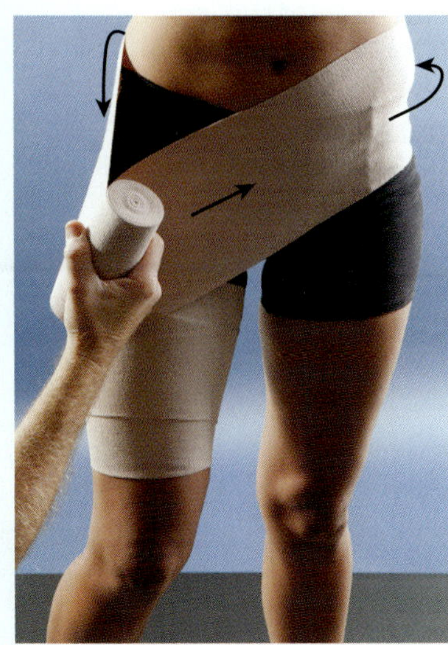

**Fig. 7–16 C**

**Fig. 7–16 D**

**STEP 4:**  Apply one circular pattern around the mid-to-proximal thigh, encircle the waist, then cross the medial proximal thigh, supporting internal rotation of the leg (Fig. 7–16E). Repeat this pattern one to two times.

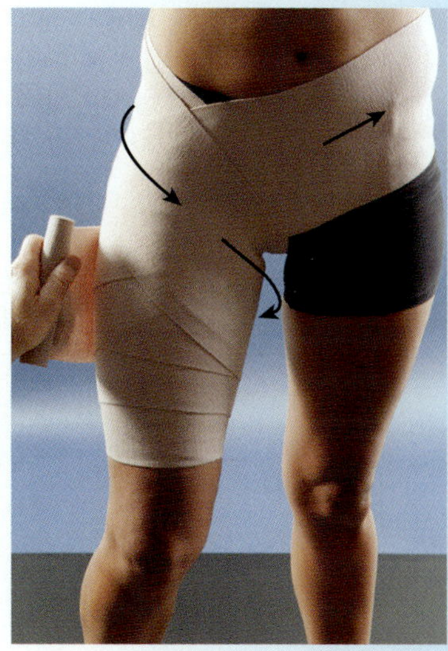

**Fig. 7–16 E**

*Steps Cont.*

**STEP 5:** Finish the wrap over the mid thigh. Anchor with Velcro, metal clips, or 1½ inch non-elastic tape for non-athletic or non-work activities.

**STEP 6:** Use 2 inch, 3 inch, or 4 inch elastic tape to anchor for athletic or work activities. Start at the lateral distal thigh and apply two to four continuous lateral-to-medial circular patterns around the thigh with moderate roll tension, again supporting internal rotation of the leg. Continue to apply the elastic tape to encircle the hip and waist with mild roll tension, across the medial proximal thigh with a moderate downward pull, then encircle the thigh and anchor on the circular tape pattern on the mid thigh (Fig. 7–16F). No additional anchors are required. When the adductor strain wrapping technique is properly applied, the patient should feel an internal rotation pull from the wrap on the leg.

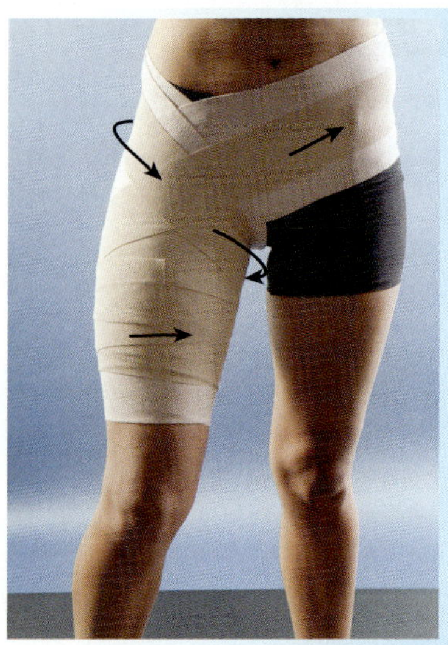

**Fig. 7–16 F**

## HIP FLEXOR STRAIN WRAP — Figure 7–17

➡ **Purpose:** The hip flexor strain technique provides compression and mild to moderate support of hip flexion when treating iliopsoas strains (Fig. 7–17).

➡ **Materials:**
• 4 inch or 6 inch width by 10 yard length elastic wrap, metal clips, 1½ inch non-elastic tape, 2 inch, 3 inch, or 4 inch elastic tape, taping scissors

➡ **Position of the patient:** Standing on a taping table, bench, or floor with the majority of the weight on the non-involved leg and the involved leg placed in a neutral position with slight knee flexion. Maintain this position during application.

➡ **Preparation:** To lessen migration, apply adherent tape spray, tape strips, or anchors directly to the skin.

➡ **Application:**

**STEP 1:** Anchor the extended end of the wrap on the mid medial thigh directly to the skin and proceed in a lateral direction around the thigh to encircle the anchor (Fig. 7–17A).

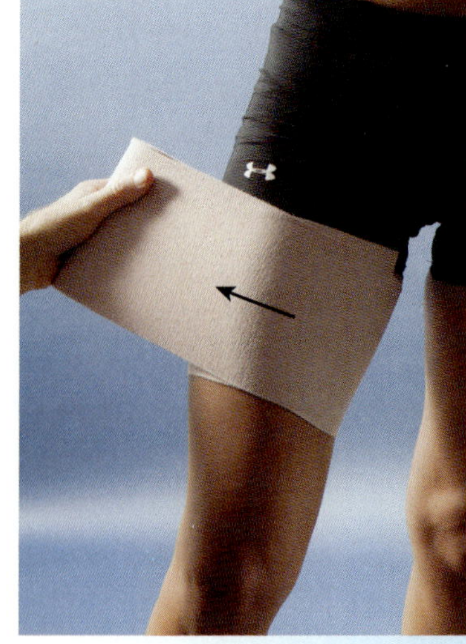

**Fig. 7–17 A**

**STEP 2:**  Continue to apply the wrap with moderate roll tension in a medial-to-lateral circular pattern. Overlap the wrap by ½ of the width and apply in a distal-to-proximal direction (Fig. 7–17B). Avoid gaps, wrinkles, and inconsistent roll tension.

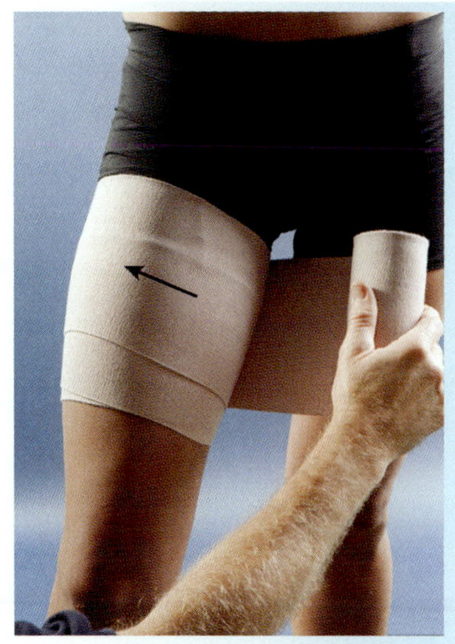

**Fig. 7–17 B**

**STEP 3:**  At the proximal thigh, apply the wrap in a medial-to-lateral direction across the lateral hip with a moderate upward pull, supporting flexion of the hip (Fig. 7–17C). Continue to encircle the waist with mild roll tension and return to the proximal thigh. Monitor roll tension to prevent constriction and irritation of the soft tissue.

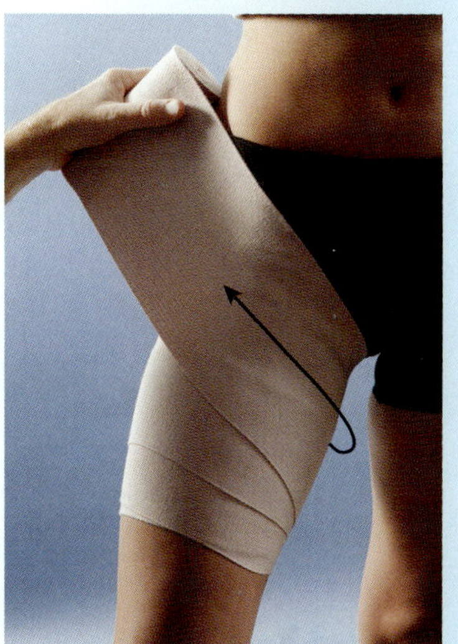

**Fig. 7–17 C**

**STEP 4:**  Apply one circular pattern around the mid-to-proximal thigh, across the lateral hip with a moderate upward pull, supporting flexion of the hip, encircle the waist, and return to the proximal thigh (Fig. 7–17D). Repeat this pattern one to two times.

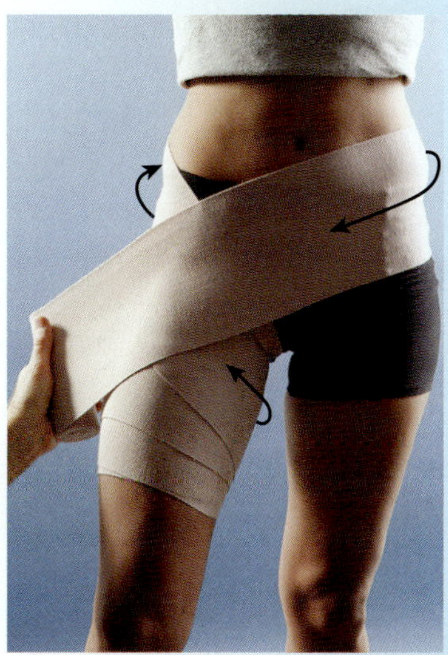

**Fig. 7–17 D**

*Steps Cont.*

**STEP 5:** Anchor the wrap over the mid thigh. Use Velcro, metal clips, or 1½ inch non-elastic tape to anchor with non-athletic or non-work activities ◀▬▬▶.

**STEP 6:** With athletic or work activities, anchor 2 inch, 3 inch, or 4 inch elastic tape on the mid medial thigh and apply two to four continuous medial-to-lateral circular patterns around the thigh with moderate roll tension. At the proximal thigh, continue to apply the elastic tape across the lateral hip with a moderate upward pull, again supporting flexion of the hip, encircle the waist with mild roll tension, and anchor on the circular tape pattern on the mid thigh (Fig. 7–17E). No additional anchors are required.

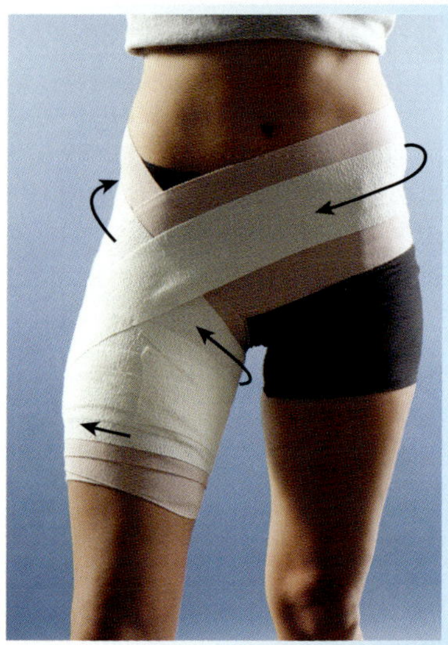

**Fig. 7–17 E**

## HIP POINTER WRAP   Figure 7–18

▶ **Purpose:** The hip pointer technique is commonly used to anchor off-the-shelf and custom-made pads to the iliac crest to absorb shock when preventing and treating contusions. Two methods are interchangeable in applying the hip pointer technique to accommodate patient preferences and available supplies; the first is illustrated here (Fig. 7–18) and the second is online at FADavis.com ◉.

### Hip Pointer Technique One

▶ **Materials:**
• 4 inch or 6 inch width by 5 yard length elastic wrap, 2 inch, 3 inch, or 4 inch elastic tape, taping scissors
▶ **Position of the patient:** Standing on a taping table, bench, or floor with the majority of the weight on the non-involved leg and the involved leg placed in a neutral position with slight knee flexion. Maintain this position during application.
▶ **Preparation:** To lessen migration, apply adherent tape spray, tape strips, or anchors directly to the skin.
▶ **Application:**

**STEP 1:** Place the pad over the injured area. Anchor the extended end of the wrap on the anterior hip directly to the skin and proceed over the pad and around the waist to encircle the anchor ◀▬▬▶ (Fig. 7–18A).

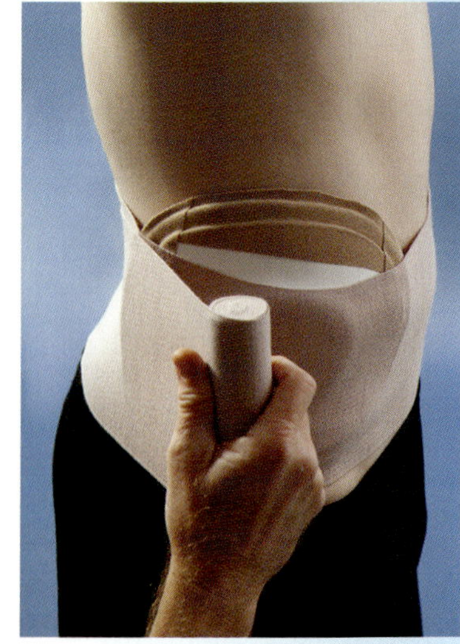

**Fig. 7–18 A**

**STEP 2:** Continue to apply the wrap with moderate roll tension over the pad and around the waist (Fig. 7–18B). Overlap the wrap by ½ of the width and avoid gaps, wrinkles, and inconsistent roll tension. Monitor roll tension to prevent constriction and irritation of the soft tissue.

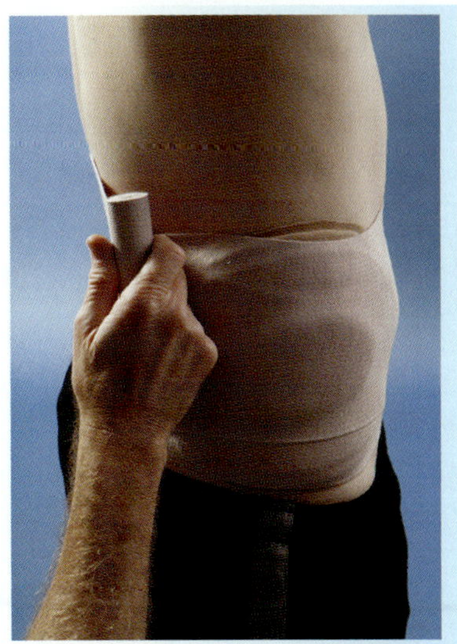

**Fig. 7–18 B**

**STEP 3:** Anchor the wrap with 2 inch, 3 inch, or 4 inch elastic tape. Apply two to three continuous circular patterns with the tape around the pad and waist with moderate roll tension ◀▥▥▶ (Fig. 7–18C). Finish the loose end of the tape on the circular tape pattern to ensure adherence. No additional anchors are required.

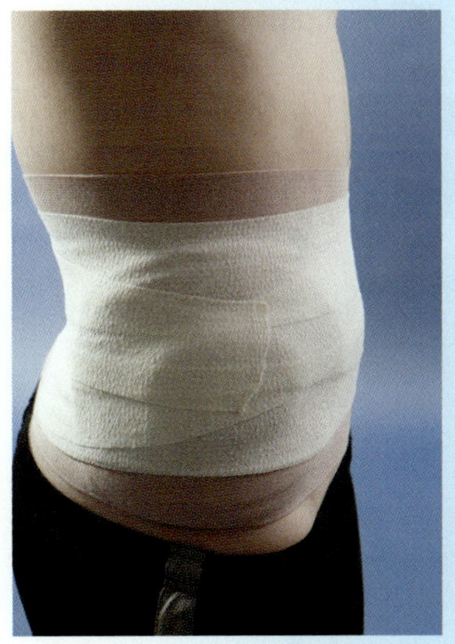

**Fig. 7–18 C**

---

**. . . IF/THEN . . .**

**IF** using the hip pointer wrap technique one or two (FADavis.com 🌐) to anchor an off-the-shelf or custom-made pad and migration occurs during activity, **THEN** consider the hip pointer taping technique; anchoring the pad directly to the skin with heavyweight elastic tape will lessen migration.

---

# Bracing Techniques

Bracing techniques provide compression and support when treating injuries and conditions of the thigh, hip, and pelvis. To provide compression, neoprene sleeves and shorts are used when treating contusions, strains, and overuse injuries and conditions. Combination braces provide compression and support for the thigh, hip, and pelvis when treating strains and overuse injuries and conditions.

## NEOPRENE SLEEVE    Figure 7–19

➡ **Purpose:** Neoprene sleeves are designed to provide compression and mild support when treating quadriceps strains and contusions, hamstrings and adductor strains, and heterotopic ossification (Fig. 7–19).

### DETAILS
Use the sleeves during rehabilitative, athletic, work, and casual activities.

➡ **Design:**
- Off-the-shelf sleeves are manufactured in universal fit designs in predetermined sizes corresponding to thigh circumference measurements.
- Several designs have an oval neoprene pad incorporated into the sleeve to provide additional compression over the injured area.
- Some designs use a contoured sleeve that wraps around the thigh. These designs are anchored with Velcro.
- Other designs have adjustable straps with Velcro closures for additional support and compression.

➡ **Position of the patient:** Sitting on a taping table or bench with the leg extended off the edge or in a chair with the knee in approximately 45 degrees of flexion.

➡ **Preparation:** Apply neoprene sleeves directly to the skin. No anchors are required.

➡ **Application:**

**STEP 1:**   Hold each side of the sleeve and place the larger end over the foot. Pull in a proximal direction until the sleeve is positioned on the thigh (Fig. 7–19). After use, clean and reuse the sleeves.

**STEP 2:**   If the design has an oval pad, position the pad over the injured area to provide additional compression.

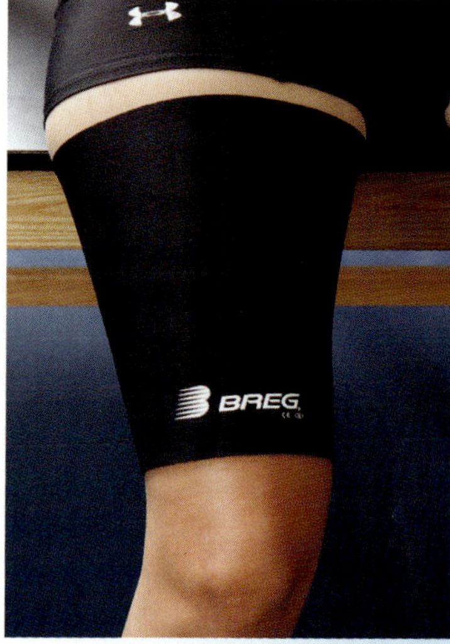

**Fig. 7–19**

## EVIDENCE SUMMARY

Neoprene thigh sleeves are commonly used following injury to provide compression and support. Neoprene sleeves are also thought to increase the temperature of the muscles, which may aid in the progression of healing. In a small study among intercollegiate athletes, researchers[14] investigated the effects of a neoprene sleeve on anterior thigh skin and intramuscular temperatures during and after exercise. During exercise, neoprene sleeves produced higher skin temperatures compared with no sleeve, but had no effect on intramuscular temperatures. Skin and intramuscular temperatures at 30 minutes postexercise remained higher with the neoprene sleeve compared to no sleeve, suggesting that neoprene sleeves may prevent tissue cooling rather than promote tissue heating.[14] The researchers[14] proposed these findings may be beneficial in the prevention and treatment of muscle strains for athletes who experience periods of inactivity during practices and competitions based on playing position or sport rules. Other researchers[15] demonstrated that a custom-made bandage, manufactured of neoprene and polyurethane foam wrapped around the thigh of healthy subjects, resulted in an increase of venous blood volume shift in cutaneous and subcutaneous tissues compared to a non-bandage condition. These findings may have been influenced by the bandage covering the skin, restricting heat elimination, elevating skin and tissue temperature, and increasing skin and tissue blood flow.[15] Further investigations are needed among different neoprene sleeves, injuries and conditions, and populations to develop the evidence base for the selection of the most appropriate design for patient care.

### Clinical Application Question 1

An outside hitter on the volleyball team sustained a second-degree hamstrings strain during a match 4 weeks ago. Her recovery has progressed without any setbacks. The therapeutic exercise program the athlete is following includes the addition of aquatic therapy. The athlete is anxious about the water and wants to have some type of support around her thigh during the exercises.

➡ **Question: What techniques can you apply to provide support?**

## NEOPRENE SHORTS　　Figure 7–20

➡ **Purpose:** Neoprene shorts provide compression and mild support when treating quadriceps, hamstrings, adductor, gluteal, and iliopsoas strains; quadriceps contusions; heterotopic ossification; greater trochanteric bursitis; and osteitis pubis (Fig. 7–20).

### DETAILS

The shorts may be used during rehabilitative, athletic, work, and casual activities.

➡ **Design:**
- Off-the-shelf shorts are manufactured in predetermined sizes and universal fit designs according to waist circumference measurements.
- The designs extend from the mid-to-distal thigh to the waist with a Velcro or elastic waistband.

➡ **Position of the patient:** Sitting in a chair or standing.

➡ **Preparation:** Apply neoprene shorts directly to the skin or over an athletic supporter or girdle. No additional anchors are required.

➡ **Application:**

**STEP 1:** To apply, place the feet into the shorts and pull in a proximal direction until the shorts are positioned on the thigh and waist (Fig. 7–20). Adjust the shorts and waistband if needed. The shorts may be washed and reused.

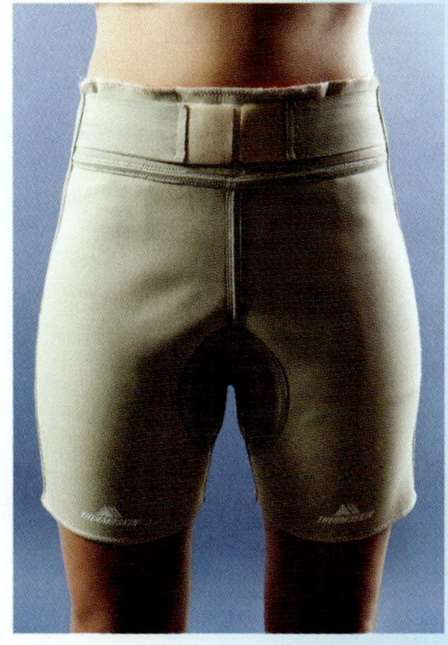

**Fig. 7–20**

## THIGH, HIP, AND PELVIS COMBINATION BRACES          Figure 7–21

➡ **Purpose:** Thigh, hip, and pelvis combination braces are used when treating quadriceps, hamstrings, adductor, and iliopsoas strains and osteitis pubis to provide compression and mild to moderate support and to limit excessive range of motion and stretch on the musculature (Fig. 7–21).

➡ **Design:**
- The braces are manufactured in universal fit designs in predetermined sizes, corresponding either to waist circumference measurements or to the height and weight of the patient.
- The designs extend from the mid-to-distal thigh to the waist and are constructed of neoprene or cotton/spandex materials. Some designs have an elastic waistband and others have an adjustable buckle at the waist.
- One design uses elastic straps with Velcro attachments to allow for several individual applications based on the injury.
- With some designs, diagonal elastic material incorporated into the brace crosses the anterior and posterior thigh, hip, and pelvis to provide compression and support.
- Some designs are available with a closed-cell foam pad to protect the thigh or iliac crest.
- Another design is manufactured with rubber tubing attached to adjustable straps. The straps allow for adjustments in the tension of the tubing.
- Some designs use a contoured neoprene strap that wraps around the waist and thigh. The strap allows for adjustments in tension.
- Other designs use neoprene straps that wrap around the thigh and lower leg to control hip flexion and extension.

➡ **Position of the patient:** Sitting in a chair or standing.

➡ **Preparation:** Apply the thigh, hip, and pelvis combination braces directly to the skin or over an athletic supporter or girdle. No additional anchors are required.

Specific instructions for fitting and application of the braces are included with each design. For proper fit and support, carefully follow the manufacturer's step-by-step procedures. The following application guidelines pertain to most braces.

➡ **Application:**

**STEP 1:** Begin by placing the feet into the shorts and pulling in a proximal direction until the brace is positioned on the thigh, hip, pelvis, and waist (Fig. 7–21A). Adjust the shorts and waistband if needed. The braces may be washed and reused.

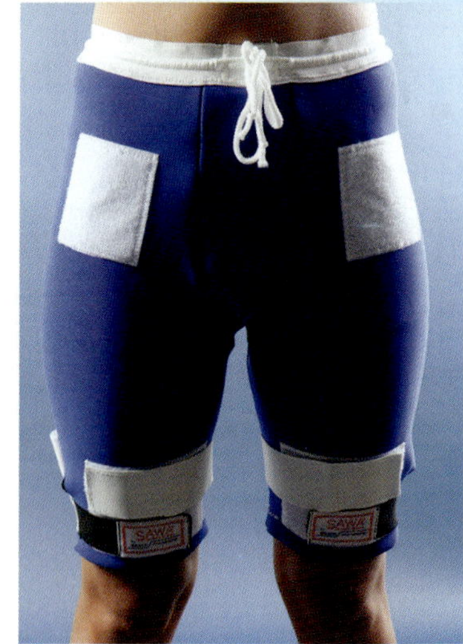

**Fig. 7–21 A**

**STEP 2:** Applying and adjusting the straps will depend on the specific brace design. When treating adductor strains, continue application of some designs by wrapping an elastic strap around the thigh, hip, pelvis, and waist in a lateral-to-medial pattern. Anchor the strap with Velcro on the thigh (Fig. 7–21B). Two elastic straps may also be applied in a crisscross pattern around the distal thighs to treat adductor strains (Fig. 7–21C). Apply an elastic strap in a vertical pattern over either the anterior thigh to treat iliopsoas strains (Fig. 7–21D) or the posterior thigh to treat hamstrings strains (Fig. 7–21E). Retighten the straps and/or reposition the shorts if necessary.

**STEP 3:** With other designs, place the feet into the shorts and pull in a proximal direction until the shorts are positioned on the thigh and waist.

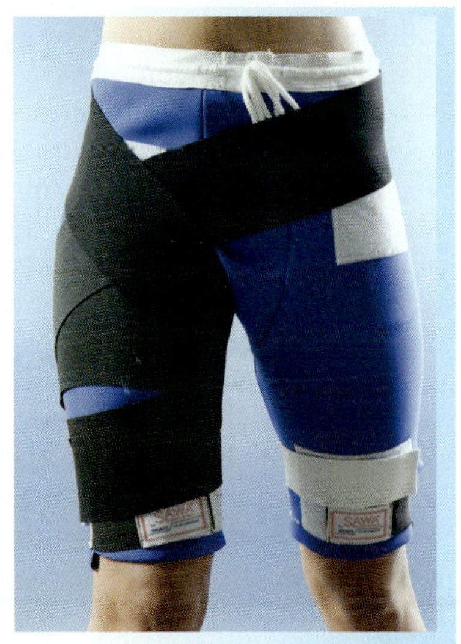

**Fig. 7–21 B**

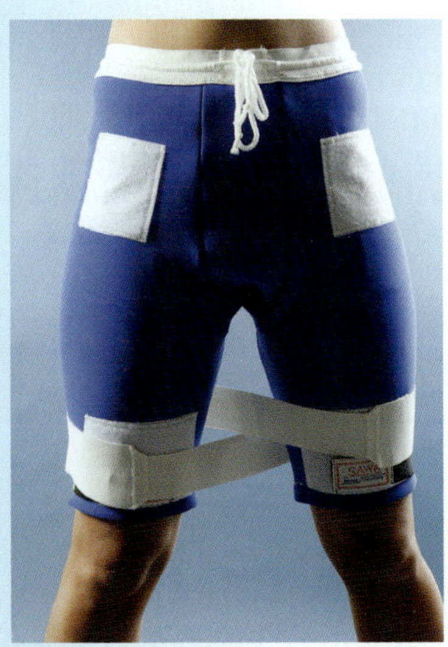

**Fig. 7–21 C**

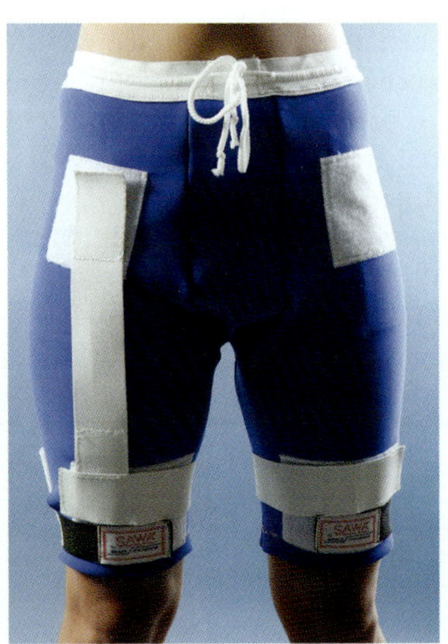

**Fig. 7–21 D**

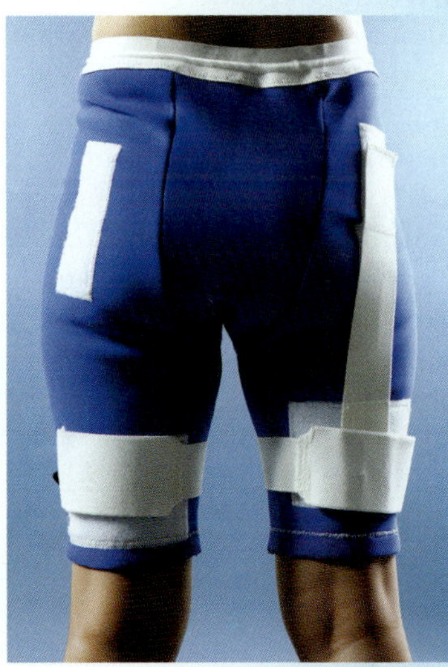

**Fig. 7–21 E**

## EVIDENCE SUMMARY

The design and use of neoprene shorts and thigh, hip, and pelvis combination braces to provide compression, support, and reduce range of motion following injury have become common in many settings.[16] However, limited investigations have examined the effectiveness of these braces on healthy and injured populations. Several researchers[17] demonstrated improvements in dynamic leg swing judgment accuracy with neoprene shorts among healthy athletes with low neuromuscular control ability. In this same study, neoprene shorts reduced accuracy scores among athletes with high neuromuscular control. Examining spandex-type shorts in various sizes among recreational athletes, researchers[18] revealed no significant differences in passive hip joint moment (passive stiffness provided by the brace) and countermovement vertical jump height when compared to loose-fitting shorts. However, medium-size spandex shorts produced significantly greater peak active hip flexion during the countermovement vertical jump. Other researchers[19] have shown spandex-type shorts had no effect on power during a single vertical jump performance; conversely, the shorts had a positive effect on repetitive jump performance. Among intercollegiate athletes in a separate study,[20] custom-made, hypercompressive neoprene and butyl rubber shorts reduced hip flexion during sprinting but did not influence speed measures compared with loose-fitting shorts. The hypercompressive shorts also produced a higher maximal countermovement vertical jump height, higher skin temperatures, and reduced longitudinal and anterior-posterior muscle oscillation during vertical jump landing. Among recreational athletes, other researchers[21] investigated the effects of spandex-type standard compression and directional (diagonal band around the waist and hips) compression shorts on electromyographic activity of the hip adductor musculature during an unanticipated run-to-cut maneuver. A significant reduction in electromyographic activity of the adductor longus was produced with the directional compression brace compared to the standard compression short. A small study[22] investigated the effects of off-the-shelf and custom-made variable compression shorts on the metabolic state of the thigh musculature through T2 weighted magnetic resonance imaging in pre- and post-submaximal running conditions. The researchers[22] proposed that T2 weighted magnetic resonance imaging represented the metabolic state and degree of muscle fatigue. Following a 30-minute submaximal treadmill running period, T2 values significantly increased in the hamstrings and hip adductors with low, mid, mid/high, and high compression and loose-fitting shorts. Compared to loose-fitting shorts, mid (approximately 15 mm Hg) and mid/high (approximately 20 mm Hg) compression shorts significantly reduced T2 values for the biceps femoris, semimembranosus, adductor longus, and adductor magnus musculature and biceps femoris, semimembranosus, and adductor longus, respectively. The researchers[22] suggested that compression shorts with 15–20 mm Hg pressure intensity over the thigh may lessen the development of muscle fatigue during a submaximal running activity.

Focusing on thigh, hip, and pelvis combination braces, researchers[16] revealed no differences between healthy brace wearers and non-brace wearers in proprioception, power, agility, speed, and aerobic capacity measures. However, combination braces were found to reduce active hip flexion and result in positive subjective evaluations regarding increased support and improved performance.[16] Examining combination braces with adjustable tension bands among recreational athletes, researchers[18] found all stiffness conditions significantly increased passive hip joint moment and the stiffest brace condition significantly reduced peak active hip flexion during a countermovement vertical jump compared to loose-fitting shorts. No significant differences in countermovement vertical jump height were found between the adjustable stiffness brace conditions and loose-fitting shorts. Further research is needed with neoprene shorts and thigh, hip, and pelvis combination braces on functional measures to determine their effectiveness in the treatment and perhaps prevention of injuries and conditions.

### ... IF/THEN ...

**IF** support is needed when treating an adductor strain for an athlete during a return to sport activities, **THEN** consider using a thigh, hip, and pelvis combination brace; neoprene shorts can be used, but a combination brace provides greater support and limits excessive range of motion because of the adjustable elastic straps and/or rubber tubing.

## ORTHOTICS

➥ **Purpose:** Orthotics provide support, absorb shock, and correct structural abnormalities when treating thigh, hip, and pelvis injuries and conditions.
- Use soft orthotic designs (see Fig. 3–18) to absorb shock and lessen stress to prevent and treat bursitis and stress fractures. Heel cups and full-length neoprene, silicone, thermoplastic rubber, polyurethane foam, and viscoelastic polymer insoles are available in off-the-shelf designs.
- Use semirigid (see Fig. 3–19) and rigid (see Fig. 3–20) orthotics to provide support and correct structural abnormalities—such as leg-length discrepancy or an increased Q angle—to treat bursitis. The designs are available off-the-shelf or custom-made.

### Clinical Application Question 2

During a baseball game, a concessionaire at the local university slipped on ice in the concession stand and immediately experienced sharp pain in the right quadriceps. Following an evaluation by a physician, the concessionaire has been receiving treatment at an out-patient orthopedic clinic for a mild quadriceps strain. Treatment has progressed normally, and he has returned to work with an elastic wrap applied to his right thigh to provide compression and support. However, the effectiveness of the wrap diminishes 1–2 hours after application.

➥ **Question: How can you manage this situation?**

# Padding Techniques

Off-the-shelf padding techniques are available in a variety of designs to prevent and treat injuries and conditions of the thigh, hip, and pelvis. Custom-made padding techniques constructed of foam and thermoplastic materials are also used with thigh, hip, and pelvis injuries and conditions. Mandatory padding of the thigh, hip, and pelvis is required with several interscholastic and intercollegiate sports. These padding techniques will be discussed further in Chapter 13.

## EVIDENCE SUMMARY

Most studies recommend using protective padding for 3–6 months upon a return to athletic activity following a thigh contusion.[23–25] Whether the pad is purchased off-the-shelf or custom-made, it should cover and protect the injured area; disperse forces to surrounding, healthy tissues; be comfortable to the patient; and remain in place during activity.[25] The pad lessens the risk of reinjury and the development of heterotopic ossification.

## OFF-THE-SHELF — Figure 7–22

➡ **Purpose:** Off-the-shelf padding techniques absorb shock and provide protection when preventing and treating quadriceps and iliac crest contusions and heterotopic ossification (Fig. 7–22). The padding techniques are available from manufacturers in a variety of designs.

### DETAILS
Off-the-shelf pads are commonly used following injury to provide shock absorption to the thigh, hip, and pelvis of athletes participating in a variety of sports. Some designs can be used prophylactically with athletes in collision and contact sports. Use the pads with athletic or work activities.

➡ **Design:**
- Individual and universal fit designs are manufactured in predetermined sizes, corresponding either to circumference measurements of the thigh or waist or the age of the patient.
- Several universal fit thigh designs are constructed of plastic inserts covered by varying thicknesses of high-density open- and closed-cell and EVA foams. The pads are contoured to the thigh; some are coated with vinyl. Universal fit hip and pelvis designs are constructed of open- and closed-cell and EVA foams (Fig. 7–22A).
- Some individual fit designs consist of a plastic material outer shell pre-molded to the contours of the thigh and hip. This outer shell is lined with open- and closed-cell foams extending in all directions to absorb shock (Fig. 7–22B).

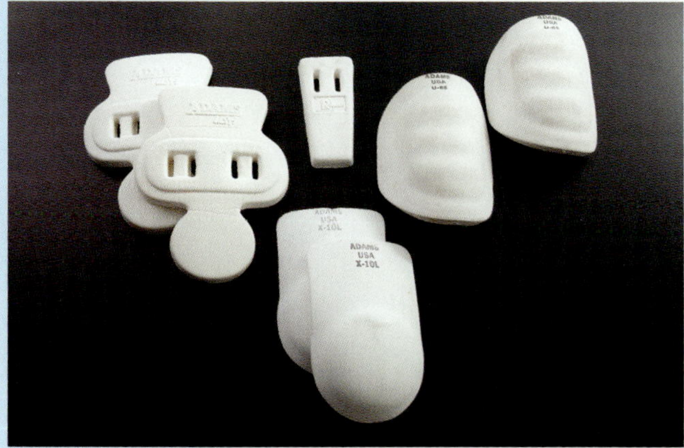

**Fig. 7–22 A** *Variety of universal fit thigh, hip, and pelvis pads.*

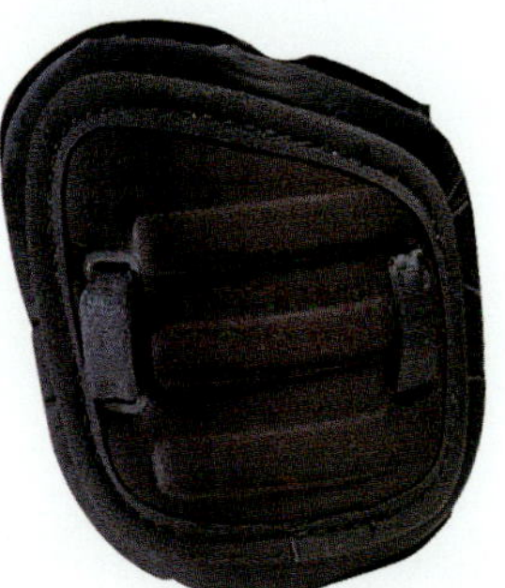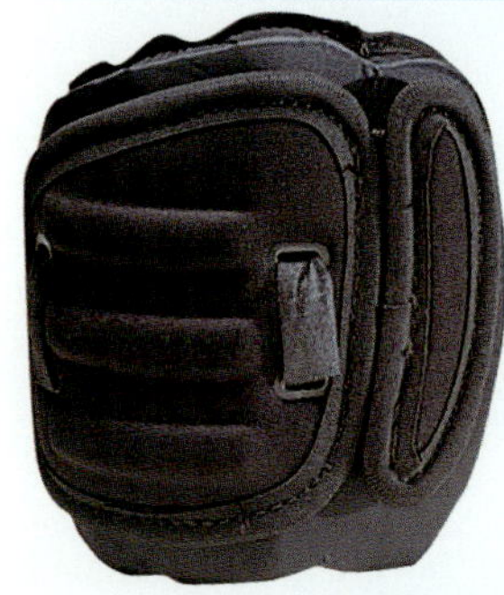

**Fig. 7–22 B** *Individual fit thigh pads. (Left) One piece. (Right) Two piece.*
*(Courtesy of Douglas Pads & Sports, Inc., Houston, TX.)*

- Other thigh and hip designs are manufactured specifically for use following injury. These pads are larger in size with additional padding to cover the thigh, hip, and pelvis (Fig. 7–22C). Some designs have neoprene straps with Velcro closures to attach the pads.
- Another thigh design consists of a high-density shell lined with foam incorporated into a neoprene sleeve.
- Some athletic pant designs, such as those for ice hockey and lacrosse, are available with pads incorporated into the thigh, hip, and pelvis area.
- Other pant designs have closed-cell foam incorporated into spandex or Lycra material shorts and are available in various lengths depending on the technique objective.

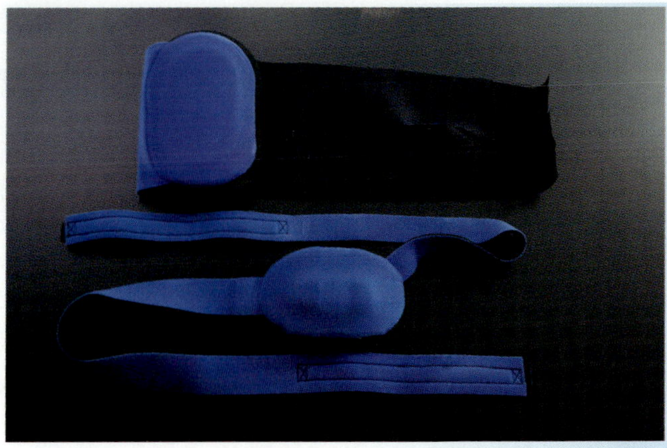

**Fig. 7–22 C** *Post-injury thigh, hip, and pelvis pads.*

➠ **Position of the patient:** Standing on a taping table, bench, or on the ground with the majority of the weight on the non-involved leg and the involved leg placed in a neutral position with slight knee flexion. Maintain this position during application.

➠ **Preparation:** Apply the off-the-shelf designs over pre-wrap or self-adherent wrap, directly to the skin, under tight-fitting clothing, or within athletic clothing.

➠ **Application:**

**STEP 1:**  With taping techniques, place the pad over the injured area and attach to the thigh over pre-wrap or self-adherent wrap with elastic tape, using the circular thigh technique (see Figs. 7–8A to D). Apply the pad directly to the skin over the iliac crest with elastic tape using the hip pointer technique (see Figs. 7–9A to D).

**STEP 2:**  The pad may also be applied directly to the skin and attached to the thigh using the quadriceps strain wrapping technique one or technique two (Fig. 7–22D). Attach the pad to the iliac crest with hip pointer wrapping technique one or technique two.

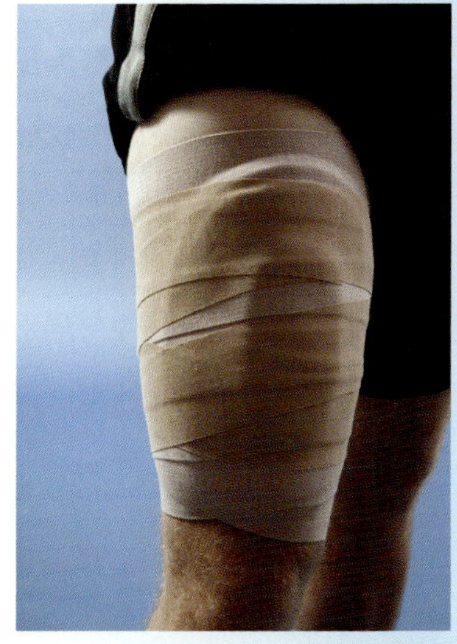

**Fig. 7–22 D**

**STEP 3:** With the strap designs, apply the pad directly to the skin and anchor the neoprene straps around the thigh or hip with Velcro (Fig. 7–22E).

**STEP 4:** The pad may also be attached to the thigh, hip, and/or pelvis by placing the pad underneath tight-fitting clothing such as spandex or Lycra shorts.

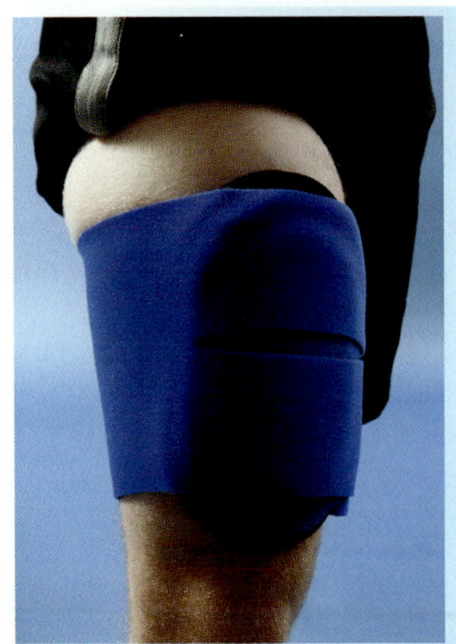

**Fig. 7–22 E**

**STEP 5:** Nylon/polyester girdles with pad pockets are available to attach the pads to the thigh, hip, and/or pelvis (Fig. 7–22F). These girdles are commonly worn by football athletes.

**Helpful Hint |**
When using off-the-shelf thigh pads in right and left designs, ensure proper placement before activity; typically, the angled side of the pad is positioned over the medial thigh.

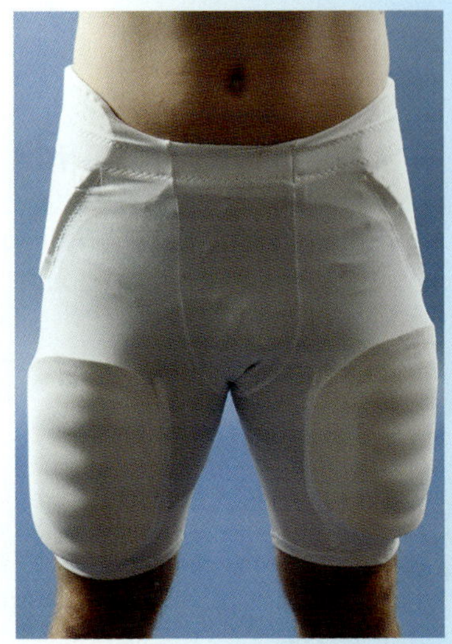

**Fig. 7–22 F**

## CUSTOM-MADE    Figure 7–23

⟹ **Purpose:** Mold thermoplastic material to absorb shock and provide protection to prevent and treat quadriceps and iliac crest contusions and heterotopic ossification (Fig. 7–23). Use these pads when off-the-shelf designs are not available.

⟹ **Materials:**
  • Paper, felt tip pen, thermoplastic material, ⅛ inch or ¼ inch foam or felt, a heating source, 2 inch or 3 inch elastic tape, an elastic wrap, soft, low-density foam, rubber cement, taping scissors

⟹ **Position of the patient:** Standing on a taping table, bench, or on the ground with the majority of the weight on the non-involved leg and the involved leg placed in a neutral position with slight knee flexion. Maintain this position during application.

⟹ **Preparation:** Design the pad with a paper pattern (see Fig. 1–10). Cut, mold, and shape the thermoplastic material on the thigh, hip, or pelvis over the injured area. Attach soft, low-density foam to the inside surface of the material (see Fig. 1–11).

⟹ **Application:**

**STEP 1:** Attach the pad to the thigh with the circular thigh taping technique, quadriceps strain wrapping technique one or technique two, or under tight-fitting clothing or an athletic girdle. Attach the pad to the iliac crest with the hip pointer taping technique, hip pointer wrapping technique one or technique two, or under tight-fitting clothing or an athletic girdle.

**STEP 2:** Consider molding and attaching a piece of thermoplastic material with cement or elastic tape to an off-the-shelf thigh, hip, or pelvis pad to provide additional protection for a contusion (Fig. 7–23).

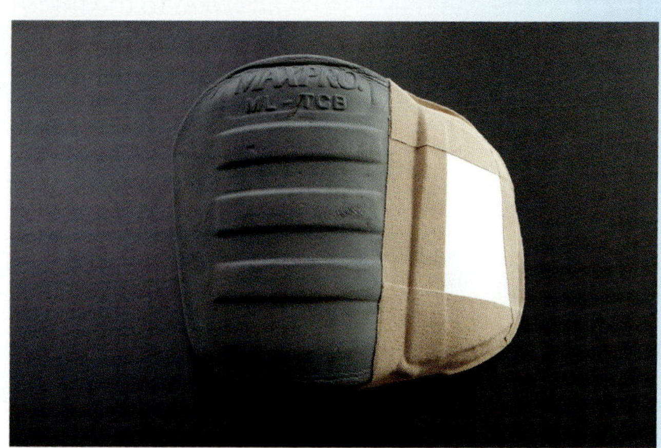

**Fig. 7–23**

## MANDATORY PADDING

The NCAA[26] and the NFHS[27] require athletes to use mandatory protective padding for the thigh, hip, and pelvis during all football practices and competitions. The majority of these pads are available in off-the-shelf designs and can be purchased in a set. The NFHS[28,29] requires the use of mandatory protective equipment for the thigh, hip, and pelvis for ice hockey and for the thigh for girls' lacrosse goalkeepers during all practices and competitions. A more in-depth discussion of these pads can be found in Chapter 13.

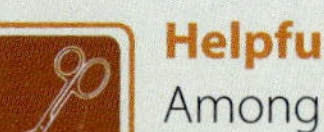

**Helpful Hint** |
Among football athletes, closely monitor the proper use and wear of mandatory thigh, hip, and pelvis padding. Many football players cut the pads to smaller sizes for additional comfort, reducing the protection provided.

### Clinical Application Question 3

With 8 minutes remaining in the Conference Championship game, the starting center on your basketball team defends against a layup and is struck in the left anterior thigh by the opponent's knee. An evaluation on the bench reveals general tenderness over the anterior quadriceps. The athlete has full bilateral range of motion, strength, and functional movement, indicating a mild contusion. Your team physician agrees.

➡ **Question: Within the limited amount of time left in the game, what techniques can you use in this situation?**

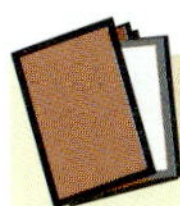

## EVIDENCE-BASED PRACTICE

Near the end of the first period, Robert Greene, a defenseman on the Davis Junior College hockey team, is pushed into the goal by an opponent while attempting to gain control of the puck. His right anterior thigh strikes the right goal post. Following stoppage of play, Julie Wells, AT, comes onto the ice to evaluate Robert. From the bench, Julie observed the mechanism of injury and begins to gather information from Robert about the injury. Following the on-ice evaluation, Robert is helped to the athletic training facility, where the team physician is waiting. In the athletic training facility, Julie questions Robert about a previous injury to his right thigh, while the team physician begins an evaluation. Robert tells Julie he has suffered two previous contusions to his right anterior thigh during the last year and a half. The team physician completes the evaluation and determines that Robert has sustained a third-degree right anterior quadriceps contusion. Robert is placed on crutches for non–weight-bearing ambulation. Julie begins treatment immediately.

After several follow-up appointments with the team physician and a comprehensive therapeutic exercise program, Robert is allowed to return to sport- and position-specific practice activities on the ice. The team physician and Julie agree that protective padding of the right thigh during these activities is warranted. Julie selects an off-the-shelf padding technique for Robert that is commonly worn by ice hockey athletes to provide protection and prevent reinjury.

Robert has progressed with his activities on the ice but recently began to notice an increase in the amount of soreness in the anterior thigh after practice. Julie performs an evaluation in the athletic training facility and finds mild swelling and point tenderness over the anterior quadriceps. Robert demonstrates bilateral strength and flexibility. Julie refers Robert to the team physician. The team physician performs an evaluation and obtains radiographs, which are negative. He is concerned about Robert's past history of injury and the possible development of heterotopic ossification. The team physician meets with Julie and recommends the following: (1) closely monitor and reduce swelling, (2) maintain strength and flexibility, and (3) consider the use of additional protective padding. The team physician allows Robert to return to practice as tolerated. Julie develops a therapeutic exercise program for Robert that includes strengthening and flexibility exercises and modalities and compression wrapping techniques for the reduction of swelling. Julie begins to

question whether the off-the-shelf ice hockey padding technique Robert is currently using is the most effective in this situation. She starts to look for a new technique to protect Robert from reinjury during practices and competitions.

1. Develop a clinically relevant question from the case in the PICO format to generate answers for the selection of a padding technique for Robert. The question should include the population or problem, the intervention, a comparison intervention (if relevant), and the clinical outcome of interest.
2. Design a search strategy and search to find the best evidence to answer the clinical question. The strategy should include relevant search terms, electronic databases, online journals, and print journals to use for the search. Discussions with your faculty, preceptor, and other health care professionals can provide evidence from expert opinion.
3. Choose three to five full text studies or reviews from your search or the chapter references. Evaluate and appraise each article to determine its value and usefulness to the case. Ask these questions for each study: (1) Are the results of the study valid? (2) What are the actual results? and (3) Are the findings clinically relevant to my patients? Prepare a summary of the evaluation with answers to the questions and rank the articles based on the evidence hierarchy in Chapter 1.
4. Integrate findings from the evidence, your clinical experience, and Robert's goals and preferences into the therapeutic exercise program for Robert. Consider which padding technique may be appropriate for Robert.
5. Evaluate the EBP process and your experience within the case. Consider these questions in the evaluation.

Was the clinical question answered?
Did the search generate quality evidence?
Was the evidence evaluated appropriately?
Was the evidence, your clinical experience, and Robert's goals and values integrated to make the clinical decision?
Did the intervention produce successful clinical outcomes for Robert?
Was the EBP experience positive for Julie and Robert?

Thigh, Hip, and Pelvis

## WRAP-UP

- Acute and chronic injuries and conditions to the thigh, hip, and pelvis can be the result of single or repeated direct forces, structural abnormalities, repetitive stress and tension, and rapid stretch, contraction, or weakness of the musculature.
- The circular thigh and hip pointer taping techniques provide support and anchor protective padding to the thigh, hip, and pelvis.
- Compression wrap techniques provide compression to control mild, moderate, and severe swelling following injury.
- The quadriceps strain wrapping techniques can be used to provide compression and support and to anchor protective padding.
- The hamstrings, adductor, and hip flexor strain wrapping techniques provide compression and support.
- The hip pointer wrapping techniques anchor protective padding to the iliac crest.
- Neoprene sleeves and shorts and thigh, hip, and pelvis combination braces are used to provide compression and support.
- Soft, semirigid, and rigid orthotics provide support, absorb shock, and correct structural abnormalities.
- Various high-density open- and closed-cell and EVA foams and plastic and thermoplastic materials absorb shock and provide protection when preventing and treating injuries and conditions.
- The NCAA and NFHS require the use of mandatory protective equipment for the thigh, hip, and pelvis in football, ice hockey, and girls' lacrosse.

## FADAVIS ONLINE RESOURCES

- Quadriceps strain wrapping technique two
- Hamstrings strain wrapping technique two
- Hip pointer wrapping technique two

## WEB REFERENCES

### SportsInjuryClinic.net
https://www.sportsinjuryclinic.net
- This website has an injury index that can be searched for treatment and rehabilitation information about a variety of thigh, hip, and pelvis injuries and conditions.

### The American Orthopaedic Society for Sports Medicine
https://www.sportsmed.org/
- This site provides access to *The American Journal of Sports Medicine,* patient newsletter, podcasts, and other educational materials.

### Sports-health
https://www.sports-health.com/

- This website allows you to search for information about a variety of thigh, hip, and pelvis injuries and conditions.

### American Medical Society for Sports Medicine Sports Medicine Today
https://www.sportsmedtoday.com/
- This site provides access to information about acute and chronic thigh, hip, and pelvis injuries and conditions.

## REFERENCES


1. Cetin, C, Sekir, U, Yildiz, Y, Aydin, T, Ors, F, and Kalyon, TA: Chronic groin pain in an amateur soccer player. Br J Sports Med 38:223–224, 2004.
2. McCulloch, PC, and Bush-Joseph, CA: Massive heterotopic ossification complicating iliopsoas tendon lengthening: A case report. Am J Sports Med 34:2022–2025, 2006.
3. Michelsson, JE, Granroth, G, and Andersson, LC: Myositis ossificans following forcible manipulation of the leg: A rabbit model for the study of heterotopic bone formation. J Bone Joint Surg Am 62:811–815, 1980.
4. Michelsson, JE, and Rauschning, W: Pathogenesis of experimental heterotopic bone formation following temporary forcible exercising of immobilized limbs. Clin Orthop Relat Res 176:265–272, 1983.
5. Brooks, JHM, Fuller, CW, Kemp, SPT, and Reddin, DB: Incidence, risk, and prevention of hamstring muscle injuries in professional rugby union. Am J Sports Med 34:1297–1306, 2006.
6. Ekstrand, J, Hägglund, M, and Waldén, M: Epidemiology of muscle injuries in professional football (soccer). Am J Sports Med 39:1226–1232, 2011.
7. Anderson, K, Strickland, SM, and Warren, R: Hip and groin injuries in athletes. Am J Sports Med 29:521–533, 2001.
8. Starkey, C, and Brown, SD: Examination of Orthopedic and Athletic Injuries, ed 4. F.A. Davis, Philadelphia, 2015.
9. Paajanen, H, Hermunen, H, and Karonen, J: Pubic magnetic resonance imaging findings in surgically and conservatively treated athletes with osteitis pubis compared to asymptomatic athletes during heavy training. Am J Sports Med 36:117–121, 2008.
10. Radic, R, and Annear, P: Use of pubic symphysis curettage for treatment-resistant osteitis pubis in athletes. Am J Sports Med 36:122–128, 2008.
11. Tibor, LM, and Sekiya, JK: Differential diagnosis of pain around the hip joint. Arthroscopy 24:1407–1421, 2008.
12. Williams, JG: Limitation of hip joint movement as a factor in traumatic osteitis pubis. Br J Sports Med 12:129–133, 1978.
13. Morris, AF: Sports Medicine: Prevention of Athletic Injuries. Wm. C. Brown Publishers, Dubuque, IA, 1984.

14. Miller, AA, Knight, KL, Feland, JB, and Draper, DO: Neoprene thigh sleeves and muscle cooling after exercise. J Athl Train 40:264–270, 2005.

15. Sommer, B, Berschin, G, and Sommer, HM: Micro-circulation under an elastic bandage during rest and exercise—Preliminary experience with the laser-Doppler spectrophotometry system O2C. J Sports Sci Med 12:414–421, 2013.

16. Berhardt, T, and Anderson, GS: Influence of moderate prophylactic compression on sport performance. J Strength Cond Res 19:292–297, 2005.

17. Cameron, ML, Adams, RD, and Maher, CG: The effect of neoprene shorts on leg proprioception in Australian football players. J Sci Med Sport 11:345–352, 2008.

18. Wannop, JW, Worobets, JT, Madden, R, and Stefanyshyn, DJ: Influence of compression and stiffness apparel on vertical jump performance. J Strength Cond Res 30:1093–1101, 2016.

19. Kraemer, WJ, Bush, JA, Bauer, JA, Triplett-McBride, NT, Paxton, NJ, Clemson, A, Koziris, LP, Mangino, LC, Fry, AC, and Newton, RU: Influence of compression garments on vertical jump performance in NCAA division I volleyball players. J Strength Cond Res 10:180–183, 1996.

20. Doan, BK, Kwon, YH, Newton, RU, Shim, J, Popper, EM, Rodgers, RA, Bolt, LR, Robertson, M, and Kraemer, WJ: Evaluation of a lower-body compression garment. J Sports Sci 21:601–610, 2003.

21. Chaudhari, AM, Jamison, ST, McNally, MP, Pan, X, and Schmitt, LC: Hip adductor activations during run-to-cut maneuvers in compression shorts: Implications for return to sport after groin injury. J Sports Sci 32:1333–1340, 2014.

22. Miyamoto, N, and Kawakami, Y: Effect of pressure intensity of compression short-tight on fatigue of thigh muscles. Med Sci Sports Exerc 46:2168–2174, 2014.

23. Ekstrand, J, and Gillquist, J: Soccer injuries and their mechanisms: A prospective study. Med Sci Sports Exerc 15:267–270, 1983.

24. Jackson, DW, and Feagin, JA: Quadriceps contusions in young athletes. J Bone Joint Surg Am 55:95–105, 1973.

25. Kaeding, CC, Sanko, WA, and Fischer, RA: Myositis ossificans: Minimizing downtime. Phys Sportsmed 23:77–82, 1995.

26. National Collegiate Athletic Association: 2014–15 Sports Medicine Handbook, ed 25. NCAA, Indianapolis, 2014. http://www.ncaapublications.com/product-downloads/MD15.pdf.

27. National Federation of State High School Associations: 2018 Football Rules Book. National Federation of State High School Associations, Indianapolis, IN, 2019.

28. National Federation of State High School Associations: 2018 Girls Lacrosse Rules Book. National Federation of State High School Associations, Indianapolis, IN, 2019.

29. National Federation of State High School Associations: 2018–19 Ice Hockey Rules Book. National Federation of State High School Associations, Indianapolis, IN, 2019.

# Part Three

# Injuries and Conditions of the Upper Body, Thorax, Abdomen, and Spine

**ICON KEY**

Helpful Hint 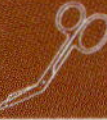

Tape may be applied directionally from either left or right 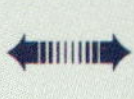

Additional resources are available at FADavis.com 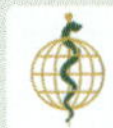

A technique video is available at FADavis.com 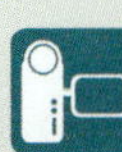

Evidence-Based Practice 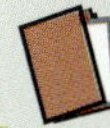

Evidence Summary 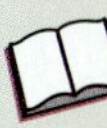

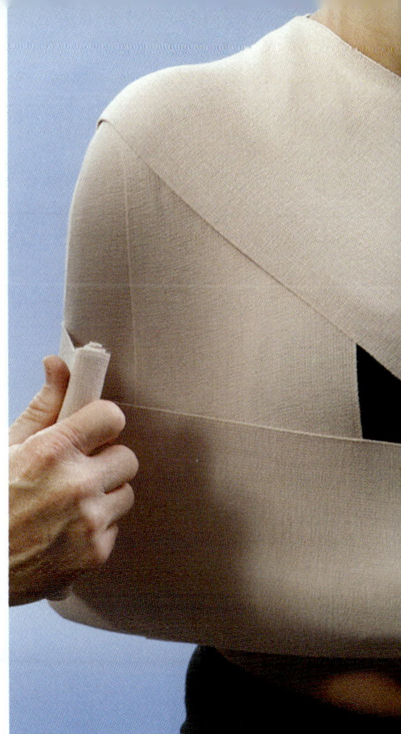

**8**

# Shoulder and Upper Arm



## INJURIES AND CONDITIONS

Acute and chronic injuries and conditions to the shoulder and upper arm can result from direct and indirect compressive forces, excessive range of motion, and repetitive stress. The structure of the shoulder allows for a considerable range of motion; the surrounding musculature provides the shoulder's main stabilization. The available range of motion and lack of stability provided by bony, ligamentous, and tendinous structures place the joint at risk for injury. A contusion, sprain, dislocation/subluxation, or fracture can result when a runner stumbles and falls to the ground on the tip of her shoulder or on the outstretched arm. Repetitive overhead movements experienced in throwing sports can cause strains and overuse injuries and conditions. Common injuries to the shoulder and upper arm include:

- Contusions
- Sprains
- Dislocations/subluxations
- Fractures
- Strains
- Ruptures
- Overuse injuries and conditions

## Contusions

Contusions to the shoulder and upper arm are caused by compressive forces and are common in athletic activities. Falling on the tip of the shoulder or experiencing a direct force to this area can cause a contusion to the distal end of the clavicle **(shoulder pointer)** (Fig. 8–1). An acute or series of repeated direct forces to the musculature of the upper arm can result in swelling, pain, and loss of range of motion. Commonly, the anterolateral aspect of the upper arm is involved, affecting the deltoid, brachialis, biceps brachii, and triceps brachii muscles and the humerus (Figs. 8–2 and 8–3). For example, a contusion to the proximal upper arm can occur when a football player cuts the sleeves off his practice jersey, allowing movement of the shoulder pad cups while running and exposing the area to a direct blow. Repeated forces can lead to the development of heterotopic ossification in a muscle or **exostosis (tackler's exostosis)** on the humerus.

## Sprains

Shoulder sprains are caused by compression and shear forces, excessive range of motion, and overuse. Forceful abduction, excessive external rotation and extension, or

241

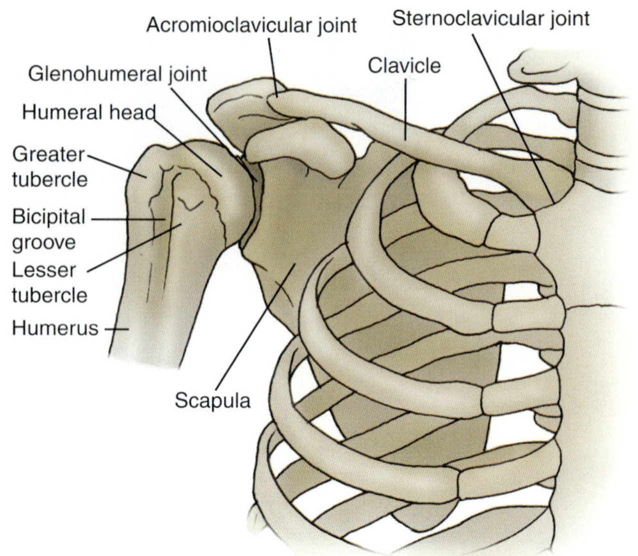


**Fig. 8–1** *Anterior view of the bones and joints of the shoulder.*

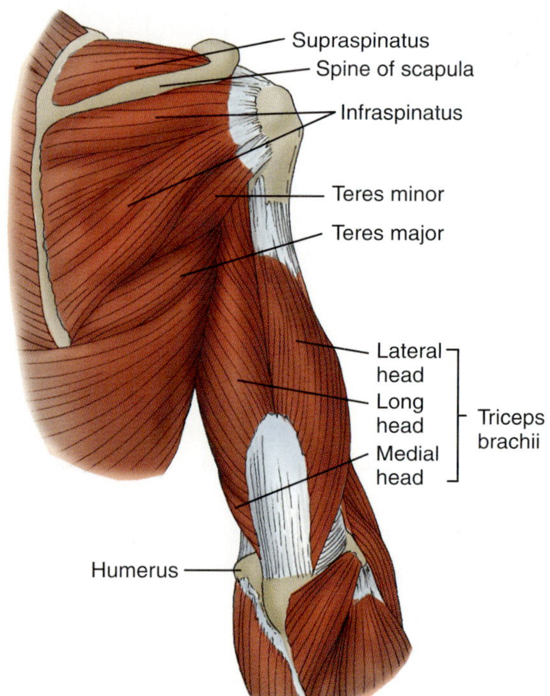


**Fig. 8–3** *Deep muscles of the posterior shoulder and upper arm.*

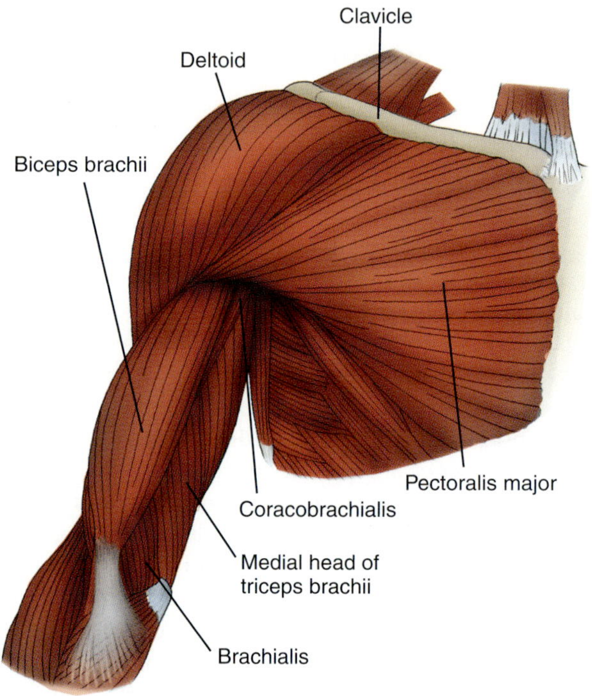


**Fig. 8–2** *Superficial muscles of the anterior shoulder and upper arm.*

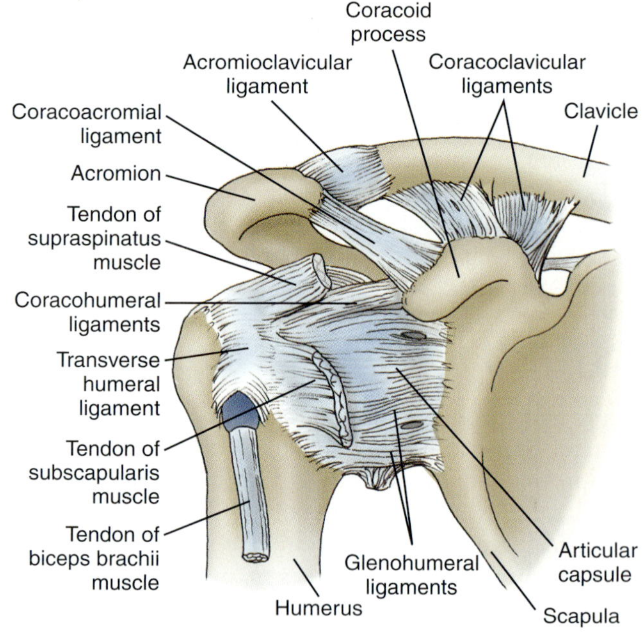


**Fig. 8–4** *Anterior view of the glenohumeral and acromioclavicular joints.*

a direct force that translates the humerus posteriorly can result in a **glenohumeral (GH) joint** sprain (Fig. 8–4). A sprain, for instance, could result from a football linebacker tackling a running back, using only the right arm and causing violent abduction, external rotation, and extension of the arm. Sprains to the **sternoclavicular (SC) joint** are caused by indirect forces placed on the clavicle, which may occur with a fall on the outstretched arm, direct compression on the lateral shoulder, or traction and torsion forces. Acromioclavicular (AC) joint sprains are the result of the acromion process being forced away from the clavicle or the clavicle being forced away from the acromion. This mechanism can occur with a fall on the outstretched hand, flexed elbow, or tip of the shoulder; direct force to the acromion; or repetitive forces and overhead activities (Fig. 8–5). AC joint sprains

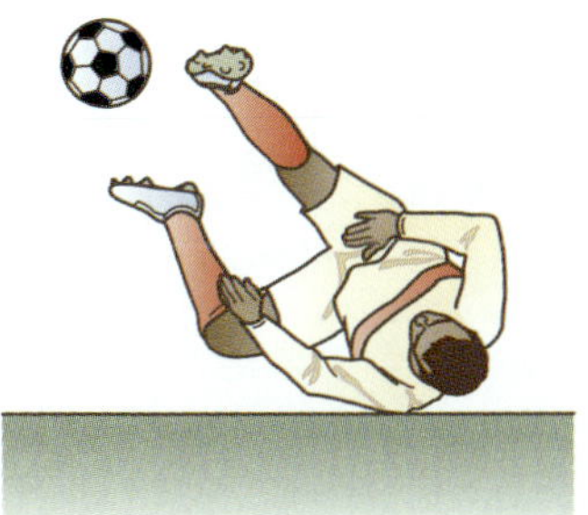

**Fig. 8–5** *Acromioclavicular (AC) joint sprain. Falling on the tip of the shoulder.*

are common in collision and contact sports as a result of being tackled or falling on the playing surface.

## Dislocations/Subluxations

Dislocations and subluxations of the GH joint are common in athletic and work activities because of the vast range of motion and minimal ligamentous support present at the joint. Both acute and chronic mechanisms are associated with these injuries. **Anterior dislocations** and **subluxations**, caused by excessive abduction, external rotation, and extension of the humerus, account for the majority of GH dislocations[1] (Fig. 8–6). This mechanism of injury is identical to the GH joint sprain mechanism. A direct force to the posterior or posterolateral shoulder can also result in an anterior dislocation and/or subluxation.

A direct force to the anterior shoulder, excessive adduction and internal rotation of the humerus, or a fall on the outstretched, internally rotated arm can result in a **posterior dislocation** and/or **subluxation.** For example, a posterior dislocation/subluxation can occur as a right-handed baseball outfielder chases a fly ball to his left and, nearing the warning track, reaches the ball with a backhanded catch, then collides with the wall, causing a longitudinal anterior force on the GH joint and excessive internal rotation of the right humerus. **Inferior dislocations** and **subluxations** are rare.

Following acute dislocations and/or subluxations, **anterior, posterior, inferior,** and **multidirectional instability** of the GH joint can develop. Due to the high occurrence of anterior dislocations/subluxations, anterior instability is more common. Instability can also be the result of chronic, repetitive forces placed on the GH joint. Repetitive forces from overhead activities, such as throwing in baseball and softball, serving in tennis, and swimming, can cause instability. Acute anterior dislocations or chronic anterior instability of the GH joint can result in a **Bankart lesion** on the anterior labrum, a **Hill-Sachs lesion** on the posterior humeral head, or a **superior labrum anteroposterior (SLAP) lesion** on the anterior and posterior superior labrum. Posterior instability is most often associated with repetitive microtrauma and can cause a **reverse Hill-Sachs lesion** on the anterior humeral head.[2] Inferior and superior instabilities are rare and limited by the bony structure of the shoulder. Acute and chronic dislocations and subluxations can also result in multidirectional instability, which is instability in more than one plane of motion at the GH joint.

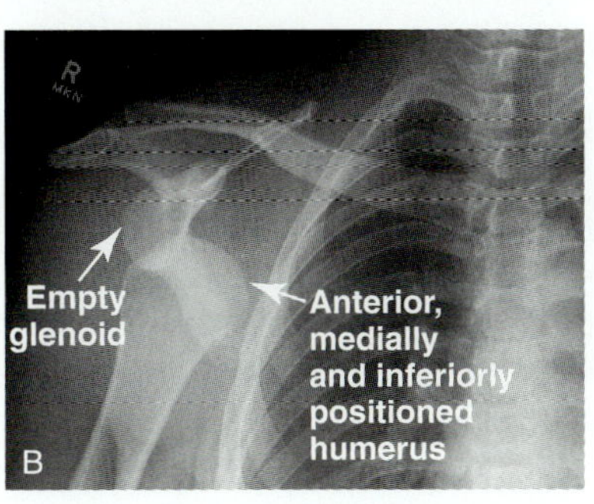


**Fig. 8–6 A** *Photograph of an anterior glenohumeral dislocation.* **B** *Dislocation of the glenohumeral joint. The head is lying anteriorly, inferiorly, and medially from its normal articulation in the glenoid fossa. (A. Courtesy of Starkey, C, and Brown, SD. Examination of Orthopedic & Athletic Injuries. 4th ed. Philadelphia, PA: F.A. Davis Company: 2015. B. Courtesy of McKinnis, LN, and Mulligan, M. Musculoskeletal Imaging Handbook. Philadelphia, PA: F.A. Davis Company: 2014.)*

# Fractures

Fractures can occur to the clavicle, scapula, and humerus. A fall on the outstretched arm or tip of the shoulder can cause a clavicular fracture, as can a direct force. The most common fracture site occurs at the middle third of the clavicle.[3] A clavicular fracture can result, for example, when a cyclist is thrown from his bike and falls to the ground on the outstretched arm. Scapular fractures are the result of a direct force, a fall on the outstretched arm, violent muscular contractions, and shoulder dislocations and subluxations. A direct force, a fall on the outstretched arm or upper arm, and shoulder dislocations can also result in a humeral fracture.

# Strains

Strains to the shoulder commonly affect the **rotator cuff** musculature, teres minor, infraspinatus, supraspinatus, and subscapularis (see Figs. 8–3 and 8–7). Injury can be caused by repetitive microtrauma and overload; shoulder impingement syndrome, with associated mechanical compression and chronic inflammation; glenohumeral instability; and falls on the outstretched arm[4] (Fig. 8–8). For example, a strain can occur in a youth league baseball pitcher as a result of repetitive throwing without appropriate recovery periods.

# Ruptures

A rupture of the biceps brachii is caused by a forceful concentric or eccentric contraction against resistance. The proximal portion of the tendon located near the bicipital groove is injured most frequently. A rupture can result, for instance, when a gymnast performs a movement on the rings with his elbows in flexion, then loses grip of the left hand, and attempts to regrip the ring as he is falling, causing a violent eccentric contraction of the left biceps brachii.

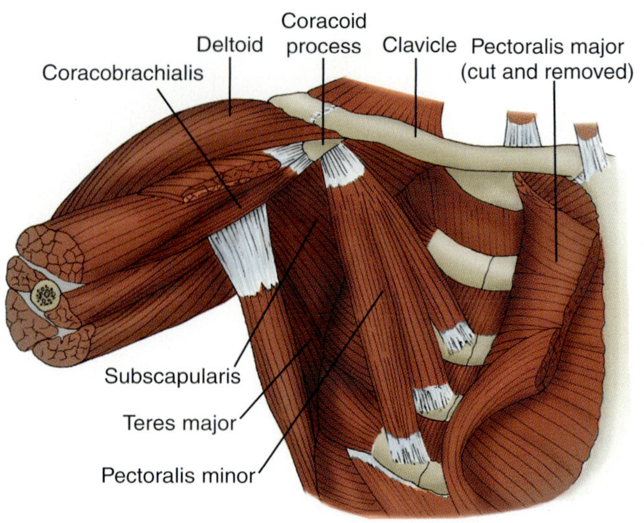


**Fig. 8–7** *Deep muscles of the anterior shoulder and upper arm.*

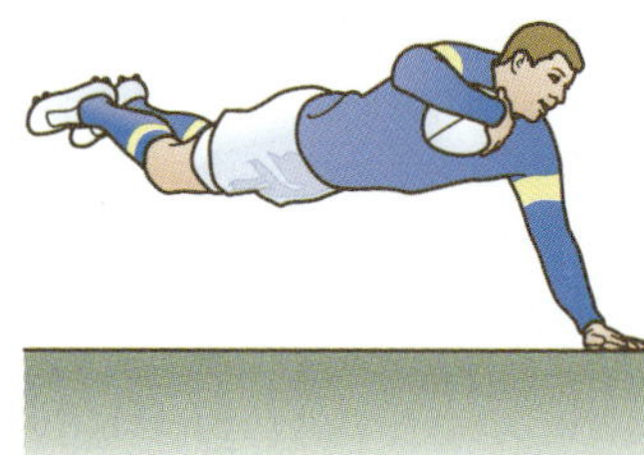

**Fig. 8–8** *Rotator cuff strain. Falling on the outstretched arm.*

# Overuse

Overuse injuries and conditions come from repetitive stress, rotator cuff pathology, and impingement. Rotator cuff or bicipital tendinitis may result from repetitive overload and stress, muscle imbalance and weakness of the rotator cuff, and shoulder impingement syndrome.

## Taping Techniques

Several taping techniques may be used to prevent and treat injuries and conditions of the shoulder and upper arm. All of the techniques are also used to anchor off-the-shelf and custom-made pads to the upper arm and/or shoulder. Protective padding techniques are illustrated in the Padding section.

### CIRCULAR UPPER ARM    Figure 8-9

➥ **Purpose:** Use the circular upper arm technique to provide mild support and anchor protective padding (Fig. 8–9). The technique is used with off-the-shelf and custom-made pads to absorb shock when preventing and treating upper arm contusions, heterotopic ossification, and exostosis.

➥ **Materials:**
• Pre-wrap or self-adherent wrap, 2 inch or 3 inch elastic tape, adherent tape spray, taping scissors

*Option:*
- 1½ inch non-elastic tape

➠ **Position of the patient:** Sitting on a taping table or bench or standing with the involved arm at the side of the body and the elbow placed in 90 degrees of flexion with moderate isometric contraction of the biceps and triceps muscles.

➠ **Preparation:** Apply adherent tape spray to the upper arm.

➠ **Application:**

**STEP 1:** Apply pre-wrap or self-adherent wrap in a circular pattern around the upper arm ◄▭▭►.

**STEP 2:** Place the pad over the injured area. Anchor 2 inch or 3 inch elastic tape directly to the distal pad (Fig. 8–9A).

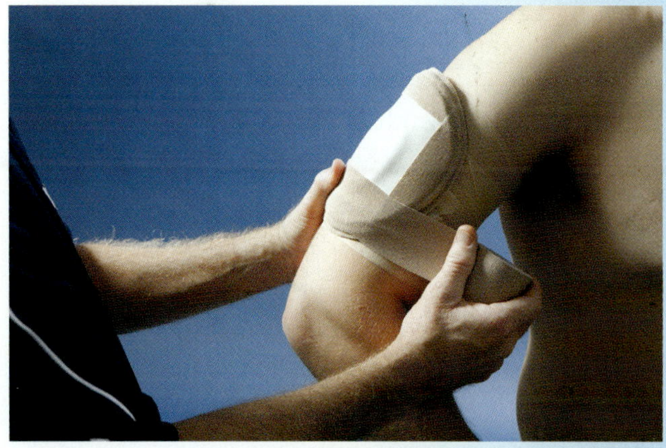

**Fig. 8–9 A**

**STEP 3:** Continue around the upper arm in a circular, distal-to-proximal pattern with moderate roll tension, overlapping the tape by ½ of its width ◄▭▭► (Fig. 8–9B). Cover the entire pad and anchor on the lateral upper arm to prevent irritation. Avoid gaps, wrinkles, and inconsistent roll tension.

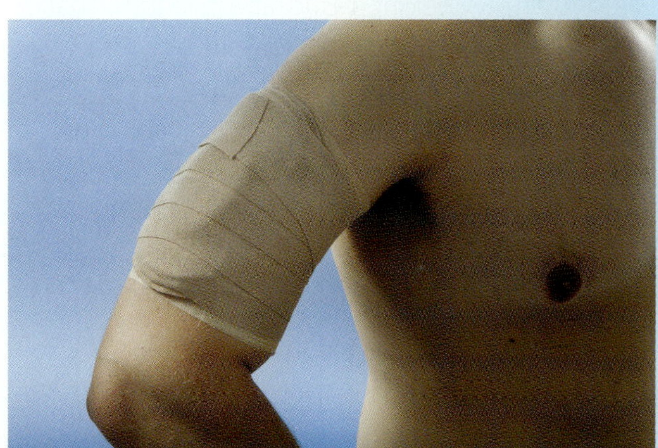

**Fig. 8–9 B**

**STEP 4:** To prevent migration of the pad, apply a distal circular strip of elastic tape with distal-to-proximal tension (Fig. 8–9C) or apply the proximal circular tape strips to the skin. No additional anchors are required.

*Option:* *Loosely apply one to two circular strips of 1½ inch non-elastic tape around the pad for additional anchors* ◄▭▭►.

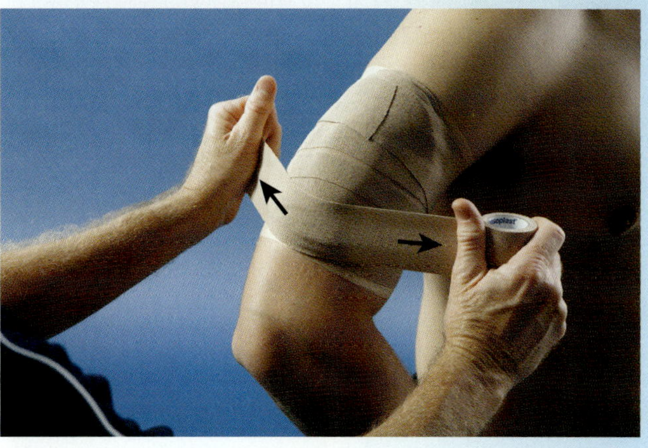

**Fig. 8–9 C**

## SHOULDER POINTER/AC JOINT SPRAIN TAPE   Figure 8-10

➠ **Purpose:** The shoulder pointer/AC joint sprain technique anchors off-the-shelf and custom-made pads to the shoulder to absorb shock when preventing and treating contusions and AC joint sprains (Fig. 8–10).

➠ **Materials:**
  • 2 inch or 3 inch heavyweight elastic tape, adherent tape spray, taping scissors

➠ **Position of the patient:** Standing with the hand of the involved arm placed on the lateral hip in a relaxed position.

➠ **Preparation:** Apply the shoulder pointer/AC joint sprain technique directly to the skin.

➠ **Application:**

**STEP 1:**   Apply adherent tape spray over the pad area and 4–6 inches beyond over the anterior and posterior shoulder. Allow the spray to dry.

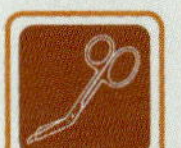

**Helpful Hint |**
You can quickly dry adherent tape spray by patting the area with a full roll of pre-wrap. When the roll begins to adhere to the skin during patting, the area is ready for application of tape.

**STEP 2:**   Cut several strips of 2 inch or 3 inch heavyweight elastic tape in lengths that will cover the pad and extend 4–6 inches beyond the pad on the two sides. Place the pad over the injured area. Anchor the first tape strip on the posterior shoulder, 4–6 inches from the edge of the pad, and pat down (Fig. 8–10A). Do not stretch the tape as the anchor is applied.

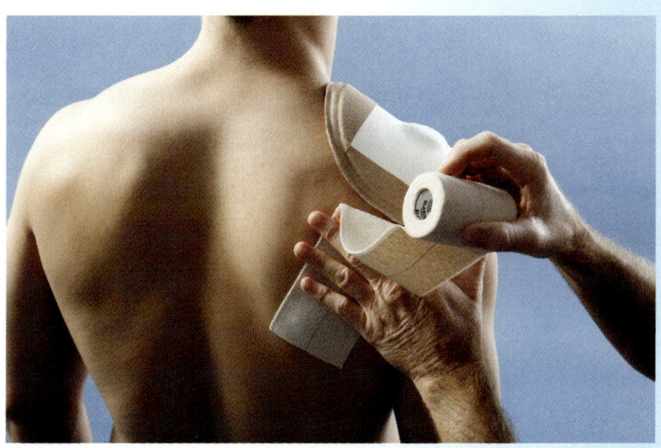

**Fig. 8–10 A**

**STEP 3:**   Continue to apply the strip to the edge of the pad. At the edge, hold the strip on the posterior shoulder with one hand and pull the strip over the pad with tension on the tape (Fig. 8–10B).

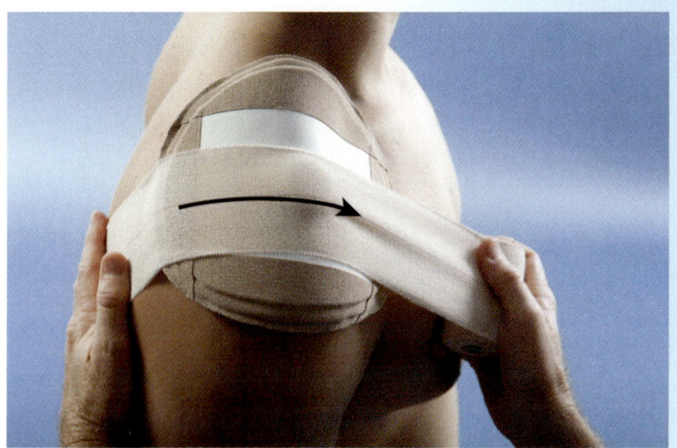

**Fig. 8–10 B**

**STEP 4:** When the strip completely covers the pad, release the tension in the tape, anchor it to the anterior shoulder, and pat down (Fig. 8–10C). Not allowing stretch in the anchor portions of the strip placed directly on the skin improves adherence of the tape. Applying tension and stretch to the portion of the strip placed over the pad secures the pad to the body. This technique can be thought of as a release-stretch-release sequence.

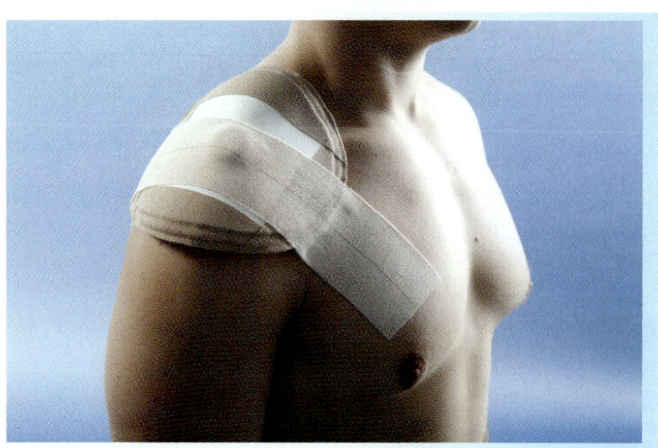

**Fig. 8–10 C**

**STEP 5:** Continue with additional strips in the same manner, overlapping each by ½ the width of the tape (Fig. 8–10D). Apply enough strips to cover the majority of the pad.

**Helpful Hint |**
To prevent skin damage from the tape adhesive, apply tape removal solvent to the skin before removing the shoulder pointer/AC joint sprain taping technique.

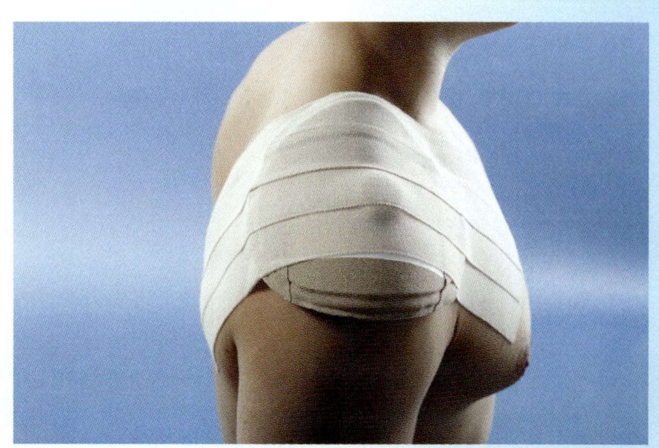

**Fig. 8–10 D**

# Wrapping Techniques

Wrapping techniques for the shoulder and upper arm provide compression, support, and immobilization. Use these techniques to prevent and treat upper arm contusions; heterotopic ossification; exostosis; shoulder pointers; GH, SC, and AC joint sprains; dislocations and subluxations; clavicular, scapular, and humeral fractures; rotator cuff strains; ruptures; and tendinitis. Wrapping techniques also attach protective pads to the shoulder and upper arm.

## UPPER ARM COMPRESSION WRAP     Figure 8-11

➠ **Purpose:** The upper arm compression wrap technique aids in reducing mild to moderate swelling following contusions and ruptures (Fig. 8–11).

➠ **Materials:**
• 2 inch, 3 inch, or 4 inch width by 5 yard length elastic wrap determined by the size of the upper arm, metal clips, 1½ inch non-elastic or 1½ inch or 2 inch elastic tape, taping scissors

*Options:*
• ¼ inch or ½ inch foam or felt
• 2 inch, 3 inch, or 4 inch width self-adherent wrap

➡ **Position of the patient:** Sitting on a taping table or bench or standing with the involved arm at the side of the body and the elbow placed in a pain-free, flexed position.

➡ **Preparation:** To lessen migration, apply adherent tape spray, tape strips, or anchors directly to the skin (see Fig. 1–7).

***Option:***
Cut a ¼ inch or ½ inch foam or felt pad and place it over the inflamed area directly to the skin to assist in controlling swelling.

➡ **Application:**

**STEP 1:** Anchor the extended end of the wrap around the distal upper arm directly to the skin and encircle the anchor ⬅▦▶ (Fig. 8–11A).

*Option:* *If an elastic wrap is not available, 2 inch, 3 inch, or 4 inch self-adherent wrap may be used.*

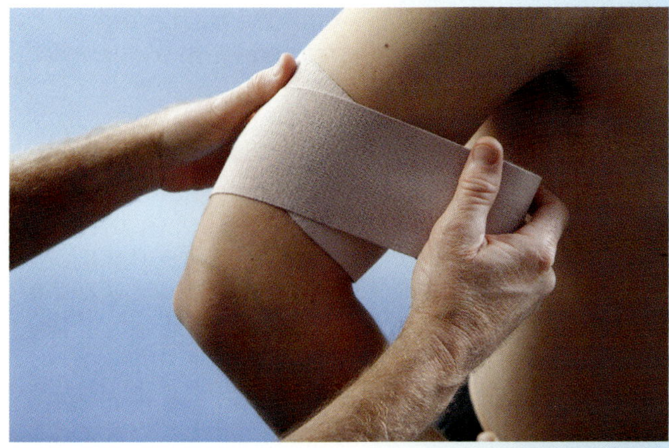

Fig. 8–11 A

**STEP 2:** Continue to apply the wrap in a spiral pattern, overlapping the wrap by ½ of its width and moving in a distal-to-proximal direction (Fig. 8–11B). Apply the greatest amount of roll tension distally and over the inflamed area and lessen the amount of roll tension as the wrap continues proximally.

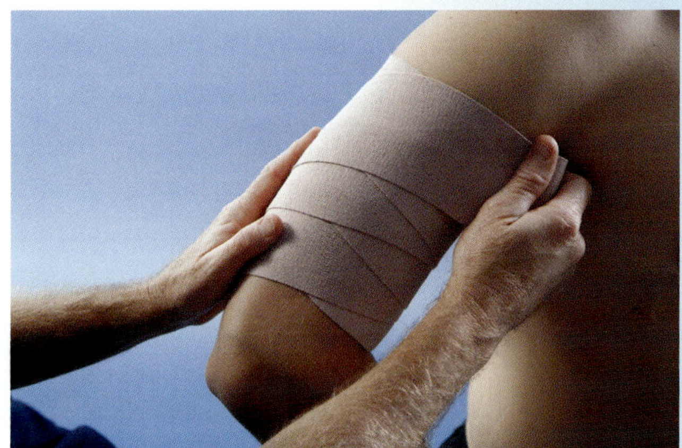

Fig. 8–11 B

**STEP 3:** Finish the wrap over the proximal upper arm. Anchor with Velcro, metal clips, or loosely applied 1½ inch non-elastic or 1½ inch or 2 inch elastic tape ⬅▦▶ (Fig. 8–11C). End the tape on the antero-lateral area to prevent irritation.

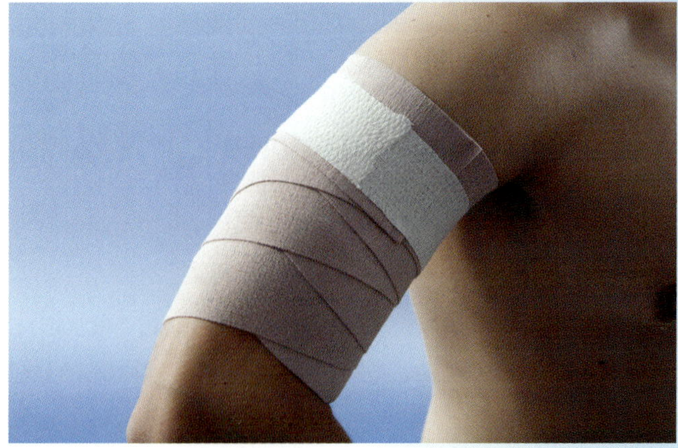

Fig. 8–11 C

## FOREARM, ELBOW, AND UPPER ARM COMPRESSION WRAP    Figure 8-12

➡ **Purpose:** Use the forearm, elbow, and upper arm compression wrap technique to control moderate to severe swelling when treating second- and third-degree upper arm contusions and ruptures. This technique prevents distal migration of post-injury swelling (Fig. 8–12).

➡ **Materials:**
- 4 inch or 6 inch width by 10 yard length elastic wrap, metal clips, 1½ inch non-elastic or 1½ inch or 2 inch elastic tape, taping scissors

*Option:*
- ¼ inch or ½ inch foam or felt

➡ **Position of the patient:** Sitting on a taping table or bench or standing with the involved arm at the side of the body and the elbow placed in a pain-free, flexed position.

➡ **Preparation:** To lessen migration, apply adherent tape spray, tape strips, or anchors directly to the skin.

*Option:*
Cut a ¼ inch or ½ inch foam or felt pad and place it over the inflamed area directly to the skin to assist in venous return.

➡ **Application:**

**STEP 1:** Anchor the elastic wrap around the wrist directly to the skin and apply the forearm compression wrap (see Fig. 9–15).

**STEP 2:** At the proximal forearm, continue the spiral wrap proximally over the elbow to the distal upper arm, overlapping the wrap by ½ of its width ◄▬► (Fig. 8–12A).

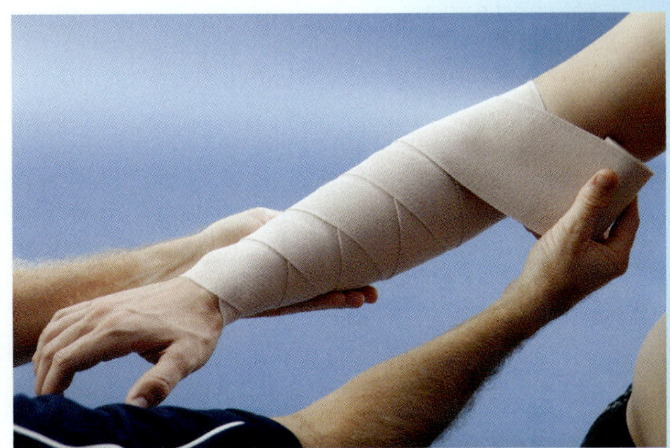

**Fig. 8–12 A**

**STEP 3:** At the distal upper arm, finish this technique with the upper arm compression wrap (Fig. 8–12B). Apply the greatest amount of roll tension distally and over the inflamed area and lessen tension as the wrap continues proximally.

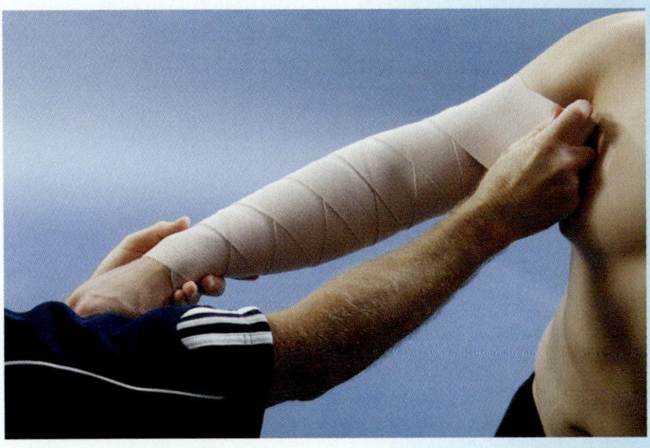

**Fig. 8–12 B**

*Steps Cont.*

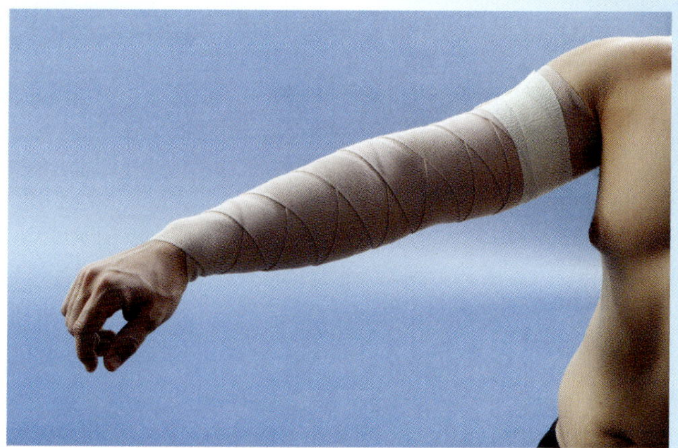

**Fig. 8–12 C**

**STEP 4:** Anchor the wrap over the proximal upper arm with Velcro, metal clips, or loosely applied 1½ inch non-elastic or 1½ inch or 2 inch elastic tape ◄▨▨▨► (Fig. 8–12C). Finish the tape on the anterolateral upper arm.

**Helpful Hint |**
Extended wear of the compression wrap may cause irritation of the skin over the cubital fossa. To prevent this irritation, place a thin foam pad over the cubital fossa underneath the wrap.

## UPPER ARM COMPRESSION SLEEVE      Figure 8–13

➠ **Purpose:** The upper arm compression sleeve technique may also be used to control mild to moderate swelling with contusions and ruptures (Fig. 8–13). This technique differs from the upper arm and forearm, elbow, and upper arm compression wrap techniques in that, after receiving instruction, the patient can apply and remove this technique without assistance.

➠ **Materials:**
• 3 inch, 3½ inch, or 4 inch width elastic sleeve determined by the size of the upper arm, taping scissors
*Option:*
• ¼ inch or ½ inch foam or felt

➠ **Position of the patient:** Sitting on a taping table or bench, or standing with the involved arm at the side of the body and the elbow placed in a pain-free, flexed position.

➠ **Preparation:** Cut a sleeve from a roll to extend from the elbow to the proximal upper arm area or from the wrist to the proximal upper arm. Cut and use a double-length sleeve to provide additional compression.
*Option:*
Cut a ¼ inch or ½ inch foam or felt pad and place it over the inflamed area to assist in controlling swelling.

➠ **Application:**

**STEP 1:** Place the hand through the sleeve and pull onto the upper arm or arm in a distal-to-proximal pattern. If using a double-length sleeve, pull the distal end over the first layer to provide an additional layer (Fig. 8–13). No anchors are required. The elastic sleeve can be cleaned and reused.

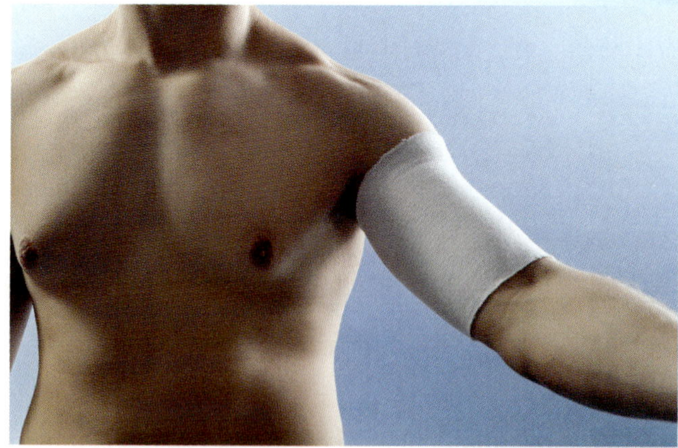

**Fig. 8–13**

## CIRCULAR UPPER ARM WRAP    Figure 8-14

➠ **Purpose:** The circular upper arm technique is used to provide compression and mild support and to anchor off-the-shelf and custom-made pads to absorb shock when preventing and treating upper arm contusions, heterotopic ossification, and exostosis (Fig. 8–14).

➠ **Materials:**
  • 3 inch, 4 inch, or 6 inch width by 5 yard length elastic wrap, 1½ inch or 2 inch elastic tape, taping scissors
  *Options:*
  • 3 inch or 4 inch width self-adherent wrap
  • 1½ inch non-elastic tape

➠ **Position of the patient:** Sitting on a taping table or bench, or standing with the involved arm at the side of the body and the elbow placed in 90 degrees of flexion with moderate isometric contraction of the biceps and triceps muscles.

➠ **Preparation:** To lessen migration, apply adherent tape spray, tape strips, or anchors directly to the skin.

➠ **Application:**

**STEP 1:**   Place the pad over the injured area. Anchor the wrap directly to the skin below the distal pad and encircle the anchor ◄▬▬▶ (Fig. 8–14A).

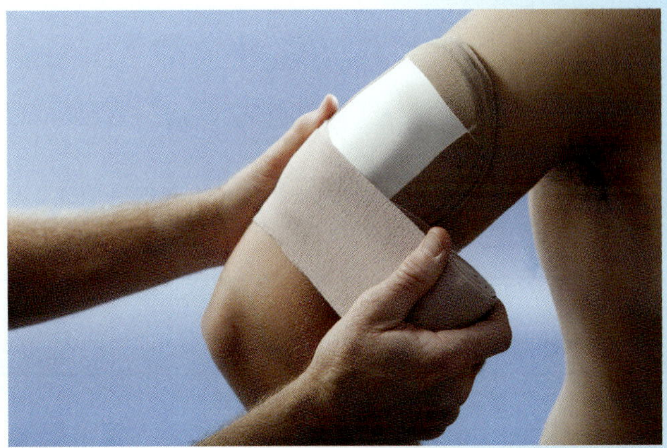

**Fig. 8–14 A**

**STEP 2:**   Continue to apply the wrap in a circular pattern with moderate roll tension, overlapping the wrap by ½ of its width, in a distal-to-proximal pattern (Fig. 8–14B). Avoid gaps, wrinkles, and inconsistent roll tension.

*Option:*   *If an elastic wrap is not available, 3 inch or 4 inch self-adherent wrap may be used.*

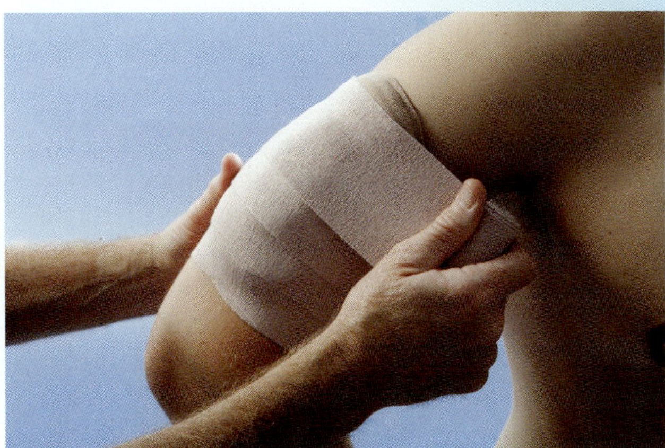

**Fig. 8–14 B**

*Steps Cont.*

**Shoulder and Upper Arm**

**STEP 3:** Completely cover the pad and finish the wrap above the proximal pad. To anchor, place 1½ inch or 2 inch elastic tape on the distal pad and apply two to three continuous distal-to-proximal circular patterns, with moderate roll tension, finishing on the tape pattern on the lateral upper arm to ensure adherence and prevent irritation ◀▬▬▶ (Fig. 8–14C). To lessen migration, apply a distal circular strip of elastic tape with distal-to-proximal tension and anchor the loose end on the circular tape pattern. The proximal portion of the elastic tape may also be applied partially on the skin.

*Option:* *Additional 1½ inch non-elastic circular strips may be applied loosely around the upper arm to anchor the pad ◀▬▬▶.*

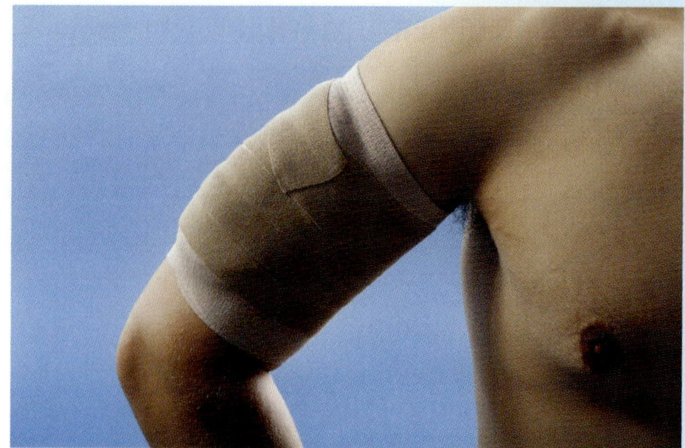

**Fig. 8–14 C**

## SHOULDER SPICA    Figure 8–15

▶ **Purpose:** The shoulder spica technique provides mild support and anchors off-the-shelf and custom-made pads to absorb shock when preventing and treating shoulder pointers and AC joint sprains (Fig. 8–15).

### DETAILS
The shoulder spica is commonly used in the treatment of many injuries and conditions to anchor ice bags to the upper arm and/or shoulder.

▶ **Materials:**
  • 4 inch or 6 inch width by 10 yard length elastic wrap, 2 inch or 3 inch elastic tape, taping scissors
▶ **Position of the patient:** Standing with the hand of the involved arm placed on the lateral hip in a relaxed position.
▶ **Preparation:** Apply the off-the-shelf or custom-made pad over the injured area directly to the skin.
▶ **Application:**

**STEP 1:** Anchor the extended end of the wrap on the mid-to-proximal lateral upper arm directly to the skin and proceed around the upper arm in a medial direction to encircle the anchor (Fig. 8–15A).

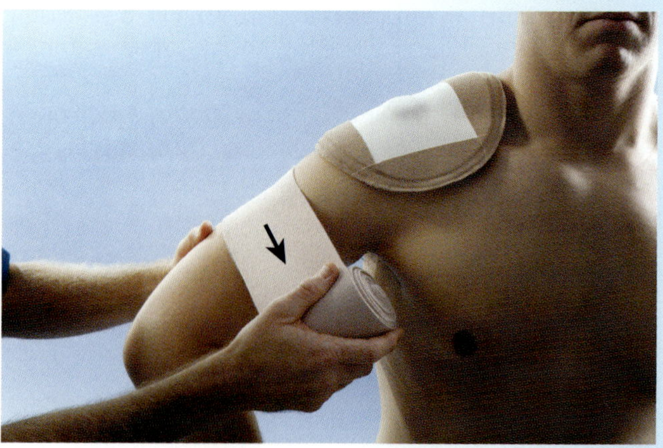

**Fig. 8–15 A**

**STEP 2:** At the posterior upper arm, continue the wrap in a medial direction over the lateral shoulder and pad, across the chest, under the axilla of the non-involved arm, then across the upper back (Fig. 8–15B). Next, continue over the lateral involved shoulder, under the axilla, and encircle the upper arm (Fig. 8–15C). Apply the wrap with moderate roll tension.

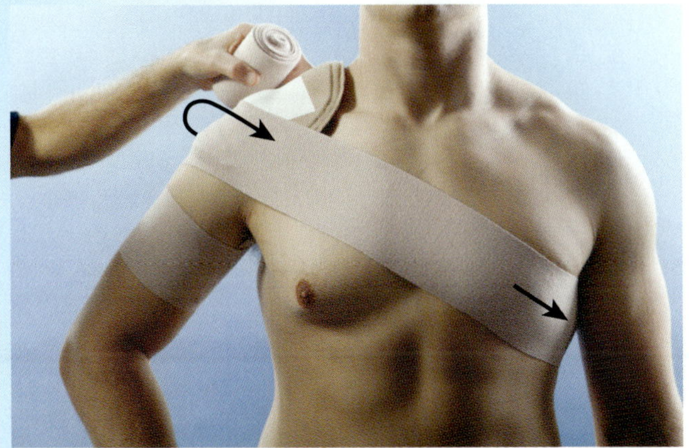

**Fig. 8–15 B**

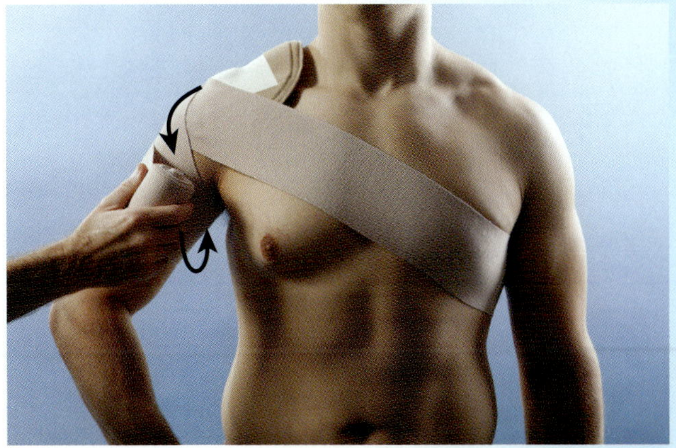

**Fig. 8–15 C**

**STEP 3:** Repeat this pattern two to four times with the wrap, overlapping slightly to cover the pad, leaving a small area in the middle of the pad exposed (Fig. 8–15D). Monitor roll tension to prevent constriction and irritation of the **axilla** areas.

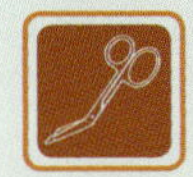

**Helpful Hint |**
Make sure you leave an exposed area in the middle of the pad because the exposed area in the spica technique will allow for the elastic tape anchor(s) to adhere directly to the pad, lessening migration.

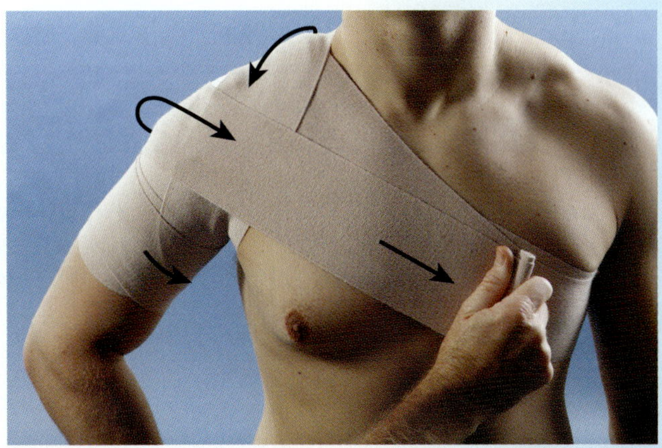

**Fig. 8–15 D**

**STEP 4:** Finish the wrap over the involved shoulder, upper back, or thorax. Anchor 2 inch or 3 inch elastic tape directly on the exposed portion of the pad (Fig. 8–15E) and apply one to two spica patterns over the wrap and pad with moderate roll tension (Fig. 8–15F).

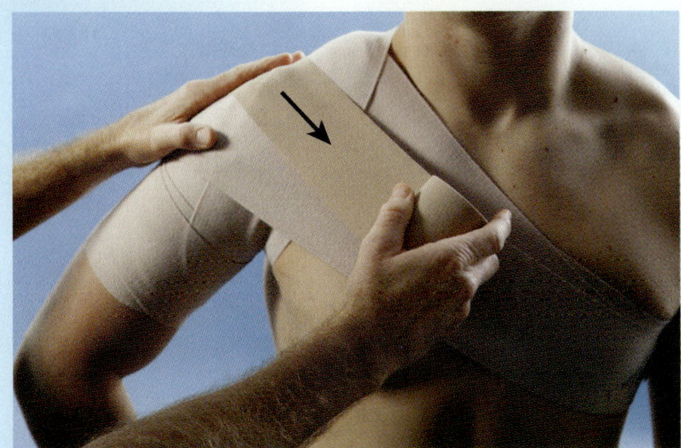

**Fig. 8–15 E**

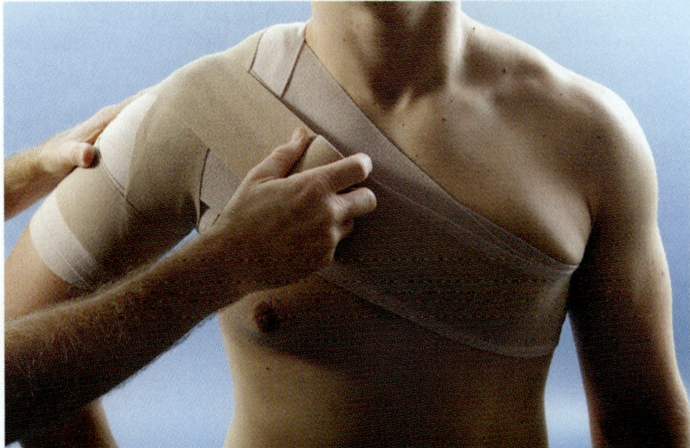

**Fig. 8–15 F**

*Steps Cont.*

**STEP 5:** Anchor the tape on the circular tape pattern over the pad (Fig. 8–15G). No additional anchors are needed.

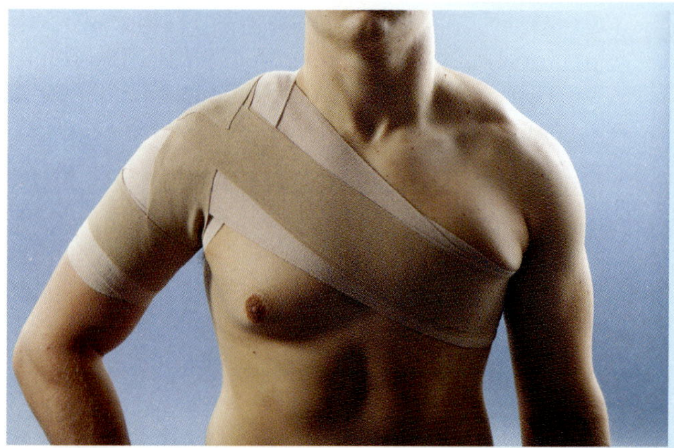

**Fig. 8–15 G**

## Clinical Application Question 1

During the first week of preseason practice, an attackman on the lacrosse team suffers a left shoulder pointer. After several days of treatment, the athlete returns to practice with an off-the-shelf pad anchored directly to the skin with elastic tape. Practice and application of the pad continue twice daily, and the adherent tape spray and tape adhesive begin to cause irritation of the skin.

➡ **Question: What techniques can you use in this situation?**

## 4 S (SPICA, SLING, SWATHE, AND SUPPORT) WRAP   Figure 8–16

➥ **Purpose:** Use the 4 S technique to provide mild to moderate support and immobilization when treating sprains, strains, dislocations, subluxations, ruptures, and stable fractures (Fig. 8–16). The 4 S wrap can replace a sling and swathe in the immediate treatment of shoulder and upper arm injuries and conditions.

➥ **Materials:**
  • 4 inch or 6 inch width by 10 yard length elastic wrap, 2 inch or 3 inch elastic tape, taping scissors

➥ **Position of the patient:** Sitting or standing with the involved arm in a pain-free position next to the body with the elbow placed in flexion.

➥ **Preparation:** Apply the 4 S wrap directly to the skin or over clothing.

➥ **Application:**

**STEP 1:** Anchor the wrap around the mid-to-proximal lateral upper arm and apply one to two shoulder *spica* patterns with moderate roll tension (Fig. 8–16A).

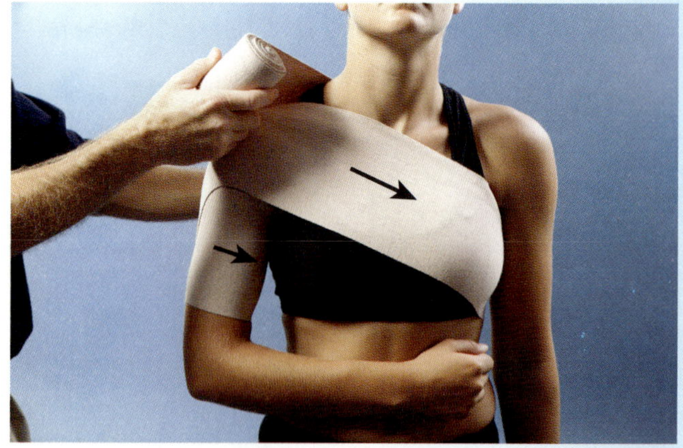

**Fig. 8–16 A**

**STEP 2:** At the involved posterior upper arm, continue the wrap over the involved shoulder, down the upper arm, under the elbow, then up the upper arm, and finish over the shoulder (Fig. 8–16B). Repeat this pattern one to two times with moderate roll tension, moving distally on the forearm with each pattern to form a *sling* (Fig. 8–16C).

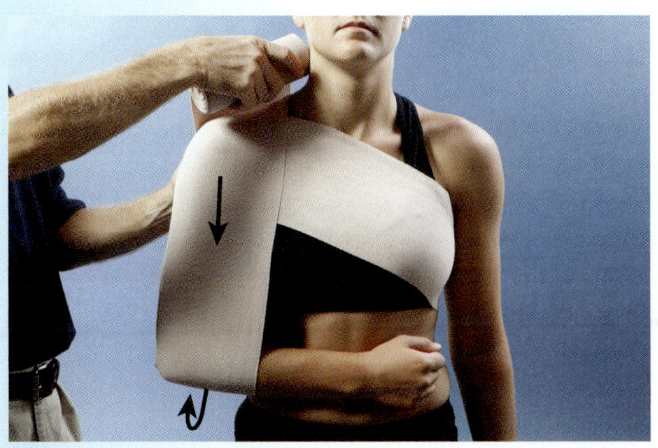

**Fig. 8–16 B**

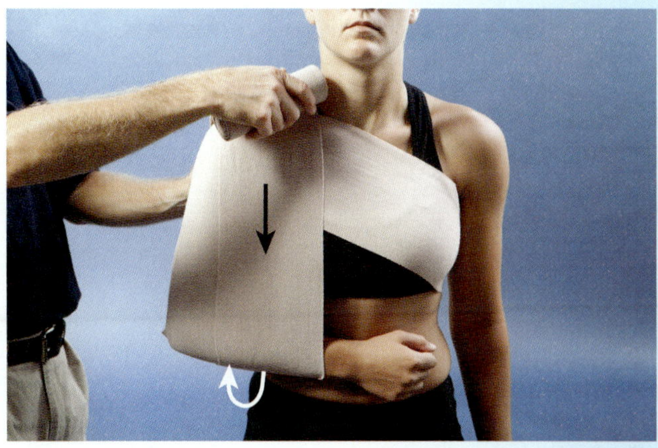

**Fig. 8–16 C**

**STEP 3:** Next, continue the wrap from the involved shoulder across the chest toward the involved hand, around the mid-to-low back, and across the distal upper arm (Fig. 8–16D). Continue to apply the wrap over the forearm, wrist, and hand, then across the mid-to-low back again with moderate roll tension (Fig. 8–16E).

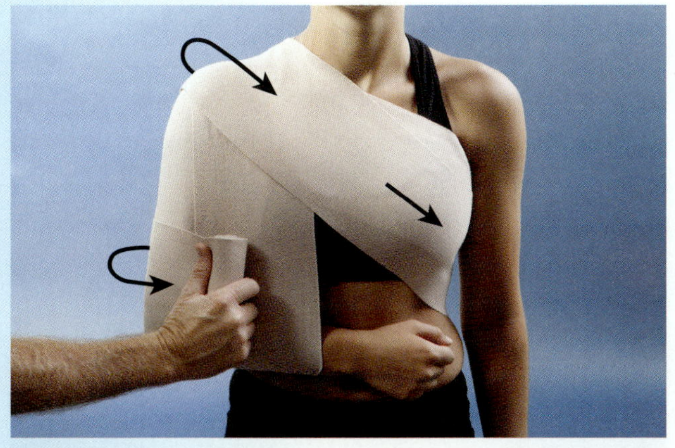

**Fig. 8–16 D**

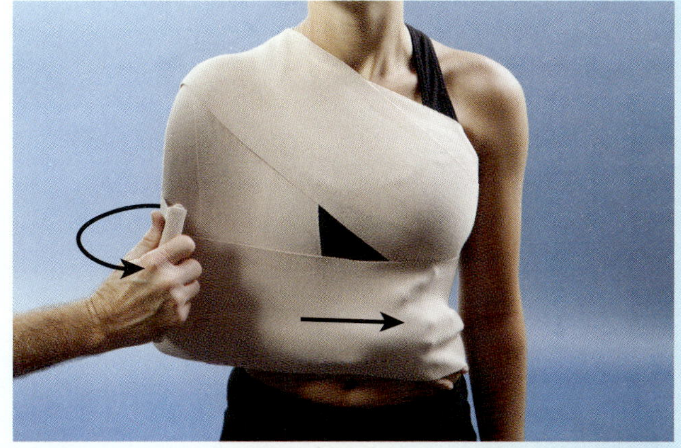

**Fig. 8–16 E**

**STEP 4:** Overlap the wrap by ½ of its width in a proximal direction and repeat the pattern one to two times. Finish over the forearm to form a *swathe* (Fig. 8–16F). Leave the fingertips exposed to monitor circulation.

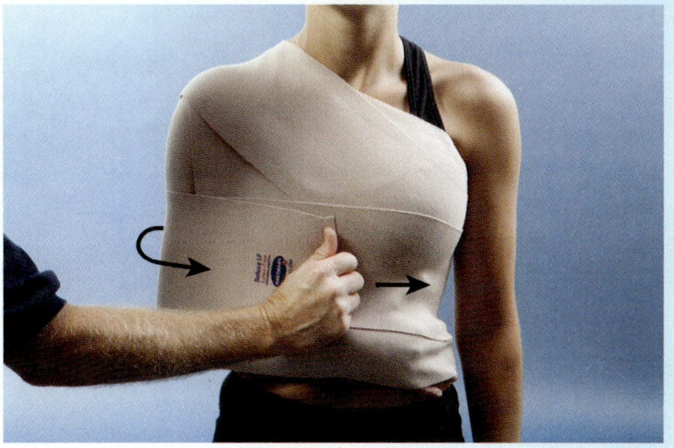

**Fig. 8–16 F**

*Steps Cont.*

**STEP 5:** Anchor 2 inch or 3 inch elastic tape over the involved shoulder and apply the spica, sling, and swathe patterns with moderate roll tension, finishing on the forearm or wrist (Fig. 8–16G). No additional anchors are required.

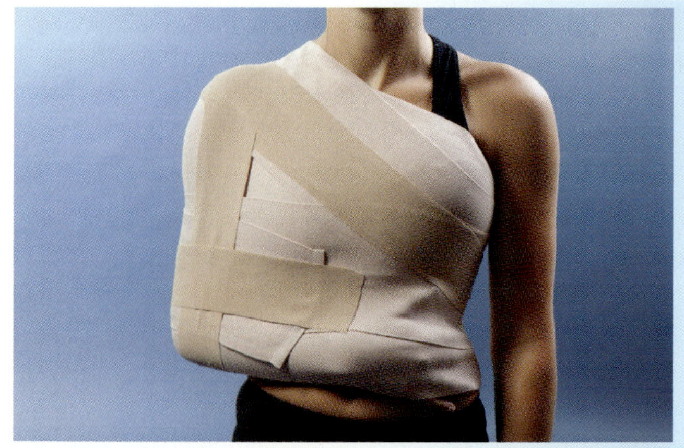

**Fig. 8–16 G**

## FIGURE-OF-EIGHT WRAP    Figure 8–17

➨ **Purpose:** The figure-of-eight technique provides mild to moderate support and immobilization when treating SC joint sprains and stable clavicular fractures (Fig. 8–17). The wrap is used in the immediate treatment of these injuries to retract the scapulae.

➨ **Materials:**
  • 4 inch or 6 inch width by 10 yard length elastic wrap, 2 inch or 3 inch elastic tape, taping scissors

➨ **Position of the patient:** Sitting or standing with the hands of the involved and non-involved arms placed in a pain-free position on the hips with elbow flexion.

➨ **Preparation:** Apply the figure-of-eight wrap directly to the skin or over clothing.

➨ **Application:**

**STEP 1:** Anchor the extended end of the wrap over the non-involved shoulder and continue in a posterior direction, under the axilla, and encircle the anchor (Fig. 8–17A).

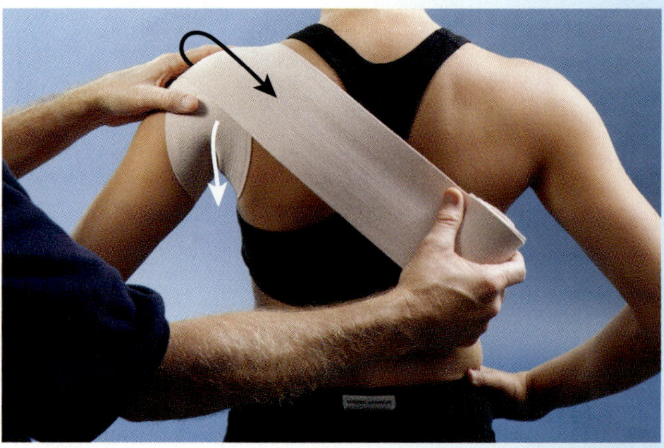

**Fig. 8–17 A**

**STEP 2:** Continue the wrap across the upper back with moderate roll tension, under the axilla of the involved shoulder, then up and across the shoulder with a moderate posterior pull (Fig. 8–17B).

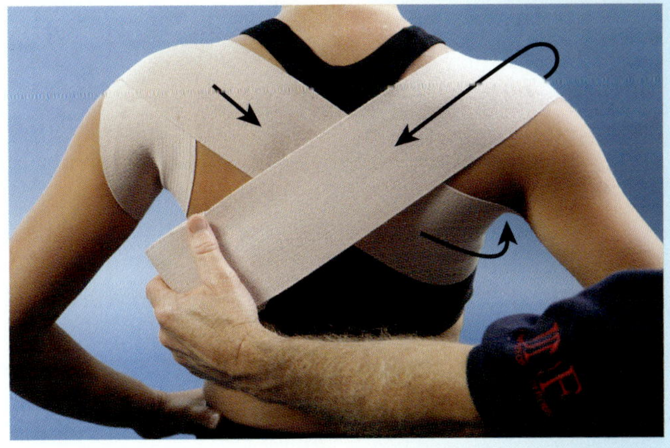

**Fig. 8–17 B**

**STEP 3:** Next, proceed from the involved shoulder across the upper back, under the axilla of the non-involved shoulder, then up and across the shoulder with a moderate posterior pull (Fig. 8–17C).

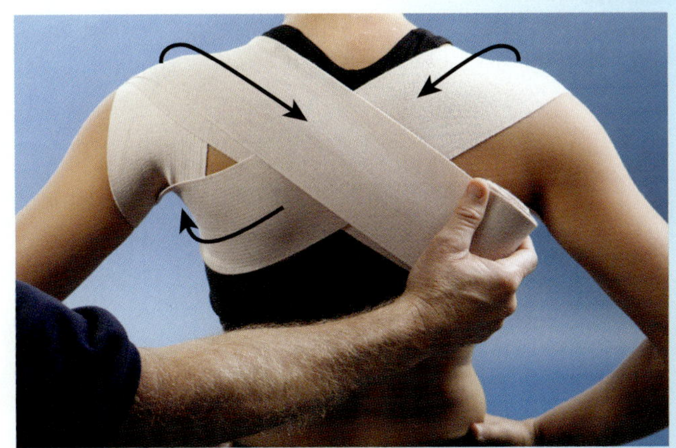

**Fig. 8–17 C**

**STEP 4:** Repeat the figure-of-eight pattern two to four times, overlapping the wrap by ⅓ of its width across the shoulders. The wrap should resemble an "X" pattern over the upper back. Monitor roll tension to prevent constriction and irritation of the axilla areas.

**STEP 5:** Anchor 2 inch or 3 inch elastic tape over the non-involved shoulder and apply one figure-of-eight pattern with moderate roll tension, again supporting retraction of the scapulae. Anchor the tape on the tape pattern on the upper back. No additional anchors are needed (Fig. 8–17D).

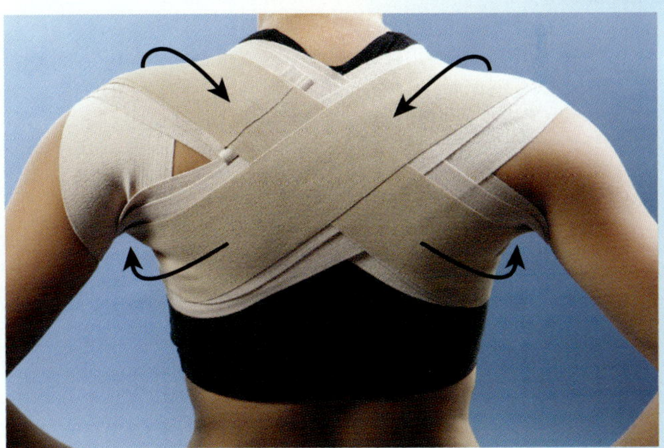

**Fig. 8–17 D**

## . . . IF/THEN . . .

**IF** a patient with a stable clavicular fracture requires support and immobilization prior to transportation to an emergency facility for further evaluation, **THEN** consider using the figure-of-eight wrap rather than a brace technique; the wrap can be applied in less time and is cost-effective in this situation, as most facilities will cut off the immobilization technique to perform an evaluation.

## SWATHE WRAP    Figure 8–18

➭ **Purpose:** Use the swathe wrap technique with slings to provide mild to moderate support and immobilization by anchoring the arm to the trunk when treating sprains, dislocations, subluxations, instabilities, lesions, fractures, strains, ruptures, and overuse injuries and conditions (Fig. 8–18).

➭ **Materials:**
  • 4 inch or 6 inch width by 10 yard length elastic wrap, metal clips, 2 inch or 3 inch elastic tape, taping scissors

➭ **Position of the patient:** Sitting or standing with the involved arm in a pain-free position next to the body with the elbow placed in flexion.

➭ **Preparation:** Place the hand, wrist, forearm, and elbow in a sling (see Figs. 8–19B and 8–19C). Apply the swathe wrap over the sling.

➭ **Application:**

**STEP 1:**    Anchor the extended end of the wrap over the elbow of the involved arm (Fig. 8–18A).

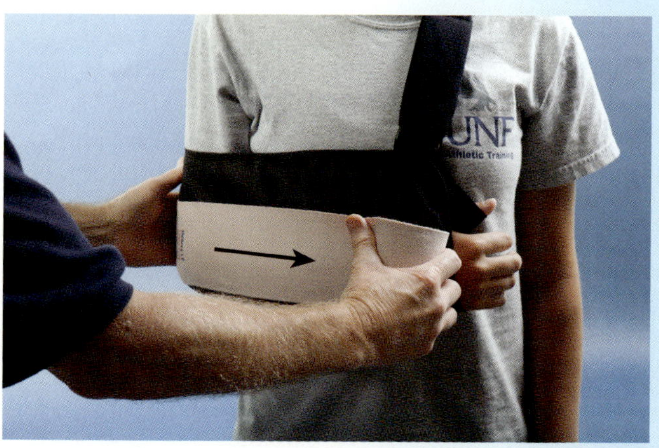

**Fig. 8–18 A**

**STEP 2:**    Apply the wrap in a lateral-to-medial pattern over the forearm, hand, and fingers with moderate roll tension. Continue around the back and return to the elbow (Fig. 8–18B).

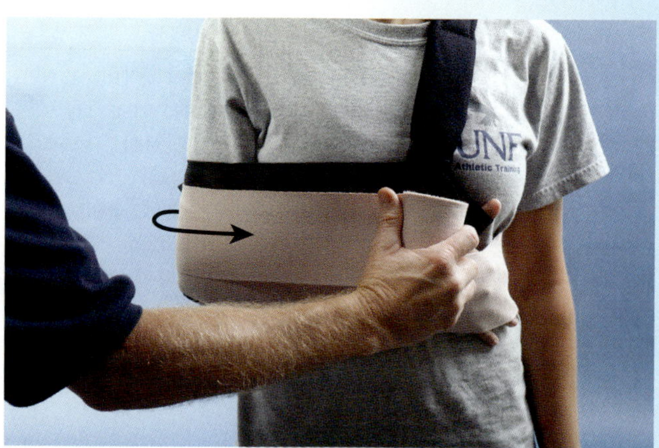

**Fig. 8–18 B**

**STEP 3:** Next, overlap the wrap by ⅓ of its width in a proximal direction and encircle the distal upper arm and trunk two to three times with moderate roll tension (Fig. 8–18C). Leave the fingertips exposed to monitor circulation.

**STEP 4:** Anchor with Velcro, metal clips, or one lateral-to-medial circular pattern on the wrap, with 2 inch or 3 inch elastic tape and moderate roll tension. No additional anchors are required.

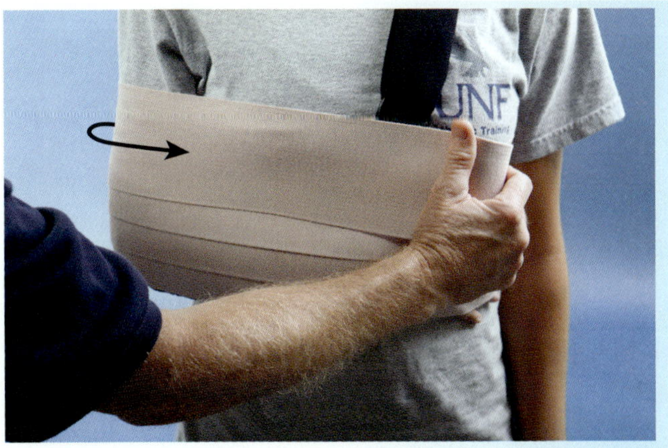

**Fig. 8–18 C**



# Bracing Techniques

Bracing techniques for the shoulder and upper arm provide support, stability, and immobilization, and limit range of motion. The designs are available off-the-shelf and custom-made and are used to prevent and treat contusions, sprains, dislocations/subluxations, fractures, strains, ruptures, and overuse injuries and conditions.

## SLINGS AND IMMOBILIZERS     Figures 8–19 and 8–20

➡ **Purpose:** Slings and immobilizers are designed to provide complete support and to immobilize the shoulder and arm following injury and surgery. Slings and immobilizers are used to treat contusions, sprains, dislocations, subluxations, instabilities, lesions, fractures, strains, ruptures, and overuse injuries and conditions. Choose the brace design according to the intended purposes of support and immobilization following injury and/or surgery.

### *Sling*

➡ **Purpose:** Slings provide complete support and immobilization of the shoulder, upper arm, elbow, forearm, wrist, and hand and are used for varying periods of time following injury and/or surgery (Fig. 8–19). Typically, slings are less expensive than the immobilizer design.

**DETAILS**
Consider applying the swathe wrap technique over the sling for additional support and immobilization of the shoulder and arm.

➡ **Design:**
- The universal fit designs are purchased in predetermined sizes according to the length of the forearm, commonly measured from the olecranon to the fifth metacarpophalangeal joint.
- The slings are constructed of a cotton, poplin, polyester/spandex, or open mesh material pouch with a closed end at the elbow and an open or closed end at the fingers. Adjustable nylon or cotton straps incorporated into the pouch through metal or plastic rings attach the sling to the body (Fig. 8–19A).
- Some designs are constructed with an adjustable pouch.

- Most designs are available with padded straps for additional comfort.
- Many designs have a loop or strap incorporated into the distal end of the pouch to provide support for the wrist, hand, and/or thumb.
- Another design uses two straps to support the proximal and distal forearm to provide immobilization.
- When properly applied, the sling immobilizes the shoulder in internal rotation against the trunk.
- With some designs, a swathe is available to provide additional support of the shoulder and arm.

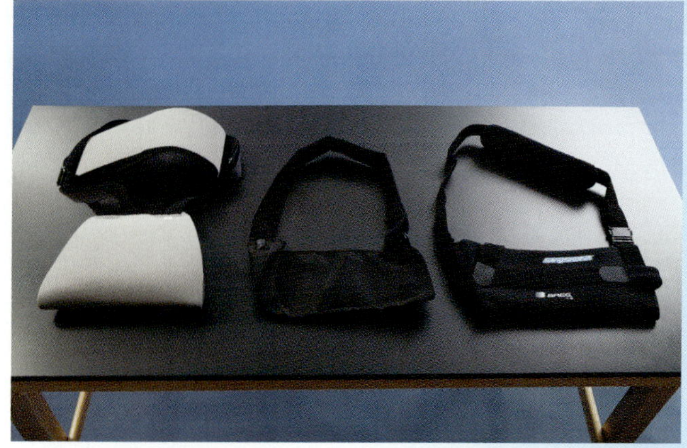

**Fig. 8–19 A**  *Slings. (Left) Sling with swathe. (Middle and Right) Universal fit slings.*

➡ **Position of the patient:** Sitting or standing with the involved arm in a pain-free position next to the body with the elbow placed in flexion.

➡ **Preparation:** Apply the sling directly to the skin or over clothing.

  Instructions for application are included with each sling. The following guidelines pertain to most designs.

➡ **Application:**

**STEP 1:**  Begin by loosening the strap on the anterior pouch.

**STEP 2:**  Place the hand, wrist, forearm, and elbow into the pouch by applying the closed end over the fingers and hand and continue pulling the pouch toward the elbow. Assistance may be required to prevent movement of the injured area (Fig. 8–19B).

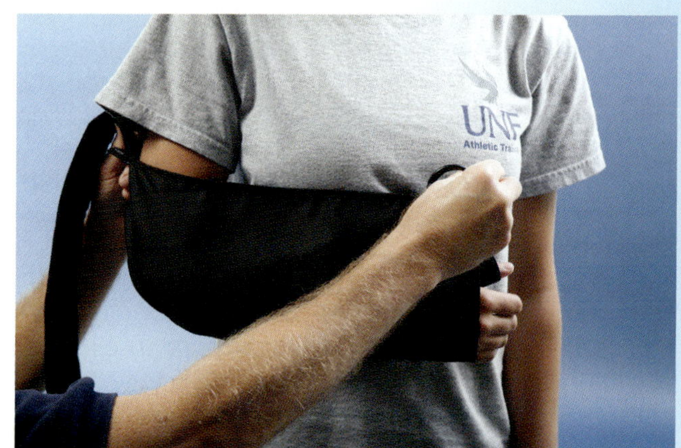

**Fig. 8–19 B**

**STEP 3:**  Position the elbow against the closed end of the pouch.

**STEP 4:**  Apply the strap located at the elbow upward across the back, over the opposite shoulder and neck, then down across the chest and through the ring on the anterior pouch (Fig. 8–19C). Adjust the tightness of the strap to achieve the desired position of the arm as indicated by a physician. Anchor the strap with Velcro or a buckle. Prevent irritation of the shoulder and/or neck with additional padding.

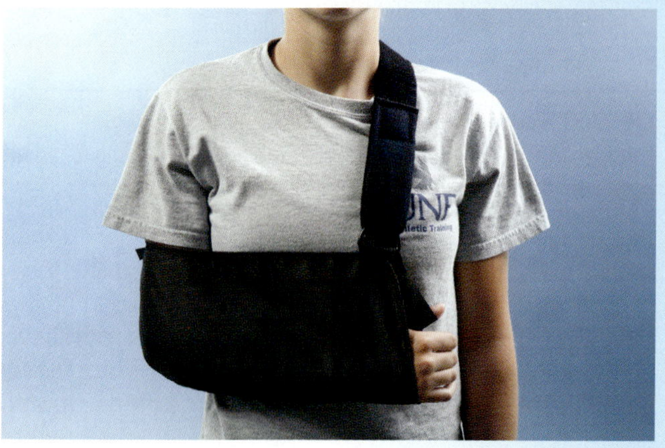

**Fig. 8–19 C**

**Helpful Hint |**
Cut a ½ inch foam or felt pad slightly wider than the strap, approximately 6–8 inches in length. Place the pad under the strap as it crosses the shoulder/neck area. A pad may also be cut and attached to the strap. First, cut the pad. Then, make two vertical cuts in the pad with taping scissors the width of the strap toward the anterior and posterior edges (Fig. 8–19D). Insert the strap through the pad and position over the shoulder/neck area (Fig. 8–19E). The pad can also be attached to the strap with self-adherent wrap.

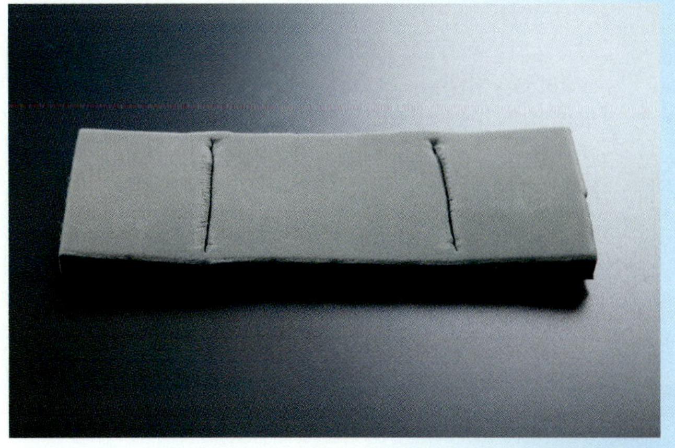

**Fig. 8–19 D**

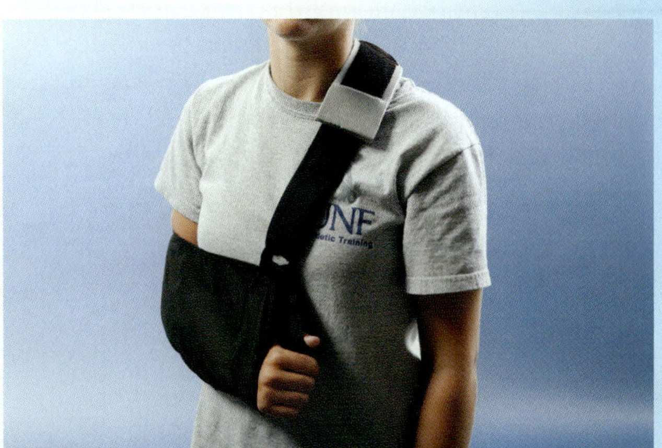

**Fig. 8–19 E**

### Immobilizer

➠ **Purpose:** Immobilizers also provide complete support and immobilization of the shoulder, upper arm, elbow, forearm, wrist, and hand (Fig. 8–20). The immobilizer is used when treating dislocations, subluxations, and postoperative procedures of the shoulder that require extended periods of immobilization in varying degrees of motion.

➠ **Design:**
- The universal fit designs are manufactured in predetermined sizes corresponding to chest circumference measurements or forearm length from the olecranon to the fifth metacarpophalangeal joint.
- The pouch and straps are constructed of soft cotton and nylon materials; most designs are available with padded straps.
- When these designs are used, a pad or inflatable air pillow is used to immobilize the shoulder in varying degrees of abduction based on the injury and/or surgical procedure (Fig. 8–20A).
- Some designs are constructed with the pouch attached to the pad or pillow. Other designs use straps to attach the forearm to the pad or pillow.
- Adjustable straps incorporated into the pouch, pad, and/or pillow attach the immobilizer to the shoulder and waist.

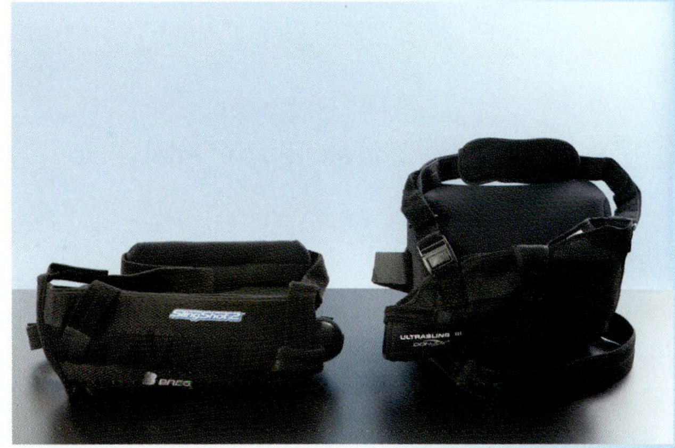

**Fig. 8–20 A** *Immobilizers.*

- Some designs have a loop or strap incorporated into the distal end of the pouch to provide support for the wrist, hand, and/or thumb. Several designs have a strap to limit posterior movement and/or internal rotation of the shoulder.

➡ **Position of the patient:** Sitting or standing with the involved arm in a pain-free position next to the body with the elbow placed in flexion.

➡ **Preparation:** Set the pad or inflatable pillow to the desired range of abduction as indicated by a physician and/or therapeutic exercise program. Apply the immobilizer directly to the skin or over clothing.
Application of the immobilizer should follow manufacturers' instructions, which are included with the brace when purchased. The following general application guidelines apply to most designs.

➡ **Application:**

**STEP 1:**    Begin application by loosening the straps and unfolding the immobilizer.

**STEP 2:**    The application of the straps and pillow will depend on the specific design. Place the hand, wrist, forearm, and elbow into the sling. Apply the shoulder strap and anchor on the anterior pouch with Velcro straps (Fig. 8–20B).

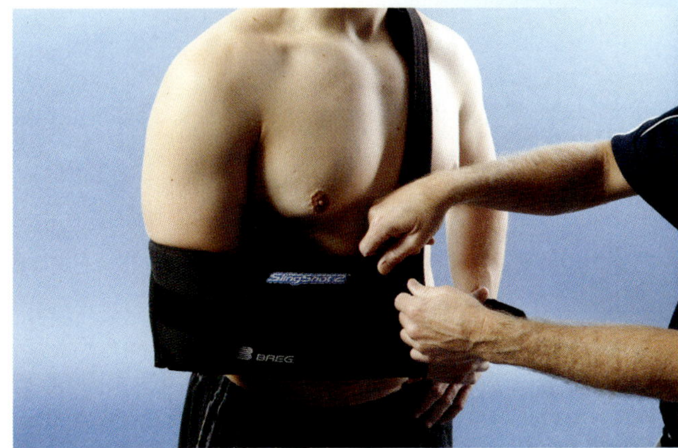

Fig. 8–20 B

**STEP 3:**    Position the pad or pillow under the involved shoulder and arm at the waistline. Attach the sling to the pad or pillow with Velcro (Fig. 8–20C).

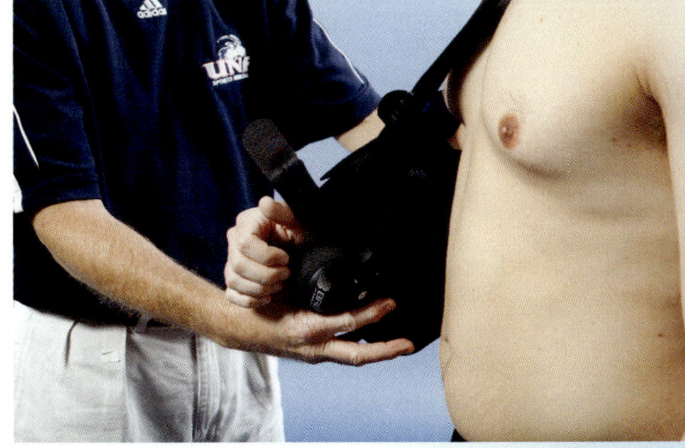

Fig. 8–20 C

**STEP 4:**    Apply the strap around the waist (Fig. 8–20D).

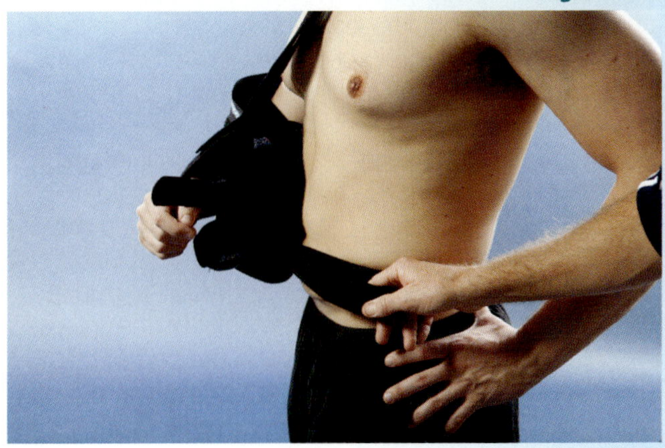

Fig. 8–20 D

**STEP 5:** Next, attach the pouch closure straps at the forearm and hand (Fig. 8–20E). Readjust the straps if needed.

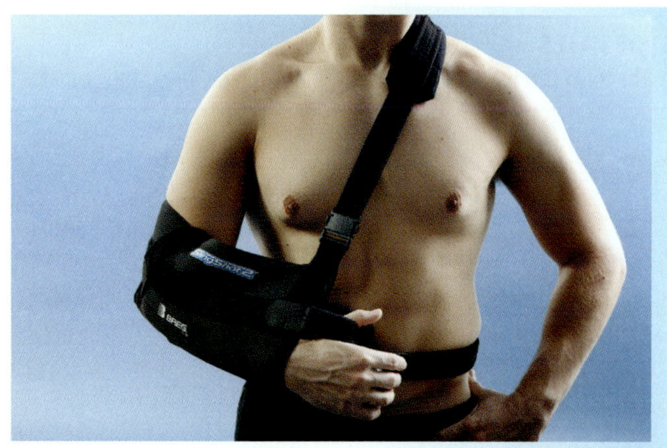

**Fig. 8–20 E**

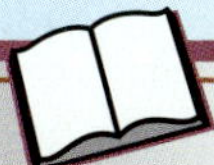

## EVIDENCE SUMMARY

Typically following a closed reduction, non-operative management of first-time anterior glenohumeral joint dislocations is a period of immobilization in a sling or immobilizer within a comprehensive rehabilitation program. The use of a sling or immobilizer brace design immobilizes the shoulder in internal rotation or internal rotation with varying degrees of abduction, respectively. Several researchers have investigated immobilization of the shoulder in external rotation to examine the effect on rates of recurrent instability. Since 2010, five evidence-based reviews[5–9] have been conducted comparing the effects of internal rotation and external rotation immobilization of the shoulder following first-time anterior glenohumeral dislocations. The results of each review demonstrated no significant differences in overall rates of recurrent subluxations and dislocations of the shoulder between immobilization methods. Among the more recent reviews, findings have revealed no significant differences in patient compliance with the immobilization interventions[9] and patient-reported quality of life[9] and shoulder instability scores.[8] Additional research is required to determine the most effective non-operative immobilization position for first-time glenohumeral dislocations to improve patient outcomes.

### . . . IF/THEN . . .

**IF** support and immobilization of the shoulder and arm in 15 degrees of abduction is required for 2 weeks following a surgical rotator cuff repair, **THEN** use the immobilizer brace, rather than the sling, because the immobilizer is designed to be worn for extended periods and to immobilize the shoulder and arm in specific ranges of abduction.

### Clinical Application Question 2

The CEO of a local architectural firm is allowed by the surgeon to begin cardiovascular activity as tolerated following a procedure to the right shoulder. An avid runner and tennis player, the CEO is currently in a postoperative sling and swathe. The surgeon recommends use of the sling and swathe for an additional 2 weeks. The CEO plans to ride a stationary bike during the lunch hour and return to work but is concerned about soiling the postoperative sling and swathe during the workout.

➡ **Question: What type of brace can you use for support and immobilization during the cardiovascular activity?**

### OFF-THE-SHELF SHOULDER STABILIZERS     Figure 8–21

➡ **Purpose:** Off-the-shelf shoulder stabilizer braces are used to provide moderate to maximal support and limit range of motion when preventing and treating sprains, dislocations, subluxations, instabilities, strains, and overuse injuries and conditions (Fig. 8–21). These braces commonly limit GH joint abduction and external rotation while allowing normal flexion, extension, and horizontal adduction. Some designs can be applied to limit several ranges of motion based on the specific needs of the patient's injury or condition.

## DETAILS
The torso vest brace may be used during athletic, work, and casual activities.

**Design:**
- The off-the-shelf braces are available in two basic designs: a torso vest with an arm cuff and an individual arm cuff.
- The torso vest braces are constructed of neoprene or polyester materials and are available in individual fit designs corresponding to chest and upper arm circumference measurements (Fig. 8–21A).
- Some vest designs attach over the torso and involved shoulder, whereas others attach over the upper abdomen and shoulders using various straps. Adjustable straps or laces are used to achieve proper fit.
- The arm cuffs of several designs are incorporated into the vest. Other designs use a plastic or metal ring to attach the arm cuff to the vest.
- Some vest designs use neoprene straps that are applied in various patterns based on the specific injury or condition.
- Torso vest braces can be worn underneath protective athletic equipment and uniforms or clothing.
- The individual arm cuff braces are manufactured in universal fit designs from neoprene, leather, or nylon in predetermined sizes according to upper arm circumference measurements or the weight of the patient (Fig. 8–21B).
- The adjustable cuff attaches to the upper arm and is anchored to the breast plate of football shoulder pads with laces, screws, or buckles.

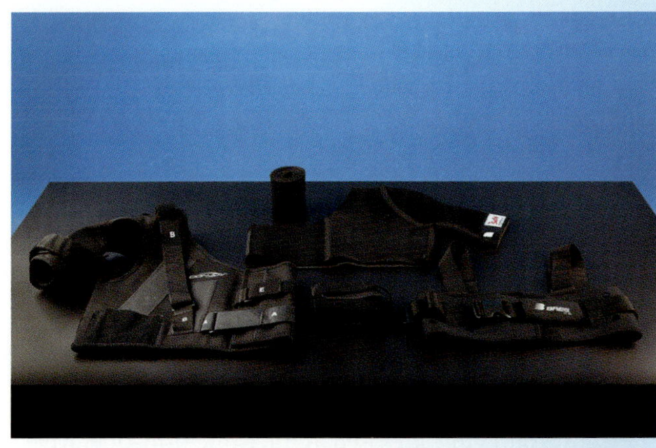

**Fig. 8–21 A** *Torso vest shoulder stabilizers.*

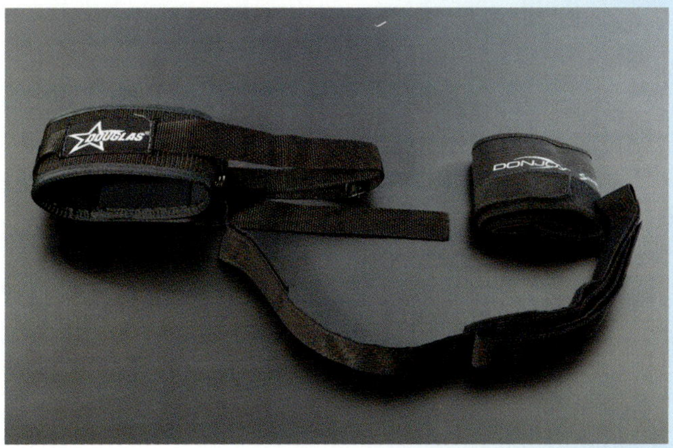

**Fig. 8–21 B** *Individual arm cuff shoulder stabilizers.*

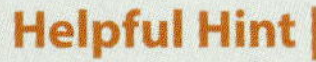

**Helpful Hint |**
When an off-the-shelf shoulder stabilizer cuff requires permanent attachment to the breast plate of football shoulder pads, first contact the manufacturer; drilling holes in the breast plate may lessen the protection provided and void the pads' warranty.

**Position of the patient:** Standing with the involved arm placed at the side of the body.

**Preparation:** Apply the torso vest design directly to the skin or over a shirt to lessen irritation. When using the individual cuff brace, anchor the cuff to the breast plate of football shoulder pads. Apply the cuff design directly to the skin or over a shirt.

Follow manufacturers' instructions, which are included with the braces when purchased, during application of these designs. The following guidelines pertain to most braces.

**⟩ Application:**

**STEP 1:**  Begin application of torso vest braces by loosening all the straps.

**STEP 2:**  When using some designs, place the involved arm into the cuff and wrap the vest around the shoulder and torso, then anchor (Fig. 8–21C).

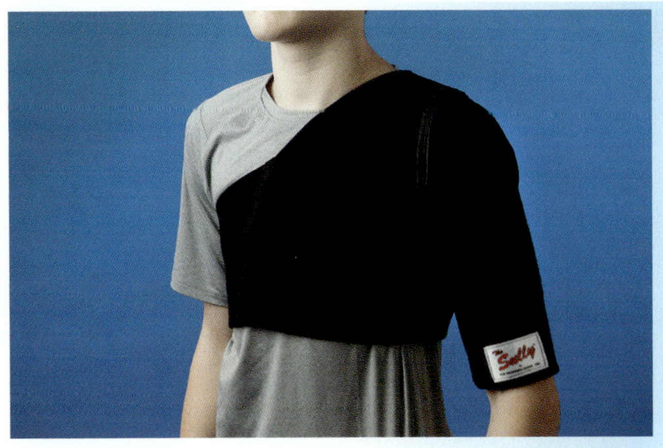

**Fig. 8–21 C**

**STEP 3:**  The application of straps will depend on the specific brace design. When treating anterior instabilities, attach the split strap on the posterior lateral involved arm. Pull the distal strap under the axilla, across the back, over the non-involved shoulder, and anchor on the torso. Next, pull the proximal strap under the axilla, across the back, and anchor on the torso (Fig. 8–21D). Two straps may be applied in an anterior and posterior pattern across the involved shoulder, back, and torso to treat multidirectional instabilities (Fig. 8–21E).

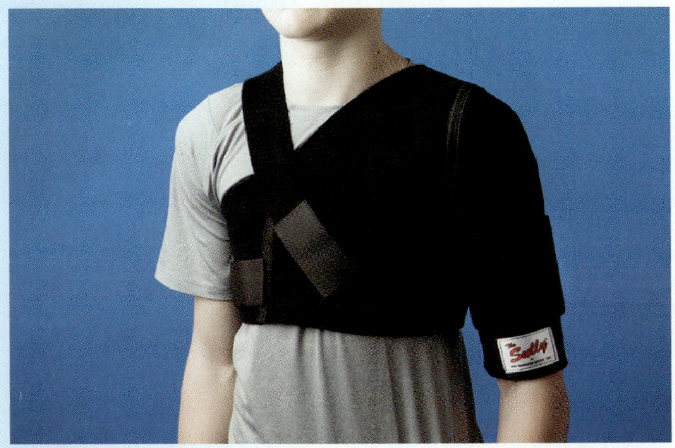

**Fig. 8–21 D**

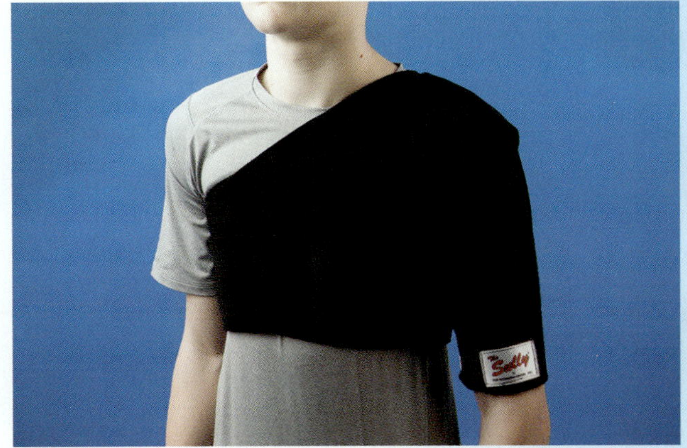

**Fig. 8–21 E**

**STEP 4:**  Apply other vest designs by placing the vest over the shoulders and around the torso, then anchor (Fig. 8–21F). Next, place the cuff around the upper arm and anchor (Fig. 8–21G).

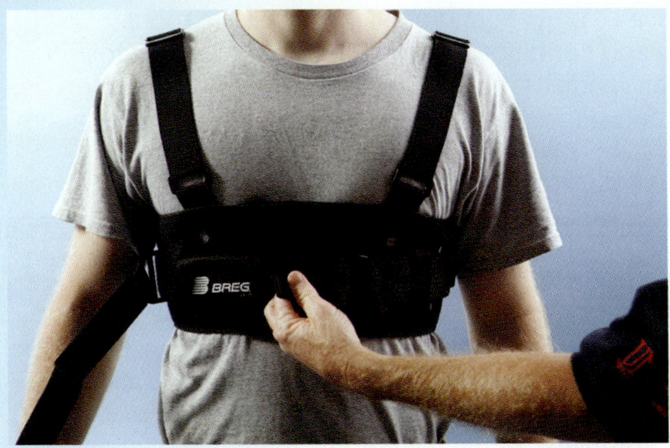

**Fig. 8–21 F**

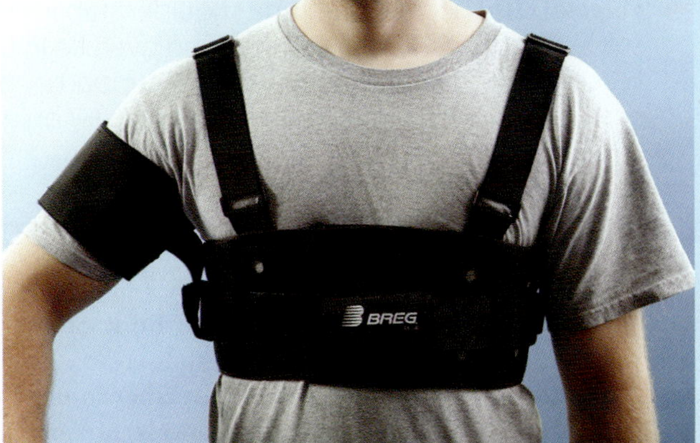

**Fig. 8–21 G**

*Steps Cont.*

**STEP 5:** When using the individual cuff designs, apply and anchor the shoulder pads. Next, apply the cuff around the proximal upper arm, superior to the belly of the biceps brachii (Fig. 8–21H).

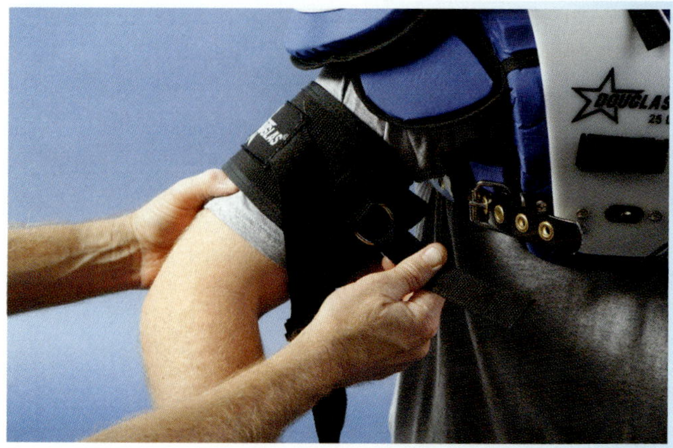

Fig. 8–21 H

**STEP 6:** Adjust the cuff and strap to limit the desired range of motion and anchor with Velcro or buckles (Fig. 8–21I).

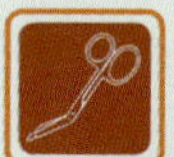

**Helpful Hint |**
Daily use of the cuff may cause irritation and pinching of the skin. To prevent this irritation, apply 3 inch or 4 inch self-adherent wrap loosely in a circular pattern around the proximal upper arm. Apply enough wrap to cover an area slightly larger than the cuff. Anchor the cuff over the wrap.

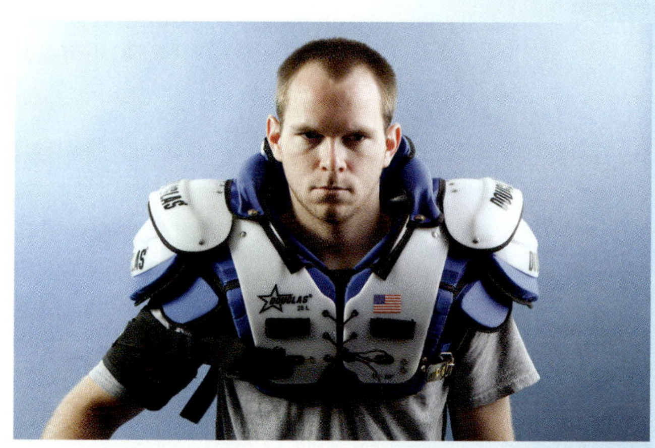

Fig. 8–21 I

## ... IF/THEN ...

**IF** limits in range of motion are required when treating GH joint instability for a football athlete, **THEN** consider using an individual cuff design; a torso vest brace can be effective, but a cuff design may be more comfortable to wear in hot and humid weather because the cuff design eliminates the need to wear a vest.

## CUSTOM-MADE SHOULDER STABILIZER

**Purpose:** Use the custom-made shoulder stabilizer brace to prevent and treat sprains, dislocations, subluxations, instabilities, strains, and overuse injuries and conditions. Custom-made shoulder stabilizer braces provide moderate to maximal support and limit range of motion. The brace can be used when off-the-shelf designs are not available. This technique and steps of application can be found at FADavis.com.

## EVIDENCE SUMMARY

Shoulder stabilizer braces are designed to limit range of motion at the GH joint, primarily abduction and external rotation, in attempts to prevent further injury. Research efforts to examine the indications for and effectiveness of shoulder stabilizer braces in restricting range of motion and preventing further injury are limited in the literature. Following exercise, several researchers[10,11] have shown a significant increase in active forward flexion, abduction, and external rotation compared to preset motion limitations among torso vest and individual cuff braces. However, postexercise external rotation in allowed abduction did not significantly increase with torso vest designs.[10] During physiological loading, other researchers[12] demonstrated torso vest and cuff designs failed to restrict preset abduction and external rotation motions. Examining active and passive range of motion, some researchers revealed that torso vest designs allowed an increase in abduction and external rotation compared to preset limitations.[13] In several studies, differences in the restriction of range of motion were found among individual torso vest and cuff brace designs.[10–13] Most important, researchers[13] have suggested that the motion limiting efficacy of shoulder stabilizing braces is enhanced when preset motion limitations are restricted or set below the protected motion minimum. Examining shoulder kinematics, a small study[14] demonstrated significant reductions in glenohumeral abduction/adduction and external rotation and scapulohumeral mediolateral rotation with a torso vest design compared with a no-brace situation among subjects with unstable shoulders.

Although a large amount of research examines the effects of taping and bracing techniques on joint-reposition sense in the lower extremities, studies examining the effects on the upper extremities are lacking. Many researchers have shown that shoulder injury and instability negatively affect passive joint-reposition sense.[15–17] Focusing on the shoulder, researchers have examined the effects of a neoprene torso vest on active joint-reposition sense.[18] The data revealed that brace wear significantly improved active joint-reposition sense at 10 degrees from full external rotation among subjects with unstable shoulders. Shoulder external rotation was limited with brace wear in subjects with stable shoulders, but no effect was found among the unstable group. The researchers[18] proposed that an increase in cutaneous input at the shoulder from the brace may have caused the improvement in active joint-reposition sense. This increase in stimulation may enhance proprioception and lessen the recurrence of dislocations or subluxations. Other researchers have also demonstrated that applying neoprene sleeves and elastic wraps and braces enhanced cutaneous stimulation.[19–21]

A limited number of studies have examined the efficacy of shoulder stabilizer braces in the prevention of recurrent shoulder instability among athletes. Several studies investigated the return to activity following an in-season traumatic anterior shoulder dislocation or subluxation injury among high school and intercollegiate athletes. Researchers[22] found 33 of 45 (73%) intercollegiate athletes returned to football, rugby, wrestling, baseball, judo, lacrosse, and boxing activities for some or the remainder of the competitive season

after completing an accelerated rehabilitation program. Off-the-shelf stabilizer braces were worn by 20 (61%) athletes in the study, and the findings showed no differences in recurrence of glenohumeral instability among braced and unbraced athletes. The specific brace design used in this study was not mentioned. Among high school and intercollegiate athletes, others[23] demonstrated that 27 of 30 (90%) athletes returned to part or all of ice hockey, football, wrestling, basketball, skiing, and gymnastic competitive seasons following a dislocation or subluxation upon completion of a rehabilitation program. A torso vest brace design was recommended for non-overhead throwing athletes and worn by 19 (70%) athletes for their return to activity. The braced athletes subjectively reported an improvement in the sense of stability and their return to activity was at or near previous levels of play. Among 11 major league amateur hockey athletes, using a torso vest brace within a therapy program consisting of rest, muscle stimulation, and weight-training resulted in no recurrence of injury.[24] All subjects had a history of shoulder dislocation or subluxation; the duration of the therapy program to return the subjects back to activity ranged from 3 to 7 weeks. Other researchers[25] have examined the efficacy of a torso vest brace within an accelerated rehabilitation program among professional soccer athletes following an in-season traumatic anterior dislocation. The subjects had no history of shoulder dislocation or subluxation, and following rehabilitation, 18 of 20 (90%) athletes returned to the competitive season approximately 40 days post-injury without pain and completed the season with no recurrence of injury.

A variety of off-the-shelf shoulder stabilizer braces are available for the treatment of GH injuries and conditions, although their effectiveness in preventing the recurrence of injury is unclear. The existing evidence and several factors[10,26] should be considered by health care professionals when selecting the specific design. First, determining the mechanism of injury will assist in identifying the specific range(s) of motion to restrict. Second, knowledge of the patient's sport or work activities will identify essential movements and force required for participation, such as an overhead motion or high strain/impact forces to the shoulder. Third, familiarity with brace designs will provide the health care professional the information needed to choose and apply the most appropriate brace to fit the needs of the patient. Additional research is needed to determine the effectiveness of these braces on active and passive range of motion, functional performance, and protection of the unstable GH joint to guide the selection and use of the most appropriate design.

## CLAVICLE BRACE    Figure 8–22

➡ **Purpose:** The clavicle brace is designed to provide moderate to maximal support and longitudinal traction to the clavicle (Fig. 8–22). Use this brace to retract the scapulae when treating SC joint sprains and clavicular fractures.

➡ **Design:**
- The braces are available in universal fit designs in predetermined sizes according to chest circumference measurements.
- The braces consist of two foam and nylon straps covered with stockinet in a figure-of-eight design, attached over the upper back with buckles, plastic rings, or Velcro closures to allow for tension adjustments.

➡ **Position of the patient:** Standing with the hands of the involved and non-involved arms placed on the hips with elbow flexion.

➡ **Preparation:** Apply the clavicle brace directly to the skin or over clothing.
   Specific instructions for application are included with each brace. The following guidelines apply to most designs.

➡ **Application:**

**STEP 1:**    Position the brace on the upper back (Fig. 8–22A).

**STEP 2:**    Apply the straps across the anterior shoulders, under the axillae, and anchor on the upper back through the buckles, rings, or closures (Fig. 8–22B).

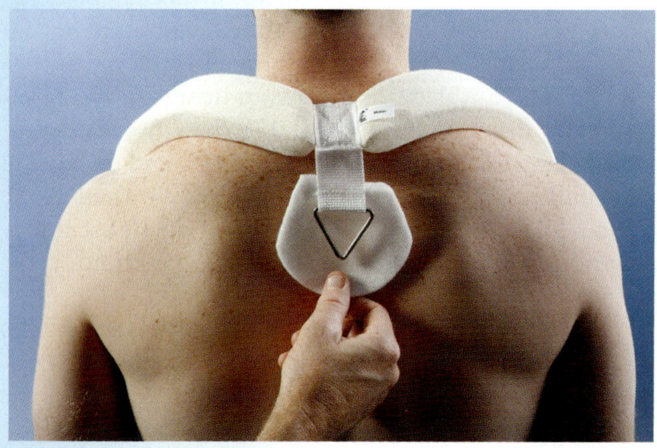

**Fig. 8–22 A**

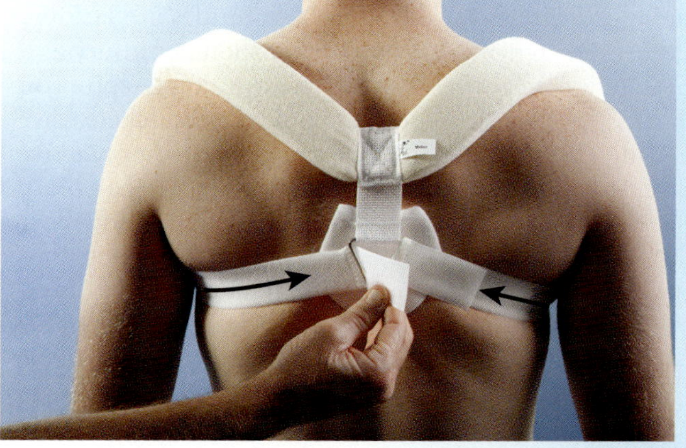

**Fig. 8–22 B**

**STEP 3:**    Adjust the straps to the desired tension, as indicated by a physician, to promote scapular retraction (Fig. 8–22C). Monitor strap tension to prevent brachial artery or nerve impingement.

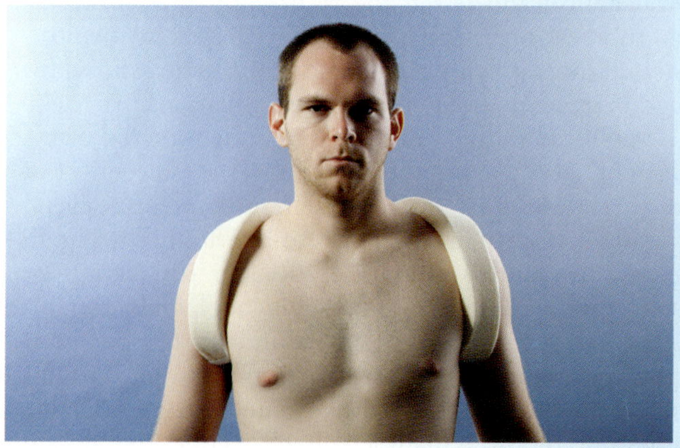

**Fig. 8–22 C**

## EVIDENCE SUMMARY

A 2016 evidence-based review[27] investigated the efficacy of sling and figure-of-eight bandage interventions in the conservative management of middle third clavicular fractures among adolescent and adult patients. Three randomized controlled trials (RCTs) of very low quality were included in the review, and pooling of the data was limited. Overall, the researchers found no significant differences between the sling and figure-of-eight bandage for visual analogue scales of pain perception at 2 weeks, rates of healing, shoulder function and cosmetic outcome scores, and time to return to school, work, or sport activities among the RCTs. An individual RCT in the review found the figure-of-eight bandage produced a greater amount of pain and discomfort for patients when compared with a sling. The insufficient evidence from this review highlights the need for further investigations of different brace designs among various populations using standardized function, healing, and pain outcome measures to identify the most effective intervention for the management of middle third clavicular fractures. Clinicians should continue to select interventions for these injuries based on their expertise and experience with brace designs and patient preferences, such as work and sport activity needs, level of comfort, and compliance.

# Padding Techniques

Use off-the-shelf and custom-made padding techniques to absorb shock and provide protection when preventing and treating shoulder and upper arm injuries and conditions. Several high school and intercollegiate sports require mandatory padding of the shoulder and upper arm. The mandatory padding techniques will be discussed in Chapter 13.

## EVIDENCE SUMMARY

Athletes participating in collision and contact sports should return to activity following an AC joint sprain with protective padding.[28] An off-the-shelf or custom-made design worn over the AC joint will dissipate impact forces and lessen the chance of reinjury.

---

### OFF-THE-SHELF    Figure 8–23

⟹ **Purpose:** Use off-the-shelf padding techniques to absorb shock and provide protection when preventing and treating AC joint sprains, shoulder pointers, and upper arm contusions, heterotopic ossification, and exostosis (Fig. 8–23).

---

### DETAILS
Each of these off-the-shelf padding techniques can be used with mandatory protective equipment; most can be worn alone.

---

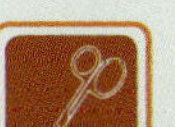

**Helpful Hint |**
When working with athletes in collision and contact sports, purchase several off-the-shelf pad designs for the shoulder and upper arm. These pads can be fitted and applied in less time than custom-made pads and can also be reused.

⟹ **Design:**
- Several padding techniques are available in individual and universal fit designs and are manufactured in predetermined sizes.
- Many AC joint designs are constructed of a thermoplastic material outer shell lined with open- and closed-cell foams with a raised area over the joint (Fig. 8–23A).
- Some of these designs can be molded to the shoulder by hand, whereas others require immersion in water to mold.
- Most designs use neoprene straps to attach the pads to the shoulder.
- Other designs are constructed of viscoelastic polymer or gel materials covered with cotton or nylon and are available in predetermined sizes (Fig. 8–23B).
- These pads are designed to be used in combination with football shoulder pads. The designs are attached to the inner lining of shoulder pads with Velcro.

- Other designs, used primarily underneath football shoulder pads, are constructed of vinyl-coated foam in a skeleton pattern or open-cell foam that covers the shoulders and upper chest and back (Fig. 8–23C).

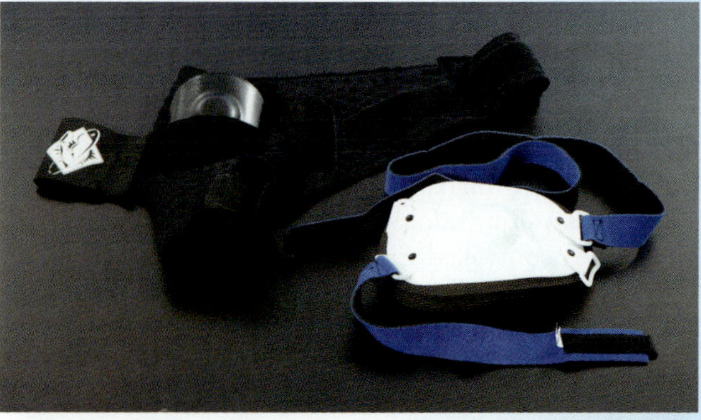

**Fig. 8–23 A** *AC joint pads. (Left) Pad in a neoprene sleeve. (Right) Pad with straps.*

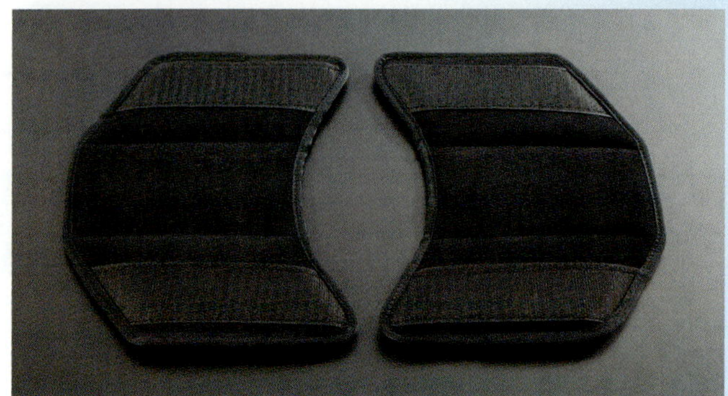

**Fig. 8–23 B** *Viscoelastic polymer pad.*

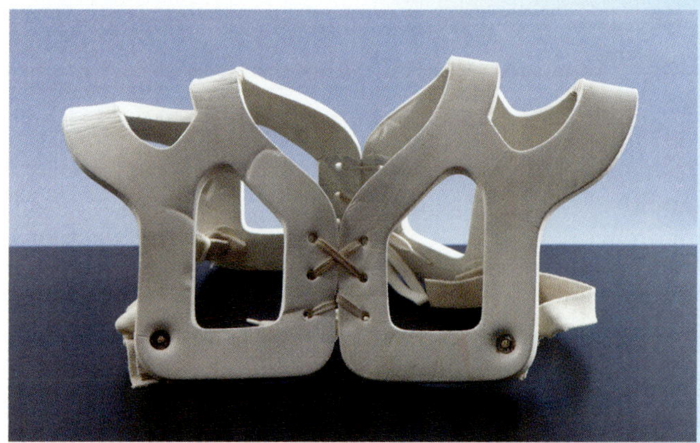

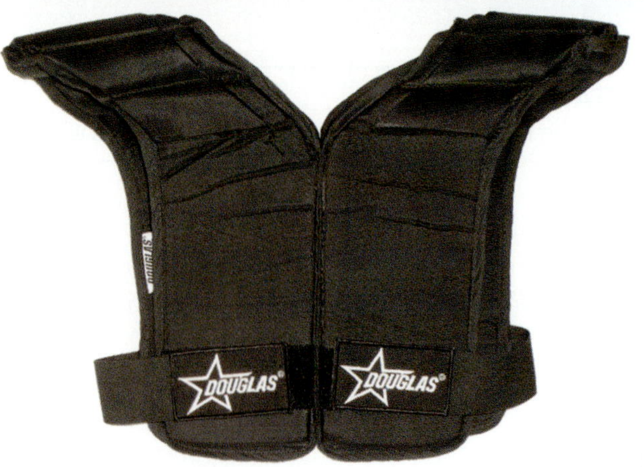

**Fig. 8–23 C** *(Top) Skeleton pad. (Bottom) Open-cell foam pad. (Courtesy of Douglas Pads & Sports, Inc., Houston, TX.)*

- The skeleton pad has anterior and posterior laces and is anchored under the axilla with elastic straps. The open-cell foam design attaches around the chest with Velcro straps.
- Upper arm designs are manufactured with high-density plastics covered by open- and closed-cell foams (Fig. 8–23D). These pads are contoured to the upper arm; some are designed to be used in combination with football shoulder pads.
- Another upper arm design consists of a high-density shell lined with foam incorporated into neoprene straps.

➠ **Position of the patient:** Standing with the hand of the involved arm placed on the lateral hip in a relaxed position.

➠ **Preparation:** Apply the off-the-shelf designs directly to the skin or over tight-fitting clothing.

➠ **Application:**

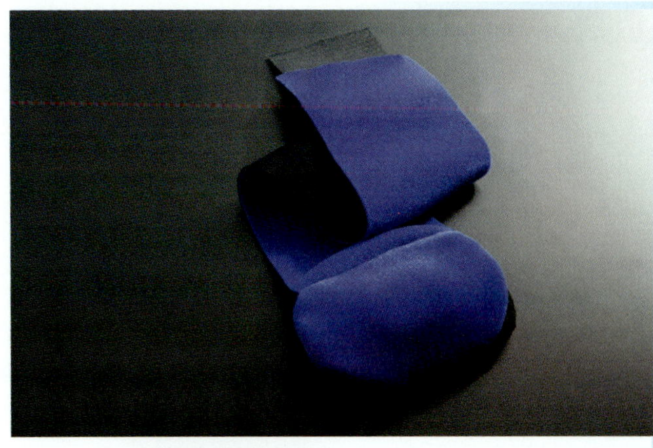

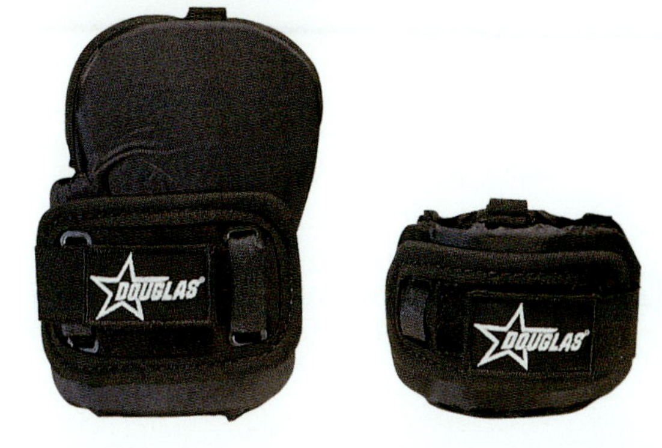


**Fig. 8–23 D** *Upper arm pads. (Top) Pad with straps. (Bottom) Pads that can be attached to football shoulder pads. (Courtesy of Douglas Pads & Sports, Inc., Houston, TX.)*

| **STEP 1:** | Begin application of neoprene strap designs by placing the pad over the injured area. When using most designs, wrap the straps around the chest and under the axilla (Fig. 8–23E). Anchor the straps with Velcro. |

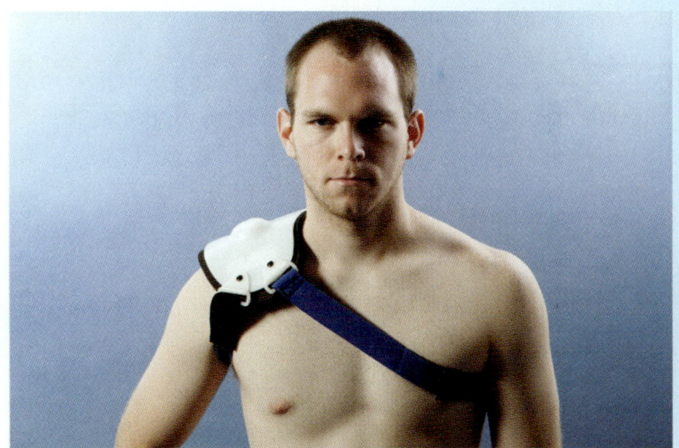

**Fig. 8–23 E**

*Steps Cont.*

**STEP 2:** Apply the viscoelastic polymer and gel material pads directly to the existing inner padding of the football shoulder pads. Determine placement of the pad and anchor with Velcro (Fig. 8–23F).

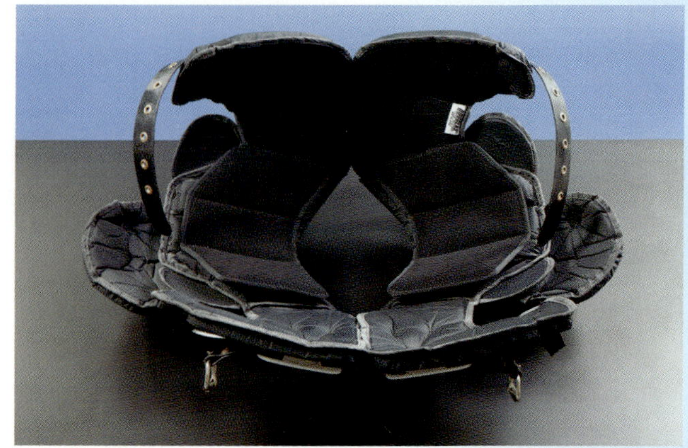

Fig. 8–23 F

**STEP 3:** Place the skeleton pad over the head and insert the arms through the openings. Pull the pad onto the shoulders, chest, and back (Fig. 8–23G).

**STEP 4:** When using the open-cell foam pad, place the pad onto the shoulders and wrap around the chest. Anchor with Velcro.

**STEP 5:** When using the upper arm pad designs, attach the pad to the cup of the football shoulder pad using the incorporated strap. Anchor the pad around the upper arm with the Velcro strap.

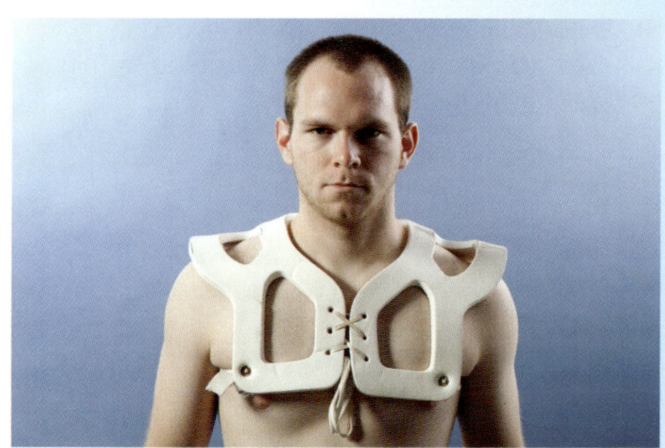

Fig. 8–23 G

**STEP 6:** When using other designs, apply the pad over the injured area and wrap the neoprene straps around the upper arm. Anchor with Velcro (Fig. 8–23H).

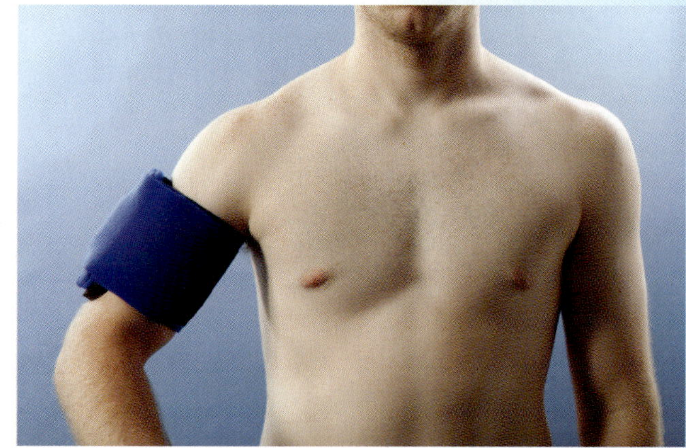

Fig. 8–23 H

### Clinical Application Question 3

Since the ninth grade, a senior linebacker on the high school football team has sustained five mild contusions to the anterolateral aspect of the left upper arm. You and the team physician have followed the athlete during this time; he has worn several different pads over the area for protection. The pad design that provides the most effective protection and is the most comfortable migrates during activity. This particular design attaches to the cup of the shoulder pad and to the upper arm with a strap.

**➡ Question: How can you manage this situation?**

## CUSTOM-MADE      Figure 8–24

- **Purpose:** Absorb shock and provide protection when preventing and treating AC joint sprains, shoulder pointers, and upper arm contusions, heterotopic ossification, and exostosis with thermoplastic material and foam (Fig. 8–24). Use these pads when off-the-shelf designs are not available.
- **Materials:**
  - Paper, felt tip pen, thermoplastic material, ⅛ inch or ¼ inch foam or felt, a heating source, 2 inch or 3 inch elastic tape, an elastic wrap, soft, low-density foam, rubber cement, taping scissors

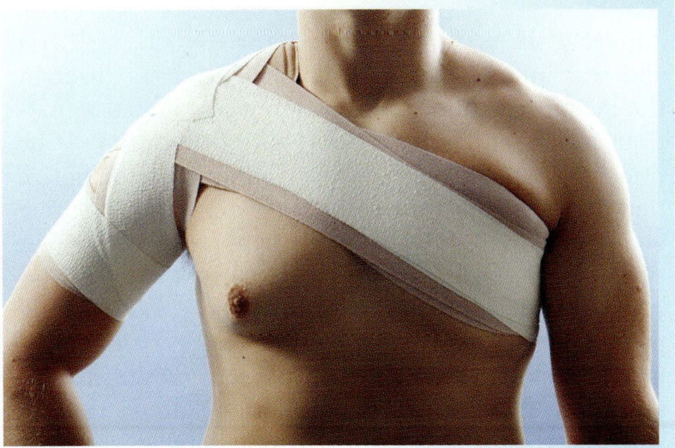

**Fig. 8–24**

- **Position of the patient:** Standing with the hand of the involved arm placed on the lateral hip in a relaxed position.
- **Preparation:** Design the pad with a paper pattern (see Fig. 1–10), then cut, mold, and shape the thermoplastic material on the shoulder or upper arm over the injured area. Attach soft, low-density foam to the inside surface of the material (see Fig. 1–11).
- **Application:**

**STEP 1:**   Attach the pad to the AC joint or tip of the shoulder with the shoulder pointer/AC joint sprain taping technique (see Figs. 8–10A–D) or the shoulder spica wrapping technique (see Figs. 8–15A–G and 8–24).

**STEP 2:**   For the upper arm, attach the pad with the circular upper arm taping (see Figs. 8–9A–C) or wrapping (see Figs. 8–14A–C) technique.

### Clinical Application Question 4

An intercollegiate baseball shortstop is struck on the acromion process of his throwing shoulder by a base runner during a double play. In the athletic training facility, you and the team physician complete an evaluation and determine that the athlete sustained a first-degree AC joint sprain. The team physician will allow a return to activity when the athlete can demonstrate full, bilateral strength and range of motion and a pre-injury throwing motion. The team physician also requests that protective padding be applied upon the athlete's return, to prevent further injury.

- **Question: What padding technique(s) are appropriate to provide protection?**

## MANDATORY PADDING

- Protective equipment is required in several high school and intercollegiate sports. The NCAA[29] and the NFHS[30] require that athletes participating in fencing, football, ice hockey, and lacrosse wear protective padding on the shoulder and/or upper arm during all practices and competitions. These pads are normally purchased off-the-shelf; many designs are constructed for specific sports and positions. Chapter 13 will provide a more in-depth discussion of these padding techniques.

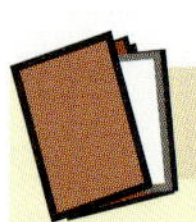

## EVIDENCE-BASED PRACTICE

Tanner is the rear tire carrier for the RN Racing Team and was injured during a pit stop. Midway through the racing schedule, Tanner Compton suffered a first-time, right glenohumeral (GH) joint dislocation. As he lifted the tire off the pit wall, Tanner did not notice that the air hose for the air impact wrench had become wrapped around the tire and his right wrist. As the rear tire changer quickly moved away from the pit wall and across the back of the race car, the air hose was violently pulled, placing an abduction, external rotation force on Tanner's right shoulder. Tanner was moved behind the pit wall and evaluated by Jordon Young, the AT with the Race Team. The evaluation showed an acute anterior GH joint dislocation. Jordon immobilized the shoulder with the 4 S wrapping technique and took Tanner to the in-field care center for further evaluation by a physician.

The orthopedist at the in-field care center obtained radiographs and reduced the shoulder. Tanner returned home with the Race Team and was scheduled for a follow-up evaluation with an orthopedic surgeon. The surgeon performed an evaluation and ordered additional radiographs and magnetic resonance imaging. The imaging studies were negative; the surgeon decided on a nonsurgical rehabilitation approach for Tanner and continued immobilization of his shoulder for 3 weeks. Tanner was placed in an immobilizer with a low inflated pillow for the extended period of immobilization.

Tanner progressed with the rehabilitation program without any delays. At post-injury week 21, he is now ready to begin functional activities. A follow-up evaluation with the surgeon demonstrates mild anterior instability of the right shoulder. Jordon designs a functional activity program, which includes lifting, carrying, and setting a 75 lb racing tire onto the rear lug nuts of a race car. These activities are performed in standing and kneeling positions and require flexion, extension, abduction, adduction, and internal and external rotation at the GH joint. The surgeon and Jordon decided that using a brace may lessen the possibility of reinjury in this phase of rehabilitation and upon his return to full activity with the Race Team. Jordon's experience with shoulder stabilizer braces is limited to those designs attached to football shoulder pads. Jordon will explore bracing techniques to find a design that will provide support and limit range of motion as part of a maintenance strengthening and flexibility program to allow Tanner a return for the remainder of the racing season. The uniform and gloves worn by Tanner on race day are constructed of flame retardant materials and may cause dehydration concerns in a hot and humid environment. Jordon will need to consider this in the selection of the bracing technique.

1. Develop a clinically relevant question from the case in the PICO format to generate answers for the selection of a bracing technique for Tanner. The question should include the population or problem, the intervention, a comparison intervention (if relevant), and the clinical outcome of interest.

2. Design a search strategy and search to find the best evidence to answer the clinical question. The strategy should include relevant search terms, electronic databases, online journals, and print journals to use for the search. Discussions with your faculty, preceptor, and other health care professionals can provide evidence from expert opinion.

3. Choose three to five full text studies or reviews from your search or the chapter references. Evaluate and appraise each article to determine its value and usefulness to the case. Ask these questions for each study: (1) Are the results of the study valid? (2) What are the actual results? and (3) Are the findings clinically relevant to my patients? Prepare a summary of the evaluation with answers to the questions and rank the articles based on the evidence hierarchy in Chapter 1.

4. Integrate findings from the evidence, your clinical experience, and Tanner's goals and preferences into the rehabilitation program for Tanner. Consider which bracing technique may be appropriate for Tanner.

5. Evaluate the EBP process and your experience within the case. Consider these questions in the evaluation.

Was the clinical question answered?

Did the search generate quality evidence?

Was the evidence evaluated appropriately?

Was the evidence, your clinical experience, and Tanner's goals and values integrated to make the clinical decision?

Did the intervention produce successful clinical outcomes for Tanner?

Was the EBP experience positive for Jordon and Tanner?

## WRAP-UP

- Shoulder and upper arm contusions, sprains, dislocations, subluxations, fractures, strains, ruptures, and overuse injuries and conditions can be caused by compressive and shear forces, excessive range of motion, forceful muscular contractions, and repetitive stresses.
- The circular upper arm and shoulder pointer/AC joint sprain taping techniques provide support and anchor protective padding.
- Elastic wraps and sleeves and self-adherent wraps provide compression and assist in reducing swelling.
- The circular upper arm and shoulder spica wrapping techniques can be used to provide support and anchor padding.
- The 4 S, figure-of-eight, and swathe wrapping techniques are used to support and immobilize the shoulder and upper arm.
- The sling, immobilizer, and clavicle bracing techniques provide support and immobilization following injury and surgery.
- Shoulder stabilizer bracing techniques are used to provide support and limit range of motion of the glenohumeral joint.
- Off-the-shelf and custom-made padding techniques constructed of open- and closed-cell foams and hard, high-density, viscoelastic polymer and gel materials absorb shock and provide protection.
- Protective padding is required for the shoulder and/or upper arm in several sports by the NCAA and NFHS.

## ⊕ FADAVIS ONLINE RESOURCES

- Custom-made shoulder stabilizer

## WEB REFERENCES

### American Academy of Orthopaedic Surgeons
https://www.aaos.org/
- This site provides access to information regarding the treatment and rehabilitation of shoulder and upper arm injuries and conditions, including the American Academy of Orthopaedic Surgeons Clinical Practice Guidelines.

### The Hughston Clinic
https://www.hughston.com/
- This site allows access to the *Hughston Health Alert* newsletter, which contains information for a variety of injuries and conditions.

### The American Orthopaedic Society for Sports Medicine
https://www.sportsmed.org/
- This site allows access to a three-dimensional animation library, videos, fact sheets, and a newsletter about shoulder injuries and conditions.

### United States National Library of Medicine
https://www.nlm.nih.gov
- This website provides access to shoulder and upper arm injury prevention, treatment, and rehabilitation information among a variety of populations.

## REFERENCES


1. Owens, BD, Campbell, SE, and Cameron, KL: Risk factors for anterior glenohumeral instability. Am J Sports Med 42:2591–2596, 2014.
2. Starkey, C, and Brown, SD: Examination of Orthopedic and Athletic Injuries, ed 4. F.A. Davis, Philadelphia, 2015.
3. Wu, CL, Chang, HC, and Lu, KH: Risk factors for nonunion in 337 displaced midshaft clavicular fractures treated with Knowles pin fixation. Arch Orthop Trauma Surg 133:15–22, 2013.
4. Meister, K, and Andrews, JR: Classification and treatment of rotator cuff injuries in the overhead athlete. J Orthop Sports Phys Ther 18:413–421, 1993.
5. Paterson, WH, Throckmorton, TW, Koester, M, Azar, FM, and Kuhn, JE: Position and duration of immobilization after primary anterior shoulder dislocation: A systematic review and meta-analysis of the literature. J Bone Joint Surg Am 92:2924–2933, 2010.
6. Vavken, P, Sadoghi, P, Quidde, J, Lucas, R, Delaney, R, Mueller, AM, Rosso, C, and Valderrabano, V: Immobilization in internal or external rotation does not change recurrence rates after traumatic anterior shoulder dislocation. J Shoulder Elbow Surg 23:13–19, 2014.
7. Liu, A, Xue, YC, Chen, Y, Bi, F, and Yan, S: The external rotation immobilisation does not reduce recurrence rates or improve quality of life after primary anterior shoulder dislocation: A systematic review and meta-analysis. Injury 45:1842–1847, 2014.
8. Braun, C, and McRobert, CJ: Conservative management following closed reduction of traumatic anterior dislocation of the shoulder. Cochrane Database Syst Rev (5);CD004962, 2019.
9. Whelan, DB, Kletke, SN, Schemitsch, G, and Chahal, J: Immobilization in external rotation versus internal rotation after primary anterior shoulder dislocation: A meta-analysis of randomized controlled trials. Am J Sports Med 44:521–532, 2016.
10. DeCarlo, M, Malone, K, Gerig, B, and Hunker, M: Evaluation of shoulder instability braces. J Sport Rehabil 4:143–150, 1996.
11. McLeod, IA, Uhl, TL, Arnold, BL, and Gansneder, BM: Effectiveness of shoulder bracing in limiting active range of motion [abstract]. J Athl Train 34(suppl):84, 1999.
12. DeSavage, M, Sitler, M, Swanik, K, Stansbury, D, and Moyer, R: Effectiveness of glenohumeral joint stability braces on restricting active shoulder range of motion during physiological loading [abstract]. J Athl Train 35(suppl):90, 2000.

13. Weise, K, Sitler, MR, Tierney, R, and Swanik, KA: Effectiveness of glenohumeral-joint stability braces in limiting active and passive shoulder range of motion in collegiate football players. J Athl Train 39:151–155, 2004.

14. Dellabiancia, F, Parel, I, Filippi, MV, Porcellini, G, and Merolla, G: Glenohumeral and scapulohumeral kinematic analysis of patients with traumatic anterior instability wearing a shoulder brace: A prospective laboratory study. Musculoskelet Surg 101(suppl 2):S159–S167, 2017.

15. Lephart, SM, Warner, JP, Borsa, PA, and Fu, FH: Proprioception of the shoulder joint in healthy, unstable, and surgically repaired shoulders. J Shoulder Elbow Surg 3:371–380, 1994.

16. Smith, RL, and Brunolli, J: Shoulder kinesthesia after anterior glenohumeral joint dislocation. Phys Ther 69:106–112, 1989.

17. Warner, JJ, Lephart, S, and Fu, FH: Role of proprioception in pathoetiology of shoulder instability. Clin Orthop 330:35–39, 1996.

18. Chu, JC, Kane, EJ, Arnold, BL, and Gansneder, BM: The effect of a neoprene shoulder stabilizer on active joint-reposition sense in subjects with stable and unstable shoulders. J Athl Train 37:141–145, 2002.

19. Khabie, V, Schwartz, MC, Rokito, AS, Gallagher, MA, Cuomo, F, and Zuckerman, JD: The effect of intraarticular anesthesia and elastic bandaging on elbow proprioception. J Shoulder Elbow Surg 7:501–504, 1998.

20. Lephart, SM, Kocher, MS, Fu, FH, Borsa, PA, and Harner, CD: Proprioception following anterior cruciate ligament reconstruction. J Sport Rehabil 1:188–196, 1992.

21. Ulkar, B, Kunduracioglu, B, Cetin, C, and Güner, RS: Effect of positioning and bracing on passive position sense of shoulder joint. Br J Sports Med 38:549–552, 2004.

22. Dickens, JF, Owens, BD, Cameron, KL, Kilcoyne, K, Allred, CD, Svoboda, SJ, Sullivan, R, Tokish, JM, Peck, KY, and Rue, JP: Return to play and recurrent instability after in-season anterior shoulder instability: A prospective multicenter study. Am J Sports Med 42:2842–2850, 2014.

23. Buss, DD, Lynch, GP, Meyer, CP, Huber, SM, and Freehill, MQ: Nonoperative management for in-season athletes with anterior shoulder instability. Am J Sports Med 32:1430–1433, 2004.

24. Sawa, TM: An alternate conservative management of shoulder dislocations and subluxations. J Athl Train 4:366–369, 1992.

25. Conti, M, Garofalo, R, Castagna, A, Massazza, G, and Ceccarelli, E: Dynamic brace is a good option to treat first anterior shoulder dislocation in season. Musculoskelet Surg 101:S169–S173, 2017.

26. Reuss, BL, Harding, WG, and Nowicki, KD: Managing anterior shoulder instability with bracing: An expanded update. Orthopedics 27:614–618, 2004.

27. Lenza, M, and Faloppa, F: Conservative interventions for treating middle third clavicle fractures in adolescents and adults. Cochrane Database Syst Rev (12);CD007121, 2016.

28. Wolfinger, CR, and Davenport, TE: Physical therapy management of ice hockey athletes: From the rink to the clinic and back. Int J Sports Phys Ther 11:482–495, 2016.

29. National Collegiate Athletic Association: 2014–15 Sports Medicine Handbook, ed 25. NCAA, Indianapolis, 2014. http://www.ncaapublications.com/productdownloads/MD15.pdf.

30. National Federation of State High School Associations: 2018–19 Ice Hockey Rules Book. National Federation of State High School Associations, Indianapolis, 2019.

# Elbow and Forearm

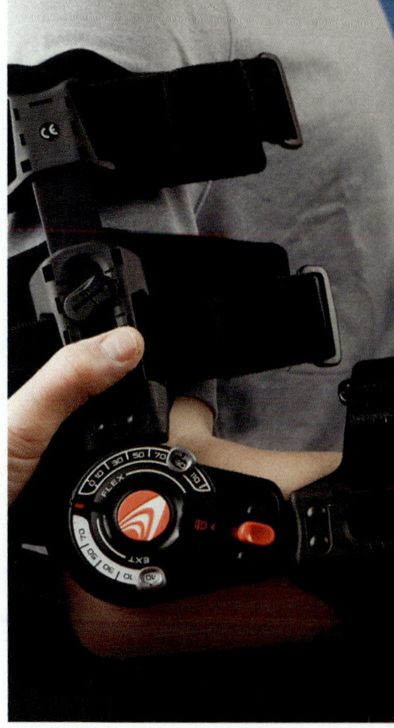

**9**



## INJURIES AND CONDITIONS

Direct forces, excessive range of motion, and repetitive and overload stresses can result in acute and chronic injuries and conditions to the elbow and forearm. Contusions, fractures, and bursitis can be caused by a direct blow or fall. Valgus, varus, and/or rotary forces can be produced during many athletic and work activities and result in a sprain, dislocation, or fracture. Overload and repetitive contractions of the musculature can lead to strains, ruptures, and overuse injuries and conditions. Common injuries to the elbow and forearm include:

- Contusions
- Sprains
- Strains
- Ruptures
- Dislocations
- Fractures
- Bursitis
- Overuse injuries and conditions
- Abrasions

## Contusions

Contusions to the elbow and forearm are caused by direct forces and commonly occur over bony prominences. The **olecranon** is frequently involved because of its exposure and lack of protection by soft tissue (Fig. 9–1). In collision and contact sports, direct blows can lead to contusions of the forearm. The ulnar side of the forearm, because of its location, is susceptible to injury as a result of contact with opponents and equipment. A contusion to the olecranon and/or ulnar forearm can occur, for instance, as a football tight end catches a pass, runs downfield with the ball in his right arm, and is tackled, receiving a blow to the right elbow and forearm from the helmet of a defensive back.

## Sprains

Sprains to the elbow are caused by acute and chronic forces. An acute valgus, varus, or rotary force or a fall on the outstretched arm causing hyperextension at the elbow can result in injury to the **ulnar collateral, radial collateral,** or **annular ligaments** (Figs. 9–1 and 9–2). Hyperextension of an elbow can take place, for instance, if the arms are extended to lessen the impact during a backward fall to the ground. More commonly, sprains to the ulnar collateral ligament are caused by repetitive

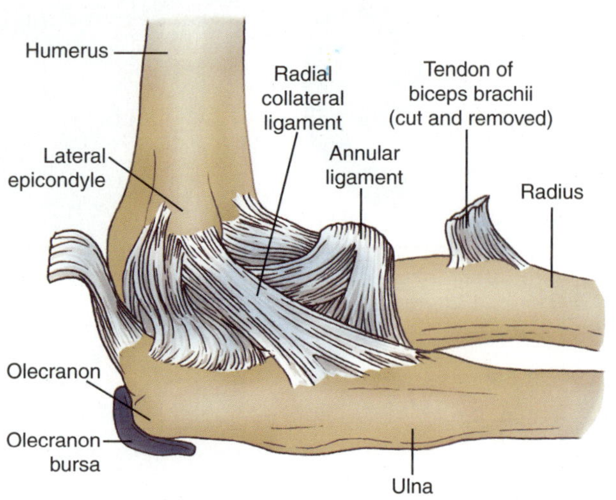

**Fig. 9–1** *Ligaments of the lateral elbow.*

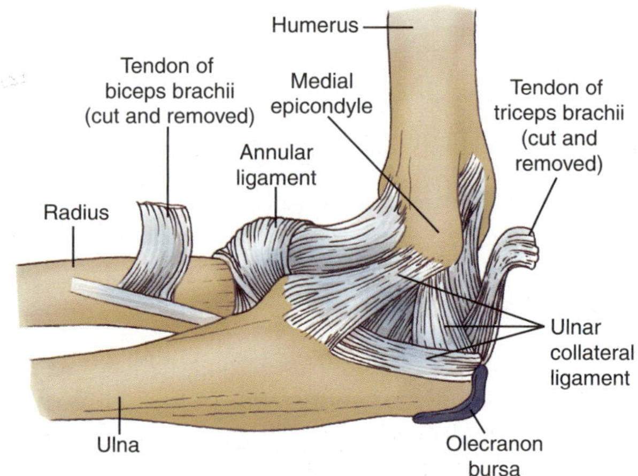

**Fig. 9–2** *Ligaments of the medial elbow.*

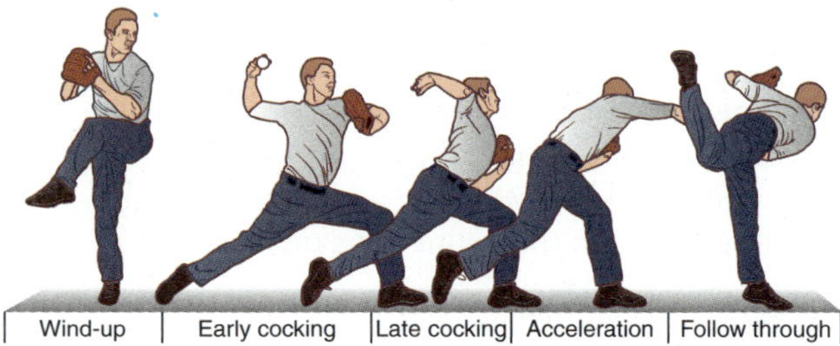

**Fig. 9–3** *Phases of the throwing motion.*

valgus forces, which occur during the overhead throwing motion.[1] For example, a baseball, softball, or tennis player with a history of medial elbow pain, indicating possible overuse, can be injured during the late cocking and early acceleration phases of the throwing motion, when valgus forces at the medial elbow are extreme (Fig. 9–3). The position of the arm against the trunk protects the elbow from varus forces; injury to the radial collateral ligament is uncommon.

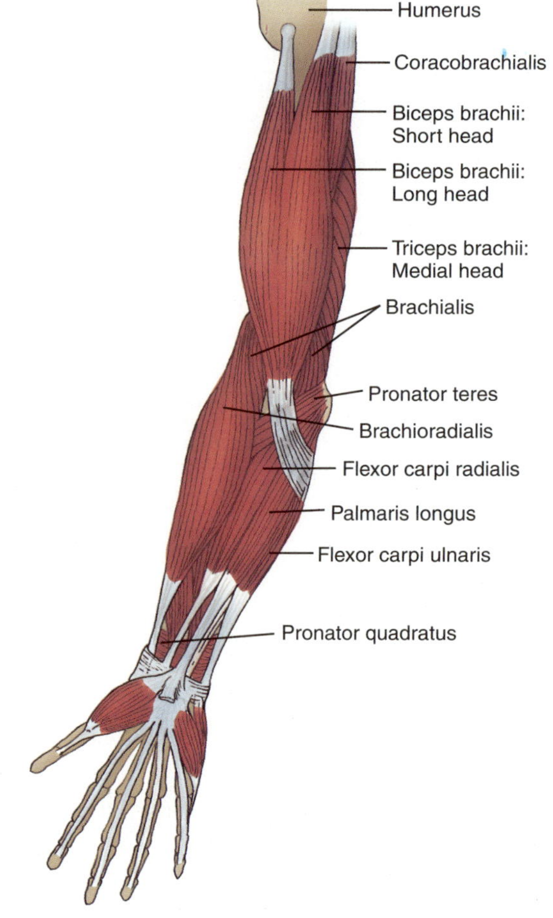

**Fig. 9–4** *Superficial muscles of the anterior upper arm, elbow, and forearm.*

## Strains

Strains of the elbow and forearm are caused by a variety of mechanisms during athletic and work activities. Brachialis, biceps brachii, and brachioradialis strains can be caused by repetitive microtrauma and overload, a fall on the outstretched arm, or a violent concentric or eccentric contraction (Fig. 9–4). A strain to the brachialis or brachioradialis can result as a construction worker attempts to catch a large box of nails, thrown from a height, with his elbows in a flexed position. This may cause a violent eccentric contraction. A strain to the triceps brachii can also result from a violent concentric or eccentric contraction (Fig. 9–5).

## Ruptures

A forceful eccentric contraction against resistance can cause a rupture of the biceps brachii. The proximal portion of the tendon is typically injured.

## Dislocations

A fall on the outstretched arm with the elbow in hyperextension, as well as valgus and rotary forces, can cause

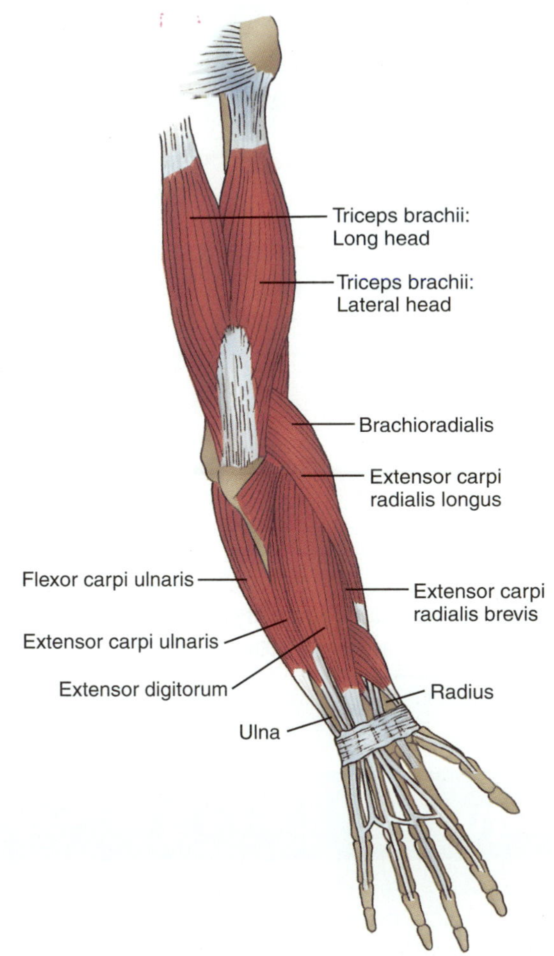

Fig. 9–5 *Superficial muscles of the posterior upper arm, elbow, and forearm.*

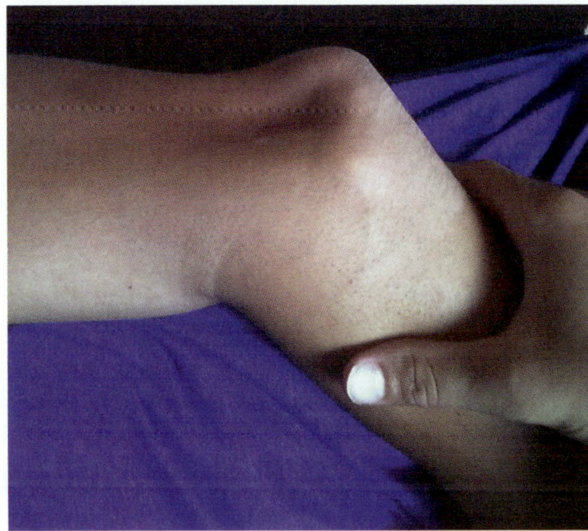

**Fig. 9–6 A** *Posterior dislocation of the elbow on inspection. (Courtesy of Starkey, C. and Brown, SD. Examination of Orthopedic & Athletic Injuries. 4th ed. Philadelphia, PA: F.A. Davis Company: 2015.)*

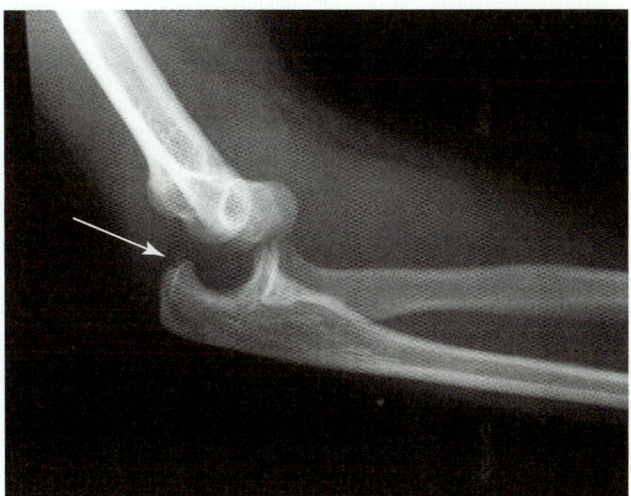

**Fig. 9–6 B** *Posterior dislocation of the elbow. Lateral radiograph showing posterior displacement (arrow) of the radius and ulna to the humeral shaft. (Courtesy of McKinnis, LN. Fundamentals of Musculoskeletal Imaging, 4th ed. Philadelphia, PA: F.A. Davis Company: 2014.)*

an elbow dislocation. With a dislocation, the ulna and/or radius can be positioned in an anterior, posterior, or lateral direction (Fig. 9–6). Dislocations are often accompanied by fractures and ligamentous and muscular trauma. For example, a dislocation can occur as a pole vaulter misses the plant of the pole, is thrown to the side of the landing pit, and lands on his right outstretched arm, causing hyperextension and rotary stress.

## Fractures

Fractures to the elbow and forearm may involve the radius, ulna, and olecranon. A fall on the outstretched arm or on a flexed elbow, direct forces, and valgus, varus, or tensile stresses can result in a fracture.

## Bursitis

The **olecranon bursa** can become inflamed through acute or chronic trauma. A fall on the flexed elbow or a direct force to the olecranon can cause acute olecranon bursitis. Repetitive compression and friction or infection can result in the development of chronic olecranon bursitis. Bursitis can be caused by activities such as wrestling without proper padding or leaning on a desktop while writing or reading.

## Overuse

Overload and repetitive stresses and faulty mechanics can cause elbow and forearm overuse injuries and conditions. **Lateral epicondylitis (tennis elbow)** can result from repetitive, eccentric overload of the wrist extensor musculature, faulty mechanics, and ill-fitting equipment. The extensor carpi radialis brevis is most commonly involved. For example, lateral epicondylitis can occur as a racquetball player participates in daily practices for several weeks without adequate rest to improve his backhand (Fig. 9–7). Repetitive wrist flexion, forearm pronation, and valgus stress at the elbow; training errors; and improper technique can cause **medial epicondylitis (golfer's elbow).** The origins of the pronator teres and flexor carpi radialis are common sites of involvement.[2] Medial epicondylitis can be caused by a youth league pitcher learning how to throw a curveball, resulting in repetitive wrist flexion and valgus stress at the elbow.

## Abrasions

Abrasions to the elbow and forearm are common in athletic activities. Rubbing and friction forces on the posterior elbow and ulnar side of the forearm during contact with athletic surfaces can result in abrasions **(turf burn).**

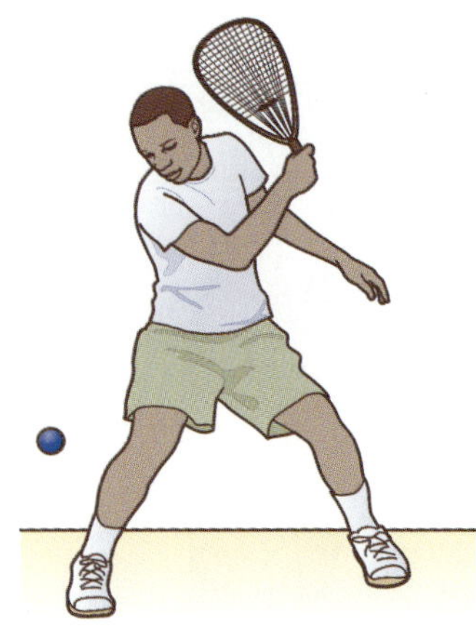

**Fig. 9–7** *Lateral epicondylitis (tennis elbow).*

---

### DETAILS
Commonly referred to as epicondylitis, the condition involves degeneration rather than the traditional inflammatory process. As a result, the term "epicondylalgia," instead of "tendinitis" or "epicondylitis," is often used to describe pain in the medial and lateral epicondyles.[3]

---

# Taping Techniques

Use taping techniques to provide support and reduce stress to the musculature and soft tissue, limit excessive range of motion, and immobilize the elbow and forearm when preventing and treating injuries and conditions. Following sprains, use several techniques to lessen excessive range of motion and immobilize the elbow and forearm. Use other techniques with overuse injuries and conditions to reduce the tension of the wrist extensor or flexor musculature during contractions. Techniques are also available to anchor protective padding to the elbow and forearm to prevent and treat contusions.

### HYPEREXTENSION — Figures 9–8 and 9–9

➠ **Purpose:** Use the hyperextension technique when treating sprains to limit hyperextension of the elbow and stretch on the soft tissues. Three interchangeable methods are available for applying the technique; the first two are illustrated here (Figs. 9–8 and Fig. 9–9) and the third is illustrated online at FADavis.com. Choose according to patient preferences.

#### Hyperextension Technique One

➠ **Materials:**
- Pre-wrap, thin foam pads, 2 inch or 3 inch heavyweight elastic tape, adherent tape spray, skin lubricant, taping scissors

**Option:**
- 4 inch or 6 inch width by 5 yard length elastic wrap

➠ **Position of the patient:** Sitting on a taping table or bench or standing with the involved arm at the side of the body. Determine the range of extension that produces pain. Stabilize the involved shoulder and place the forearm in supination. Support the posterior elbow and place a hand on the wrist. Slowly move the elbow into extension until pain occurs. Once painful range of motion is determined, place the involved elbow in a pain-free range and maintain this position during application. Also, maintain a moderate isometric contraction of the upper arm and forearm musculature.

➠ **Preparation:** Shave the arm from the proximal upper arm to mid forearm. Apply this technique directly to the skin or over one layer of pre-wrap. Place thin foam pads over the cubital fossa to prevent irritation. A skin lubricant may also be used. Apply adherent tape spray from the proximal upper arm to the mid forearm.

➠ **Application:**

**STEP 1:** Apply two anchors of 2 inch or 3 inch heavyweight elastic tape around the proximal upper arm and the mid forearm with a mild amount of roll tension ◄▓▓► (Fig. 9–8A).

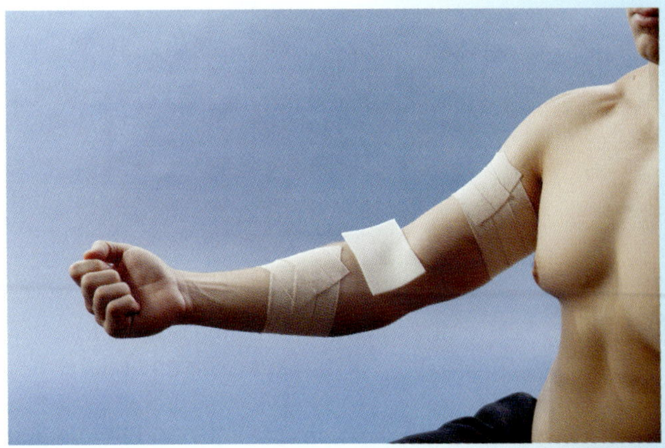

**Fig. 9–8 A**

**STEP 2:** Using 2 inch or 3 inch heavyweight elastic tape, anchor on the proximal lateral upper arm, continue distally across the cubital fossa, and anchor the strip on the medial mid forearm (Fig. 9–8B). Monitor the pain-free position of the elbow and apply the tape with moderate roll tension.

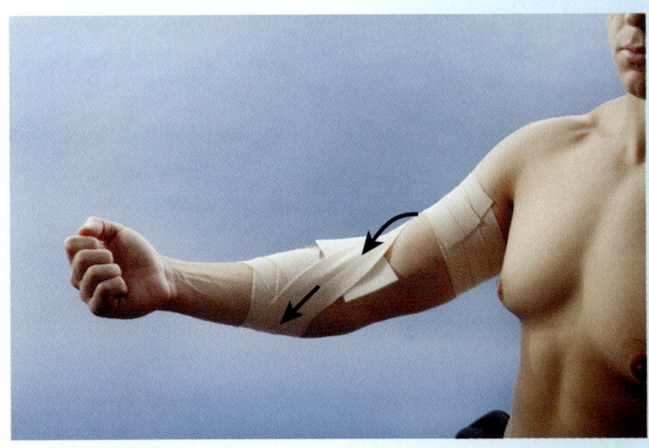

**Fig. 9–8 B**

**STEP 3:** Apply another strip of 2 inch or 3 inch heavyweight elastic tape from the proximal medial upper arm, across the cubital fossa, and anchor on the lateral mid forearm (Fig. 9–8C). These strips should form an "X" over the cubital fossa.

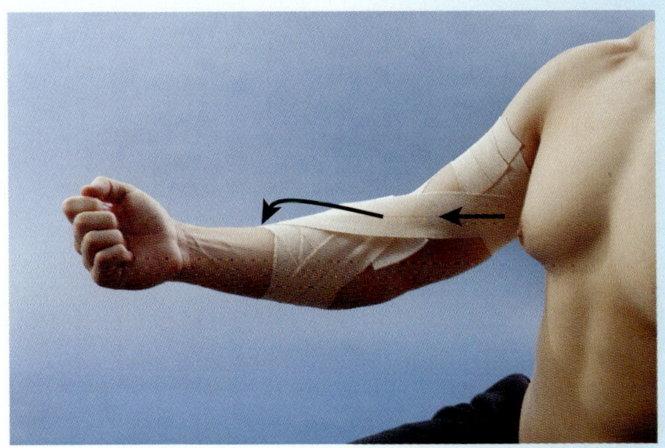

**Fig. 9–8 C**

*Steps Cont.*

**STEP 4:** Begin the next strip on the anterior proximal upper arm, across the cubital fossa, and anchor on the anterior mid forearm (Fig. 9–8D). These strips can be repeated, overlapping by ⅓ of the tape width to provide additional support.

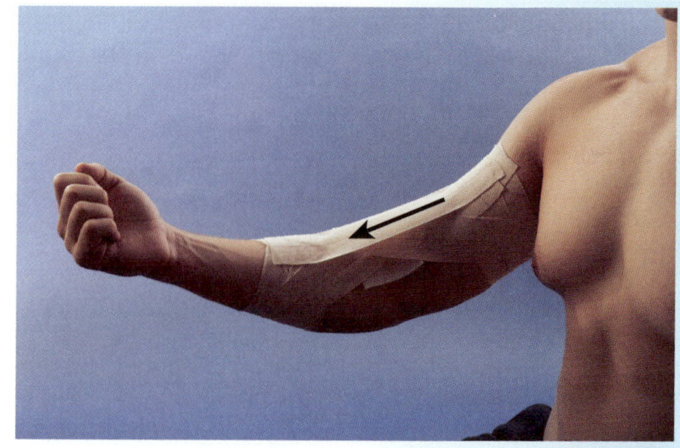

Fig. 9–8 D

**STEP 5:** At the proximal upper arm and mid forearm, apply three to four circular closure patterns with 2 inch or 3 inch heavyweight elastic tape, overlapping each by ½ of the tape width with mild tension ◄━━━━► (Fig. 9–8E). The closure patterns should not enclose or cause constriction of the cubital fossa. Non-elastic tape anchors are not necessary.

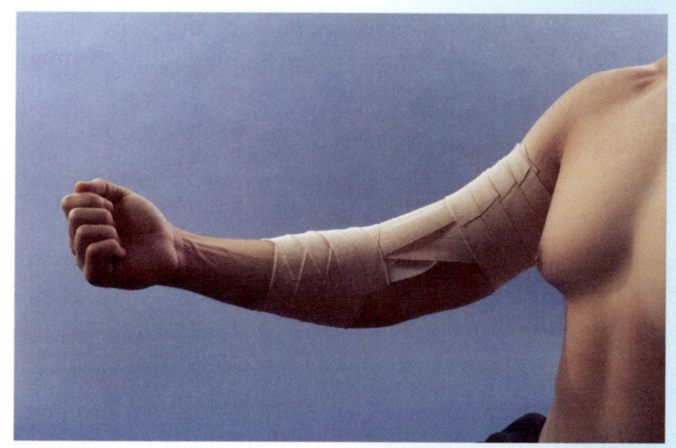

Fig. 9–8 E

*Option:* *Apply a 4 inch or 6 inch width by 5 yard length elastic wrap in a circular pattern with moderate roll tension in a proximal-to-distal direction over the technique to lessen migration and unraveling of the tape ◄━━━━►. Anchor with 2 inch or 3 inch elastic tape in a circular pattern with mild roll tension. Finish the anchor on the anterior mid forearm to prevent irritation from the tape ◄━━━━► (Fig. 9–8F).*

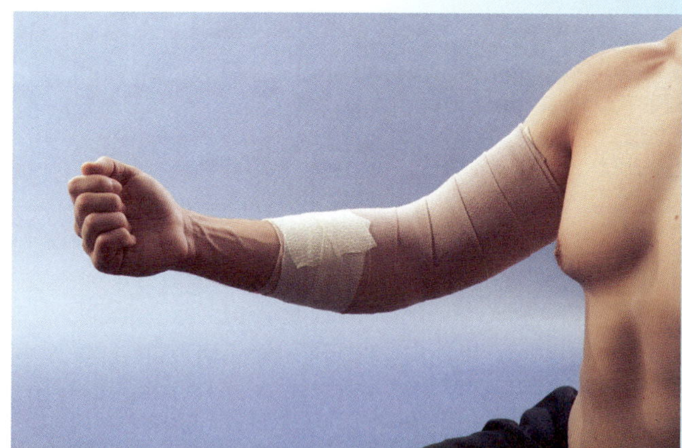

Fig. 9–8 F

**Helpful Hint |**
Improper application of elbow and/or forearm taping, wrapping, bracing, and/or padding techniques can compress soft tissues and the radial, median, and ulnar nerves as they superficially cross the elbow. This will affect the sensory distribution of the nerves. If numbness occurs in the hand, fingers, and/or thumb following application, immediately remove the technique and monitor the condition.

### *Hyperextension Technique Two*

➤ **Materials:**
- Pre-wrap, thin foam pads, 2 inch or 3 inch heavyweight elastic tape, adherent tape spray, skin lubricant, taping scissors

***Option:***
- 4 inch or 6 inch width by 5 yard length elastic wrap

➤ **Position of the patient:** Sitting on a taping table or bench or standing with the involved arm at the side of the body. Determine the range of extension that produces pain. Once determined, place the involved elbow in a pain-free range and maintain this position during application. Maintain a moderate isometric contraction of the upper arm and forearm musculature.

➤ **Preparation:** Shave the arm from the proximal upper arm to mid forearm. Apply the technique directly to the skin or over one layer of pre-wrap. Place thin foam pads over the cubital fossa to prevent irritation. A skin lubricant may also be used. Apply adherent tape spray from the proximal upper arm to the mid forearm.

➤ **Application:**

**STEP 1:** Apply anchors as illustrated in Figure 9–8A.

**STEP 2:** Anchor a strip of 2 inch or 3 inch heavyweight elastic tape on the medial anterior proximal upper arm, continue across the cubital fossa, and anchor on the medial anterior mid forearm (Fig. 9–9A). Apply the strip with a moderate amount of roll tension. Monitor the pain-free position of the elbow.

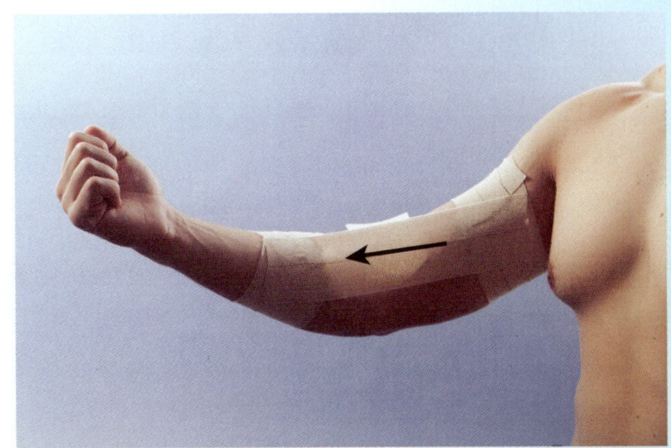

**Fig. 9–9 A**

**STEP 3:** Place the next strip of 2 inch or 3 inch heavyweight elastic tape on the anterior proximal upper arm, overlapping the first by ½ of the tape width, across the cubital fossa, and anchor on the anterior mid forearm (Fig. 9–9B).

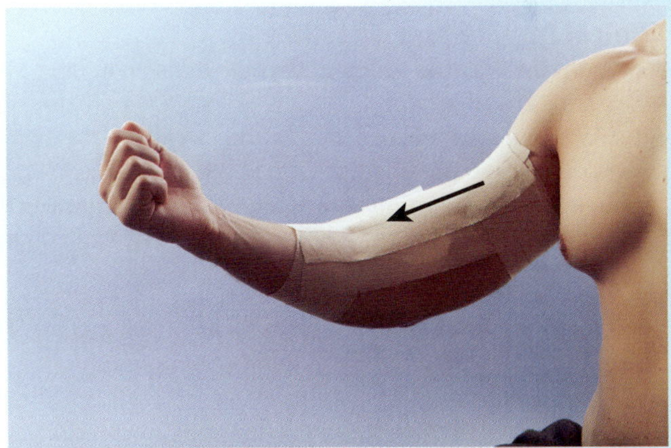

**Fig. 9–9 B**

*Steps Cont.*

**Elbow and Forearm**

**STEP 4:** Apply a strip, overlapping the second strip by ½ of its width, from the lateral anterior proximal upper arm, continue across the cubital fossa, and anchor on the lateral anterior mid forearm (Fig. 9–9C).

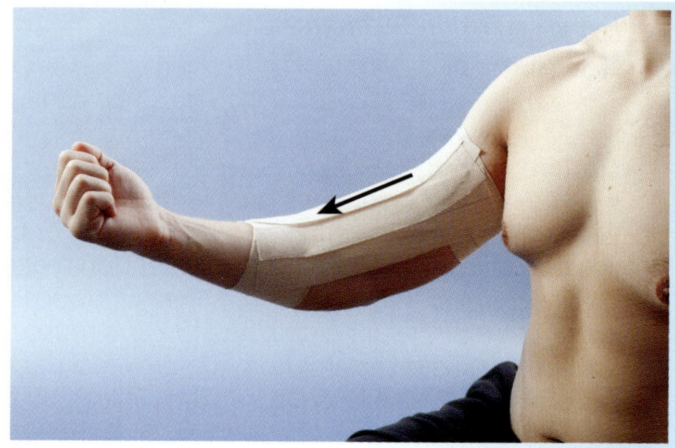

Fig. 9–9 C

**STEP 5:** Apply three to four circular closure patterns with mild tension around the proximal upper arm and mid forearm with 2 inch or 3 inch heavyweight elastic tape ◄▬▬► (Fig. 9–9D). Anchors of non-elastic tape are not required. Monitor the cubital fossa for constriction.

*Option:* *Consider applying a 4 inch or 6 inch width by 5 yard length elastic wrap with moderate roll tension in a circular pattern in a proximal-to-distal direction over the technique to prevent migration and unraveling of the tape ◄▬▬►. Anchor with elastic tape and finish on the anterior mid forearm ◄▬▬►.*

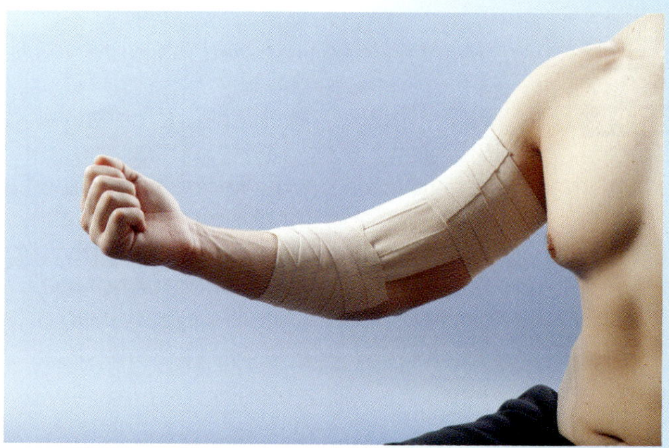

Fig. 9–9 D

---

### Clinical Application Question 1

A high school wrestler suffered a hyperextension injury to his right elbow several weeks ago. He has completed rehabilitation and returned to practice with a hyperextension taping technique on the elbow to prevent further injury. After 45 minutes of practice, the "X" and longitudinal elastic tape strips that cross the cubital fossa begin to tear from the edges, decreasing the effectiveness of the technique.

➠ **Question: What options are available in this situation?**

---

## LATERAL EPICONDYLITIS STRAP    Figures 9–10 and 9–11

➠ **Purpose:** The strap technique is used when treating lateral epicondylitis to reduce the tension or pull of the wrist extensor musculature at its origin on the lateral epicondyle of the humerus. These straps can be made from taping materials or purchased off-the-shelf. The off-the-shelf designs are illustrated in the Bracing section. Two interchangeable methods are illustrated in the application of the technique; the different methods accommodate patient preferences and available supplies.

### *Lateral Epicondylitis Strap Technique One*

➤ **Materials:**
 • Pre-wrap or self adherent wrap, 1 inch or 2 inch heavyweight elastic tape, taping scissors
➤ **Position of the patient:** Sitting on a taping table or bench or standing with the involved arm at the side of the body, the involved elbow placed in slight flexion, and the forearm in a neutral position.
➤ **Preparation:** Apply the technique directly to the skin or over pre-wrap or self-adherent wrap.
➤ **Application:**

**STEP 1:** Anchor 1 inch or 2 inch heavyweight elastic tape on the lateral forearm approximately ¾ of an inch distal from the lateral epicondyle of the humerus (Fig. 9–10A). Continue around the forearm in a circular, lateral-to-medial pattern and return to the anchor position (Fig. 9–10B).

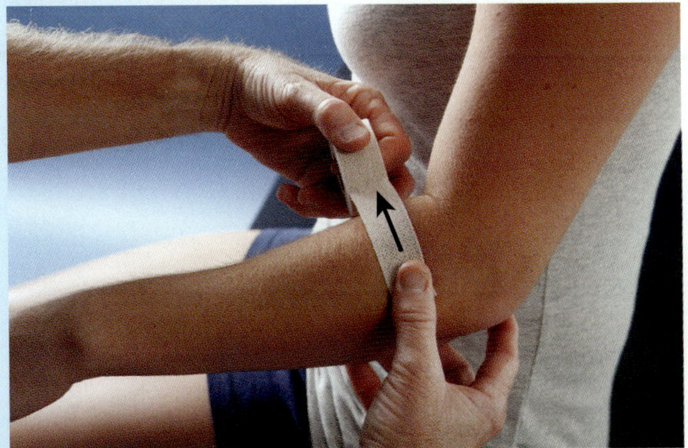
**Fig. 9–10 A**

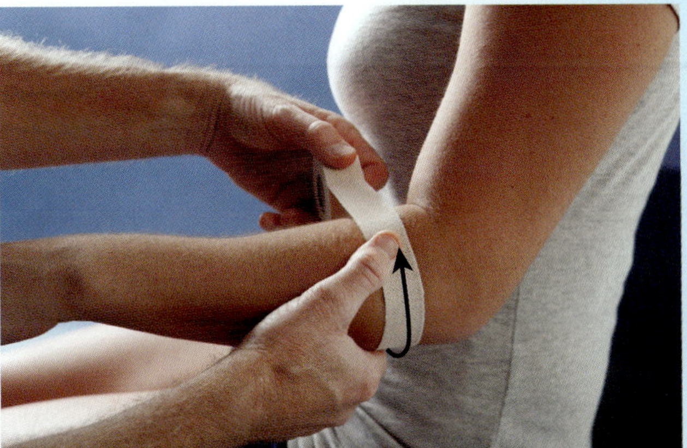
**Fig. 9–10 B**

**STEP 2:** Without overlapping, continue to apply the tape around the forearm with three to four continuous circular patterns and finish on the lateral forearm (Fig. 9–10C). Additional non-elastic tape strips are not necessary.

**Helpful Hint |**
The roll tension of the elastic tape to achieve proper tension and relief of pain will vary among patients. Check the tension of the tape by allowing the patient to perform a previously painful activity. Readjust the tension of the tape if necessary.

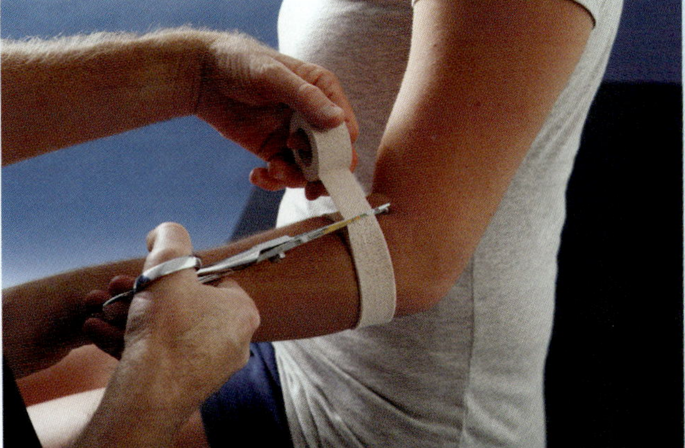
**Fig. 9–10 C**

## EVIDENCE SUMMARY

The exact positioning of a taping material strap or off-the-shelf brace on the proximal forearm is critical but not adequately addressed in the literature.[4] Several studies suggest a position ¾ of an inch distal to the lateral epicondyle of the humerus.[5,6]

### Lateral Epicondylitis Strap Technique Two

➠ **Materials:**
  • Pre-wrap or self-adherent wrap, 1 inch non-elastic tape
➠ **Position of the patient:** Sitting on a taping table or bench or standing with the involved arm at the side of the body, the involved elbow placed in slight flexion, and the forearm in a neutral position.
➠ **Preparation:** Apply the technique directly to the skin or over pre-wrap or self-adherent wrap.
➠ **Application:**

**STEP 1:** Place 1 inch non-elastic tape on the lateral forearm approximately ¾ of an inch distal from the lateral epicondyle of the humerus (Fig. 9–11) and continue around the forearm in a circular, lateral-to-medial pattern, returning to the anchor position. Roll tension will vary among patients.

**STEP 2:** Continue with three to four continuous circular patterns around the forearm, without overlapping, and anchor on the lateral forearm. Additional anchors are not necessary. Readjust the tension of the tape if necessary.

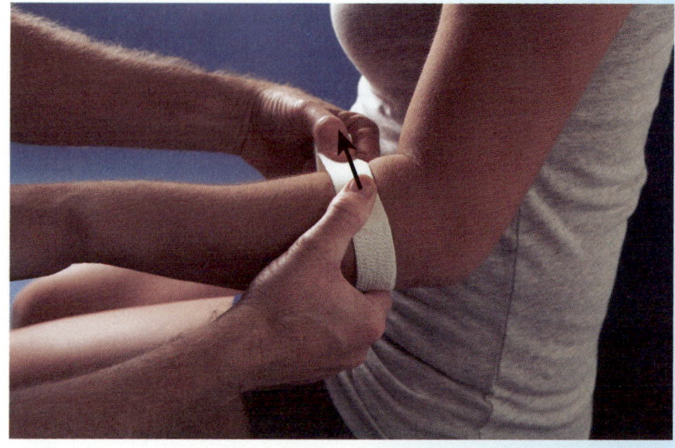

**Fig. 9–11**

## CIRCULAR FOREARM    Figure 9–12

➠ **Purpose:** The circular forearm technique provides mild support and anchors off-the-shelf and custom-made pads to absorb shock when preventing and treating forearm contusions (Fig. 9–12).
➠ **Materials:**
  • Pre-wrap or self-adherent wrap, 2 inch or 3 inch elastic tape, adherent tape spray, taping scissors
  *Option:*
  • 1½ inch non-elastic tape
➠ **Position of the patient:** Sitting on a taping table or bench or standing with the involved arm at the side of the body and the involved elbow placed in slight flexion. Maintain a moderate isometric contraction of the forearm musculature.
➠ **Preparation:** Apply adherent tape spray to the forearm.
➠ **Application:**

**STEP 1:** Apply pre-wrap or self-adherent wrap in a circular pattern around the forearm ⬅▥▥▥▶.

**STEP 2:** Place the pad over the injured area. Anchor 2 inch or 3 inch elastic tape directly to the distal lateral pad and encircle the anchor (Fig. 9–12A).

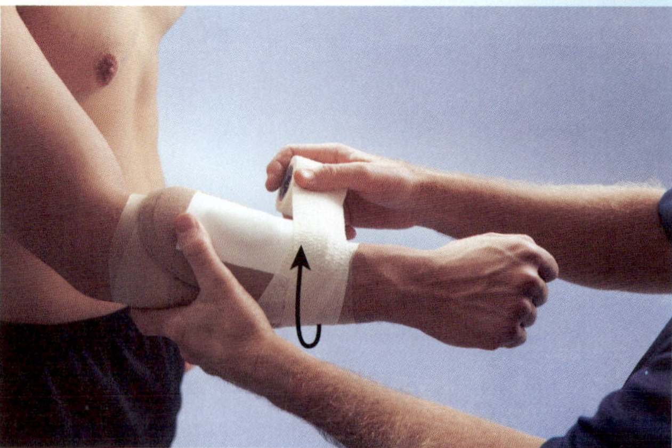

**Fig. 9–12 A**

**STEP 3:** Continue to apply the tape in a circular, lateral-to-medial direction around the forearm with moderate roll tension, overlapping the tape by ½ of its width (Fig. 9–12B). Apply the tape in a distal-to-proximal pattern and cover the entire pad.

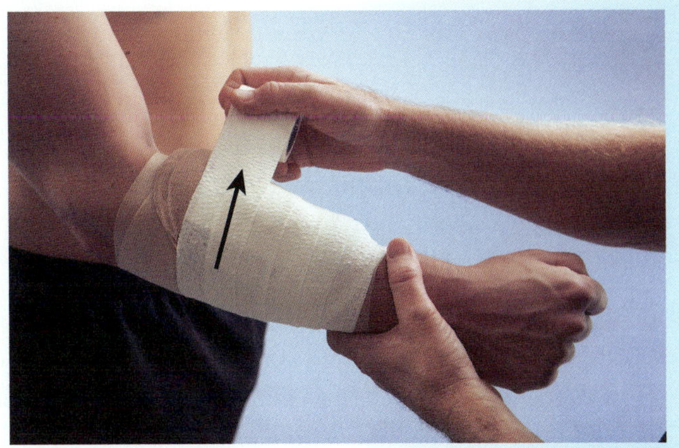

**Fig. 9–12 B**

**STEP 4:** Anchor the tape on top of the pad on the circular pattern (Fig. 9–12C). Avoid gaps, wrinkles, and inconsistent roll tension. To lessen migration of the pad, apply the proximal circular tape strips to the skin.

*Option:* *Loosely apply one to two circular anchors of 1½ inch non-elastic tape around the pad, ending on top of the pad ◄▦▦▦▶.*

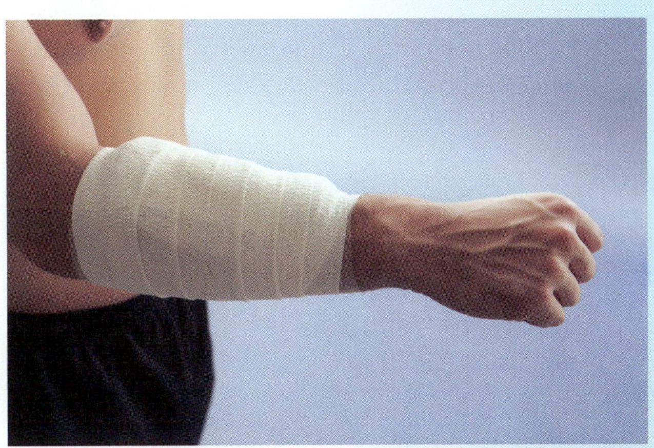

**Fig. 9–12 C**

## 🌐 FIGURE-OF-EIGHT ELBOW TAPE

**Purpose:** Use the figure-of-eight elbow technique to provide mild support and anchor protective padding. Use the technique with off-the-shelf and custom-made padding to absorb shock when preventing or treating elbow contusions and olecranon bursitis. Protective padding techniques are illustrated in the Padding section. This technique and steps of application can be found on FADavis.com.

## POSTERIOR SPLINT     Figure 9–13

**Purpose:** The posterior splint technique is used to immobilize the elbow when treating dislocations, following a reduction and postoperative procedures (Fig. 9–13). This technique is identical to the posterior splint illustrated in Chapter 4 (see Fig. 4–10) with regard to the materials used. Two interchangeable methods are available for the application of the technique to accommodate available supplies; the first is illustrated here (Fig. 9–13) and the second is illustrated online at FADavis.com. 🌐

---

### DETAILS
Periods of immobilization are normally determined by a physician following evaluation of the patient. Complete immobilization can be provided by cast technicians and physicians using rigid cast tape applied over stockinet.

### Design:
- Off-the-shelf rigid splints are available in pre-cut and padded designs. The splints are constructed of several layers of rigid fiberglass material and covered with fabric and foam padding in 2, 3, 4, and 5 inch widths by 10, 12, 15, 30, 35, and 45 inch lengths.

### Posterior Splint Technique One

### Materials:
- Off-the-shelf rigid, padded splint, gloves, water, towel, two 4 inch width by 10 yard length elastic wraps, metal clips, 1½ inch non-elastic tape or 2 inch self-adherent wrap

**Position of the patient:** Sitting on a taping table or bench with the involved arm at the side of the body and the forearm in a neutral position or prone on a taping table or bench with the involved arm extended off the edge and the forearm in a neutral position. Place the elbow in the desired range of flexion as indicated by a physician. Maintain this position during application.

**Preparation:** Mold and apply the padded splint directly to the skin.

**Application:**

**STEP 1:**   Remove the splint from the package and immerse in water of 70° to 75°F to begin the chemical reaction. Submerge the splint the length of time it takes to squeeze the splint once or twice. Remove the splint and place lengthwise on a towel.

**STEP 2:**   Quickly roll the splint and towel together to remove excess water (Fig. 9–13A).

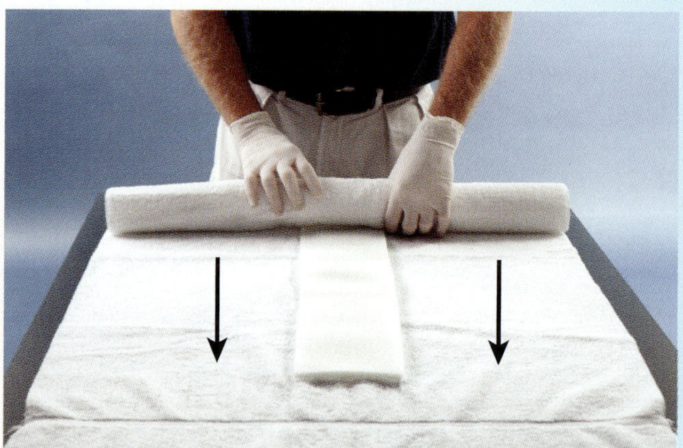

Fig. 9–13 A

**STEP 3:**   Apply the splint from the proximal posterior upper arm to the wrist (Fig. 9–13B).

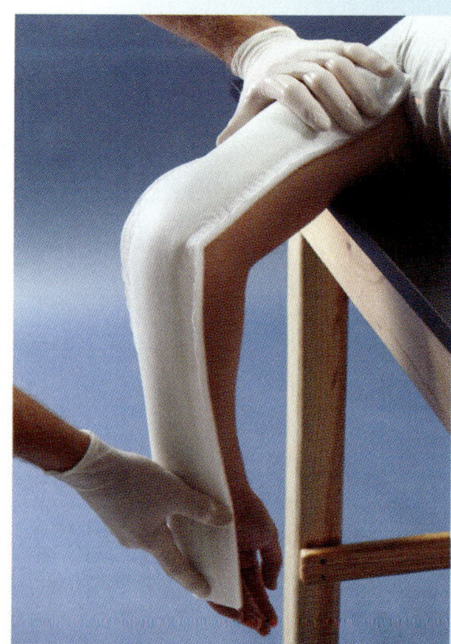

Fig. 9–13 B

**STEP 4:** Mold the splint to the body contours with the application of a 4 inch width by 10 yard length elastic wrap in a spiral pattern with moderate roll tension ◄▬▬► (Fig. 9–13C). Continue to mold and shape the splint with the hands. Monitor the position of elbow flexion. After 10–15 minutes, the fiberglass should be cured; remove the elastic wrap.

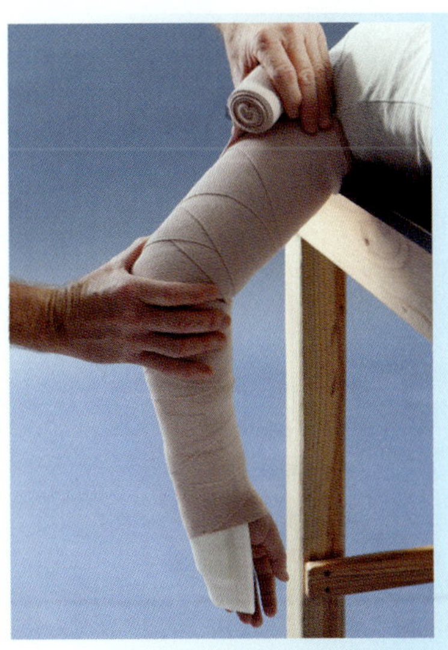

**Fig. 9–13 C**

**STEP 5:** Using another 4 inch width by 10 yard length elastic wrap, attach the splint to the upper arm, elbow, forearm, and wrist in a spiral, distal-to-proximal pattern with moderate roll tension ◄▬▬► (Fig. 9–13D). Anchor the wrap with metal clips, or loosely applied 1½ inch non-elastic tape or 2 inch self-adherent wrap. The patient may need a sling for daily activities.

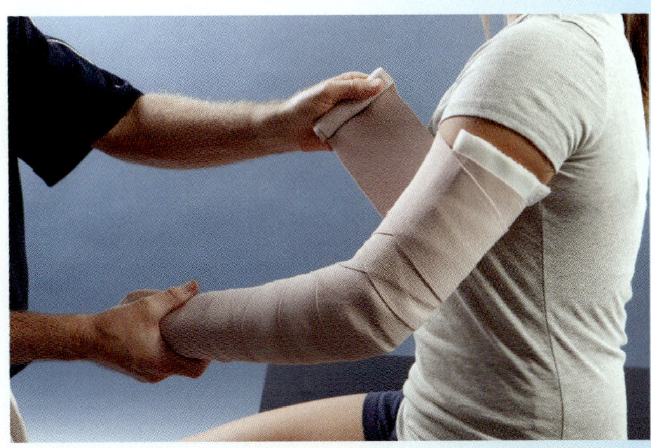

**Fig. 9–13 D**

# Wrapping Techniques

Use wrapping techniques to provide compression and support and to anchor protective padding to the elbow and forearm when preventing and treating contusions, sprains, strains, ruptures, dislocations, and olecranon bursitis. There are five compression wrapping techniques that provide mechanical pressure over the upper arm, elbow, forearm, wrist, and hand following injury. Choose a technique based on the amount of swelling and effusion present.

## ELBOW COMPRESSION WRAP    Figure 9–14

▬► **Purpose:** Apply the elbow compression wrap technique when treating contusions, sprains, strains, ruptures, dislocations, and olecranon bursitis of the elbow to control mild to moderate swelling and effusion (Fig. 9–14).

➠ **Materials:**
- 4 inch or 6 inch width by 5 yard length elastic wrap, metal clips, 1½ inch non-elastic or 2 inch or 3 inch elastic tape, taping scissors

***Options:***
- ¼ inch or ½ inch foam or felt
- 3 inch or 4 inch width self-adherent wrap
- ¼ inch or ½ inch open-cell foam

➠ **Position of the patient:** Sitting on a taping table or bench or standing with the involved arm at the side of the body and the involved elbow placed in a pain-free, flexed position.

➠ **Preparation:** To lessen migration, apply adherent tape spray, tape strips, or anchors directly to the skin (see Fig. 1–7).

***Option:***
Cut a ¼ inch or ½ inch foam or felt pad and place it over the inflamed area directly to the skin to assist in venous return.

➠ **Application:**

**STEP 1:**  Apply the extended end of the wrap around the mid forearm directly to the skin and encircle the anchor ◄▬► (Fig. 9–14A).

*Option:*  *If an elastic wrap is not available, 3 inch or 4 inch self-adherent wrap may be used.*

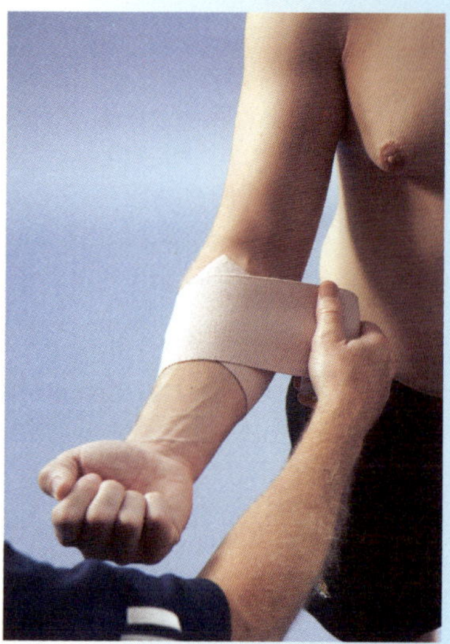

**Fig. 9–14 A**

**STEP 2:**  Continue to apply the wrap in a spiral pattern, moving in a distal-to-proximal direction, and overlapping the wrap by ½ of its width (Fig. 9–14B). Apply the greatest amount of roll tension distally and over the inflamed area and lessen roll tension as the wrap continues proximally.

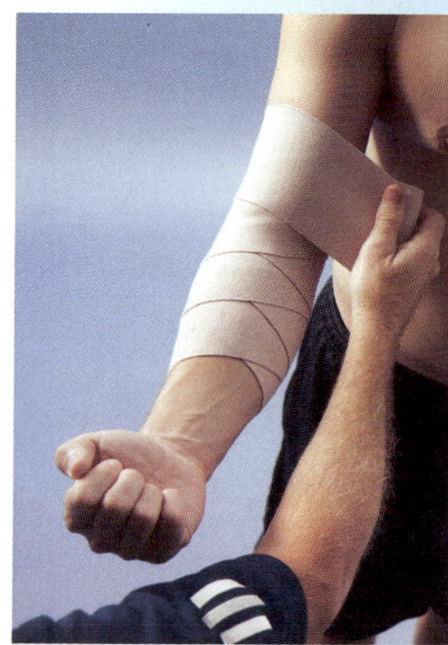

**Fig. 9–14 B**

**STEP 3:** Finish the spiral pattern over the mid upper arm and anchor with Velcro, metal clips, or loosely applied 1½ inch non-elastic or 2 inch or 3 inch elastic tape ◀▦▶ (Fig. 9–14C). Finish the tape on the anterior upper arm to prevent irritation.

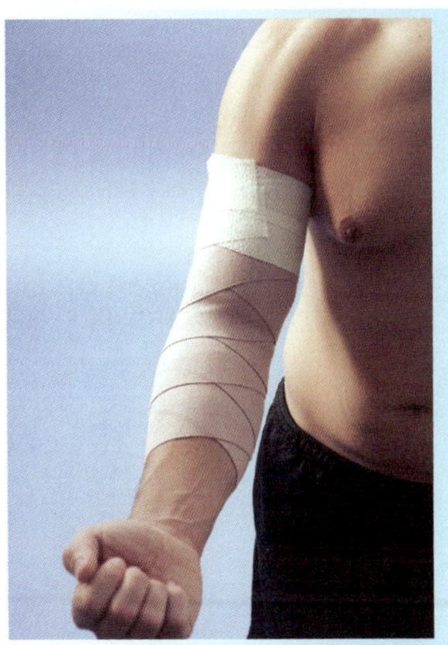

**Fig. 9–14 C**

*Option:* *A ¼ inch or ½ inch open-cell foam pad may be placed over the posterior elbow, extending from the lateral humeral epicondyle to the medial humeral epicondyle, for additional compression around the olecranon process (see Fig. 9–28A). The pad is particularly useful when treating olecranon bursitis. Apply the pad directly on the skin and cover with the compression wrap (Fig. 9–14D).*

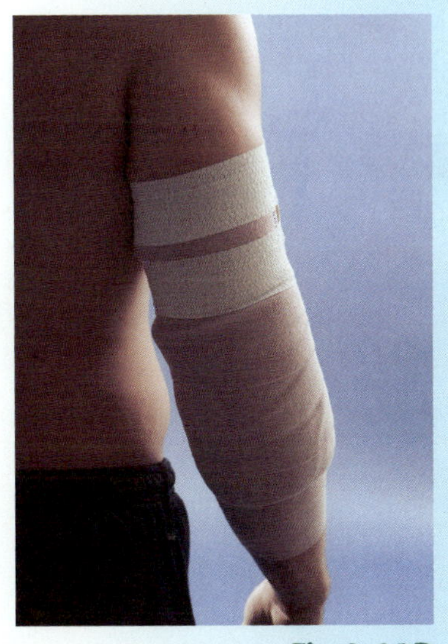

**Fig. 9–14 D**

## | FOREARM COMPRESSION WRAP    Figure 9–15

➠ **Purpose:** Use the forearm compression wrap technique to control mild to moderate swelling when treating forearm contusions and strains (Fig. 9–15).

➠ **Materials:**
- 2 inch, 3 inch, or 4 inch width by 5 yard length elastic wrap, metal clips, 1½ inch non-elastic or 2 inch or 3 inch elastic tape, taping scissors

*Options:*
- ¼ inch or ½ inch foam or felt
- 2 inch, 3 inch, or 4 inch width self-adherent wrap

➠ **Position of the patient:** Sitting on a taping table or bench or standing with the involved arm at the side of the body and the involved elbow placed in a pain-free, flexed position.

➠ **Preparation:** To lessen migration, apply adherent tape spray, tape strips, or anchors directly to the skin.
*Option:*
Cut a ¼ inch or ½ inch foam or felt pad and place it over the inflamed area directly to the skin to assist in controlling swelling.

➠ **Application:**

**STEP 1:**   Anchor the extended end of the wrap around the wrist directly to the skin and encircle the anchor ◀▥▥▥▶ (Fig. 9–15A).

*Option:*   *If an elastic wrap is not available, 2 inch, 3 inch, or 4 inch self-adherent wrap may be used.*

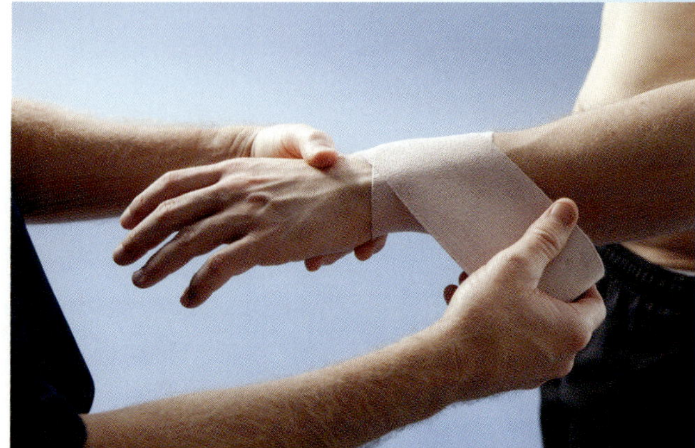

Fig. 9–15 A

**STEP 2:**   Using a spiral pattern, apply the wrap in a distal-to-proximal direction (Fig. 9–15B). Overlap the wrap by ½ of its width; apply the greatest amount of roll tension distally and over the inflamed area.

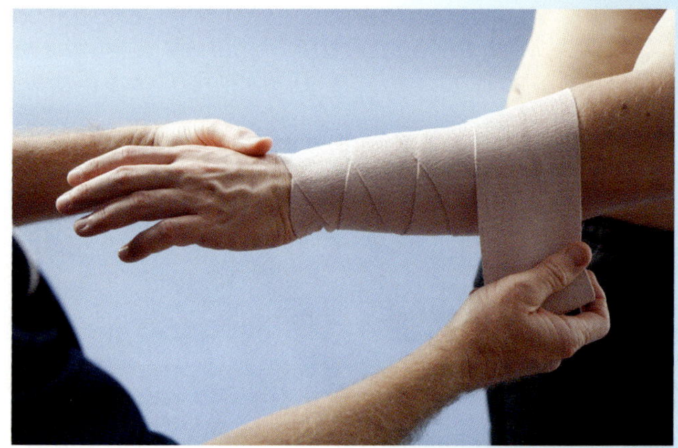

Fig. 9–15 B

**STEP 3:**   Finish the wrap at the proximal forearm (Fig. 9–15C).

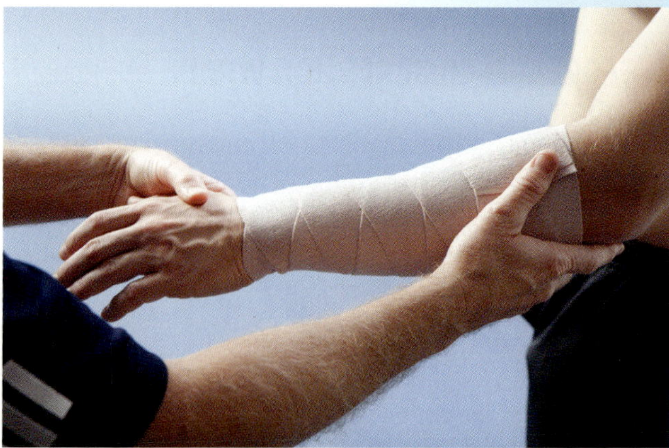

Fig. 9–15 C

**STEP 4:** Anchor the wrap over the proximal forearm with Velcro, metal clips, or loosely applied 1½ inch non-elastic or 2 inch or 3 inch elastic tape, finishing on the anterolateral proximal forearm ◀▦▦▶ (Fig. 9–15D).

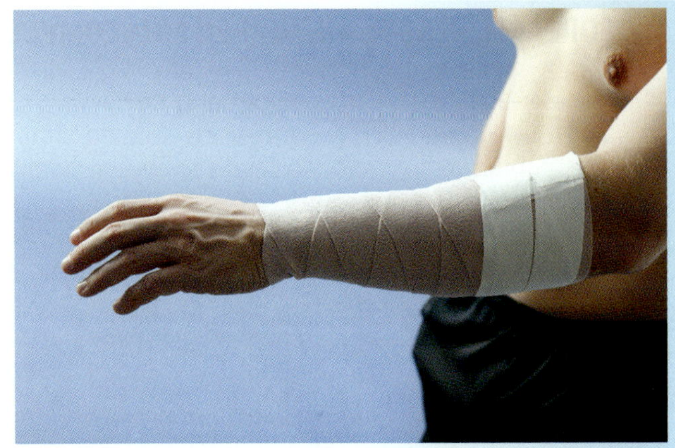

**Fig. 9–15 D**

## HAND, WRIST, AND FOREARM COMPRESSION WRAP    Figure 9–16

▥▶ **Purpose:** Use the hand, wrist, and forearm compression wrap technique to control moderate to severe swelling when treating second- and third-degree forearm contusions and strains. The technique prevents distal migration of post-injury swelling (Fig. 9–16).

▥▶ **Materials:**
- 3 inch or 4 inch width by 5 yard length elastic wrap, metal clips, 1½ inch non-elastic or 2 inch or 3 inch elastic tape, taping scissors

*Option:*
- ¼ inch or ½ inch foam or felt

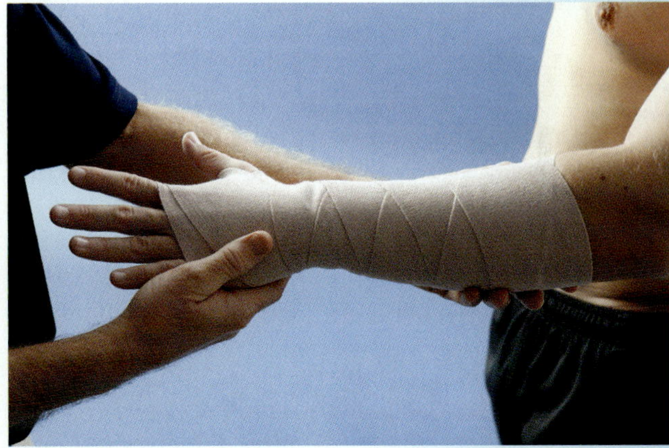

**Fig. 9–16**

▥▶ **Position of the patient:** Sitting on a taping table or bench or standing with the involved arm at the side of the body and the involved elbow placed in a pain-free, flexed position.

▥▶ **Preparation:** To lessen migration, apply adherent tape spray, tape strips, or anchors directly to the skin.

*Option:*
Cut a ¼ inch or ½ inch foam or felt pad and place it over the inflamed area directly to the skin to assist in venous return.

▥▶ **Application:**

**STEP 1:** Anchor the wrap in a circular pattern on the dorsal surface of the hand just distal to the MCP joints of fingers two through five and apply the hand and wrist compression wrap technique (see Fig. 10–15).

**STEP 2:** At the wrist, finish the technique with the forearm compression wrap (see Figs. 9–15 and 9–16).

**STEP 3:** Anchor over the proximal forearm with Velcro, metal clips, or loosely applied 1½ inch non-elastic or 2 inch or 3 inch elastic tape ◀▦▦▶. End the tape on the anterolateral proximal forearm.

## FOREARM, ELBOW, AND UPPER ARM COMPRESSION WRAP    Figure 9–17

➡ **Purpose:** Use the forearm, elbow, and upper arm compression wrap technique when treating second- and third-degree elbow contusions, sprains, strains, ruptures, dislocations, and olecranon bursitis. The technique controls moderate to severe swelling and prevents distal migration of post-injury swelling (Fig. 9–17).

➡ **Materials:**
- 4 inch or 6 inch width by 10 yard length elastic wrap, metal clips, 1½ inch non-elastic or 2 inch or 3 inch elastic tape, taping scissors

  *Options:*
- ¼ inch or ½ inch foam or felt
- ¼ inch or ½ inch open-cell foam

➡ **Position of the patient:** Sitting on a taping table or bench or standing with the involved arm at the side of the body and the involved elbow placed in a pain-free, flexed position.

➡ **Preparation:** To lessen migration, apply adherent tape spray, tape strips, or anchors directly to the skin.

  *Option:*
  Cut a ¼ inch or ½ inch foam or felt pad and place it over the inflamed area directly to the skin to assist in controlling swelling.

➡ **Application:**

**STEP 1:** This wrap technique for the elbow and forearm is identical to the compression technique for the upper arm illustrated in Figure 8–12. Apply the greatest amount of roll tension distally and lessen tension as the wrap continues proximally. This technique may be started with a circular pattern just distal to the MCP joints of the fingers; apply the hand and wrist compression wrap technique (Fig. 9–17).

*Option:* *Consider using a ¼ inch or ½ inch open-cell foam pad over the posterior elbow for additional compression to assist in venous return.*

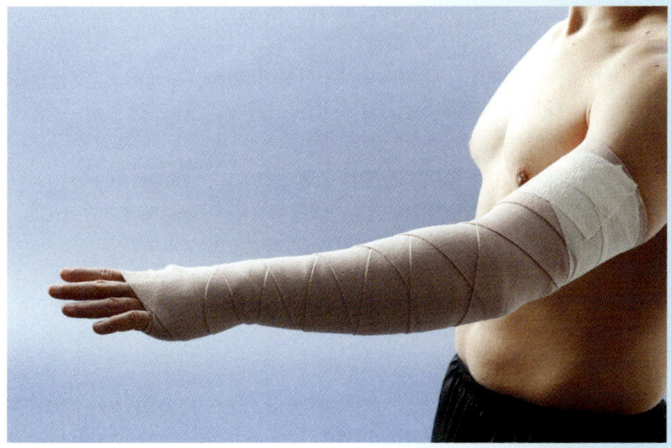

**Fig. 9–17**

## ELBOW AND FOREARM COMPRESSION SLEEVE    Figure 9–18

➡ **Purpose:** Use the elbow and forearm compression sleeve technique to control mild to moderate swelling and effusion when treating elbow and forearm contusions, sprains, strains, ruptures, dislocations, and olecranon bursitis (Fig. 9–18). Following proper instruction, the patient can apply and remove this compression technique without assistance.

➡ **Materials:**
- 3 inch, 3½ inch, or 4 inch width elastic sleeve determined by the size of the upper arm and forearm, taping scissors

  *Options:*
- ¼ inch or ½ inch foam or felt
- ¼ inch or ½ inch open-cell foam

➡ **Position of the patient:** Sitting on a taping table or bench or standing with the involved arm at the side of the body and the involved elbow placed in a pain-free, flexed position.

➡ **Preparation:** Cut a sleeve from a roll to extend from the mid forearm to the mid upper arm, wrist to the proximal forearm, MCP joints of the hand to the proximal forearm, wrist to the proximal upper arm, or the MCP joints of the hand to the proximal upper arm. Cut and use a double-length sleeve to provide additional compression.

***Option:***
Cut a ¼ inch or ½ inch foam or felt pad and place it over the inflamed area directly to the skin to assist in controlling swelling.

➡ **Application:**

**STEP 1:**   Apply the sleeve over the fingers and pull onto the forearm, elbow, and/or upper arm in a distal-to-proximal pattern (Fig. 9–18A). If using a technique that includes the hand, cut a small hole in the sleeve for the thumb using taping scissors (Fig. 9–18B). When using a double-length sleeve, pull the distal end over the first layer to provide an additional layer. No anchors are required; the sleeve can be cleaned and reused.

*Option:*   *A ¼ inch or ½ inch open-cell foam pad may be cut and placed over the posterior elbow for additional compression.*

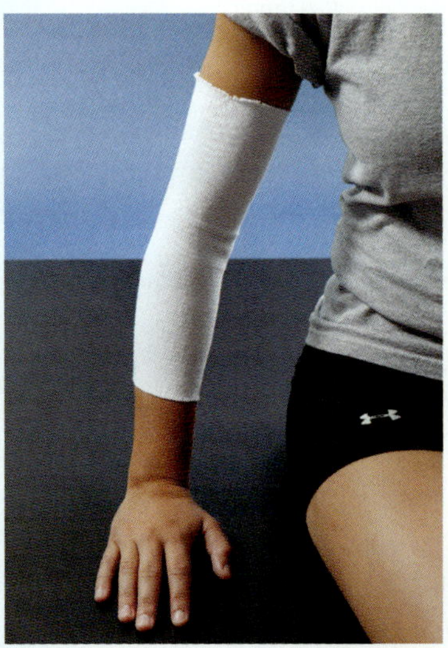

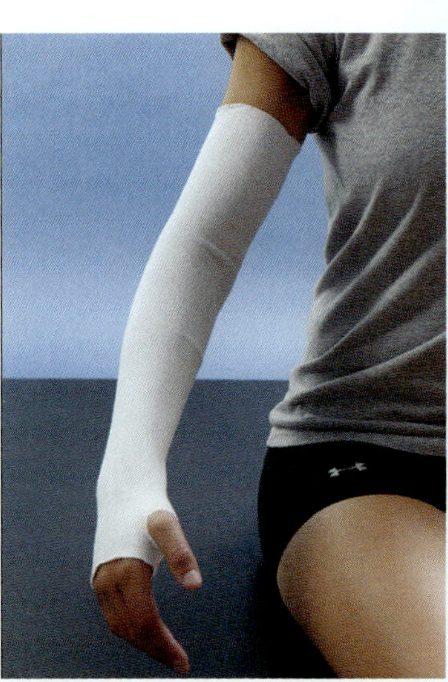

**Fig. 9–18 A**        **Fig. 9–18 B**

---

### Clinical Application Question 2

A sniper on the SWAT team has been practicing for an upcoming national competition. One of the events requires him to be in a prone position on his elbows for extended periods of time. He begins to develop pain in the right posterior elbow and is evaluated by a physician. The sniper is diagnosed with right elbow olecranon bursitis and allowed to continue practice if the condition does not worsen.

➡ **Question: What techniques can you use to treat the condition?**

---

## CIRCULAR ELBOW WRAP        Figure 9–19

➡ **Purpose:** Use the circular elbow technique to provide compression and mild support and to anchor off-the-shelf and custom-made pads that absorb shock when preventing and treating elbow contusions and olecranon bursitis (Fig. 9–19).

➡ **Materials:**
  • 3 inch, 4 inch, or 6 inch width by 5 yard length elastic wrap, 2 inch or 3 inch elastic tape, taping scissors
  *Options:*
  • 3 inch, 4 inch, or 6 inch width self-adherent wrap
  • 1½ inch non-elastic tape
➡ **Position of the patient:** Sitting on a taping table or bench or standing with the involved arm at the side of the body and the involved elbow placed in slight flexion. Maintain a moderate isometric contraction of the upper arm and forearm musculature.
➡ **Preparation:** To lessen migration, apply adherent tape spray, tape strips, or anchors directly to the skin.
➡ **Application:**

**STEP 1:**  Place the pad over the injured area. Anchor the extended end of the wrap directly to the skin below the distal pad and encircle the anchor ⬅▮▮▮▶ (Fig. 9–19A).

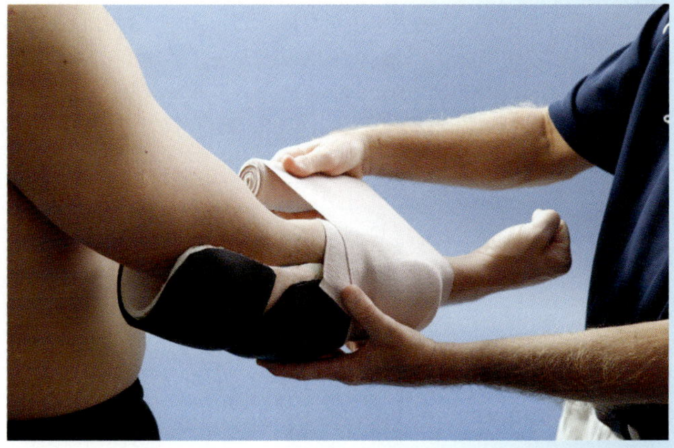

**Fig. 9–19 A**

**STEP 2:**  In a circular pattern with moderate roll tension, continue to apply the wrap in a distal-to-proximal pattern, overlapping the wrap by ½ of its width (Fig. 9–19B). Completely cover the pad with the wrap and finish on the upper arm. Avoid gaps, wrinkles, and inconsistent roll tension.

*Option:*  *If an elastic wrap is not available, 3 inch, 4 inch, or 6 inch self-adherent wrap may be used.*

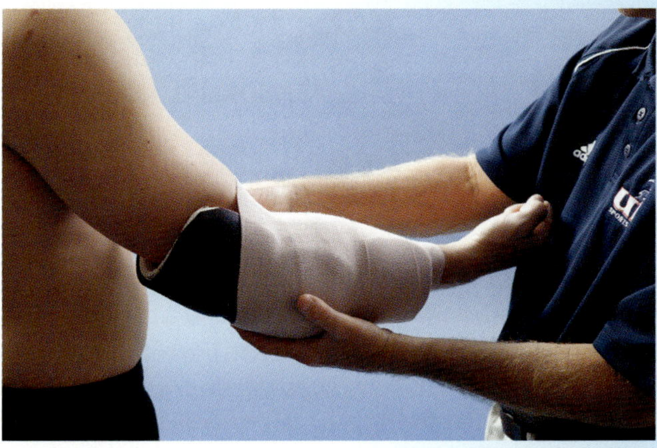

**Fig. 9–19 B**

**STEP 3:** Anchor 2 inch or 3 inch elastic tape on the loose end of the wrap and apply two to three circular patterns, with moderate roll tension, and finish on the tape pattern on the lateral upper arm to prevent irritation ◀▦▶ (Fig. 9–19C). For additional support and to lessen migration of the pad, anchor 2 inch or 3 inch elastic tape on the proximal lateral forearm and apply the figure-of-eight taping technique.

*Option:* *Loosely apply one to two 1½ inch non-elastic tape circular strips over the elastic tape around the upper arm to anchor ◀▦▶. Finish the tape on the lateral upper arm.*

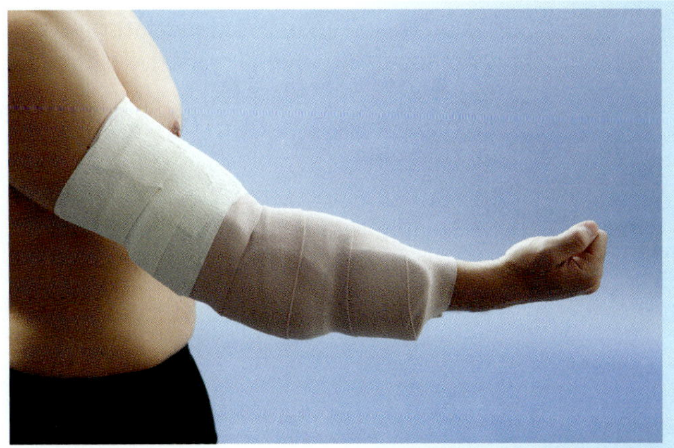

**Fig. 9–19 C**

## CIRCULAR FOREARM WRAP — Figure 9–20

➡ **Purpose:** The circular forearm technique provides compression and mild support and attaches off-the-shelf and custom-made pads to the forearm to absorb shock when treating contusions (Fig. 9–20).

➡ **Materials:**
• 2 inch, 3 inch, or 4 inch width by 5 yard length elastic wrap, 2 inch or 3 inch elastic tape, taping scissors
*Options:*
• 2 inch, 3 inch, or 4 inch width self-adherent wrap
• 1½ inch non-elastic tape

➡ **Position of the patient:** Sitting on a taping table or bench or standing with the involved arm at the side of the body and the involved elbow placed in flexion. Maintain a moderate isometric contraction of the forearm musculature.

➡ **Preparation:** To lessen migration, apply adherent tape spray, tape strips, or anchors directly to the skin.

➡ **Application:**

**STEP 1:** Apply the pad over the injured area. Anchor the wrap directly to the skin below the distal pad on the lateral forearm and encircle the anchor in a lateral-to-medial direction (Fig. 9–20A).

*Option:* *If an elastic wrap is not available, 2 inch, 3 inch, or 4 inch self-adherent wrap may be used.*

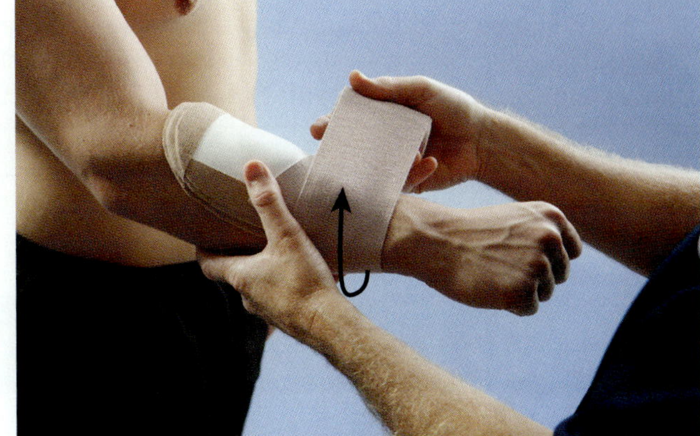

**Fig. 9–20 A**

*Steps Cont.*

**STEP 2:** Continue the wrap in a circular, lateral-to-medial pattern, overlapping by ½ of its width with moderate roll tension, in a distal-to-proximal pattern (Fig. 9–20B). Cover the pad with the wrap and finish on the proximal forearm. Avoid gaps, wrinkles, and inconsistent roll tension.

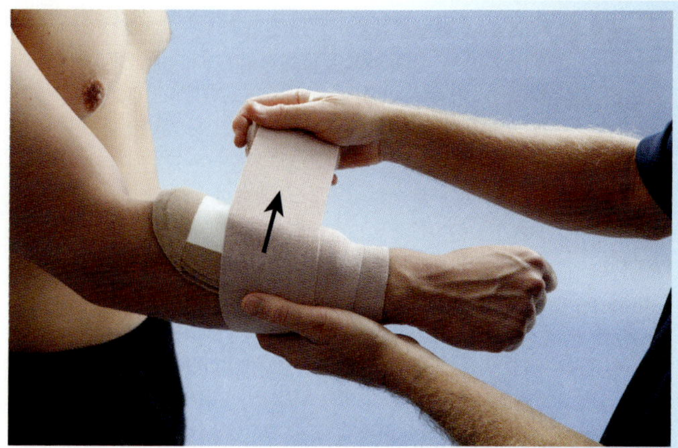

**Fig. 9–20 B**

**STEP 3:** To anchor, apply 2 inch or 3 inch elastic tape on the proximal lateral pad and apply two to three lateral-to-medial circular patterns, with moderate roll tension, finishing on the tape pattern on the proximal lateral forearm to prevent irritation (Fig. 9–20C).

*Option:* *Apply one to two 1½ inch non-elastic tape circular strips loosely over the elastic tape around the proximal forearm to anchor* ◀▬▬▶. *End the anchors on the lateral forearm.*

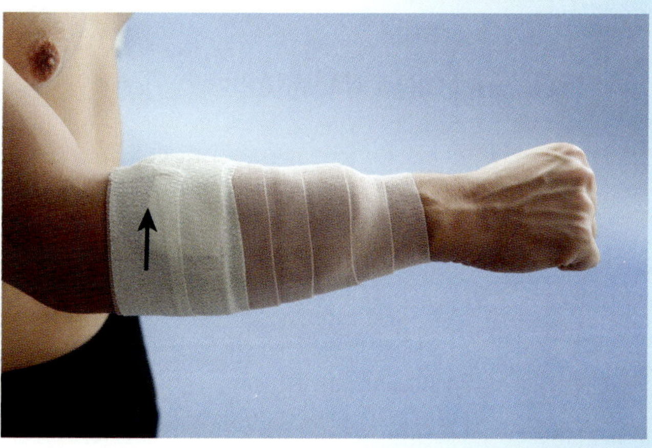

**Fig. 9–20 C**

---

**. . . IF/THEN . . .**

**IF** a compression wrap is needed following an injury to the elbow, **THEN** carefully consider the injury and technique objective(s) prior to application. When treating severe swelling and effusion, using the elbow compression wrap may allow swelling/effusion to migrate distally into the hand, while the forearm, elbow, and upper arm compression wrap provides compression from the wrist or distal MCP joints to the proximal upper arm, lessening distal migration.

## Bracing Techniques

Several bracing techniques for the elbow and forearm are available in off-the-shelf and custom-made designs. Some bracing techniques are used following sprains, dislocations, and postoperative procedures to provide immobilization, support, and compression and to limit range of motion. Other bracing techniques can be used to provide compression and correct structural abnormalities when treating overuse injuries and conditions.

## | **REHABILITATIVE**    Figure 9–21

**Purpose:** Rehabilitative braces provide immobilization, mild to moderate support, and protected range of motion when treating elbow sprains, dislocations, and postoperative procedures (Fig. 9–21). These designs can replace a plaster or fiberglass cast or splint. The braces are removable, allowing for treatment and rehabilitation, and have adjustable range of motion to control and support early movement.

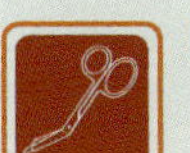

### DETAILS
Consider using this design in combination with several compression wrapping techniques (see Figs. 9–14, 9–17, and 9–18).

**Design:**
  • The braces are available in universal fit and right or left styles in predetermined sizes, corresponding to mid upper arm circumference measurements or length of the forearm.
  • Most designs are constructed of foam, polyethylene, or elastic material in upper arm and forearm wraps or cuffs, with unilateral or bilateral aluminum bars. Some of the wraps or cuffs are **malleable**.
  • In some designs, the bars are incorporated into plastic materials that are attached directly to the wraps or cuffs; other designs use Velcro straps to attach the bars.
  • Other designs have telescoping bars to assist with comfort and size adjustments.
  • The single polycentric hinge on most designs allows for control and locking of range of motion. Easy-to-use dials for quick range of motion settings are available with some designs.
  • Straps incorporated into the aluminum bars anchor the brace to the upper arm and forearm.
  • Some designs are available with a detachable sling.
  • Other designs have a bar and/or cuff incorporated into the distal end of the brace to provide support and immobilization of the wrist and hand.

**Position of the patient:** Sitting on a taping table or bench with the involved elbow in a pain-free range of motion.

**Preparation:** Set the brace range of motion at the desired settings of flexion and extension as indicated by a physician and/or therapeutic exercise program. Apply the brace directly to the skin or over a shirt.
   Specific instructions for applying the braces are included with each design. The following general application guidelines apply to most designs.

> **Helpful Hint |**
> Following application of the brace, check the actual range of flexion and extension with a goniometer to ensure the correct settings.

**Application:**

**STEP 1:**    Begin application by loosening the straps and unfolding the brace.

**STEP 2:**    Position the brace over the involved upper arm, elbow, and forearm. Align the hinge(s) with the joint line and the bar(s) along the medial and/or lateral upper arm and forearm (Fig. 9–21A). With some designs, adjust the telescoping bars to the length of the upper arm and forearm. Reposition or mold the wraps or cuffs if necessary.

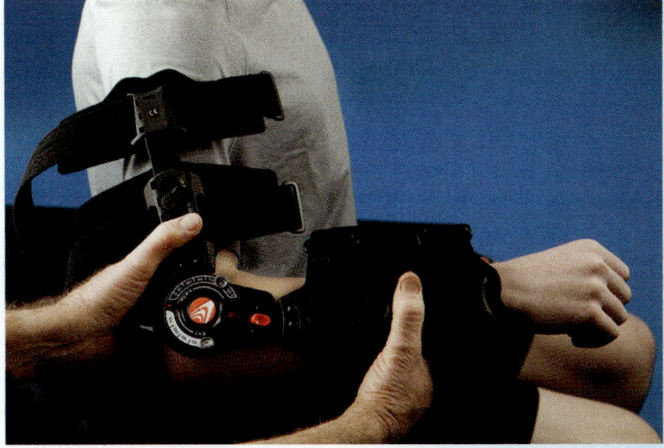

**Fig. 9–21 A**

*Steps Cont.*

**STEP 3:** Anchor the wraps or cuffs around the upper arm and forearm. At the proximal forearm, pull the strap tight and anchor. Next, anchor the distal upper arm strap. Continue to anchor the remaining straps in this alternating pattern (Fig. 9–21B).

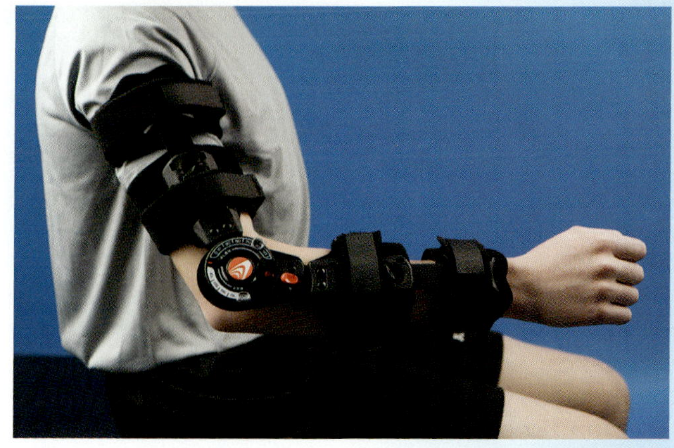

Fig. 9–21 B

**STEP 4:** When using sling designs, apply the strap located at the posterior elbow or anterior upper arm upward over the opposite shoulder and neck, then down across the chest to the distal brace or wrist, and anchor (Fig. 9–21C).

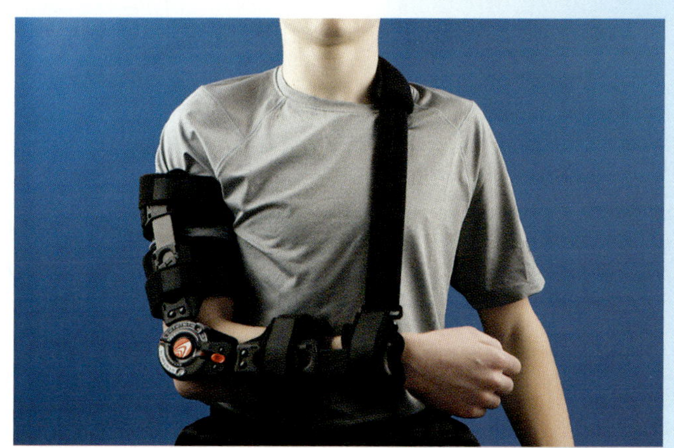

Fig. 9–21 C

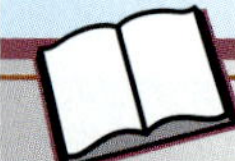

## EVIDENCE SUMMARY

A small randomized trial[7] examined the effects of rehabilitative braces and plaster splints in the postoperative management of active patients following elbow medial or lateral collateral ligament reconstruction. The findings showed a significant decrease in visual analogue scales of pain perception in the brace group at postoperative weeks 2, 6, and 12 compared with the splint group. Rehabilitative braces also produced significantly greater improvements in mid arm circumference measurements and grip strength at weeks 2, 6, 12, and 24 and weeks 2 and 6, respectively. Rehabilitative braces are frequently used with elbow injuries to provide immobilization and protected range of motion. Although the evidence in the literature to support or refute the use of these braces is limited, positive patient outcomes have been demonstrated. Additional research is needed among various populations to determine the most effective brace design based on the injury or surgical procedure and patient goals and preferences.

| **FUNCTIONAL** | Figure 9–22 |

➡ **Purpose:** Functional braces are designed to provide moderate stability to the elbow when treating sprains, dislocations, and postoperative procedures (Fig. 9–22). The designs are commonly used following injury to the ulnar collateral, radial collateral, or annular ligaments to control valgus, varus, rotary, and hyperextension stresses.

**DETAILS**

Functional braces are commonly used to provide elbow stability for athletes in sports such as field hockey, football, ice hockey, lacrosse, and wrestling but can also be useful with work and casual activities. The nonpliable materials of the brace must be padded to meet NCAA[8] and NFHS[9] rules.

➡ **Design:**
- These braces are available in off-the-shelf and custom-made designs in universal and right or left styles.
- Off-the-shelf designs are constructed in predetermined sizes corresponding to mid upper arm circumference measurements. Small size adjustments may be made during wear.
  - Most designs consist of a one-piece neoprene sleeve with medial and lateral hinged aluminum bars. Proximal and distal pockets or pouches anchor the bars to the sleeve. Nylon straps with Velcro closures for the upper arm provide additional support to the bars and anchor the brace.
  - Many designs are available with an adjustable upper arm portion, an open cubital fossa cut-out, and epicondyle pads located under the hinge(s).
  - Most off-the-shelf designs have polycentric hinges that allow for range of motion control. A hyperextension block is also available.
  - Most designs use additional straps across the cubital fossa to prevent hyperextension.
  - Many off-the-shelf braces are available with posterior elbow padding for additional protection.
- Custom-made designs are manufactured for a specific patient following casting of the upper arm, elbow, and forearm by a manufacturer's representative or orthopedic technician. Following brace construction, adjustments in size are limited.
  - Custom-made braces are similar to custom-made functional knee designs (see Fig. 6–20) and consist of a frame or shell, epicondyle pads, liners, and straps.
  - The frames are manufactured of carbon composite, aluminum, or carbon/graphite laminate materials with monocentric or polycentric hinges that allow for control over range of motion. Most designs contain a hyperextension block.
  - Epicondyle pads and liners are constructed of suede or chamois. Some designs have pneumatic pads to enhance fit and comfort. Nylon straps with Velcro closures anchor the brace.
  - An off-the-shelf design of this brace is available in a right or left style and is constructed in predetermined sizes corresponding to mid upper arm and elbow circumference measurements.
➡ **Position of the patient:** Sitting on a taping table or bench or standing with the involved arm at the side of the body and the involved elbow placed in slight flexion.
➡ **Preparation:** Set the brace range of motion at the desired settings of flexion and extension. Apply functional braces directly to the skin. Loosen all straps.

    Instructions for application of functional braces are included with each design. For proper application and use, follow the step-by-step procedure. The following general application guidelines apply to most functional designs.
➡ **Application:**

**STEP 1:** Apply most sleeve designs by placing the larger end over the fingers and hand. Pull the sleeve in a proximal direction until the hinges are centered over the joint line (Fig. 9–22A). When using upper arm wrap designs, encircle the upper arm and anchor this portion with Velcro.

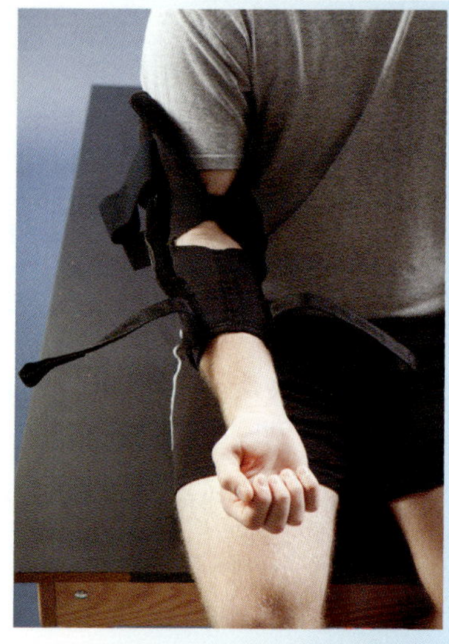

Fig. 9–22 A

**STEP 2:** The application of straps will depend on the specific sleeve design. Apply most straps by pulling the straps tight and anchoring with Velcro (Fig. 9–22B).

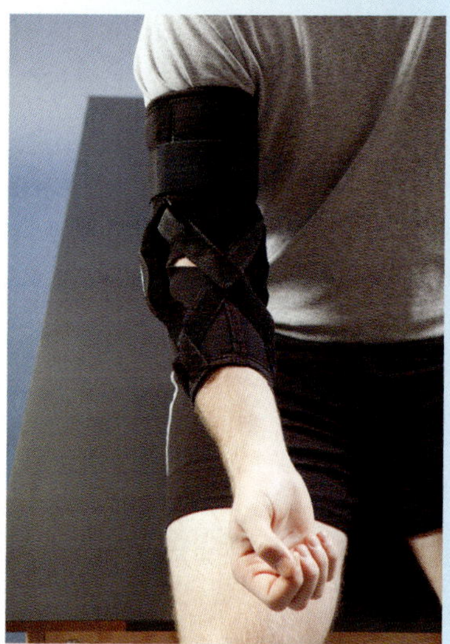

Fig. 9–22 B

**STEP 3:** Begin application of custom-made designs by pulling the brace onto the upper arm, elbow, and forearm in a distal-to-proximal direction (Fig. 9–22C). Position the hinges approximately ½ inch superior to the joint line.

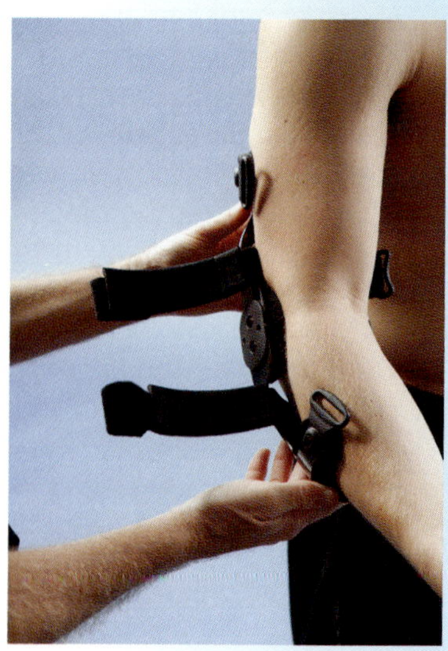

Fig. 9–22 C

**STEP 4:** The application of straps will depend on the specific brace design. When using some designs, anchor the proximal, anterior forearm strap (Fig. 9–22D), then the distal, anterior upper arm strap (Fig. 9–22E).

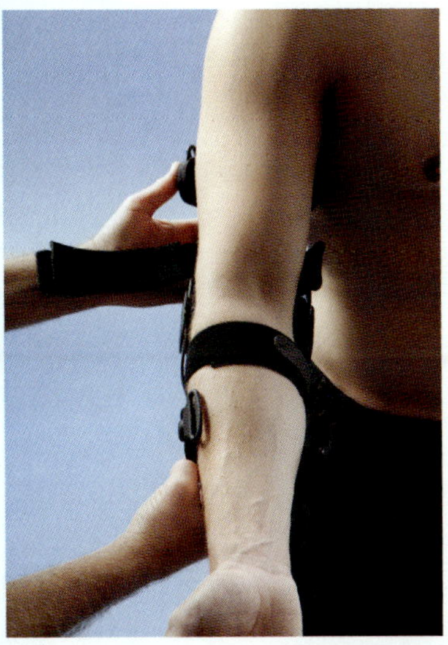

**Fig. 9–22 D**

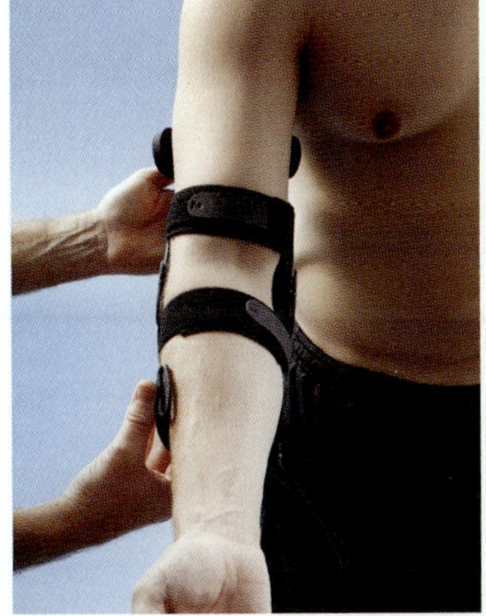

**Fig. 9–22 E**

**STEP 5:** Next, anchor the proximal, anterior upper arm strap (Fig. 9–22F). Continue and anchor the distal, anterior forearm strap (Fig. 9–22G).

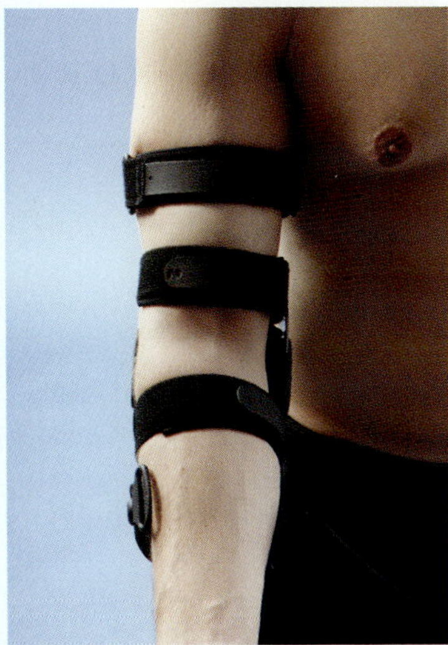

**Fig. 9–22 F**

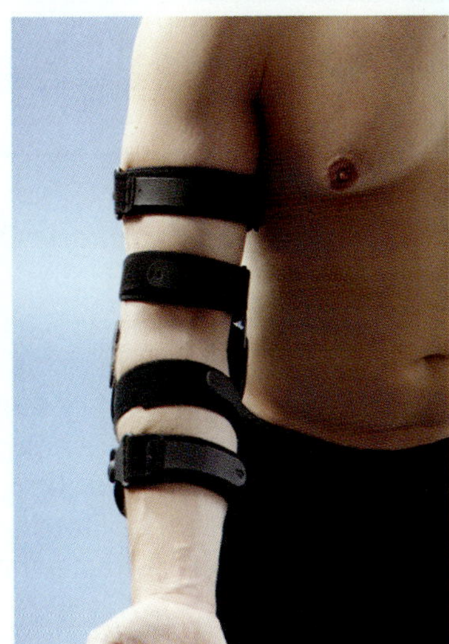

**Fig. 9–22 G**

*Steps Cont.*

**STEP 6:**   Last, anchor the posterior upper arm strap (Fig. 9–22H).

**STEP 7:**   Allow the patient to actively flex and extend the elbow to ensure proper fit. Retighten the straps and/or reposition the brace if necessary.

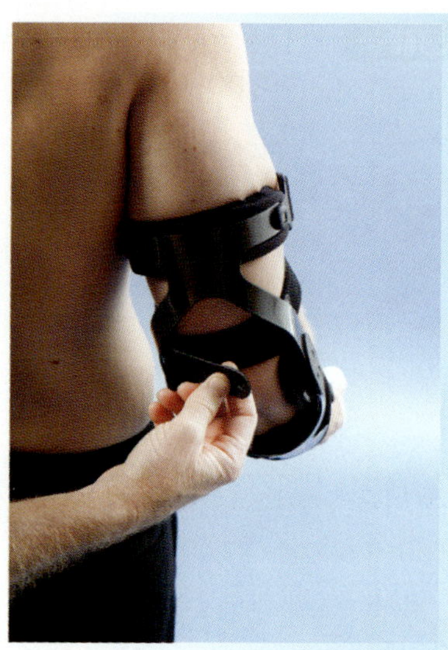

**Fig. 9–22 H**

## NEOPRENE SLEEVE WITH HINGED BARS   Figure 9–23

➡ **Purpose:** Neoprene sleeves with hinged bars designed for the knee (see Fig. 6–22) may be used to provide compression and mild to moderate support when treating elbow sprains, dislocations, and postoperative procedures. Use this technique when off-the-shelf elbow brace designs are not available or resources do not permit the purchase of these designs. Two methods are available for the application of the technique to accommodate patient preferences and available supplies; the first is illustrated here (Fig. 9–23), and the second is illustrated online at FADavis.com.

### DETAILS
Use the braces during rehabilitative, athletic, work, and casual activities. Apply padding to all nonpliable materials, commonly the hinges, to meet NCAA and NFHS rules.

### Neoprene Sleeve with Hinged Bars Technique One

➡ **Materials:**
  • Off-the-shelf neoprene sleeve with hinged bars
  *Option:*
  • 2 inch or 3 inch elastic tape or self-adherent wrap, taping scissors
➡ **Position of the patient:** Sitting on a taping table or bench or standing with the involved arm at the side of the body and the involved elbow placed in slight flexion.
➡ **Preparation:** Set the brace range of motion at the desired settings of flexion and extension. Apply neoprene sleeves with hinged bars directly to the skin. Loosen the straps.
➡ **Application:**

**STEP 1:**  Apply the larger end of the brace over the fingers and hand. Continue to pull in a proximal direction over the elbow. Position the hinges over the joint line and the patellar cut-out over the olecranon (Fig. 9–23A).

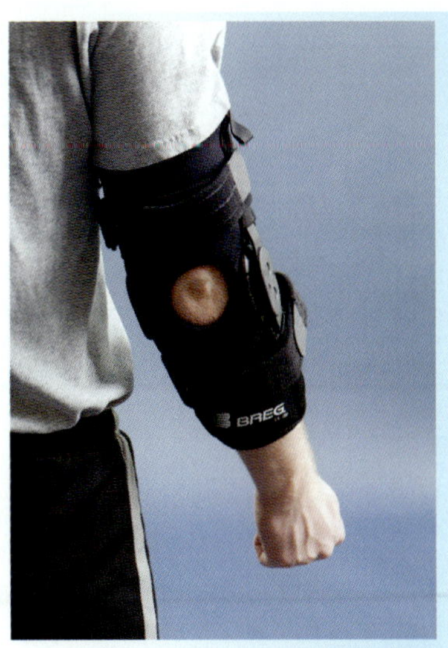

**Fig. 9–23 A**

**STEP 2:**  Tighten the straps and anchor with Velcro (Fig. 9–23B).

*Option:*  *Apply additional anchors with 2 inch or 3 inch elastic tape or self-adherent wrap in a circular pattern with moderate roll tension around the upper arm and forearm.*

**Helpful Hint |**
Neoprene sleeves with hinged bar braces for the knee are manufactured in predetermined sizes corresponding to thigh, knee, and/or lower leg circumference measurements. Because of the difference in girth measurements with the upper arm and forearm, off-the-shelf knee braces in sizes of XS, S, and M are typically required for use on the elbow.

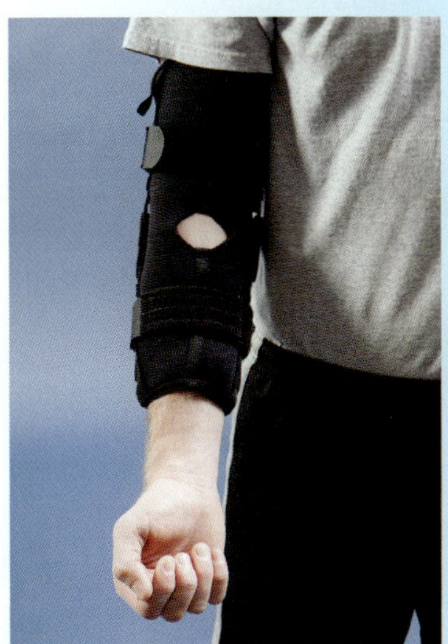

**Fig. 9–23 B**

## EVIDENCE SUMMARY

Functional elbow braces are commonly used to provide support, limit hyperextension, and protect healing tissues following injury. While several off-the-shelf and custom-made designs are available, there are limited investigations to determine the efficacy of these braces. Among healthy athletes, several researchers[10] demonstrated off-the-shelf braces failed to restrict active and passive extension during physiological loading compared to preset limitations. However, these same designs prevented full extension when preset to a 30 degree extension limit. The findings also revealed significant differences among the individual off-the-shelf designs in restricting elbow extension. The researchers[10] suggested the motion limiting effectiveness of off-the-shelf elbow braces can be enhanced when the preset limit is set below the protected motion minimum. A cadaveric study[11] evaluated the efficacy of an off-the-shelf design in the stabilization of specimens with simulated lateral collateral ligament injury. Using a simulator to produce active and passive elbow extension, investigators found the brace did not increase the stability of the elbow compared to non-braced specimens.

The use of functional elbow braces in the prevention of injury has been investigated in two small studies. Among high school baseball athletes, researchers examined the effects of a functional design on medial elbow joint space opening,[12] shoulder and elbow passive range of motion,[13] and grip strength.[13] Using a repetitive throwing activity simulating pitching, researchers[12] found no significant changes in ulnohumeral joint space opening measured by ultrasound imaging in the brace condition following 20, 40, 60, 80, and 100 pitches.

Brace wear was also shown to significantly reduce joint space opening when compared to a non-brace situation after 60, 80, and 100 pitches. Using the same repetitive throwing activity, other researchers[13] found no significant differences in shoulder and elbow passive range of motion following 20, 40, 60, 80, and 100 pitches and grip strength following 100 pitches with the use of a functional brace compared to a non-brace control. While these limited findings appear to support the use of functional braces in the prevention of elbow injuries among baseball athletes, NCAA and NFHS rules governing the use of braces should be reviewed prior to use in practices and competitions. Further research is needed with off-the-shelf and custom-made braces to determine the effects of different designs, construction materials, and fit on support and restriction of excessive valgus, varus, rotary, and hyperextension stresses during athletic and work activities to guide clinical decisions.

---

### ...IF/THEN...

**IF** using the neoprene sleeve with hinged bars technique one and the distal end is not snugly fitted on the forearm, allowing migration, **THEN** consider the application of technique two. The heavyweight elastic tape will conform to the upper arm and forearm and securely anchor the bars.

---

### ...IF/THEN...

**IF** application of hyperextension taping technique one, two, or three is not effective in limiting hyperextension during a return to activity following a sprain, **THEN** consider using a functional brace or neoprene sleeve with hinged bars technique one or two to provide greater support and limits in hyperextension.

---

### Clinical Application Question 3

At the end of a busy day, a window cleaner stepped off the scaffolding and caught his foot on several safety straps. The cleaner fell to the ground and landed on the right outstretched arm, sustaining a posterior elbow dislocation and third-degree ulnar collateral ligament sprain. Following surgery and rehabilitation, he returns to work. The surgeon recommends bracing for the elbow for the next 5 months to provide support.

➡ **Question: What bracing techniques are appropriate in this situation?**

---

## EPICONDYLITIS STRAP          Figure 9–24

➡ **Purpose:** Many epicondylitis strap brace designs are available to lessen tension on the wrist extensor or flexor musculature when treating lateral or medial epicondylitis (Fig. 9–24). These designs are commonly referred to as counterforce braces.[14]

### DETAILS
Use the straps with athletic, work, or casual activities.

➡ **Design:**
- Purchase the straps off-the-shelf in universal styles and predetermined sizes corresponding to proximal forearm circumference measurements. Several designs are available in universal sizes.
- Most designs are manufactured of neoprene or foam composite materials with a D-ring Velcro closure.
- Some designs are constructed of a non-elastic foam material.
- The straps contain a conformed neoprene, foam, air cell, viscoelastic, gel, padded plastic, or padded plastic/metal buttress incorporated into the strap.
- Other designs are available with gel packs that can be removed and heated and/or cooled to provide treatment to the wrist extensor and/or flexor musculature.
- Some braces are designed specifically for lateral or medial epicondylitis, while other braces can be positioned for both conditions.

➡ **Position of the patient:** Sitting on a taping table or bench or standing with the involved arm at the side of the body, the involved elbow placed in slight flexion, and the forearm in a neutral position.

➡ **Preparation:** Apply epicondylitis straps directly to the skin. No anchors are required.

➡ **Application:**

**STEP 1:**  Apply lateral epicondylitis designs by placing the buttress on the lateral forearm approximately ¾ of an inch distal from the lateral epicondyle of the humerus (Fig. 9–24A).

**STEP 2:**  Wrap the strap snugly around the proximal forearm and/or through the D-ring and anchor (Fig. 9–24B).

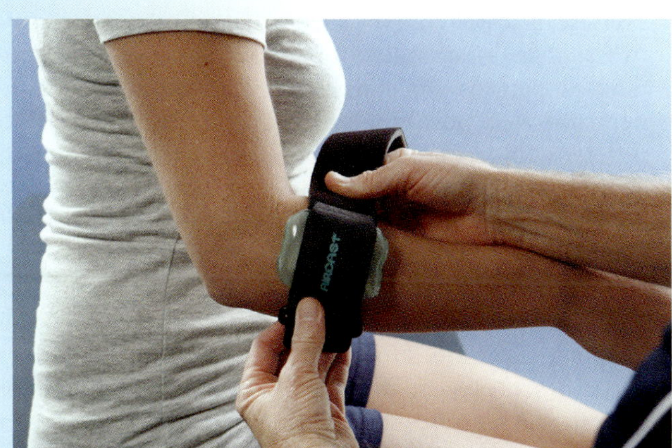

**Fig. 9–24 A**

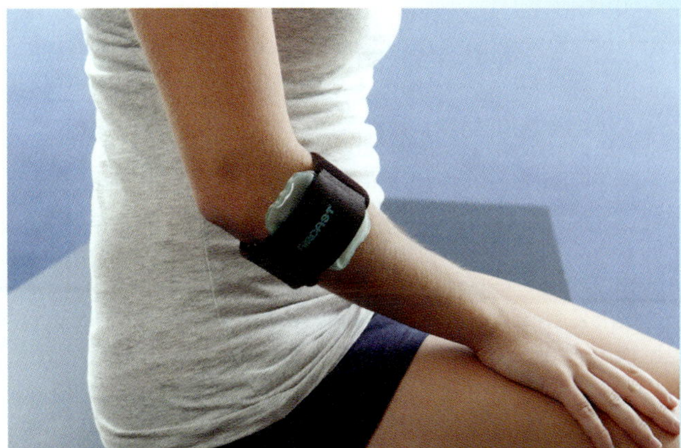

**Fig. 9–24 B**

**STEP 3:**  Apply medial epicondylitis designs by positioning the buttress on the medial forearm just distal from the medial epicondyle of the humerus (Fig. 9–24C).

**STEP 4:**  Wrap and anchor the strap (Fig. 9–24D).

**STEP 5:**  Allow the patient to perform a previously painful activity. Readjust the tension of the strap if necessary.

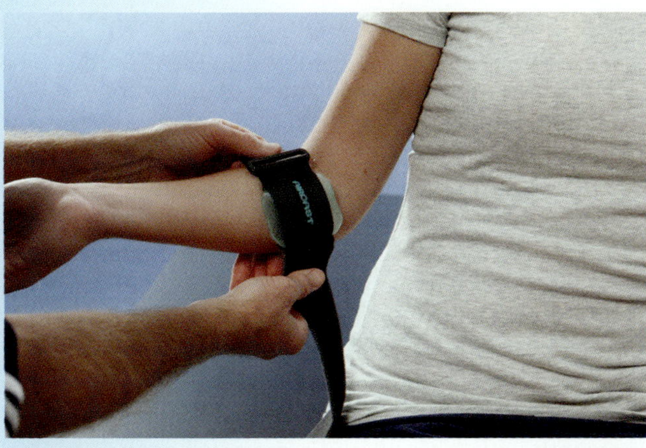

**Fig. 9–24 C**

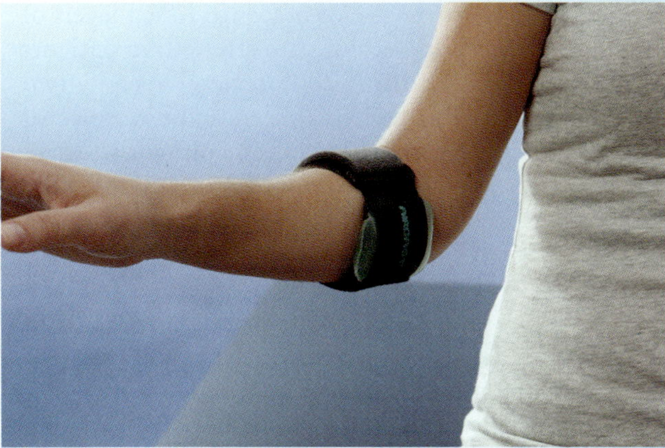

**Fig. 9–24 D**

### Clinical Application Question 4

A javelin thrower on the track and field team has been receiving treatment for lateral epicondylitis over the past 3 weeks. He has returned to activity with the use of a counterforce brace to lessen the pain associated with the throwing motion. After a few days of wearing the brace during practice, the brace loosens and the pain returns to the lateral forearm. He has worn taping material straps, but they were not effective in lessening the symptoms.

➡ **Question: What can be done in this situation?**

## EVIDENCE SUMMARY

A bracing technique for the forearm was first introduced in 1971[15]; over 40[16] various interventions have been used individually and in combination for the treatment and rehabilitation for lateral epicondylitis, or epicondylalgia. Numerous studies have been conducted to investigate the effects of counterforce bracing techniques, and the results have produced contradictory findings.

Several theoretical mechanisms of action for the braces are presented in the literature. Many researchers[5,17–19] have suggested that braces lessen tension at the proximal musculotendinous junction by reducing muscular expansion and decreasing the force of muscular contractions. Other researchers[6,20,21] believe the braces broaden the area for the common extensor tendon origin, artificially creating a second, wider muscle origin. This broadening may direct stress to healthy tissues or the band, decreasing stress on the lateral epicondyle.

Initial evidence-based reviews have examined the efficacy of braces for the treatment of lateral epicondylitis. In a 2002 review,[22] five studies among patients with lateral epicondylitis revealed no significant differences in pain and grip strength with the use of braces compared with conservative treatment, injection therapy, and anti-inflammatory cream and when the braces were used as an adjunct to manual therapy, therapeutic ultrasound, and anti-inflammatory cream. A 2004 review[23] included 11 studies and found inconclusive evidence to support the use of braces to lessen levels of pain and increase grip and forearm strength in patients with lateral epicondylitis. A 2005 review[24] of only two studies produced insufficient evidence for the use of braces in the treatment of lateral epicondylitis. These reviews appear to provide no definitive evidence for the efficacy of braces, perhaps as a result of variations in outcome measures, intervention durations, and brace designs.

Since 2005, several studies have been conducted to investigate the effects of braces on pain and strength of the forearm musculature among patients with lateral epicondylitis. The effects of braces and a taping technique on pain associated with lateral epicondylitis have produced mixed results. Researchers[25] have demonstrated no significant effects on pressure pain threshold during mechanical application of pressure at the lateral epicondyle with the use of a forearm and forearm/elbow brace compared with a no-brace situation. Other researchers found no significant changes in visual analogue scales of pain perception between braces, ultrasound therapy, and laser therapy at 2 and 6 week periods[26] and between braces, a therapeutic exercise protocol, and combination of both interventions at 1 year.[27] Examining Kinesio Taping with therapeutic exercise and a brace in combination with therapeutic exercise, researchers[28] revealed no significant differences in visual analogue scales of pain perception at 2, 4, and 6 week periods. In contrast, several researchers have demonstrated positive outcomes with brace use. Two different forearm/elbow brace designs were shown to significantly reduce visual analogue scales of pain perception when compared to a wrist splint and placebo.[29] Other investigators[30] found two different forearm/elbow brace designs significantly reduced visual analogue scales of pain perception when compared with a no-brace situation. However, no significant differences in pain scores were revealed between the two brace designs.[30] A significant reduction in pain was produced at 6 weeks following the use of a wrist extension splint compared with an elbow brace design.[31] Examining pain at rest and during movement, researchers[32] found that a forearm brace and wrist splint resulted in significant improvements in pain at 2 and 6 week follow-up periods. At rest, a forearm brace in combination with forearm/upper arm strengthening significantly reduced patient-reported severity of pain scores at 2 weeks and frequency of pain scores at 6 and 12 week periods compared to a placebo brace and forearm/upper arm strengthening.[33] Other researchers[34] found significant reductions in visual analogue scales of pain perception following 4 week use of a spiral forearm splint designed to restrict wrist extension and limit forearm supination and pronation. The application of a diamond-shaped taping technique has been shown to significantly reduce visual analogue scales of pain perception compared to a no-tape situation.[35] The taping technique consisted of four strips of non-elastic tape anchored directly on the skin in a diamond pattern around the lateral epicondyle.

Studies examining the effects of bracing and taping on pain-free grip strength among subjects with lateral epicondylitis have produced conflicting findings. Researchers[25] found no significant changes in grip strength with forearm and forearm/elbow braces when compared with a no-brace situation. Other researchers[26] examined the effects of braces, therapeutic exercise, and combination of both interventions and showed no changes in grip strength at 2 and 6 week periods. A small study[28] found no significant differences in grip strength with Kinesio Taping in combination with therapeutic exercise compared to a brace and therapeutic exercise at 2, 4, and 6 week periods. Examining forearm braces of varying widths, researchers[36] demonstrated a significant reduction in grip strength with a 2.5 cm design compared to 5.5 cm, 7.5 cm, and 12.0 cm braces. In contrast, others[34] demonstrated that a spiral forearm splint significantly increased grip strength following 4 weeks of wear. Investigating a forearm brace and wrist splint, researchers[32] demonstrated significant improvements in grip strength following 6 weeks of brace wear and 2 and 6 weeks of splint wear. Other researchers[30] found significant improvements in grip strength with two different forearm/elbow brace designs compared with a no-brace situation. No significant differences were demonstrated between the two brace designs. A forearm and placebo brace, both in combination with therapeutic exercise, were shown to significantly improve grip strength at 26 weeks.[33] However, no significant differences were found between the forearm and placebo brace. With a diamond taping technique, grip strength was significantly increased compared to a no-tape situation.[35]

Electromyographic investigations of the forearm musculature with brace wear have produced positive findings. Examining a group of tennis players without symptoms of lateral epicondylitis, researchers demonstrated lower electromyographic activity of the extensor carpi ulnaris and extensor carpi radialis among the brace group than among the unbraced group during backhand and serve strokes.[37] Brace wear has also been shown to significantly reduce electromyographic activity of the extensor carpi radialis brevis and extensor digitorum communis in normal subjects, as compared with controls.[5] Researchers[38] found a significant reduction in electromyographic activity of the extensor carpi radialis brevis with two forearm brace designs compared with no-brace among normal subjects. Other researchers[36] demonstrated significant reductions in electromyographic activity of the extensor carpi radialis and extensor digitorum communis with a 2.5 cm width brace compared to 5.5 cm, 7.5 cm, and 12.0 cm designs during a maximum grip contraction task among healthy subjects. Despite these findings, reductions in electromyographic activity associated with counterforce bracing have not been shown to correlate with clinical improvement of lateral epicondylitis.[4]

Several studies have examined the effect of brace wear on functional outcomes among various populations. Researchers[33] found significant improvements in patient-reported elbow stiffness and function scores at 26 weeks with a forearm brace in combination with therapeutic exercise compared to a placebo brace and therapeutic exercise among patients with lateral epicondylitis. During a submaximal and maximal grip task with healthy subjects, 5.5 cm and 12.0 cm width braces significantly decreased wrist range of motion when compared to 2.5 cm and 7.5 cm brace designs.[36] Other researchers[30] demonstrated a significant improvement in finger dexterity scores with a forearm brace compared to a no-brace situation among patients with lateral epicondylitis.

Recommendations on when and how to apply counterforce braces when treating lateral epicondylitis vary in the literature. Several investigators suggest using the braces in the acute phase of treatment,[15,18] only during painful activities,[15] during all activities if moderate symptoms are present, and all the time (excluding sleep) if severe symptoms are present,[39] and when symptoms have resolved[17] for a 1-year period.[15] Most researchers agree that counterforce bracing is an adjunct to a comprehensive treatment program.[4]

The amount of tension with which the brace should be applied on the forearm remains unknown. In previous studies, application tension has been described with the terms "comfortably"[6,15] and "snugly"[5,39] in regard to the fit on the proximal forearm. Some researchers have suggested that an application pressure of 40–50 mm Hg may provide the optimal mechanical effect.[4] Note that excessive tension of the brace can cause edema and anterior interosseous nerve syndrome, affecting intraneural blood flow and causing deep forearm pain and weakness of the hand musculature.[40] As previously mentioned in the Taping section of this chapter, positioning of the brace ¾ of an inch distal to the lateral epicondyle appears to be the preferred placement on the forearm for treating lateral epicondylitis.[5,6] No specific application recommendations for medial epicondylitis were found in the literature.

While the research has shown mixed results with regard to the effectiveness of counterforce bracing when treating lateral epicondylitis, counterforce bracing continues to be used. The existing evidence can be incorporated with clinician experience and patient preferences to guide clinical decisions for treatment and rehabilitation interventions. Additional high-quality randomized controlled trials with standardized outcome measures and intervention durations among different forearm and forearm/elbow brace designs can provide the necessary evidence to improve patient care. Further investigations are necessary to examine application tension and position, optimal periods of application, and the long-term clinical effects of the braces.

## NEOPRENE SLEEVE    Figure 9–25

**Purpose:** Neoprene sleeves provide compression and mild support when preventing and treating contusions, sprains, strains, ruptures, dislocations, bursitis, abrasions, and overuse injuries and conditions (Fig. 9–25).

### DETAILS
Use the sleeves during rehabilitative, athletic, work, and casual activities.

**Design:**
- The off-the-shelf sleeves are manufactured in universal fit designs in predetermined sizes corresponding to elbow joint circumference measurements.
- Most designs extend from the mid upper arm to the mid forearm. Some designs extend to the distal forearm for additional support and protection.
- Many designs are constructed with protective padding incorporated into the posterior elbow.
- Other designs contain viscoelastic polymer pads incorporated into the sleeve to provide additional compression to the wrist flexor and/or extensor musculature.
- Some designs have a lateral and/or medial epicondylitis strap incorporated with a Velcro closure.

**Position of the patient:** Sitting on a taping table or bench or standing with the involved arm at the side of the body and the involved elbow placed in slight flexion.

**Preparation:** Apply neoprene sleeves directly to the skin. No anchors are required.

**Application:**

**STEP 1:**  Hold each side of the sleeve and apply the larger end over the fingers and hand. Pull in a proximal direction until the sleeve is positioned on the elbow (Fig. 9–25).

**STEP 2:**  Apply epicondylitis sleeve designs by positioning the pad(s) or buttress, then wrap and anchor the straps.

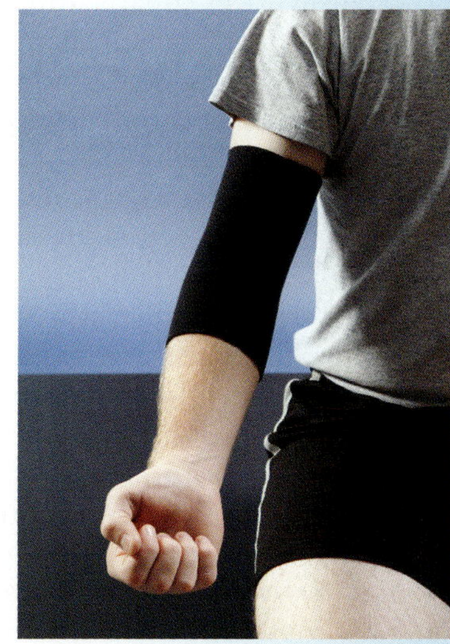

**Fig. 9–25**

## SLINGS

**Purpose:** Slings provide support and immobilization when treating elbow and forearm injuries and conditions.
- Use slings (see Fig. 8–19) to treat sprains, strains, ruptures, dislocations, fractures, bursitis, and overuse injuries and conditions; this technique can be used postoperatively as well.

# Padding Techniques

➡ Off-the-shelf and custom-made padding techniques provide shock absorption and protection when preventing and treating elbow and forearm injuries and conditions. Padding for the elbow and/or forearm is mandatory with several interscholastic and intercollegiate sports. These mandatory techniques will be discussed further in Chapter 13.

## OFF-THE-SHELF     Figures 9–26 and 9–27

➡ **Purpose:** Off-the-shelf padding techniques are available in a variety of designs to provide shock absorption and protection. Use these techniques when preventing and treating contusions, bursitis, abrasions, and overuse injuries and conditions. Many of these padding designs are similar to the techniques illustrated in Chapter 6 (see Figs. 6–26 and 6–27). Following is a description of two basic designs.

### Soft, Low-Density

**DETAILS**

Soft, low-density pads are commonly used to provide shock absorption to the elbow and forearm of athletes in sports such as baseball, basketball, field hockey, football, ice hockey, lacrosse, softball, volleyball, and wrestling. The pads may also be used in work and casual activities.

➡ **Design:**
- The pads are available in universal fit designs in predetermined sizes based on upper arm, forearm, or elbow joint circumference measurements or weight of the patient (Fig. 9–26A).
- Many designs are manufactured of high-impact open- and closed-cell foams, covered with polyester/spandex or woven fabric materials with Velcro closure elastic straps.
- Some pads are constructed of woven fabric and neoprene materials, with the neoprene located on the medial aspect of the elbow and forearm to provide an adherent surface for athletic equipment.
- Other designs incorporate high-impact foam over the posterior elbow in a neoprene or cloth sleeve.

➡ **Position of the patient:** Sitting on a taping table or bench or standing with the involved arm at the side of the body and the involved elbow placed in slight flexion.

➡ **Preparation:** Apply the soft, low-density designs directly to the skin or over tight-fitting clothing.

➡ **Application:**

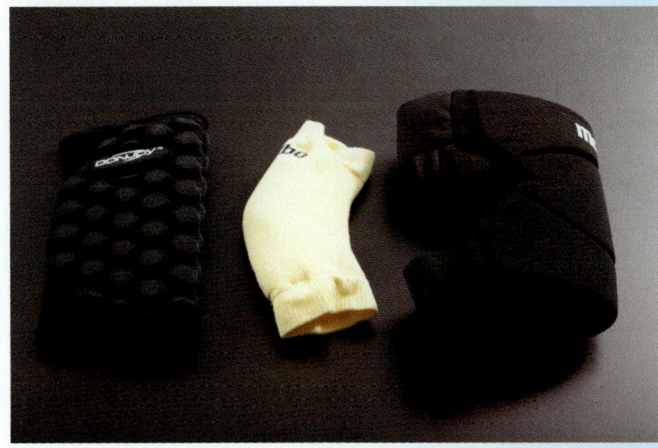

**Fig. 9–26 A** *Variety of soft, low-density pads.*

**STEP 1:**  Place the larger end of the pad over the fingers and hand. Pull in a proximal direction onto the elbow and/or forearm (Fig. 9–26B). When using some designs, anchor the straps.

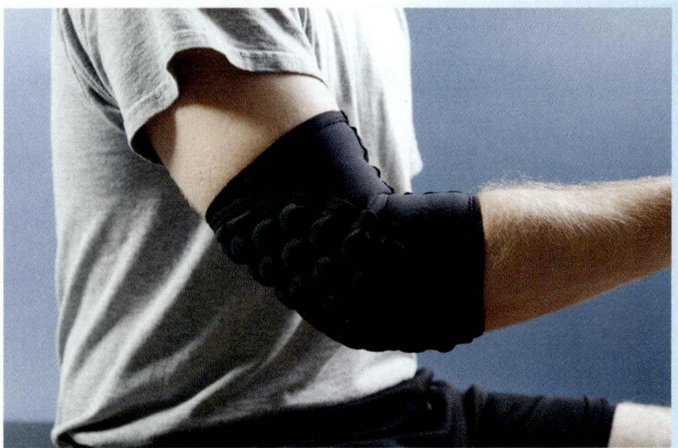

**Fig. 9–26 B**

### Hard, High-Density

---

**DETAILS**
Hard, high-density pads are commonly used to provide shock absorption to the elbow and forearm of athletes in sports such as baseball, basketball, field hockey, football, ice hockey, lacrosse, skiing, softball, volleyball, and wrestling. The pads may also be used in work and casual activities.

---

⟶ **Design:**
- These pads are available in universal and right or left styles corresponding to upper arm, forearm, or elbow joint circumference measurements or age of the patient (Fig. 9–27A).
- Many designs consist of a polycarbonate or plastic outer shell lined with open- and closed-cell foams incorporated into vinyl or woven fabric materials. These pads are pre-molded to the contours of the upper arm, elbow, and forearm.
- Most pads are designed with protective materials covering the medial and lateral upper arm, elbow, and forearm to provide additional protection.
- Some pads are one-piece designs, while other pads are three-piece to allow for maximum range of motion and comfort.

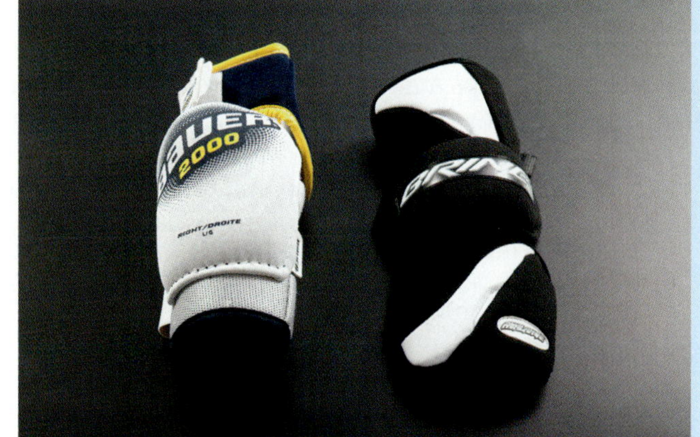

**Fig. 9–27 A** *Variety of hard, high-density pads. (Left) Ice hockey. (Right) Lacrosse.*

- The designs are available in a variety of lengths depending on the technique objective.
- Hard, high-density pads are attached to the upper arm, elbow, and forearm with various adjustable nylon straps with Velcro or buckle closures.
- Another design uses a polycarbonate cup lined with foam that attaches to the hinges of functional elbow braces to protect the olecranon.

⟶ **Position of the patient:** Sitting on a taping table or bench or standing with the involved arm at the side of the body and the involved elbow placed in slight flexion.

⟶ **Preparation:** Apply the hard, high-density designs directly to the skin or over tight-fitting clothing.

⟶ **Application:**

**STEP 1:** Apply the pad over the posterior elbow. The application of straps will depend on the specific design. Normally, pull the straps across the anterior upper arm and forearm and anchor on the pad with Velcro or buckle closures (Fig. 9–27B). Readjust the straps if necessary for proper fit.

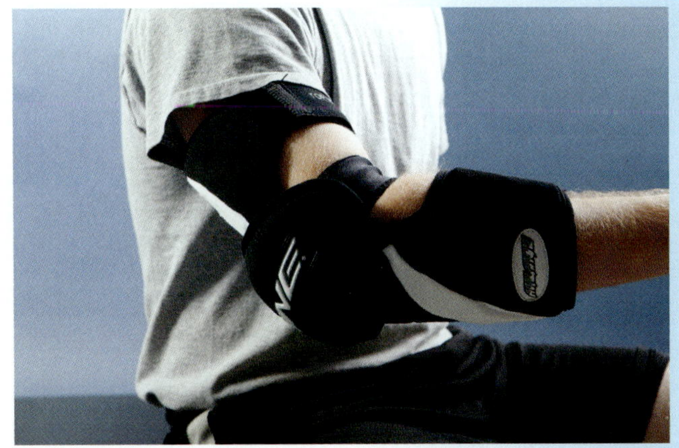

**Fig. 9–27 B**

## COMPRESSION WRAP PAD    Figure 9–28

➡ **Purpose:** Use the compression wrap pad to reduce mild, moderate, or severe swelling and effusion when treating elbow contusions, sprains, strains, ruptures, dislocations, and bursitis (Fig. 9–28).
➡ **Materials:**
 • ¼ inch or ½ inch open-cell foam, taping scissors
➡ **Position of the patient:** Sitting on a taping table or bench or standing with the involved arm at the side of the body and the involved elbow placed in a pain-free, flexed position.
➡ **Preparation:** Apply the pad directly to the skin.
➡ **Application:**

**STEP 1:** Extend the pad across the posterior elbow, from the lateral humeral epicondyle to the medial humeral epicondyle, and approximately 3 inches proximally and distally from the olecranon (Fig. 9–28A).

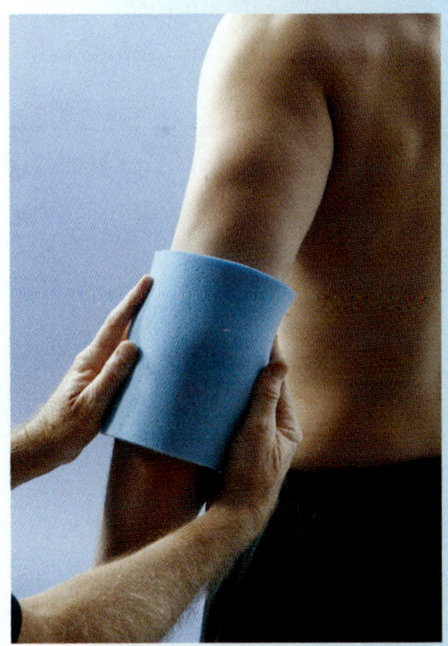

**Fig. 9–28 A**

*Steps Cont.*

**STEP 2:** Place the pad over the posterior elbow and apply the compression wrap technique to anchor (see Figs. 9–14, 9–17, 9–18, and 9–28B).

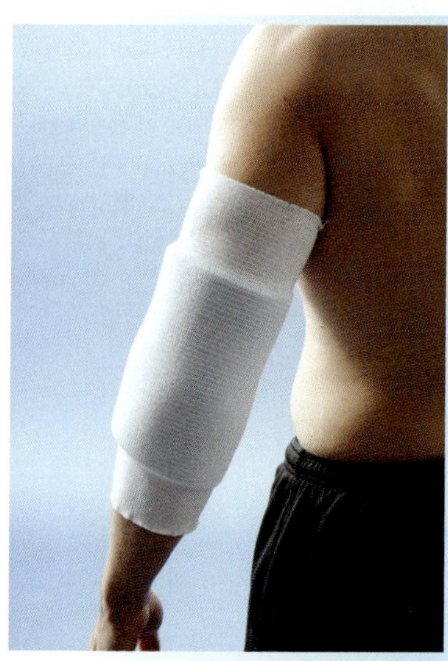

**Fig. 9–28 B**

## ⊕ CUSTOM-MADE

➡ **Purpose:** Use thermoplastic material to construct custom-made pads to absorb shock and provide protection when preventing and treating elbow and forearm contusions. This technique and steps of application can be found on FADavis.com.

## MANDATORY PADDING

The NCAA[8] and NFHS[9] require athletes to use protective padding for the elbow and/or forearm during all fencing, field hockey, ice hockey, and lacrosse practices and competitions. These padding techniques are available in a variety of off-the-shelf designs. A further discussion of these techniques can be found in Chapter 13.

### Clinical Application Question 5

During rehabilitation of her left knee at the local out-patient orthopedic clinic, a landscape supervisor discusses the problems she is experiencing with her elbow pads. Each weekend when she is rollerblading, the pads slide down onto her forearms. She exchanged the pads and was fitted with another pair at the sporting goods store. The next weekend, these pads also slid down onto her forearms. She is annoyed about the pads and is considering not using any protective equipment for her elbows.

➡ **Question: How can you manage this situation?**

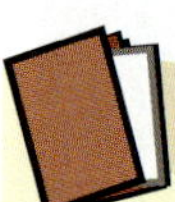

## EVIDENCE-BASED PRACTICE

In the second competition of the season, Leo Reagan, a veteran bull rider on the circuit, is thrown from a bull during his first-round ride. Leo was able to release his right hand from the bull rope around the bull but fell to the ground on the left outstretched arm, sustaining a left posterolateral elbow dislocation. Jay Patrick, the AT traveling with the circuit, evaluated Leo. Jay immobilized the left elbow, and Leo was transported to a local hospital by EMS. In the emergency room, an orthopedic surgeon performed an evaluation, including imaging studies, and then successfully reduced the elbow. The studies revealed no fractures but showed a second-degree sprain to the ulnar collateral ligament. The surgeon immobilized Leo's left elbow in 90 degrees of flexion and allowed him to return home for a follow-up evaluation with a local orthopedic surgeon.

The next day, Leo is evaluated by the orthopedic surgeon in his hometown. The surgeon reviewed the previous imaging studies, conducted a clinical evaluation, and agreed with the initial diagnosis. The surgeon believed Leo could return to his previous activities, following a nonsurgical rehabilitation approach. Leo remained immobilized in 90 degrees of elbow flexion for 3 additional days and began rehabilitation at Power Orthopedic Clinic. Five days post-injury, the immobilization was discontinued. The surgeon was concerned about moderate ulnar collateral ligament laxity and recommended that Leo be protected against valgus and hyperextension stress at the elbow during this phase of rehabilitation. Jay and the surgeon select an off-the-shelf functional bracing technique for Leo.

Leo tolerates the rehabilitation without problems and has increased flexibility, strength, and dynamic stability of the elbow and surrounding joints. The surgeon is satisfied with Leo's healing and progress and allows a progression into bull riding activities around 11 weeks post-injury. Jay is not sure about the fit and stability of the off-the-shelf functional bracing technique Leo used during rehabilitation. Leo has an increased carrying angle, cubitus valgus, caused by his high school and intercollegiate experiences as a baseball pitcher. During the rehabilitation, this condition, at times, affected the positioning of the brace hinges over the joint line during elbow flexion and extension. The rehabilitation program also resulted in an increase in the girth of Leo's upper arm and forearm musculature. Leo's left arm is the free hand during bull riding and is subjected to violent flexion and extension at the elbow. Jay knows that proper brace application and fit are critical to protect Leo from further injury. Jay and the surgeon decide to investigate available functional bracing techniques to choose the most effective design for Leo.

Leo returns to competitive bull riding using the bracing technique selected for him. During his first week back, he falls several times on his left elbow. Each time, the left elbow was in a flexed position in the brace. Pain and swelling are present over the posterior elbow. Leo is evaluated by a physician and diagnosed with acute olecranon bursitis. The physician allows Leo to continue bull riding activities if protected from further injury. Jay has access to and experience with multiple padding techniques for this situation. He has also recently received information on a cutting-edge padding design specifically manufactured for use with bracing techniques. Jay plans to spend some time to search for the best technique to protect Leo's elbow.

1. Develop two clinically relevant questions from the case in the PICO format to generate answers for the selection of a: (1) bracing technique for bull riding activities and (2) padding technique for olecranon bursitis for Leo. The questions should include the population or problem, the intervention, a comparison intervention (if relevant), and the clinical outcome of interest.

2. Design a search strategy and search to find the best evidence to answer the clinical questions. The strategies should include relevant search terms, electronic databases, online journals, and print journals to use for the search. Discussions with your faculty, preceptor, and other health care professionals can provide evidence from expert opinion.

3. Choose two to three full text studies or reviews from each of your searches or the chapter references. Evaluate and appraise each article to determine its value and usefulness to the case. Ask these questions for each study: (1) Are the results of the study valid? (2) What are the actual results? and (3) Are the findings clinically relevant to my patients? Prepare a summary of the evaluation with answers to the questions and rank the articles based on the evidence hierarchy in Chapter 1.

4. Integrate findings from the evidence, your clinical experience, and Leo's goals and preferences into the case. Consider which bracing and padding techniques may be appropriate for each situation.

5. Evaluate the EBP process and your experience within the case. Consider these questions in the evaluation.

Were the clinical questions answered?
Did the searches generate quality evidence?
Was the evidence evaluated appropriately?
Was the evidence, your clinical experience, and Leo's goals and values integrated to make the clinical decisions?
Did the interventions produce successful clinical outcomes for Leo?
Was the EBP experience positive for Jay and Leo?

**Elbow and Forearm**

## WRAP-UP

- Acute and chronic injuries and conditions to the elbow and forearm are caused by direct forces, abnormal ranges of motion, forceful muscular contractions, and overload and repetitive stresses.
- The hyperextension taping technique reduces range of motion of the elbow.
- The lateral epicondylitis strap taping and epicondylitis bracing techniques lessen tension of the wrist extensors and/or flexors on the humeral epicondyles.
- The circular forearm and figure-of-eight taping techniques provide support and anchor protective padding.
- Posterior splints and slings provide immobilization following injury/surgery.
- Elastic wraps and sleeves provide compression to control swelling and effusion.
- The circular elbow and forearm wrapping techniques can be used to support and anchor protective padding.
- Rehabilitative braces provide support, immobilization, and protective range of motion, while functional braces provide stability following injury/surgery.
- The neoprene sleeve and sleeve with hinged bars bracing techniques provide compression and support to the elbow.
- Soft, low-density and hard, high-density off-the-shelf and custom-made padding techniques provide shock absorption, protection, and compression.
- The NCAA and NFHS require the use of mandatory protective equipment for the elbow and/or forearm in several sports.

## FADAVIS ONLINE RESOURCES

- Hyperextension taping technique three
- Figure-of-eight elbow taping technique
- Posterior splint technique two
- Neoprene sleeve with hinged bars technique two
- Custom-made pad

## WEB REFERENCES

### American Sports Medicine Institute

http://www.asmi.org
- This site provides you access to an online library and other educational materials.

### The Hughston Clinic

https://www.hughston.com
- This site allows access to the *Hughston Health Alert* newsletter and online articles about a variety of elbow and forearm injuries and conditions.

### American Academy of Orthopaedic Surgeons

https://www.aaos.org/
- This site provides access to information regarding the treatment and rehabilitation of elbow and forearm injuries and conditions, including the American Academy of Orthopaedic Surgeons Clinical Practice Guidelines.

### Medscape

https://www.medscape.com/
- This site provides access to information about acute and chronic elbow and forearm injuries and conditions.

## REFERENCES

1. Watson, JN, McQueen, P, and Hutchinson, MR: A systematic review of ulnar collateral ligament reconstruction techniques. Am J Sports Med 42:2510–2516, 2014.
2. Ciccotti, MC, Schwartz, MA, and Ciccotti, MG: Diagnosis and treatment of medial epicondylitis of the elbow. Clin Sports Med 23:693–705, 2004.
3. Starkey, C, and Brown, SD: Examination of Orthopedic and Athletic Injuries, ed 4. F.A. Davis, Philadelphia, 2015.
4. Meyer, NJ, Pennington, W, Haines, B, and Daley, R: The effect of the forearm support band on forces at the origin of the extensor carpi radialis brevis: A cadaveric study and review of literature. J Hand Ther 15:179–185, 2002.
5. Snyder-Mackler, L, and Epler, M: Effect of standard and Aircast tennis elbow bands on integrated electromyography of forearm extensor musculature proximal to the bands. Am J Sports Med 17:278–281, 1989.
6. Wadsworth, CT, Nielson, DH, Burns, LT, Krull, JD, and Thompson, CG: Effect of the counterforce armband on wrist extension and grip strength and pain in subjects with tennis elbow. J Orthop Sports Phys Ther 11:192–197, 1989.
7. Merolla, G, Bianchi, P, and Porcellini, G: Efficacy, usability, and tolerability of a dynamic elbow orthosis after collateral ligament reconstruction: A prospective randomized study. Musculoskelet Surg 98:209–216, 2014.
8. National Collegiate Athletic Association: 2014–15 Sports Medicine Handbook, ed 25. NCAA, Indianapolis, 2014. http://www.ncaapublications.com/product-downloads/MD15.pdf.
9. National Federation of State High School Associations: 2018 Field Hockey Rules Book. National Federation of State High School Associations, Indianapolis, 2019.
10. Lake, AW, Sitler, MR, Stearne, DJ, Swanik, CB, and Tierney, R: Effectiveness of prophylactic hyperextension

elbow braces on limiting active and passive elbow extension prephysiological and postphysiological loading. J Orthop Sport Phys 35:837–843, 2005.

11. Manocha, RH, King, GJW, and Johnson, JA: In vitro kinematic assessment of a hinged elbow orthosis following lateral collateral ligament injury. J Hand Surg Am 43:123–132, 2018.

12. Hattori, H, Akasaka, K, Otsudo, T, Takei, K, and Yamamoto, M: The effects of elbow bracing on medial elbow joint space gapping associated with repetitive throwing in high school baseball players. Orthop J Sports Med 5:2017. doi: 10.1177/2325967117702361.

13. Hattori, H, Akasaka, K, Otsudo, T, Hall, T, Amemiya, K, and Mori, Y: Use of an elbow brace during repetitive pitching does not cause an increased mechanical burden on the throwing arm. PMR: 2019. doi: 10.1002/pmrj.12083.

14. Nirschl, RP: The etiology and treatment of tennis elbow. J Sports Med 2:308–328, 1974.

15. Froimson, AI: Treatment of tennis elbow with forearm support band. J Bone Joint Surg 53:183–184, 1971.

16. Luk, JKH, Tsang, RCC, and Leung, HB: Lateral epicondylitis: Midlife crisis of a tendon. Hong Kong Med J 20:145–151, 2014.

17. Galloway, M, DeMaio, M, and Mangine, R: Rehabilitative techniques in the treatment of medial and lateral epicondylitis. Orthopedics 15:1089–1096, 1992.

18. Gellman, H: Tennis elbow (lateral epicondylitis). Orthop Clin North Am 23:75–82, 1992.

19. Jansen, CW, Olson, SL, and Hasson, SM: The effect of use of a wrist orthosis during functional activities on surface electromyography of the wrist extensors in normal subjects. J Hand Ther 10:283–289, 1997.

20. Kivi, P: The etiology and conservative treatment of humeral epicondylitis. Scand J Rehabil Med 15:37–41, 1982.

21. Nirschl, RP: Tennis elbow. Orthop Clin North Am 4:787–800, 1973.

22. Struijs, PAA, Smidt, N, Arola, H, van Dijk, CN, Buchbinder, R, and Assendelft, WJJ: Orthotic devices for the treatment of tennis elbow. Cochrane Database Syst Rev (1);CD001821, 2002.

23. Borkholder, CD, Hill, VA, and Fess, EE: The efficacy of splinting for lateral epicondylitis: A systematic review. J Hand Ther 17:181–199, 2004.

24. Bisset, L, Paungmali, A, Vicenzino, B, and Beller, E: A systematic review and meta-analysis of clinical trials on physical interventions for lateral epicondylagia. Br J Sports Med 39:411–422, 2005.

25. Bisset, LM, Collins, NJ, and Offord, SS: Immediate effects of 2 types of braces on pain and grip strength in people with lateral epicondylalgia: A randomized controlled trial. J Orthop Sports Phys Ther 44:120–128, 2014.

26. Öken, Ö, Kahraman, Y, Ayhan, F, Canpolat, S, Yorgancioglu, ZR, and Öken, ÖF: The short-term efficacy of laser, brace, and ultrasound treatment in lateral epicondylitis: A prospective, randomized, controlled trial. J Hand Ther 21:63–68, 2008.

27. Struijs, PAA, Korthals-de Bos, IBC, van Tulder, MW, van Gijk, CN, Bouter, LM, and Assendelft, WJJ: Cost effectiveness of brace, physiotherapy, or both for treatment of tennis elbow. Br J Sports Med 40:637–643, 2006.

28. Phadke, S, and Desai, S: Effectiveness of Kinesiotape versus counterforce brace as an adjunct to occupational therapy in lateral epicondylitis. Indian J Physiother Occup Ther 11:42–46, 2017.

29. Sadeghi-Demneh, E, and Jafarian, F: The immediate effects of orthoses on pain in people with lateral epicondylalgia. Pain Res Treat 2013:353597. doi: 10.1155/2013/353597.

30. Barati, H, Zarezadeh, A, MacDermid, JC, and Sadeghi-Demneh, E: The immediate sensorimotor effects of elbow orthoses in patients with lateral elbow tendinopathy: A prospective crossover study. J Shoulder Elbow Surg 28:e10–e17, 2019.

31. Garg, R, Adamson, GJ, Dawson, PA, Shankwiler, JA, and Pink, MM: A prospective randomized study comparing a forearm strap brace versus a wrist splint for the treatment of lateral epicondylitis. J Shoulder Elbow Surg 19:508–512, 2010.

32. Altan, L, and Kanat, E: Conservative treatment of lateral epicondylitis: Comparison of two different orthotic devices. Clin Rheumatol 27:1015–1019, 2008.

33. Kroslak, M, Pirapakaran, K, and Murrell, GAC: Counterforce bracing of lateral epicondylitis: A prospective, randomized, double-blinded, placebo-controlled trial. J Shoulder Elbow Surg 28:288–295, 2019.

34. Najafi, M, Arazpour, M, Aminian, G, Curran, S, Madani, SP, and Hutchins, SW: Effect of a new hand-forearm splint on grip strength, pain, and function in patients with tennis elbow. Prosthet Orthot Int 40:363–368, 2016.

35. Shamsoddini, A, and Hollisaz, MT: Effects of taping on pain, grip strength and wrist extension force in patients with tennis elbow. Trauma Mon. 18:71–74, 2013.

36. Marcolino, AM, Fonseca, MC, Leonardi, NT, Barbosa, RI, Neves, LM, and de Jesus Guirro, RR: The influence of different non-articular proximal forearm orthoses (brace) widths in the wrist extensors muscle activity, range of motion and grip strength in healthy volunteers. J Back Musculoskelet Rehabil 30:145–151, 2017.

37. Groppel, JL, and Nirschl, RP: A mechanical and electromyographical analysis of the effects of various joint counterforce braces on the tennis player. Am J Sports Med 14:195–200, 1986.

38. Yoon, JJ, and Bae, H: Change in electromyographic activity of wrist extensor by cylindrical brace. Yonsei Med J 54:220–224, 2013.

39. Priest, JD: Tennis elbow: The syndrome and a study of average players. Minn Med 59:367–371, 1976.

40. Enzenauer, RJ, and Nordstrom, DM: Anterior interosseous nerve syndrome associated with forearm band treatment of lateral epicondylitis. Orthopedics 14:788–790, 1991.

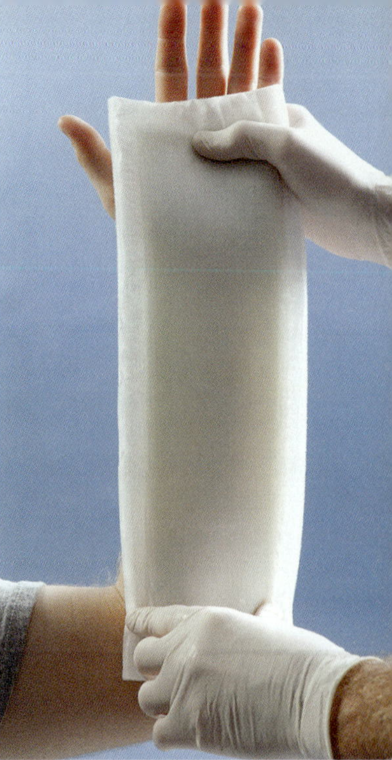

# Wrist





## INJURIES AND CONDITIONS

Acute and chronic injuries and conditions to the wrist may result from compressive forces, excessive range of motion, and repetitive stresses. Normal range of motion and stability of the wrist are required for participation in most athletic, work, and casual activities. Loss of range of motion as a result of contusions, sprains, fractures, dislocations, and overuse injuries and conditions can be caused by compressive forces, a fall on the outstretched arm, excessive range of motion, and/or repetitive stresses. Sprains, fractures, and dislocations can occur due to excessive range of motion and shearing forces and can result in loss of wrist stability. Common injuries to the wrist include:

- Contusions
- Sprains
- Triangular fibrocartilage complex
- Fractures
- Dislocations
- Ganglion cysts
- Overuse injuries and conditions

## Contusions

While uncommon, contusions to the wrist do occur; they may be caused by compressive forces. Athletes participating in sports that utilize a stick can be injured as a result of being struck on the wrist by an opponent. Although mandatory gloves normally protect the wrist, an ice hockey forward, for example, can be struck with a stick during a shot on goal.

## Sprains

Sprains to the wrist are common in athletic and work activities and are caused by several mechanisms. A fall on the outstretched arm, rotary forces, and abnormal ranges of motion can result in injury to the ligamentous and capsular tissues of the distal **radioulnar** and **radiocarpal joints** (Fig. 10–1). For example, a wrestler may sprain his wrist during a takedown when he lands on the outstretched arm and hyperextends his wrist (Fig. 10–2).

## Triangular Fibrocartilage Complex (TFCC)

Injury to the **TFCC** can be caused by a fall on the outstretched arm, rotary stress, and excessive range of motion. Athletic participation with the upper extremity in a closed kinetic chain position increases the risk of injury[1] (Fig. 10–3). Excessive forces and abnormal ranges of motion placed on the wrist during gymnastic floor exercises, for instance, can contribute to a TFCC injury.

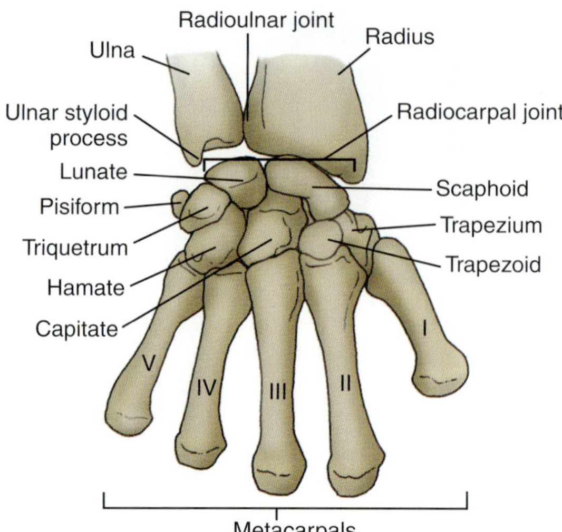



**Fig. 10–1**  *Dorsal view of the bones and joints of the wrist.*

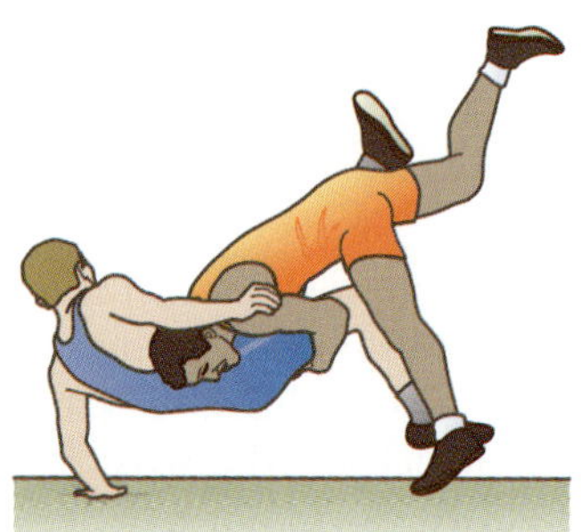

**Fig. 10–2**  *Wrist sprain.*

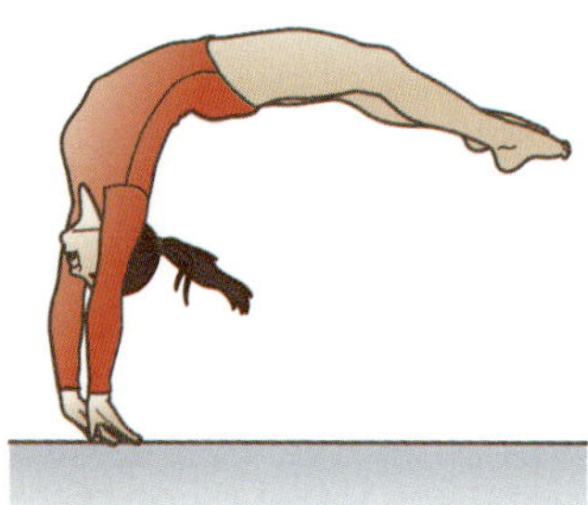

**Fig. 10–3**  *Upper extremity closed kinetic chain movement.*

## Fractures

Fractures to the distal radius can be the result of a fall on the outstretched arm. A fall on the outstretched arm and shearing forces can cause fractures of the scaphoid and hamate (Fig. 10–4).

## Dislocations

Dislocations of the wrist can occur at the distal radioulnar joint and may be associated with a fracture and soft tissue injury. The causes include excessive extension, pronation, and supination.

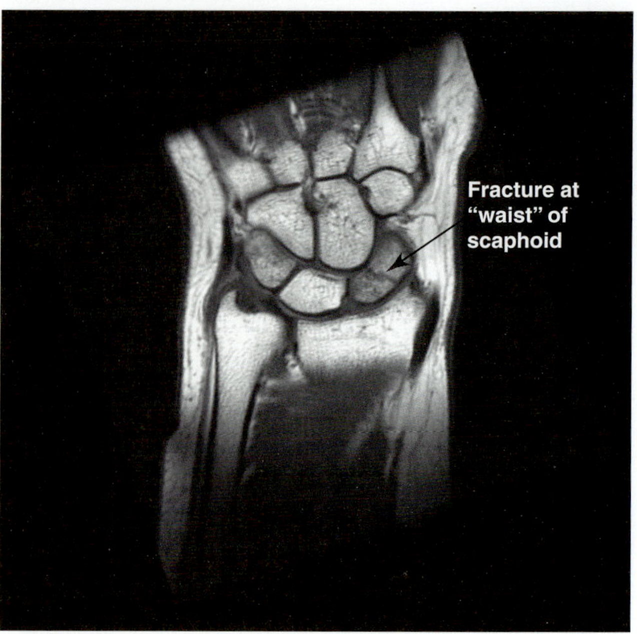



**Fig. 10–4**  *T1-weighted coronal MRI of the wrist. A fracture is evident as the low-signal-intensity line across the waist of the scaphoid. (Courtesy of McKinnis, LN. Fundamentals of Musculoskeletal Imaging, 4th ed. Philadelphia, PA: F.A. Davis Company: 2014.)*

## Ganglion Cysts

**Ganglion cysts** may form on the dorsal or **palmar** wrist following a sprain or repetitive hyperextension. A dorsal cyst is more commonly seen. For example, a cyst can develop in a competitive weightlifter as a result of daily training, which can cause repetitive hyperextension and overload.

## Overuse

Overuse injuries and conditions are caused by excessive, repetitive stress to the wrist. Repetitive pressure on the palmar aspect of the wrist and palms during athletic and work activities may cause flexor digitorum tendinitis (Fig. 10–5). Flexor carpi radialis and flexor carpi ulnaris tendinitis may be the result of excessive flexion often seen in sports involving a racquet. Excessive gripping and radial and ulnar deviation can cause **de Quervain's tenosynovitis.** Excessive use of a hammer, which requires constant gripping and repetitive wrist motion, can result in tenosynovitis. Nerve entrapment and compression syndromes are caused by repetitive wrist flexion and extension, direct forces, structural abnormalities, and repetitive compression and can affect the median, ulnar, and/or radial nerves. Compression of the median nerve is referred to as **carpal tunnel syndrome**[2] (Fig. 10–6). The excessive wrist flexion and extension experienced in rowing, for example, can lead to carpal tunnel syndrome.

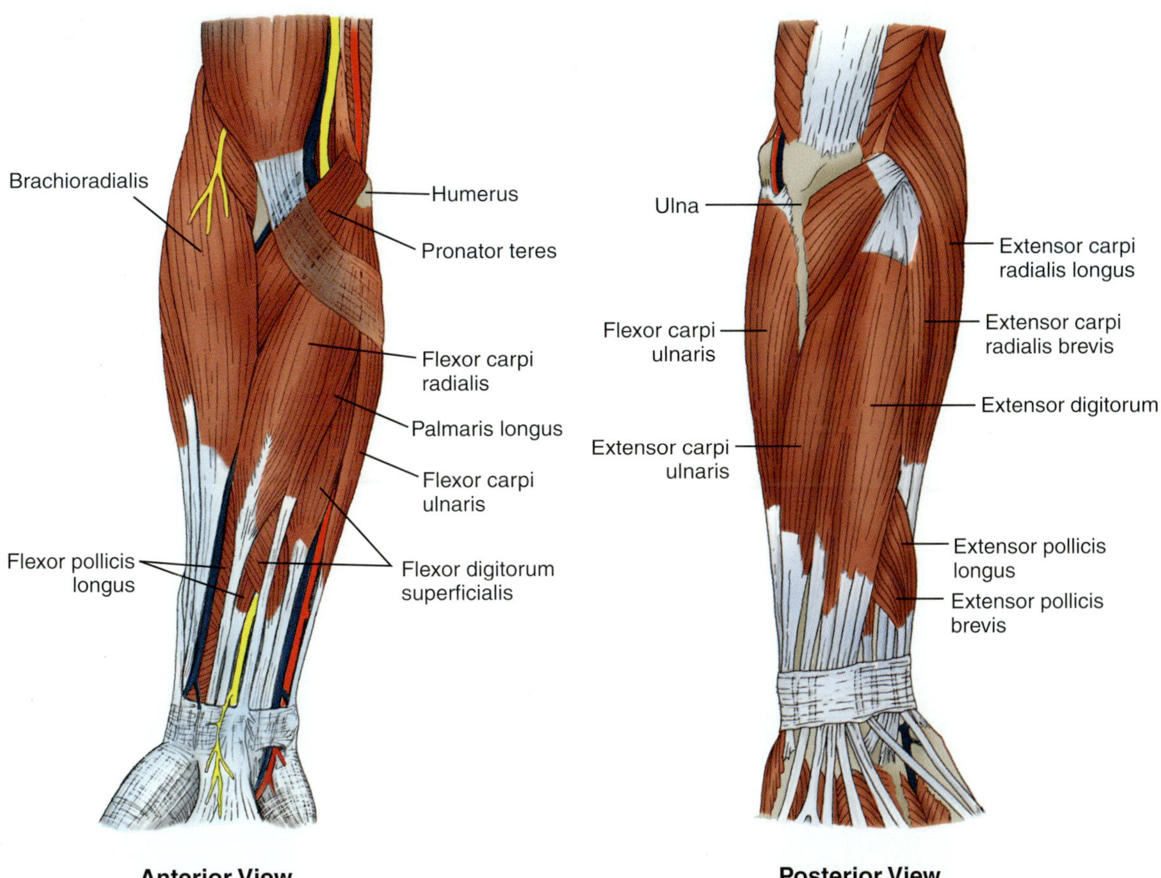


**Fig. 10–5** *Superficial muscles of the forearm and wrist.*

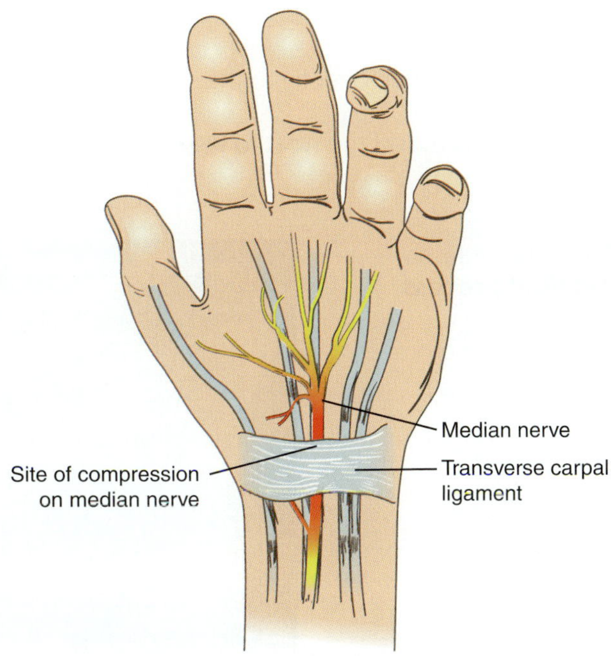


**Fig. 10–6** *Carpal tunnel syndrome.*

# Taping Techniques

Several taping techniques provide support, limit range of motion, and anchor protective padding to the wrist. Many techniques are used to prevent and treat sprains, TFCC injury, fractures, and dislocations and to provide support and lessen excessive range of motion. With proper application, these techniques provide varying amounts of support; the application of the same technique on two patients may produce different outcomes. Consider the purpose of the technique, the injury, the patient, and the activity when deciding which technique to use. Other taping techniques are used to immobilize the wrist or anchor protective padding. Note that many of these techniques may be used for hand and thumb injuries and conditions as indicated.

## CIRCULAR WRIST      Figure 10–7

➠ **Purpose:** Use the circular wrist technique to provide mild support, limit range of motion, and anchor protective padding to the wrist. Use this technique when preventing and treating contusions, sprains, fractures, and dislocations. Protective padding techniques are illustrated in the Padding section.

➠ **Materials:**
- 1½ inch or 2 inch non-elastic tape

*Options:*
- Pre-wrap or self-adherent wrap
- 2 inch or 3 inch elastic tape, taping scissors

➠ **Position of the patient:** Sitting on a taping table or bench with the wrist in a neutral position and the fingers in abduction.

> **Helpful Hint |**
> Maintain a neutral position of the wrist by having the patient place his or her extended, abducted fingers into your abdomen area. This position also lessens movement of the patient's arm during application.

➠ **Preparation:** Apply the circular wrist technique directly to the skin.
*Option:*
Apply pre-wrap or self-adherent wrap around the wrist to lessen irritation ⬅▬▬➡.

➠ **Application:**

**STEP 1:**   Anchor 1½ inch or 2 inch non-elastic tape over the **ulnar styloid process** (Fig. 10–7A).

*Option:*   *Use 2 inch or 3 inch elastic tape to provide additional support.*

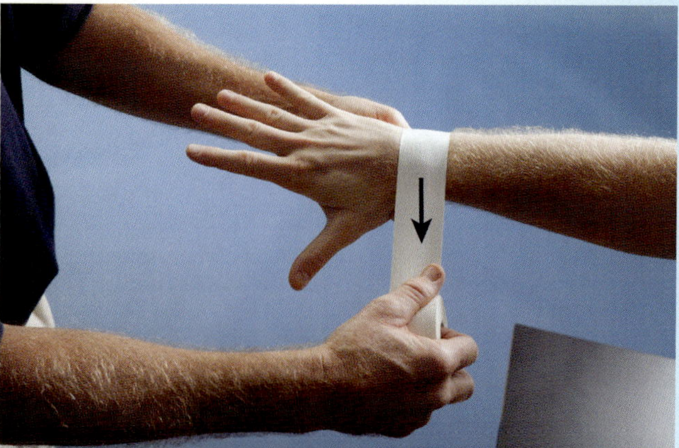

**Fig. 10–7 A**

**STEP 2:** Continue to apply the tape using a moderate amount of roll tension in a circular, lateral-to-medial direction around the wrist and return to the anchor (Fig. 10–7B).

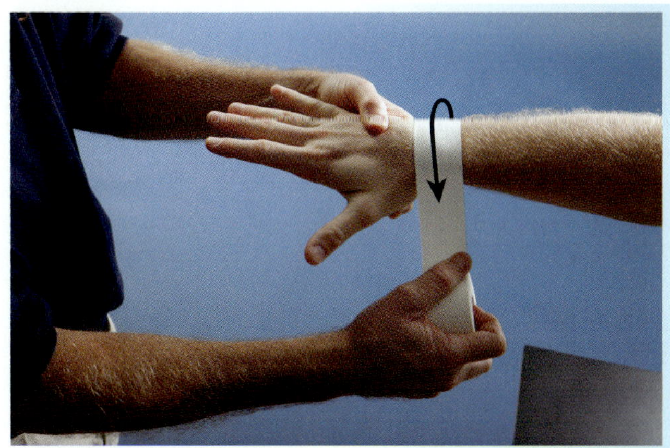

**Fig. 10–7 B**

**STEP 3:** Apply four to five additional circular strips around the wrist, either directly over the last strip or overlapping by ½ of the width of the tape (Fig. 10–7C). Apply the strips in an individual or continuous pattern with moderate roll tension.

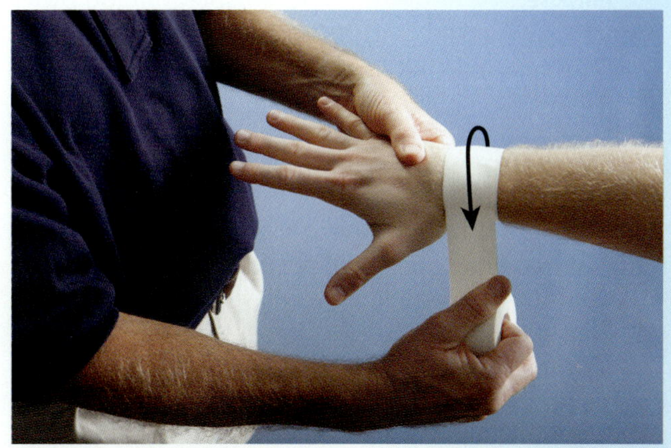

**Fig. 10–7 C**

*Option:* *Use 2 inch or 3 inch elastic tape for circular strips around the proximal hand and palm to provide additional support or anchor protective padding (Fig. 10–7D). These strips should not cause constriction of the thumb and hand.*

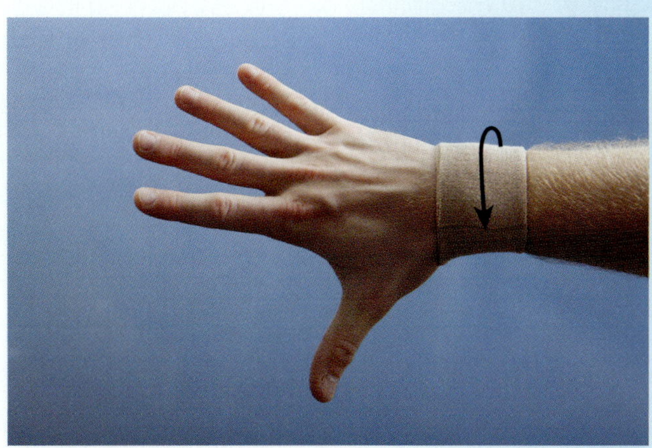

**Fig. 10–7 D**

*Steps Cont.*

**Wrist**

**STEP 4:** Finish the circular pattern over the dorsum of the wrist to prevent unraveling from contact with equipment during activity (Fig. 10–7E).

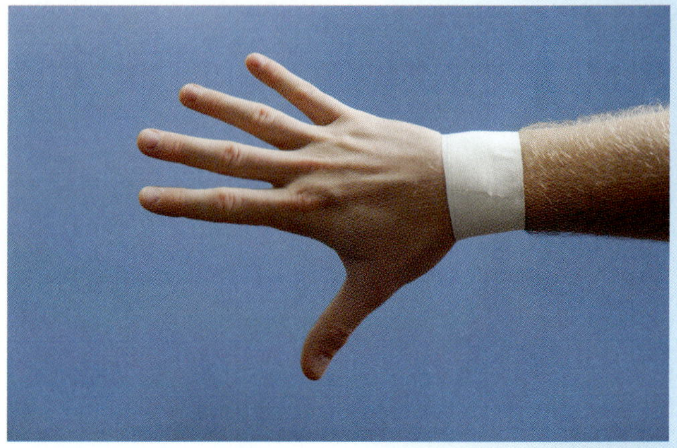

Fig. 10–7 E

## FIGURE-OF-EIGHT TAPE — Figure 10–8

➡ **Purpose:** The figure-of-eight wrist technique provides mild to moderate support, limits range of motion, and anchors custom-made braces and off-the-shelf and custom-made padding when preventing and treating contusions, sprains, TFCC injury, fractures, and dislocations (Fig. 10–8).

➡ **Materials:**
- 1½ inch or 2 inch non-elastic tape

*Options:*
- Pre-wrap
- 1½ inch or 2 inch elastic tape or self-adherent wrap, taping scissors

➡ **Position of the patient:** Sitting on a taping table or bench with the wrist and hand in a neutral position and the fingers in abduction.

➡ **Preparation:** Apply the figure-of-eight technique directly to the skin.

*Option:*

Apply pre-wrap around the hand and wrist to lessen irritation ◄▦►.

➡ **Application:**

**STEP 1:** Anchor 1½ inch non-elastic tape over the ulnar styloid process and encircle the wrist in a lateral-to-medial direction with moderate roll tension.

*Option:* *Consider using 1½ inch or 2 inch elastic tape or self-adherent wrap to prevent constriction of the hand.*

**STEP 2:** At the ulnar styloid process, proceed in a medial direction over the dorsum of the hand (Fig. 10–8A), continue over the **thenar web space,** then across the distal palm (Fig. 10–8B). The tape may need to be partially creased when covering the thenar web space to prevent constriction. Apply the tape with moderate roll tension and remain proximal to the **metacarpophalangeal (MCP) joints** of the hand.

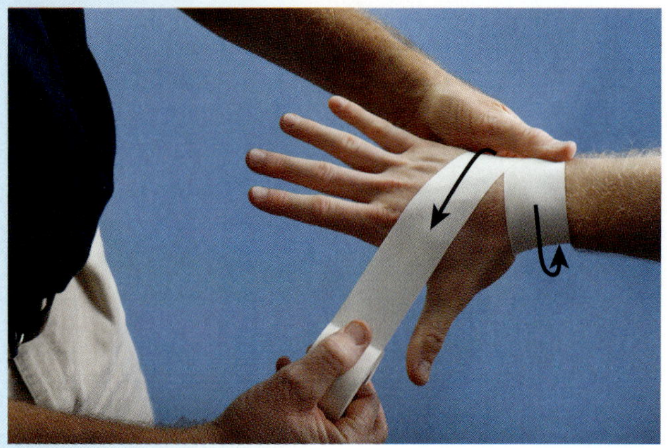

Fig. 10–8 A

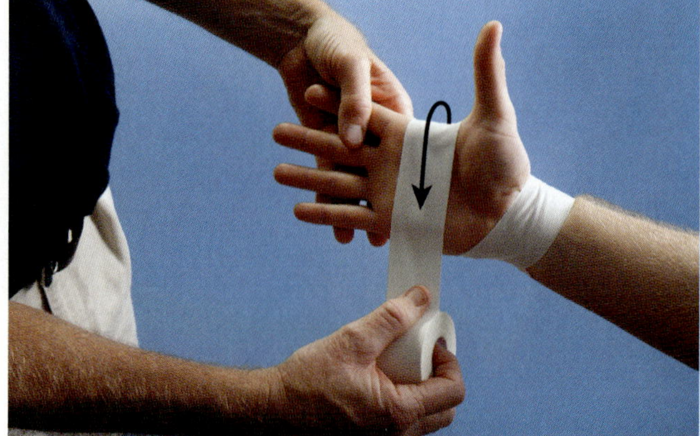

Fig. 10–8 B

**STEP 3:** Next, continue from the fifth metacarpal over the dorsum of the hand to the distal radius (Fig. 10–8C), around the wrist, and return to the ulnar styloid process with moderate roll tension (Fig. 10–8D).

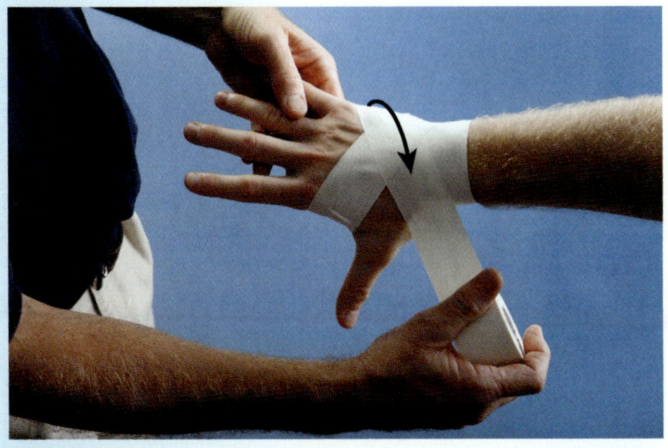

**Fig. 10–8 C**

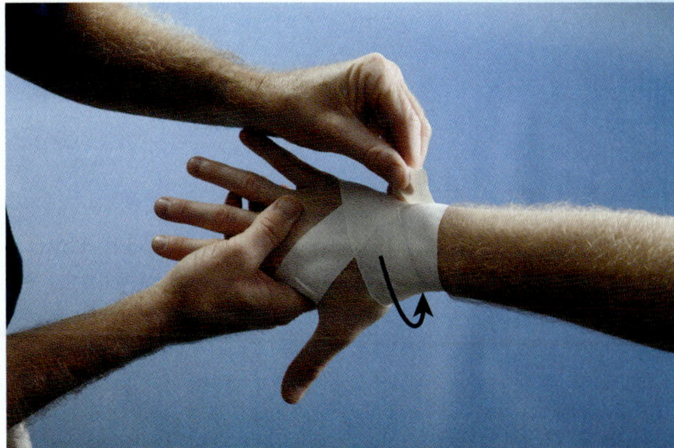

**Fig. 10–8 D**

**STEP 4:** Repeat the figure-of-eight pattern, overlapping by ⅓ of the tape width, and anchor on the dorsal wrist (Fig. 10–8E). The pattern should not cause constriction of the hand and thumb.

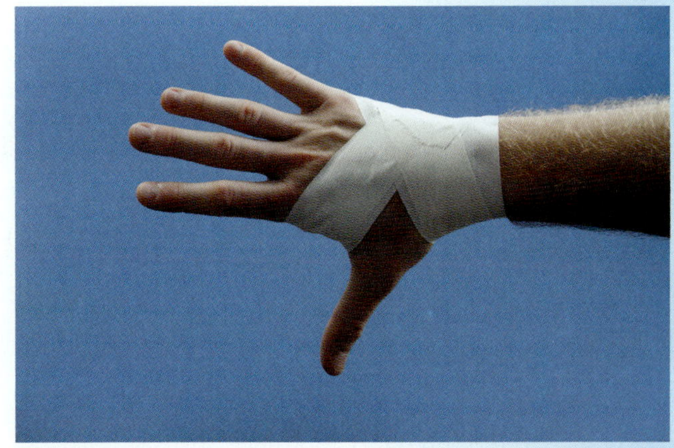

**Fig. 10–8 E**

## FAN TAPE    Figure 10–9

➡ **Purpose:** Use the fan technique to provide moderate support and limit excessive flexion and extension when preventing and treating sprains, TFCC injury, fractures, and dislocations (Fig. 10–9).

➡ **Materials:**
 • 1½ inch or 2 inch non-elastic and elastic tape, taping scissors
 ***Option:***
 • Pre-wrap or self-adherent wrap, adherent tape spray

➡ **Position of the patient:** Sitting on a taping table or bench with the wrist in a neutral position and the fingers in abduction. Determine painful range(s) of motion by placing the forearm on a table. Position the elbow in 90 degrees of flexion and the wrist over the edge of the table with the dorsal hand facing the floor.

To determine painful flexion, stabilize the forearm, place a hand on the dorsal fingers, and slowly move the hand and wrist into flexion until pain occurs. Place a hand on the palmar fingers and slowly move the hand and wrist into extension to determine painful extension. Once painful range(s) of motion is (are) determined, place the wrist in a pain-free range and maintain this position during application.

**Preparation:** Apply the fan technique directly to the skin.

**Option:**

Apply adherent tape spray and pre-wrap or self-adherent wrap around the hand and wrist to provide additional adherence and lessen irritation.

**Application:**

**STEP 1:** Apply an anchor of 1½ inch or 2 inch non-elastic tape around the distal hand, just proximal to the MCP joints, and an anchor around the distal forearm with mild roll tension (Fig. 10–9A).

*Option:* *Consider using 1½ inch or 2 inch elastic tape for the hand and forearm anchors to prevent constriction.*

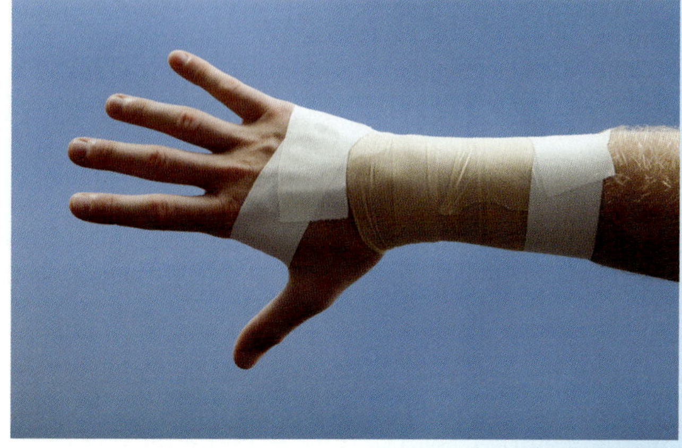

Fig. 10–9 A

**STEP 2:** To limit wrist flexion, anchor 1½ inch or 2 inch non-elastic tape on the dorsal lateral hand, proceed in a proximal direction across the hand and wrist, and anchor on the distal forearm (Fig. 10–9B). Monitor the pain-free position of the wrist and apply the tape with moderate roll tension.

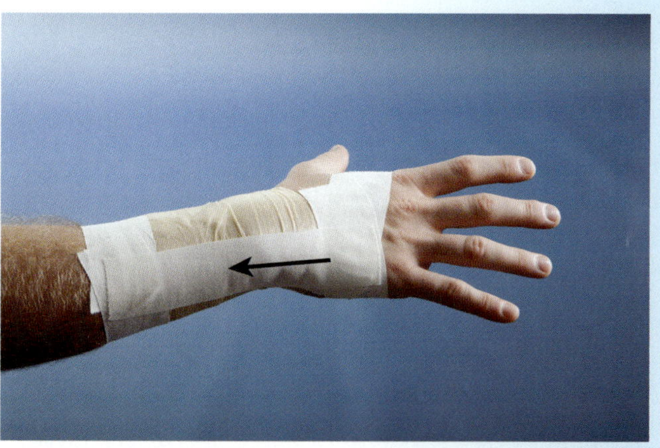

Fig. 10–9 B

**STEP 3:** Start the next strip on the dorsal hand by overlapping the first by ⅓ of the tape width. Continue across the hand and wrist, and anchor on the distal forearm (Fig. 10–9C).

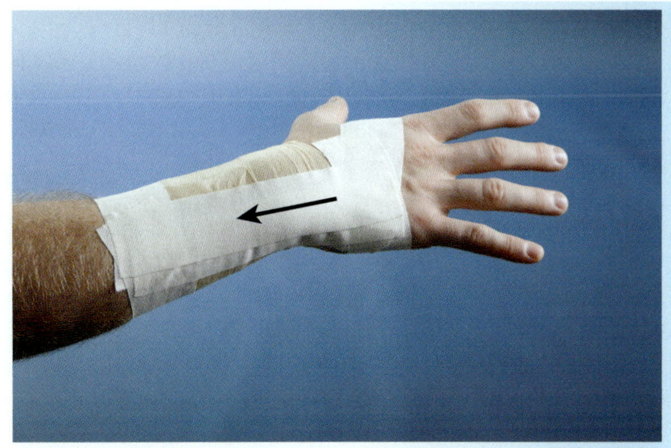

**Fig. 10–9 C**

**STEP 4:** Continue to apply four to five additional strips in this overlapping pattern with moderate roll tension (Fig. 10–9D). Apply enough strips to cover the dorsal hand. The fan should not constrict the thumb. The length from the distal hand to the distal forearm can be measured and a one-piece fan made.

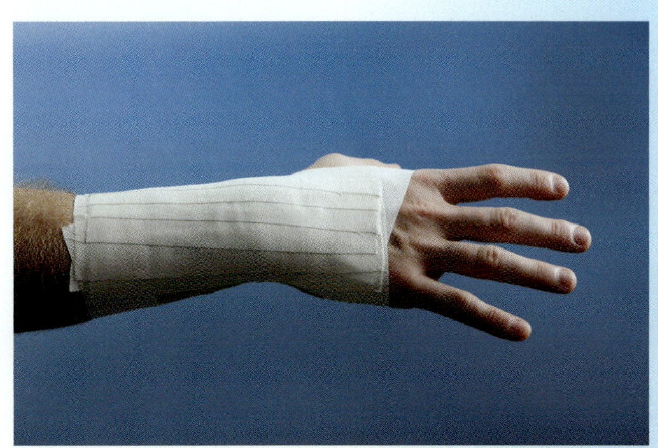

**Fig. 10–9 D**

### Helpful Hint |

On a taping table or bench, apply a strip of 1½ inch or 2 inch non-elastic tape of a length measured from the distal hand to the distal forearm. Continue to apply strips, overlapping by ⅓ of the tape width, until a 3 inch to 4 inch width fan is constructed. Smooth and adhere the strips together with the hands. Begin to remove the fan by pulling the first strip off the table or bench.

Make two fans by applying strips twice the length measured from the hand to the forearm. Continue to apply the overlapping strips and remove the fan from the table or bench. Bring the non-adherent ends together and cut the fan in half. Use one strip on the dorsal hand and the other on the palmar hand.

*Steps Cont.*

**STEP 5:** To limit wrist extension, anchor a strip of 1½ inch or 2 inch non-elastic tape on the palmar lateral hand; continue across the hand and wrist with moderate roll tension, and anchor on the distal forearm (Fig. 10–9E). Repeat the overlapping strips in a distal-to-proximal fashion (Fig. 10–9F). Monitor the pain-free position of the wrist.

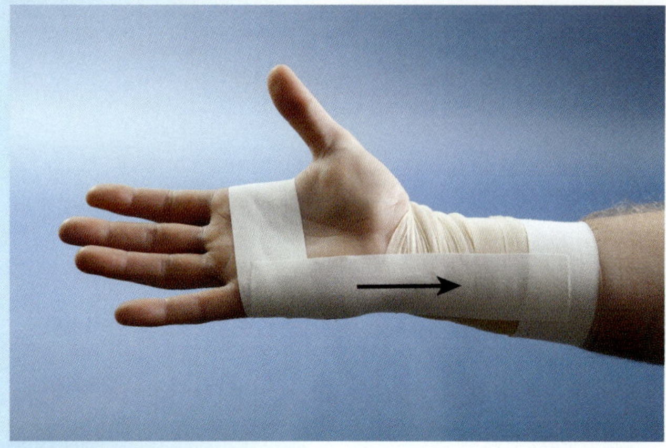

Fig. 10–9 E

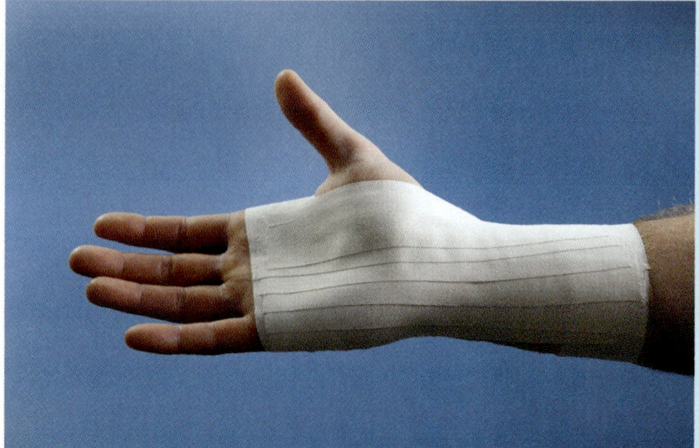

Fig. 10–9 F

**STEP 6:** At the distal hand and forearm, apply two to four closure strips with 1½ inch or 2 inch non-elastic or elastic tape with moderate roll tension ◀▥▶ (Fig. 10–9G). The closure strips should not cause constriction of the thumb. Partially crease the tape over the thenar web space if necessary.

**STEP 7:** Use a dorsal and palmar fan to limit multi-directional motion. The circular wrist or figure-of-eight technique may be applied to anchor the strips and provide additional support.

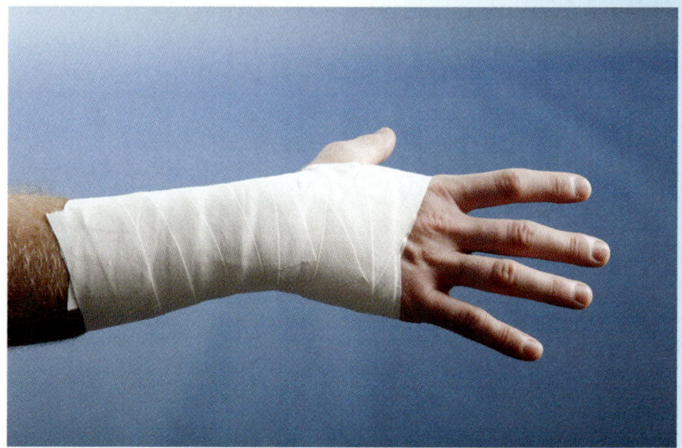

Fig. 10–9 G

## STRIP TAPE     Figures 10–10 and 10–11

➡ **Purpose:** The strip tape technique provides moderate support and limits excessive flexion and extension when preventing and treating sprains, TFCC injury, fractures, and dislocations. Two interchangeable methods are illustrated in the application of the technique. Choose according to patient preferences and available supplies.

### Strip Tape Technique One

➡ **Materials:**
  • 1½ inch or 2 inch non-elastic and elastic tape, 4 inch width heavy resistance exercise band, taping scissors
  **Option:**
  • Pre-wrap or self-adherent wrap, adherent tape spray

➡ **Position of the patient:** Sitting on a taping table or bench with the wrist in a neutral position and the fingers in abduction. Determine painful range(s) of motion. Once the range is determined, place the wrist in a pain-free range and maintain this position during application.

➡ **Preparation:** Apply strip tape technique one directly to the skin.
  **Option:**
  Apply adherent tape spray and pre-wrap or self-adherent wrap around the hand and wrist to provide additional adherence and lessen irritation ◀▥▶.

➡ **Application:**

**STEP 1:** Apply anchors as illustrated in Figure 10–9A.

**STEP 2:** To limit wrist flexion, anchor a piece of 4 inch width heavy resistance exercise band over the dorsal hand with 1½ inch or 2 inch elastic tape with mild roll tension ◄▬▬►. Leave approximately 2–3 inches of the band extending distally beyond the anchor (Fig. 10–10A).

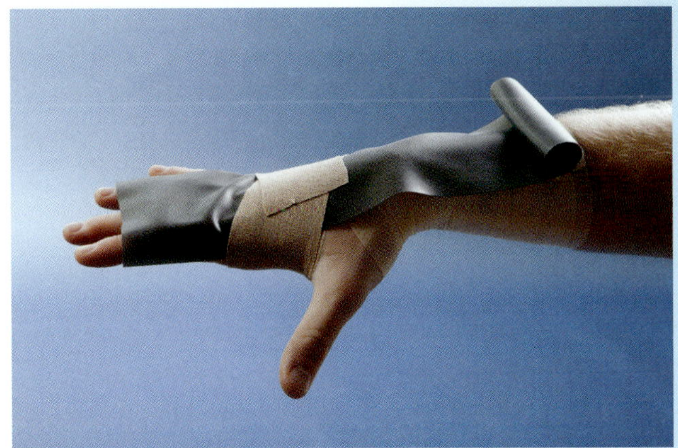

Fig. 10–10 A

**STEP 3:** Pull the band proximally with moderate tension across the hand and wrist, and anchor with mild roll tension on the distal forearm with 1½ inch or 2 inch elastic tape ◄▬▬► (Fig. 10–10B). Monitor the pain-free position of the wrist and cut the band approximately 2–3 inches beyond the anchor. A second piece of elastic exercise band may be applied directly over the first for additional support.

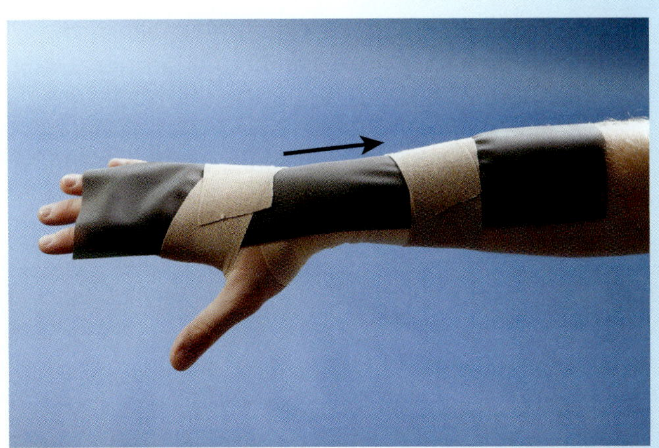

Fig. 10–10 B

**STEP 4:** To limit wrist extension, anchor the 4 inch heavy resistance exercise band with 1½ inch or 2 inch elastic tape on the palmar hand with mild roll tension, leaving approximately 2–3 inches of the band extending distally ◄▬▬►. Pull the band across the hand and wrist with moderate tension and anchor on the distal forearm ◄▬▬► (Fig. 10–10C). Cut the band approximately 2–3 inches beyond the anchor. Monitor the pain-free position of the wrist. Apply a second piece of elastic exercise band if necessary.

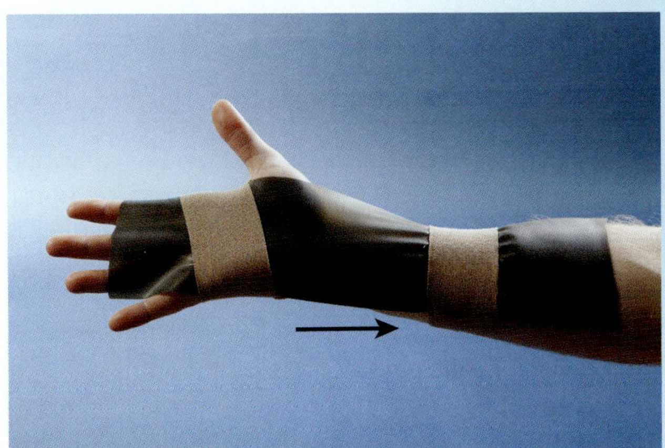

Fig. 10–10 C

*Steps Cont.*

**Wrist**

**STEP 5:** Fold the excess band over the distal hand and forearm anchors and apply two to three circular closure strips in an individual or continuous pattern with 1½ inch or 2 inch non-elastic or elastic tape ◄▥▥▥► (Fig. 10–10D). Apply the tape with moderate roll tension.

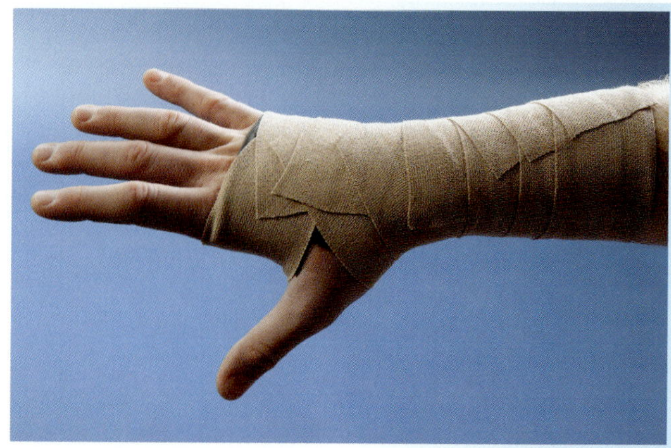

**Fig. 10–10 D**

**STEP 6:** Use the circular wrist or figure-of-eight technique to anchor the exercise band and provide additional support (Fig. 10–10E). Monitor the thumb and thenar web space to prevent constriction. To limit multidirectional motion, apply a dorsal and palmar elastic exercise band.

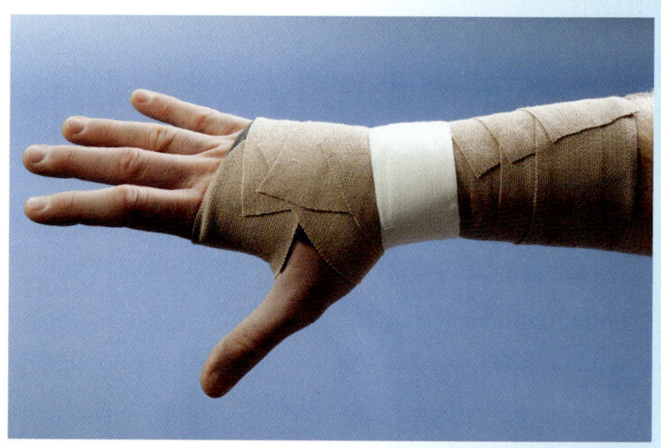

**Fig. 10–10 E**

### Strip Tape Technique Two

▥► **Materials:**
- 1½ inch or 2 inch non-elastic and elastic tape, 2 inch or 3 inch width heavyweight moleskin, taping scissors

*Option:*
- Pre-wrap or self-adherent wrap, adherent tape spray

▥► **Position of the patient:** Sitting on a taping table or bench with the wrist in a neutral position and the fingers in abduction. Determine painful range(s) of motion. Once the range is determined, place the wrist in a pain-free range and maintain this position during application.

▥► **Preparation:** Apply this strip tape technique directly to the skin.

*Option:*
Apply adherent tape spray and pre-wrap or self-adherent wrap around the hand and wrist to provide additional adherence and lessen irritation ◄▥▥▥►.

▥► **Application:**

**STEP 1:** Apply anchors as illustrated in Figure 10–9A.

**STEP 2:** Measure and cut a strip of 2 inch or 3 inch heavyweight moleskin from the distal hand to the distal forearm anchors.

**STEP 3:** To limit wrist flexion, apply the moleskin strip on the dorsal hand, pull the strip across the hand and wrist with moderate tension, and attach on the distal forearm (Fig. 10–11A). Monitor the pain-free position of the wrist.

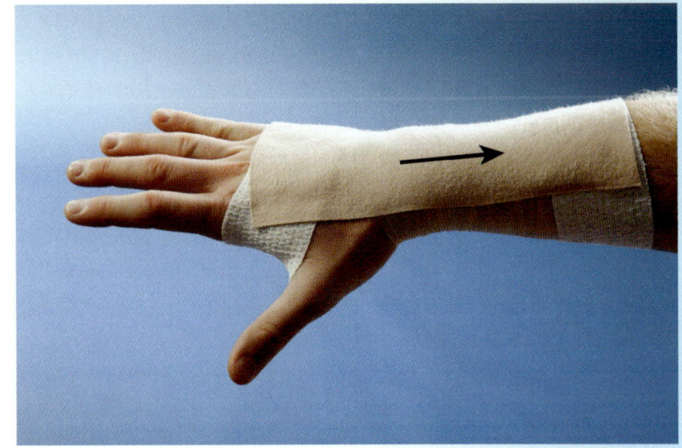

**Fig. 10–11 A**

**STEP 4:** Anchor the moleskin with mild tension on the distal hand and forearm with 1½ inch or 2 inch elastic tape ⬅▥▥▥▶ (Fig. 10–11B).

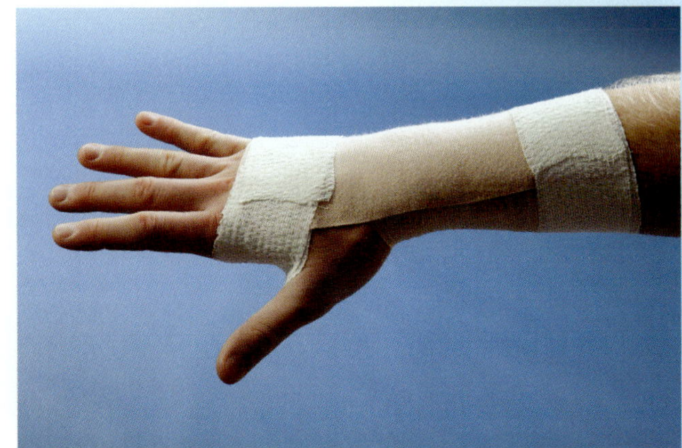

**Fig. 10–11 B**

**STEP 5:** To limit wrist extension, apply a moleskin strip on the palmar hand, continue over the hand and wrist with moderate tension, and anchor on the distal forearm (Fig. 10–11C). Anchor on the distal hand and forearm with 1½ inch or 2 inch elastic tape with mild roll tension ⬅▥▥▥▶ (Fig. 10–11D). Monitor the pain-free position of the wrist.

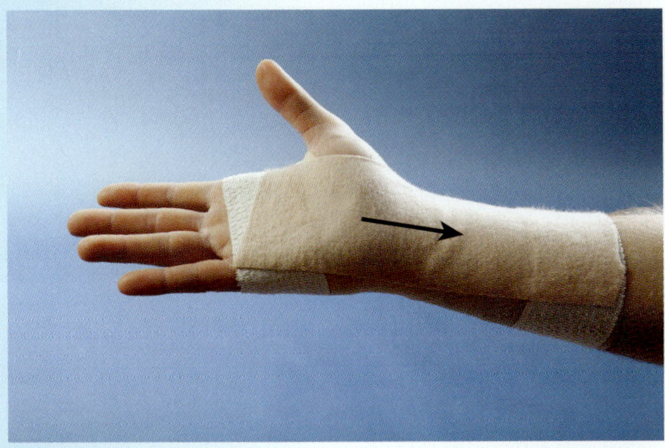

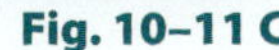

**Fig. 10–11 C**

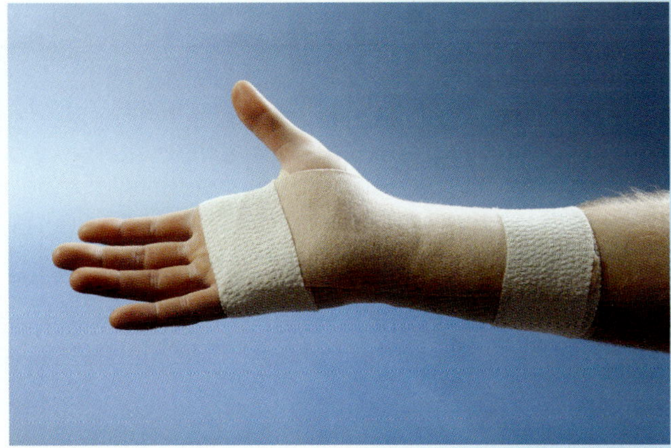

**Fig. 10–11 D**

*Steps Cont.*

**STEP 6:** Apply two to three individual or continuous circular closure strips with moderate roll tension around the hand and forearm with 1½ inch or 2 inch non-elastic or elastic tape ◄▬▬► (Fig. 10–11E).

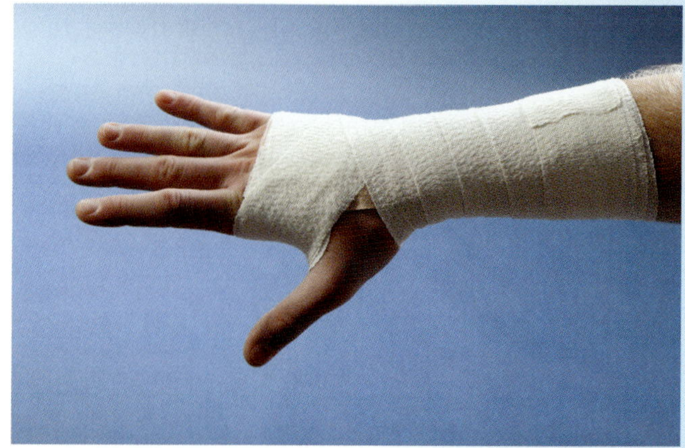

**Fig. 10–11 E**

**STEP 7:** Anchor the moleskin and provide additional support with the application of the circular wrist or figure-of-eight technique (Fig. 10–11F). Monitor the thumb and thenar web space to prevent constriction. Use both moleskin strips to limit multidirectional motion.

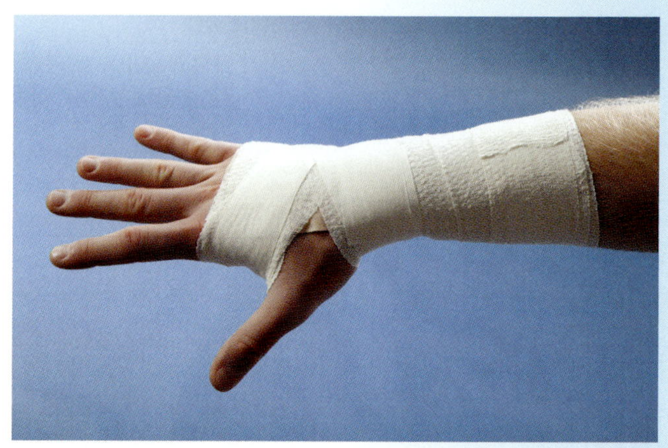

**Fig. 10–11 F**

## "X" TAPE　　Figure 10–12

▬► **Purpose:** The "X" technique provides moderate support and limits excessive flexion and extension when preventing and treating sprains, TFCC injury, fractures, and dislocations (Fig. 10–12).

▬► **Materials:**
- 1½ inch or 2 inch non-elastic and elastic tape, taping scissors

*Option:*
- Pre-wrap or self-adherent wrap, adherent tape spray

▬► **Position of the patient:** Sitting on a taping table or bench with the wrist in a neutral position and the fingers in abduction. Determine painful range(s) of motion. Once the range is determined, place the wrist in a pain-free range and maintain this position during application.

▬► **Preparation:** Apply the "X" technique directly to the skin.

*Option:*

Apply adherent tape spray and pre-wrap or self-adherent wrap around the hand and wrist to provide additional adherence and lessen irritation ◄▬▬►.

▬► **Application:**

**STEP 1:**  Apply anchors as illustrated in Figure 10–9A.

**STEP 2:**  To limit wrist flexion, anchor 1½ inch or 2 inch non-elastic tape at an angle on the dorsal hand proximal to the second MCP joint. Continue across the hand and wrist with moderate roll tension, and anchor on the lateral distal forearm (Fig. 10–12A). Monitor the pain-free position of the wrist.

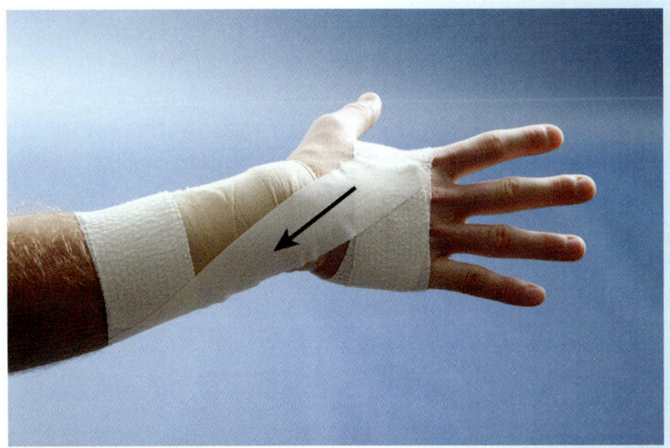

Fig. 10–12 A

**STEP 3:**  Apply the next strip on the dorsal hand proximal to the fifth MCP joint; proceed across the hand and wrist, and finish on the medial distal forearm (Fig. 10–12B).

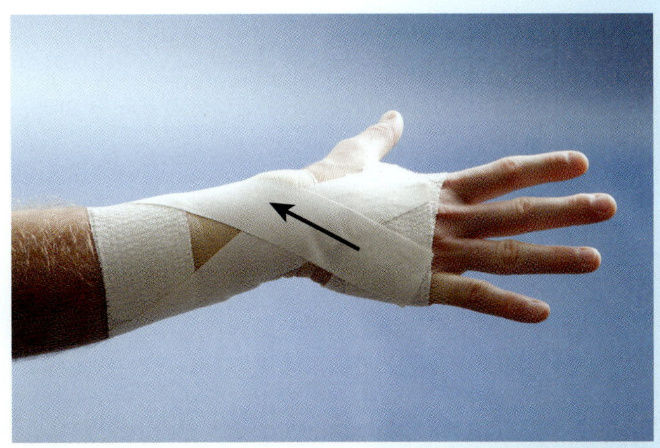

Fig. 10–12 B

**STEP 4:**  Overlap the tape by ⅓ of the width and apply two to four additional strips in the "X" pattern with moderate roll tension (Fig. 10–12C). Monitor the pain-free position of the wrist.

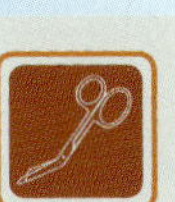

**Helpful Hint |**
Pre-make the "X" strip on a taping table or bench after determining the length from the distal hand to the distal forearm. Smooth and adhere the≈tape on the countertop, then place on the patient. Trim any excess tape with taping scissors.

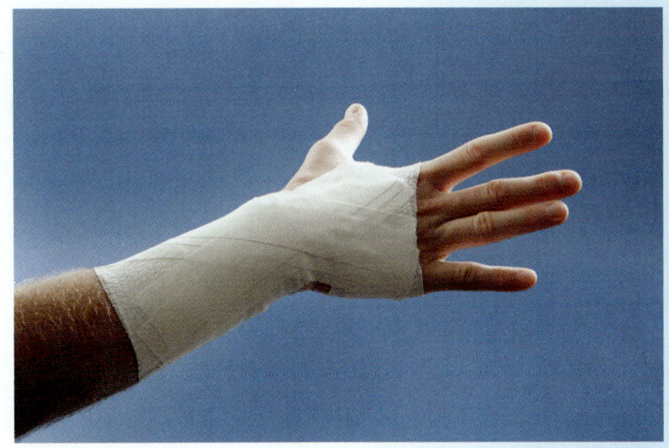

Fig. 10–12 C

*Steps Cont.*

**STEP 5:** To limit wrist extension, place 1½ inch or 2 inch non-elastic tape proximal to the second MCP joint at an angle on the palmar hand. Continue across the hand and wrist, and anchor on the medial distal forearm with moderate roll tension (Fig. 10–12D).

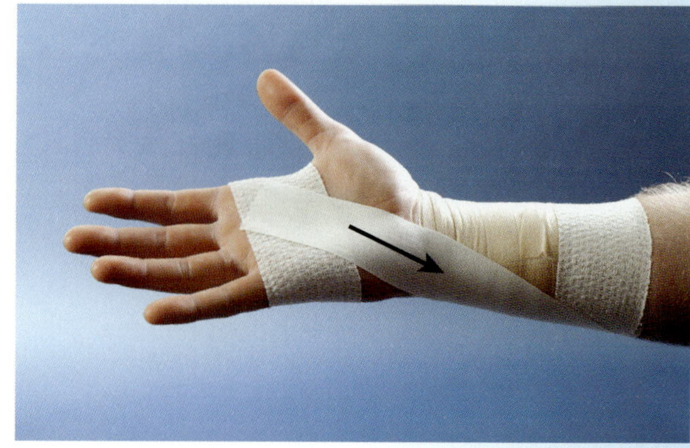

Fig. 10–12 D

**STEP 6:** Apply a strip on the palmar hand proximal to the fifth MCP joint, across the hand and wrist, and anchor on the lateral distal forearm (Fig. 10–12E).

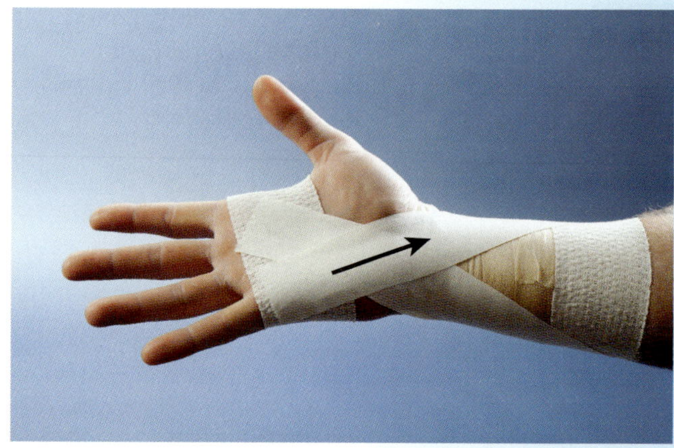

Fig. 10–12 E

**STEP 7:** Apply two to four additional strips, overlapping by ⅓ of the tape width, in the "X" pattern with moderate roll tension (Fig. 10–12F). Monitor the pain-free position of the wrist.

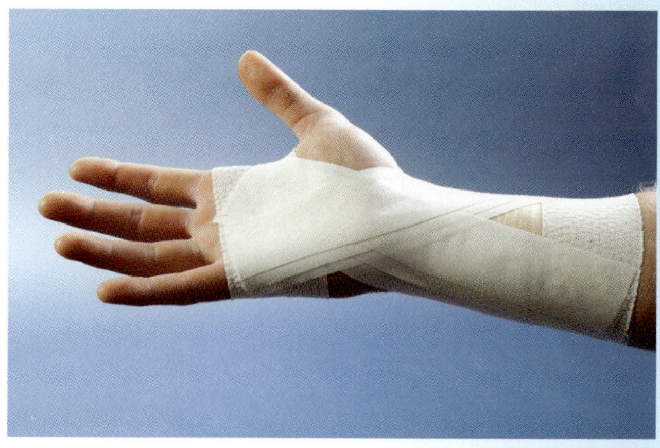

Fig. 10–12 F

**STEP 8:** Place two to four closure strips with moderate roll tension in a circular pattern around the hand and forearm, using 1½ inch or 2 inch non-elastic or elastic tape ◀▦▦▶ (Fig. 10–12G).

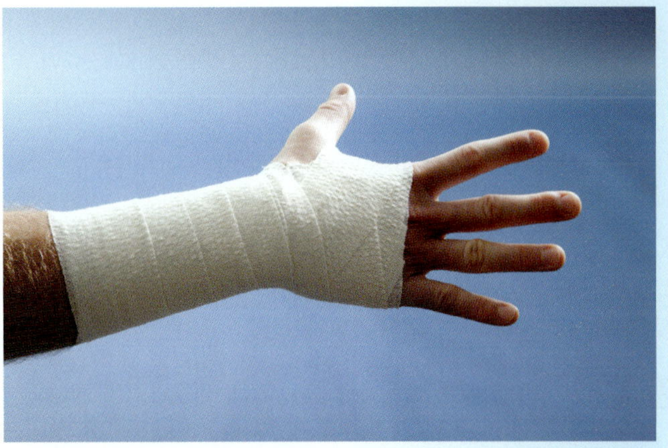

Fig. 10–12 G

**STEP 9:** Apply the circular wrist or figure-of-eight technique to anchor the strips and provide additional support (Fig. 10–12H). Monitor the thumb and thenar web space to prevent constriction. Use the dorsal and palmar "X" strips to limit multi-directional motion.

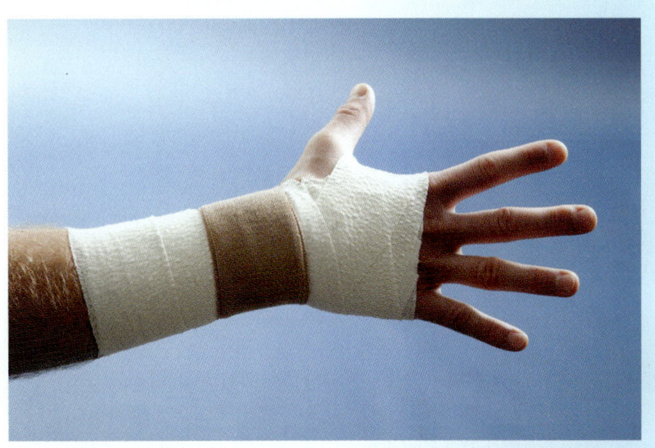

Fig. 10–12 H

## Clinical Application Question 1

About midway through the Australian Rules Football season, a half forward suffers a right wrist sprain caused by a fall during a match. Following a period of rehabilitation, he is allowed to return to activity with an off-the-shelf functional brace that has been approved for use. During the first match, the half forward falls on his right outstretched arm but continues to play.

➠ **Question: What taping techniques can you apply at halftime to provide additional stability?**

### . . . IF/THEN . . .

**IF** an athlete asks for the wrists to be taped and she or he has no history of injury, **THEN** consider applying the non-elastic tape circular wrist technique; it provides mild support, is quick to apply, and requires less expensive non-elastic tape.

## WRIST SEMIRIGID CAST   Figure 10–13

➠ **Purpose:** The semirigid cast technique provides maximum support and limits wrist range of motion when treating sprains, TFCC injury, fractures, and dislocations (Fig. 10–13). The cast should be applied by qualified health care professionals. The cast may be used during athletic and work activities, removed, and then used again.

**Wrist**

➠ **Materials:**
- 2 inch or 3 inch semirigid cast tape, gloves, water, self-adherent wrap, ⅛ inch foam or felt, 2 inch elastic tape, taping scissors

*Option:*
- Thermoplastic material, a heating source

➠ **Position of the patient:** Sitting on a taping table or bench with the hand and wrist in the position to be immobilized, as indicated by a physician, and the fingers in abduction.

➠ **Preparation:** Apply ⅛ inch foam or felt over bony prominences and palmar surface of the thumb to lessen the occurrence of irritation.

➠ **Application:**

**STEP 1:** Apply two to three layers of self-adherent wrap to the hand, wrist, and distal forearm with mild to moderate roll tension ◄▬▬► (Fig. 10–13A). The wrap may be applied in a figure-of-eight pattern.

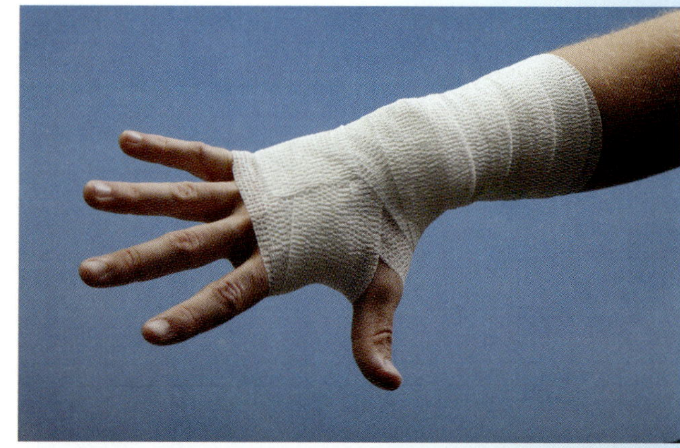

**Fig. 10–13 A**

**STEP 2:** With 2 inch or 3 inch semirigid cast tape, anchor on the distal lateral forearm and apply circular, lateral-to-medial patterns with moderate roll tension in a proximal-to-distal direction, overlapping the tape by ⅓–⅔ of its width (Fig. 10–13B).

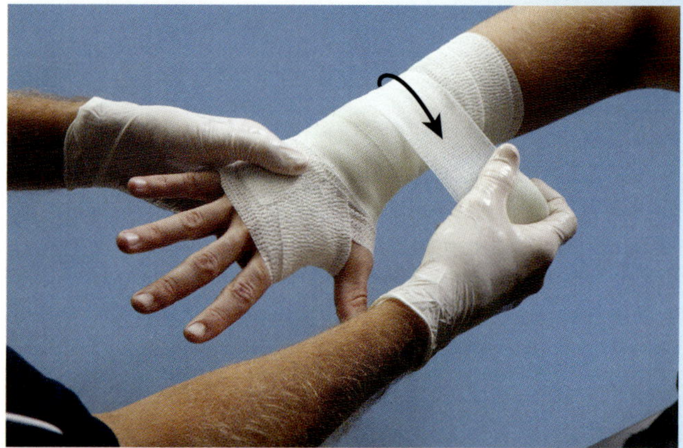

**Fig. 10–13 B**

**STEP 3:** At the wrist, continue to apply the tape in a figure-of-eight pattern with moderate roll tension involving the hand and wrist (Fig. 10–13C). Apply the tape proximal to the MCP joints of fingers two through five. Depending on the patient's size, the cast tape may need to be creased or partially cut when covering the thenar web space to prevent constriction.

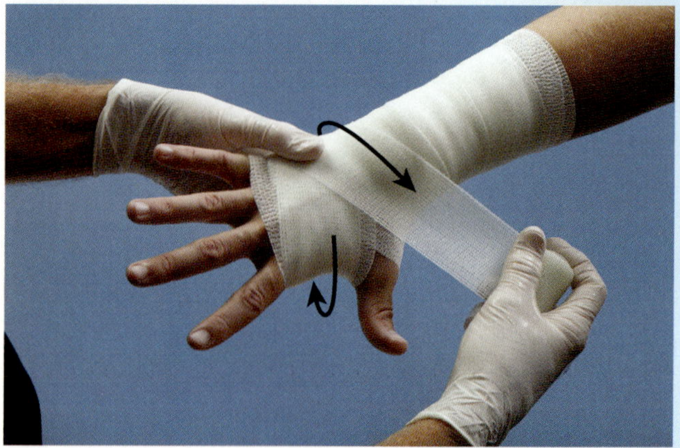

**Fig. 10–13 C**

*Option:*     *Mold and incorporate thermoplastic material over the dorsal and/or palmar hand and wrist to provide additional support (Fig. 10–13D).*

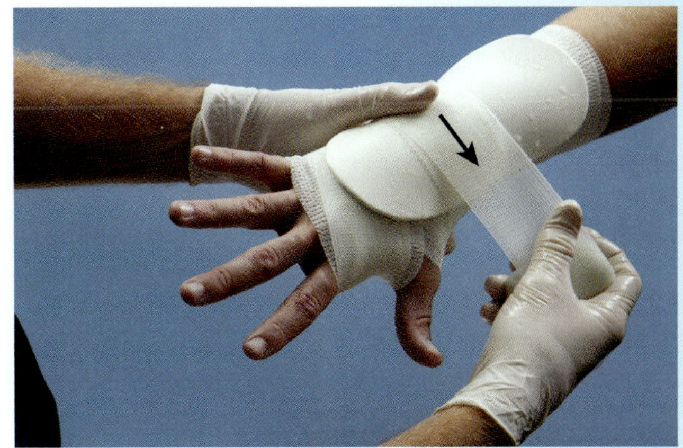

Fig. 10–13 D

**STEP 4:**     Continue to alternate figures-of-eight with circular patterns around the hand, wrist, and distal forearm, overlapping the tape by ⅓–⅔ of its width (Fig. 10–13E).

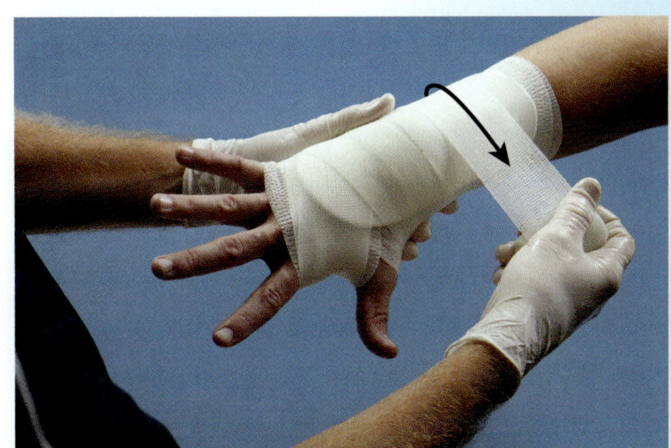

Fig. 10–13 E

**STEP 5:**     Finish the tape pattern on the dorsal wrist/distal forearm and smooth and mold the cast with the hands (Fig. 10–13F).

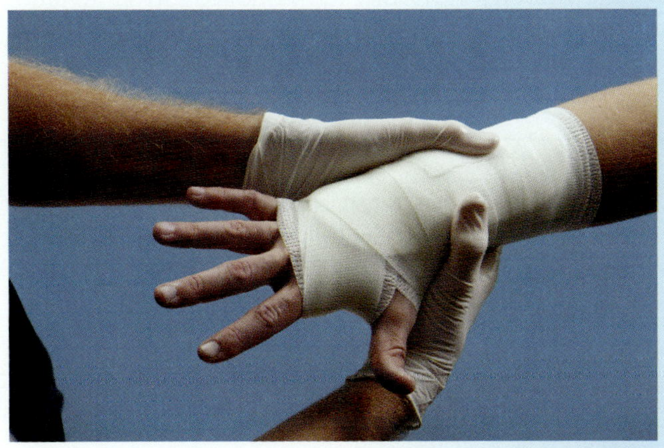

Fig. 10–13 F

*Steps Cont.*

**STEP 6:** Cover the semirigid cast with closed-cell, slow-recovery foam or similar material of at least ½ inch thickness for all athletic practices and competitions (see Fig. 10–21A–B).

**STEP 7:** Remove the cast by cutting with taping scissors along the ulnar or radial aspect of the cast (Fig. 10–13G). Choose the side that is opposite from the injured area.

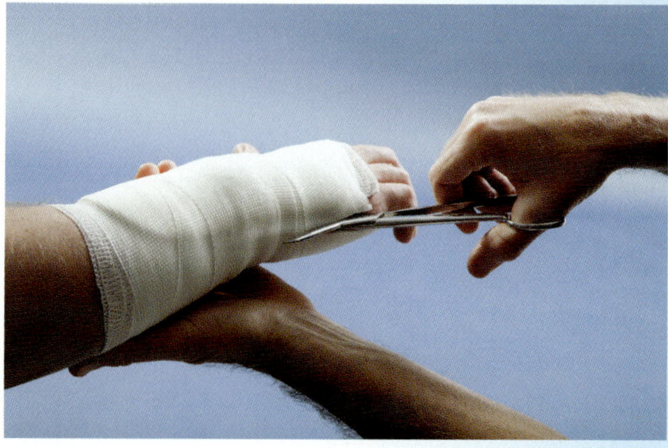

Fig. 10–13 G

**STEP 8:** To reuse, apply two to three layers of self-adherent wrap to the hand, wrist, and distal forearm ⬅▬▶. Place the cast on the hand, wrist, and forearm, and anchor with 2 inch elastic tape or self-adherent wrap with moderate roll tension in a circular pattern ⬅▬▶ (Fig. 10–13H).

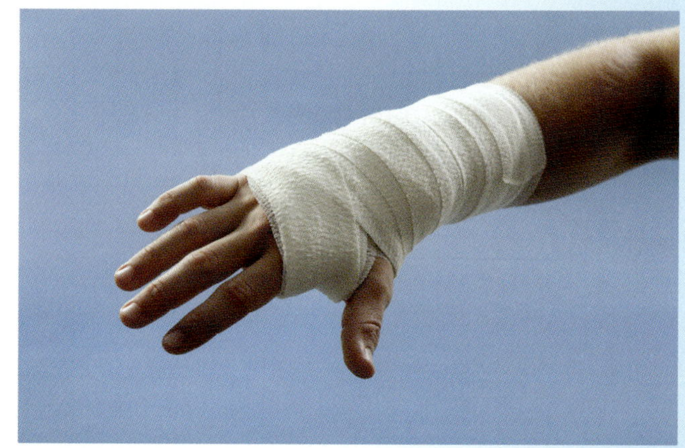

Fig. 10–13 H

## POSTERIOR SPLINT    Figure 10–14

**Purpose:** The posterior splint technique is used to immobilize the wrist and hand when treating sprains, TFCC injury, fractures, dislocations, and overuse injuries and conditions (Fig. 10–14). Use the splint as temporary immobilization prior to further evaluation by a physician. This technique is applied with the same materials listed in Chapter 9 (see Fig. 9–13). Two methods are interchangeable in applying the posterior splint technique to accommodate available supplies; the first is illustrated here (Fig. 10–14), and the second is online at FADavis.com ✿.

### DETAILS
Periods of immobilization are normally determined by a physician following evaluation of the patient. Cast technicians and physicians can provide complete immobilization with rigid cast tape applied over stockinet.

**Design:**
- Purchase off-the-shelf rigid splints in pre-cut and padded designs. The splints are manufactured of several layers of rigid fiberglass material, covered with fabric and foam padding in 2, 3, 4, and 5 inch widths by 10, 12, 15, 30, 35, and 45 inch lengths.

### Posterior Splint Technique One
**Materials:**
- Off-the-shelf rigid, padded splint, gloves, water, towel, two 4 inch width by 5 yard length elastic wraps, metal clips, 1½ inch non-elastic tape or 2 inch self-adherent wrap

➡ **Position of the patient:** Sitting on a taping table or bench with the hand and wrist in a neutral position. Place the wrist in the desired range of flexion or extension as indicated by a physician. Maintain this position during application.

➡ **Preparation:** Mold and apply the padded splint directly to the skin.

➡ **Application:**

**STEP 1:** Remove the splint from the package and immerse in water of 70° to 75°F. Submerge the splint the length of time to squeeze the splint once or twice. Remove the splint from the water and place lengthwise on a towel. Quickly roll the splint and towel together to remove excess water (Fig. 10–14A).

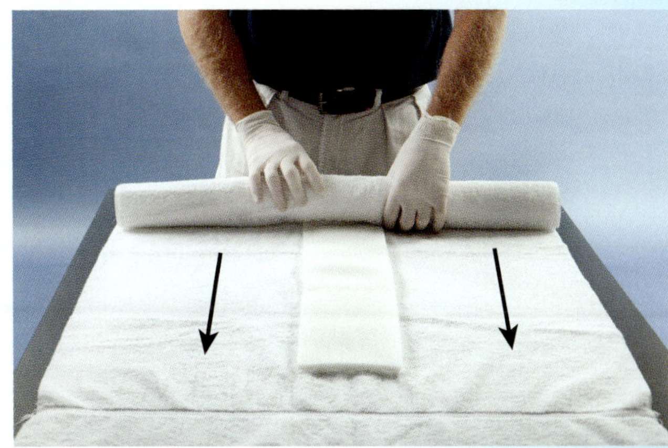

**Fig. 10–14 A**

**STEP 2:** Apply the splint from just proximal to the MCP joints of fingers two through five to the mid to proximal forearm (Fig. 10–14B). The splint is most commonly used on the palmar aspect of the hand, wrist, and forearm.

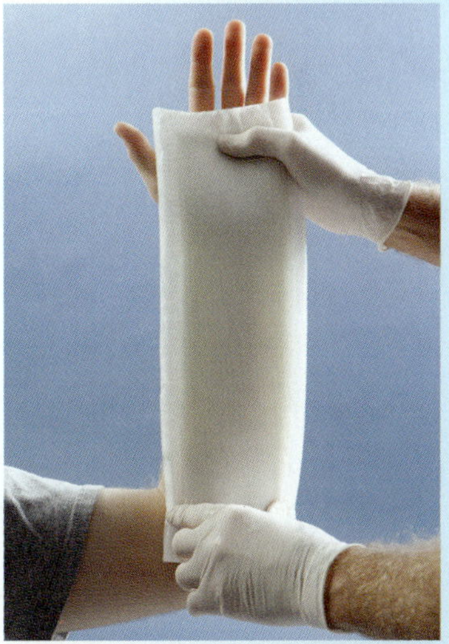

**Fig. 10–14 B**

**STEP 3:** Apply a 4 inch width by 5 yard length elastic wrap in a spiral pattern with moderate roll tension to mold the splint to the contours of the hand, wrist, and forearm ◀▪▪▪▪▶ (Fig. 10–14C). Mold and shape the splint with the hands. Monitor the position of wrist flexion or extension. After 10–15 minutes, the fiberglass should be cured; remove the elastic wrap.

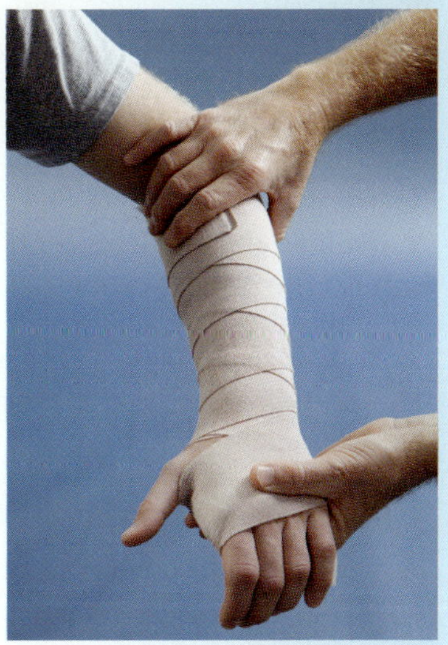

**Fig. 10–14 C**

*Steps Cont.*

**STEP 4:**  Attach the splint to the hand, wrist, and forearm with another 4 inch width by 5 yard length elastic wrap with moderate roll tension using a distal-to-proximal spiral pattern ◀▬▬▶ (Fig. 10–14D). Anchor the wrap with metal clips, or loosely applied 1½ inch non-elastic tape or 2 inch self-adherent wrap. A sling may be required for daily activities.

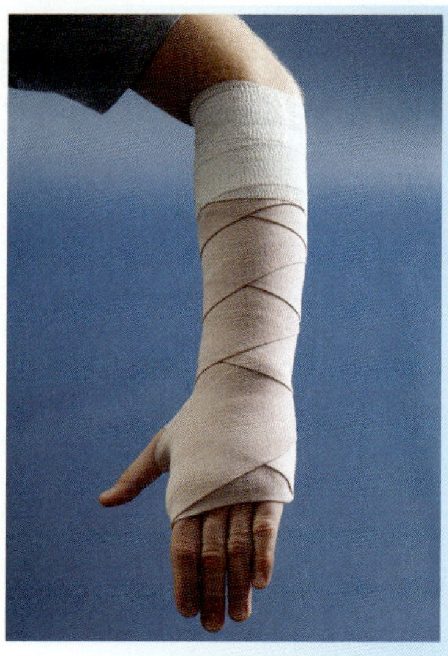

**Fig. 10–14 D**

# Wrapping Techniques

Use wrapping techniques to provide compression to assist in controlling swelling following soft tissue injuries and conditions. Use elastic and self-adherent wraps also to anchor protective padding and braces when preventing and treating contusions, sprains, fractures, dislocations, and overuse injuries and conditions. These techniques can also be used for hand injuries and conditions as indicated.

## HAND AND WRIST COMPRESSION WRAP     Figure 10–15

➡ **Purpose:** The hand and wrist compression wrap technique provides pressure and lessens mild, moderate, or severe swelling and inflammation when treating contusions, sprains, dislocations, and ganglion cysts (Fig. 10–15).

➡ **Materials:**
  • 2 inch, 3 inch, or 4 inch width by 5 yard length elastic wrap, metal clips, 1½ inch non-elastic or 1½ inch or 2 inch elastic tape, ⅛ inch or ¼ inch foam or felt, taping scissors
  *Options:*
  • 1½ inch, 2 inch, or 3 inch width self-adherent wrap
  • ¼ inch or ½ inch open-cell foam

➡ **Position of the patient:** Sitting on a taping table or bench with the wrist and hand in a pain-free position and the fingers in abduction.

➡ **Preparation:** Because of the irregular shape of the hand and wrist, place ⅛ inch or ¼ inch foam or felt over the inflamed area directly to the skin to assist in venous return. The pad is particularly useful for providing compression following aspiration of a ganglion cyst.

➡ **Application:**

**STEP 1:** Anchor the extended end of the elastic wrap on the dorsal surface of the hand just distal to the MCP joints of fingers two through five and encircle the hand ◀▦▶ (Fig. 10–15A).

*Option:* *If an elastic wrap is not available, 1½ inch, 2 inch, or 3 inch self-adherent wrap may be used.*

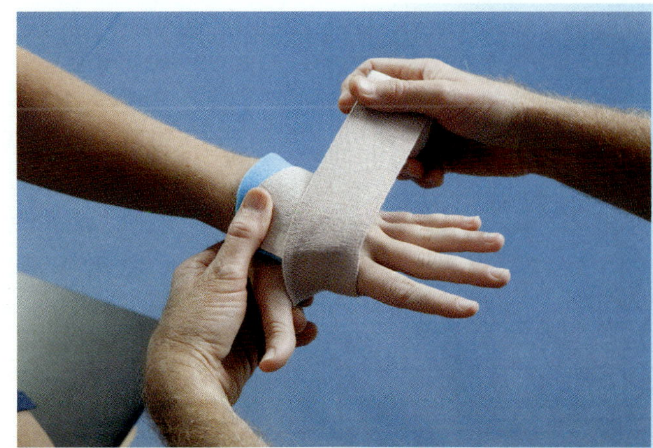

**Fig. 10–15 A**

**STEP 2:** Continue around the hand over the thenar web space, overlapping the wrap by ⅓–½ of its width (Fig. 10–15B).

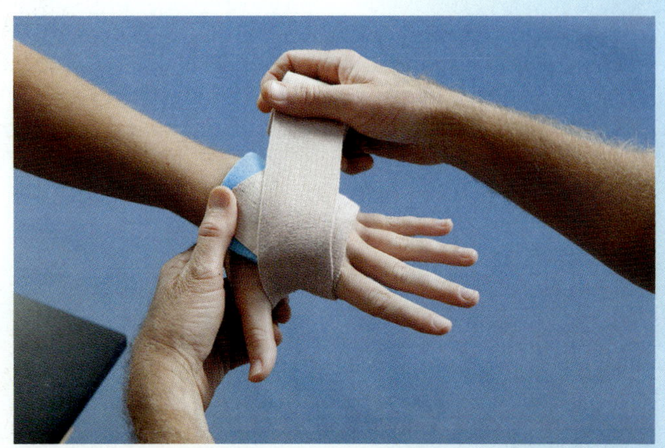

**Fig. 10–15 B**

**STEP 3:** Next, proceed across the dorsal hand, encircle the wrist, then across the dorsal hand, and encircle the hand in a figure-of-eight pattern (Fig. 10–15C).

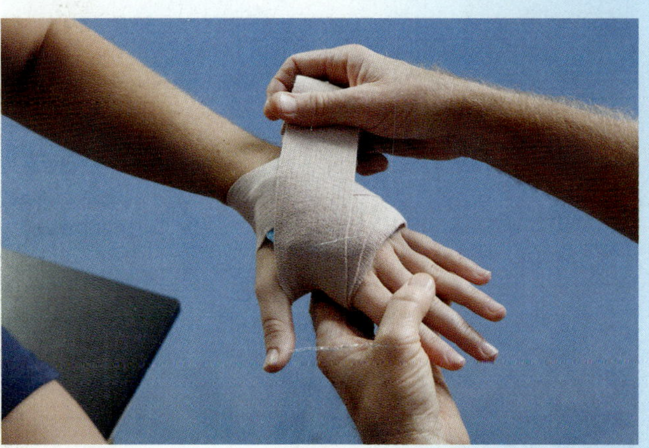

**Fig. 10–15 C**

*Steps Cont.*

**STEP 4:** Repeat the figure-of-eight pattern, overlapping by ⅓–½ of the wrap width (Fig. 10–15D). Cover all exposed areas. Roll tension is greatest distally and lessens proximally.

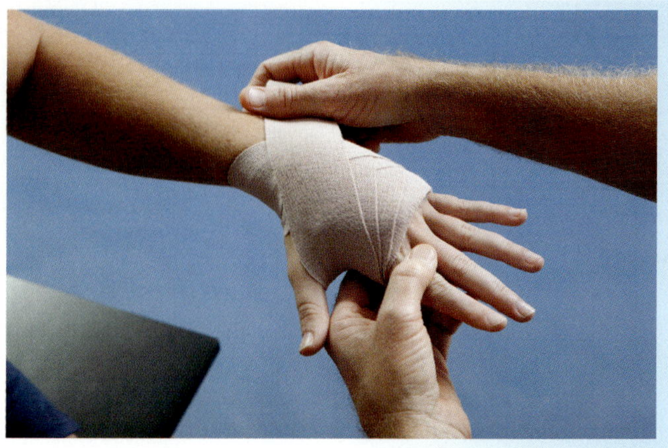

Fig. 10–15 D

**STEP 5:** At the wrist, continue the wrap in a distal-to-proximal direction over the distal forearm in a spiral pattern. Anchor over the dorsum of the distal forearm with Velcro, metal clips, or loosely applied 1½ inch non-elastic or 1½ inch or 2 inch elastic tape ◄▦▦► (Fig. 10–15E). In order to lessen migration, apply a figure-of-eight pattern loosely through the hand with 1½ inch or 2 inch elastic tape or self-adherent wrap ◄▦▦► (Fig. 10–15F).

*Option:* *A ¼ inch or ½ inch open-cell foam pad may be placed over the dorsal hand, extending from the MCP joints to the wrist, for additional compression (see Fig. 11–27). Apply the pad directly on the skin and cover with the compression wrap.*

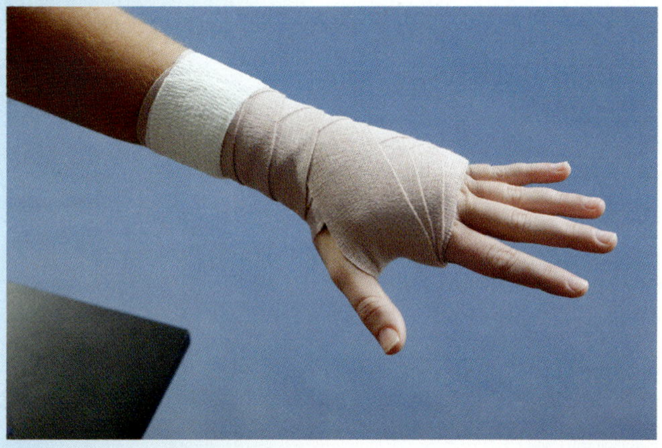

Fig. 10–15 E

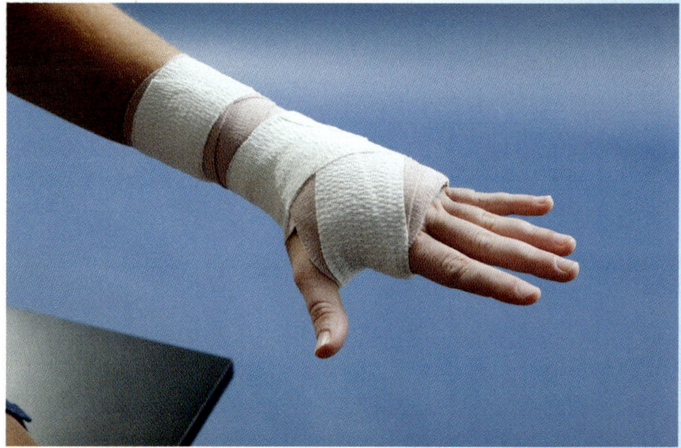

Fig. 10–15 F

## FIGURE-OF-EIGHT WRAP     Figure 10–16

▦► **Purpose:** Use the figure-of-eight wrist technique to provide compression and mild support and to anchor custom-made braces and protective padding when preventing and treating contusions, sprains, TFCC injury, fractures, dislocations, and overuse injuries and conditions (Fig. 10–16).

▦► **Materials:**
  • 2 inch, 3 inch, or 4 inch width by 5 yard length elastic wrap, metal clips, 1½ inch non-elastic or 1½ inch or 2 inch elastic tape, taping scissors
  **Option:**
  • 1½ inch, 2 inch, or 3 inch width self-adherent wrap

➠ **Position of the patient:** Sitting on a taping table or bench with the wrist and hand in a neutral position and the fingers in abduction.

➠ **Preparation:** To lessen migration, apply adherent tape spray, tape strips, or anchors directly to the skin (see Fig. 1–7).

➠ **Application:**

**STEP 1:**  Place the brace or pad over the injured area.

**STEP 2:**  Anchor the elastic wrap directly to the skin over the ulnar styloid process and apply the figure-of-eight taping technique with moderate roll tension (Fig. 10–16A).

*Option:*  *If an elastic wrap is not available, 1½ inch, 2 inch, or 3 inch self-adherent wrap may be used.*

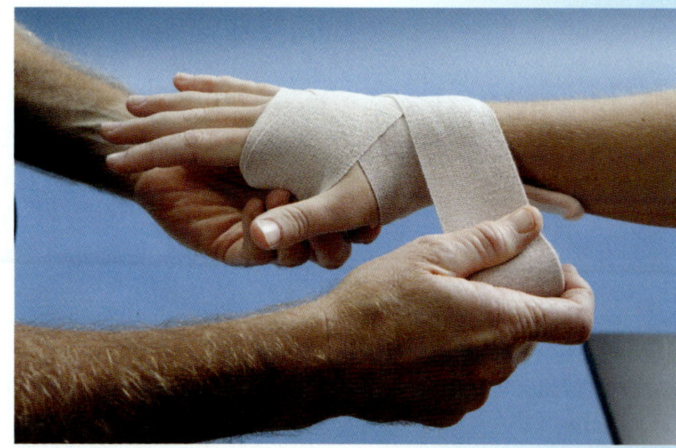

**Fig. 10–16 A**

**STEP 3:**  Finish the wrap and anchor over the wrist or distal forearm with Velcro, metal clips, or loosely applied 1½ inch non-elastic or 1½ inch or 2 inch elastic tape ◀▬▬▶ (Fig. 10–16B). A figure-of-eight pattern may be applied loosely through the hand with 1½ inch or 2 inch elastic tape or self-adherent wrap for additional support.

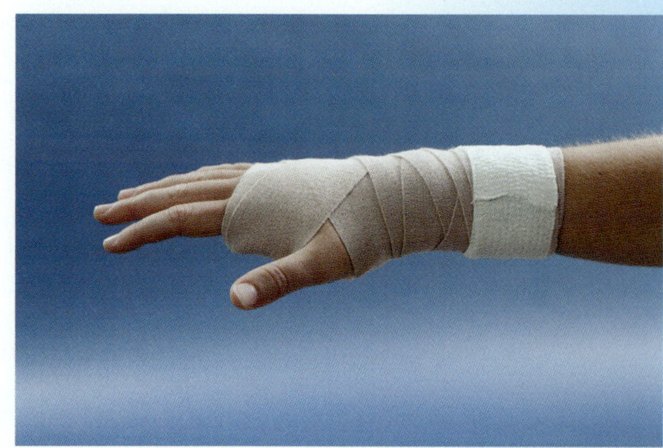

**Fig. 10–16 B**

**. . . IF/THEN . . .**

**IF** using an elastic or self-adherent wrap to control swelling over the dorsal hand and wrist following a contusion, **THEN** consider applying the hand and wrist compression wrap; this technique, along with a foam or felt pad, provides compression over a greater area than the figure-of-eight wrap.

# Bracing Techniques

Off-the-shelf and custom-made braces are available for the wrist in a variety of designs. The braces can be classified into three categories: prophylactic, rehabilitative, and functional. Use these bracing techniques to prevent and treat acute and chronic injuries and conditions. Note that several of these braces are also used for hand and thumb injuries and conditions.

## PROPHYLACTIC        Figure 10–17

➡ **Purpose:** Prophylactic braces are designed to prevent or reduce the severity of wrist injuries (Fig. 10–17). These braces, referred to as wrist guards, provide moderate support and are primarily used to protect the wrist from sprains, TFCC injury, fractures, and dislocations.

### DETAILS
Prophylactic braces are commonly used to provide wrist stability for patients in sports such as biking, in-line skating, skiing, and snowboarding but can also be useful with work and casual activities. Most braces can be used either under or over athletic and work gloves. Prophylactic braces may be used in combination with the circular wrist (Fig. 10–7), figure-of-eight (Fig. 10–8), fan (Fig. 10–9), strip (Figs. 10–10 and 10–11), and "X" (Fig. 10–12) taping techniques to provide additional stability.

➡ **Design:**
- Off-the-shelf prophylactic braces are available in universal fit and right or left styles in predetermined sizes corresponding to wrist circumference measurements or width from the second to the fifth MCP joint.
- The braces are constructed in circumferential and open designs in different lengths based on the amount of protection desired.
- Most designs are manufactured of a nylon mesh material outer shell with an EVA foam or gel pad and moisture-resistant lining.
- Some braces have a high-density plastic or aluminum palmar and/or dorsal bar(s) incorporated into the outer shell to limit wrist flexion and/or extension.
- Other designs are constructed with a plastic, leather, or Kevlar palmar pad that covers the entire or proximal palm.
- Most prophylactic braces are attached to the hand, wrist, and forearm through nylon straps with Velcro closures.
- Some designs allow for unrestricted finger and thumb range of motion, while other designs are available in a glove design.

➡ **Position of the patient:** Sitting on a taping table or bench with the wrist and hand in a neutral position.

➡ **Preparation:** Apply the brace directly to the skin or over a glove.
   Follow the manufacturer's instructions that are included with the braces when purchased during the application of prophylactic designs. The following guidelines apply to most prophylactic designs.

➡ **Application:**

**STEP 1:**    Begin application by loosening the straps and unfolding the brace.

**STEP 2:**    Place the brace onto the involved hand, wrist, and forearm. Align the bar(s) on the dorsal and/or palmar aspect of the hand, wrist, and forearm (Fig. 10–17A). Reposition the brace if necessary.

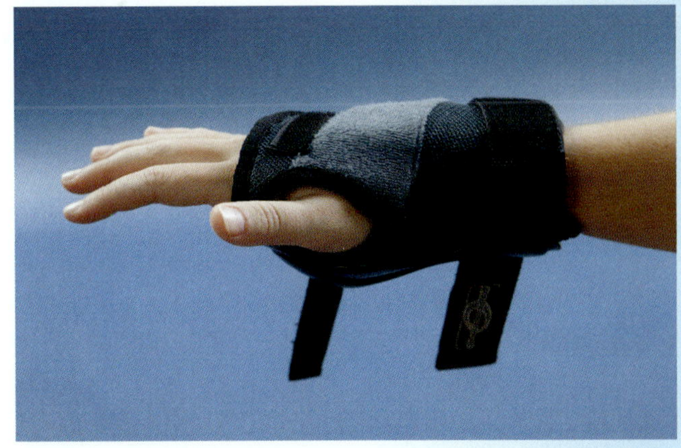

Fig. 10–17 A

**STEP 3:**    Wrap the outer shell around the hand, wrist, and forearm. Continue with most designs by pulling the straps tight and anchoring with Velcro (Fig. 10–17B).

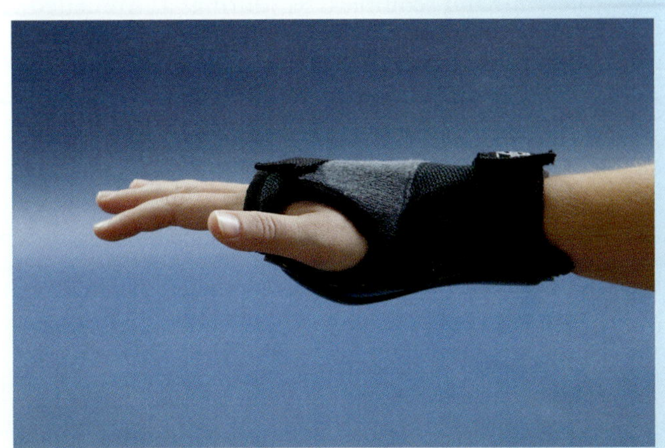

Fig. 10–17 B

## EVIDENCE SUMMARY

Several studies have described the high incidence of wrist injury among snowboarders[3,4] and in-line skaters.[5,6] Off-the-shelf wrist guards are used by many in attempts to protect against or lessen the severity of injury. A position statement from the Canadian Paediatric Society[7] recommends that physicians provide in-office guidance to families regarding the use of wrist guards for snowboarding activities. Although the effects of prophylactic knee and ankle bracing techniques are well documented, limited investigations in the literature have examined the effectiveness of wrist guards.

The researchers who have examined the protective value of off-the-shelf wrist guards have produced positive findings. Cadaveric studies have revealed differences in injury patterns with the use of guards. Using a fast, gravity-driven load, guards provided protection against capsular disruption, carpal fractures, and ligamentous injury compared to non-braced specimens.[8] Examining braced and non-braced specimens with a servohydraulic load simulating a fall on the outstretched hand, investigators found guards reduced dorsal and volar distal radius bone strain and increased energy absorption.[9] A significant reduction in wrist dorsiflexion was found with guard use during the application of a compressive load compared to a control group.[10] During a simulated fall on a snowy surface, specimens fitted with guards required a significantly greater force to produce fracture than specimens without guards.[11] Other investigations revealed no significant differences in the force required to produce fracture using a quasistatic load among braced and non-braced specimens.[12] In a separate study, researchers[13] used a manual drop test method and wrist/hand model to simulate a fall on the outstretched hand in braced and non-braced conditions. Off-the-shelf and custom-made guards significantly decreased peak impact force and peak deceleration compared to non-braced models.

An evidence-based review[14] conducted in 2007 examined the efficacy of wrist guards in the prevention of injuries among snowboarders. The findings among six studies revealed a significant reduction in the risk of wrist fractures and sprains and overall injury to the wrist with brace use. Some evidence indicated that wrist guards may reduce the risk of shoulder injury. However, other data suggested brace use may increase the risk of finger and elbow-shoulder injuries. Based on the various wrist guards in the studies,[14] determination of the most effective design was not possible.

The prophylactic effects of a wrist guard are determined by many factors, one being the amount of energy absorbed by the materials of the guard. Some researchers demonstrated that off-the-shelf designs provided limited impact force attenuation on the hand[15] and forearm/hand complex[16,17] during a simulated fall. Others[17] found off-the-shelf braces effective in force attenuation on the elbow. A guard too rigid may produce high stress loads at the distal and/or proximal end(s) of the brace. Researchers have reported forearm fractures associated with the use of rigid guards with in-line skaters.[18] The optimal wrist guard should absorb the maximum amount of energy without the production of these high stress points.[19]

Overall, most[8,11,19–24] researchers agree that using prophylactic wrist guards in snowboarding and in-line skating activities can lower the incidence and severity of injuries. However, further research is needed to understand fully the mechanism of wrist injury, the different guard designs and materials, and the functional role of wrist guards to provide a framework for future guard design.[8,11] The existing literature and evidence can be utilized by health care professionals to guide clinical decisions for the prevention of wrist injuries.

## ...IF/THEN...

**IF** a prophylactic brace is needed to lessen wrist flexion, extension, and ulnar and radial deviation, **THEN** consider a circumferential design, which will provide greater support than an open design.

## REHABILITATIVE      Figure 10–18

➠ **Purpose:** Rehabilitative braces are designed to provide compression, immobilization, and mild to moderate support. The braces also limit range of motion and correct structural abnormalities when treating sprains, TFCC injury, fractures, dislocations, tendinitis, tenosynovitis, nerve entrapment and compression syndromes, and postoperative procedures (Fig. 10–18). The braces can replace rigid casting and be removed to accommodate treatment and rehabilitation. Rehabilitative brace designs may be used with the hand and wrist compression wrap technique.

➠ **Design:**
- Off-the-shelf universal fit and right or left style rehabilitative braces are available in predetermined sizes based on wrist circumference measurements or width from the second to the fifth MCP joint.
- The circumferential and open designs are available in various lengths depending on the technique objective.
- Some braces are non-elastic in design while others are elastic.
- Most non-elastic designs are constructed with an outer shell of polyester/cotton or foam laminate, nylon/fiber, canvas, soft leather, perforated suede, or plastic, and lined with nylon, cotton or suede stockinet, or polypropylene felt.
  - Non-elastic braces have dorsal, palmar, and/or ulnar aluminum or plastic bar(s) incorporated into the outer shell to lessen wrist flexion, extension, and/or ulnar and radial deviation. Many of these are malleable as well as removable.
  - Some of these designs contain an adjustable air bladder system for additional compression and support.
  - The non-elastic braces are anchored to the hand, wrist, and forearm with adjustable D-ring closures, pull-tab laces, and Velcro straps.
- Elastic designs consist of a cotton, nylon, polyester, or neoprene material outer shell with a polypropylene felt, cotton, or Lycra material lining.
  - Most of these designs are available with adjustable dorsal and/or palmar aluminum or plastic bar(s) attached to the outer shell.
  - Several designs contain a viscoelastic polymer pad incorporated into the palmar aspect of the brace to lessen compressive forces.
  - D-ring closures, laces, and Velcro straps attach the braces to the hand, wrist, and forearm.
- Some non-elastic and elastic designs allow unrestricted motion of the fingers and thumb while other designs are available with an attached thumb spica to place the thumb in a neutral position.

## DETAILS

The non-elastic braces are commonly used to immobilize the wrist in a neutral or **cock-up position;** most designs allow for adjustments in fit depending on the injury or condition. Although most elastic designs also immobilize the wrist in a neutral or cock-up position, limited range of motion is allowed.

➠ **Position of the patient:** Sitting on a taping table or bench with the involved hand and wrist in a pain-free range of motion.

➠ **Preparation:** Apply the brace directly to the skin.

   Instructions for the application of rehabilitative braces are included with each brace when purchased. The following guidelines pertain to most designs.

➠ **Application:**

**STEP 1:**   Loosen the straps and unfold the brace.

**STEP 2:**   Apply the brace onto the involved hand, wrist, and forearm. Align the bar(s) on the dorsal and/or palmar aspect of the hand, wrist, and forearm (Fig. 10–18A). Remold and reposition the bars if necessary.

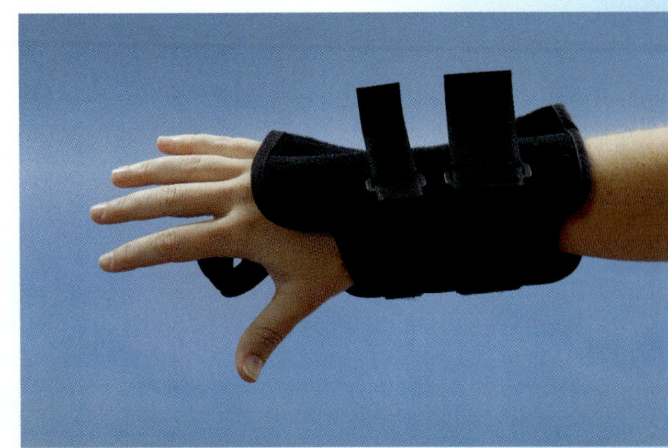

**Fig. 10–18 A**

**STEP 3:**   Wrap the outer shell around the hand, wrist, and forearm. The application of straps will depend on the specific brace design. Begin application of most designs by pulling the strap through the hand and anchoring. Next, pull the most distal wrist strap and anchor. Continue in a proximal direction and anchor the remaining straps (Fig. 10–18B). When using other designs, pull the tab lacing closure(s) tight and anchor. The patient may require a sling for daily activities.

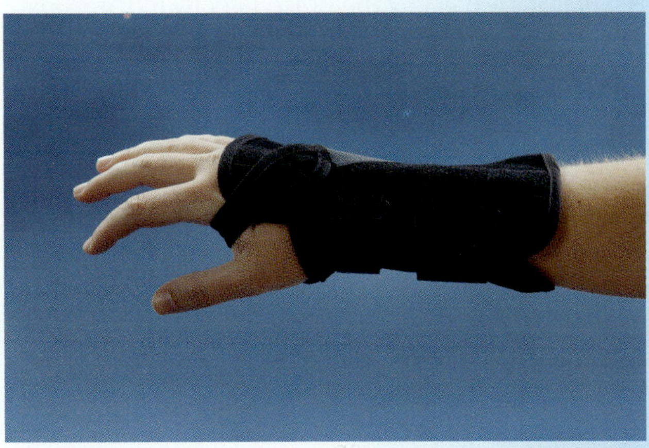

**Fig. 10–18 B**

### Clinical Application Question 2

A retired circus clown is seen in a local out-patient orthopedic clinic for treatment of de Quervain's tenosynovitis of the left wrist. He was placed in an off-the-shelf thumb, hand, and wrist brace by a physician 1 week ago and restricted from his daily fly-fishing activities. The retired clown complains of itching underneath the brace; upon removal, mild redness and swelling are present on the dorsal left wrist. The physician originally ordered the brace to be worn for 3 weeks.

➠ **Question: How can you manage this situation?**

## FUNCTIONAL    Figure 10–19

➠ **Purpose:** Functional braces provide compression and moderate stability to the wrist when preventing and treating sprains, TFCC injury, fractures, dislocations, tendinitis, tenosynovitis, nerve entrapment and compression syndromes, and postoperative procedures (Fig. 10–19).

### DETAILS
Functional braces are commonly used to provide wrist stability for athletes in sports such as baseball, basketball, diving, fencing, field hockey, football, gymnastics, ice hockey, lacrosse, soccer, skiing, softball, volleyball, and wrestling but can also be useful with work and casual activities. Functional braces are commonly used following injury and may be used in combination with the circular wrist, figure-of-eight, fan, strip, and "X" taping techniques to provide additional stability.

➠ **Design:**
- Off-the-shelf functional braces are available in universal and right or left styles, corresponding to wrist circumference measurements or width from the second to the fifth MCP joint.
- These braces are available in circumferential and open designs of various lengths and are commonly lower profile in construction and lighter in weight than rehabilitative braces.
- Some designs are constructed of neoprene with adjustable, interchangeable dorsal and/or palmar foam insert(s) or aluminum bar(s) to restrict excessive range of motion.
- Other braces are manufactured of a cotton/elastic, nylon, or polyester material outer shell with a Lycra, cotton stockinet, or polypropylene felt lining. Adjustable dorsal and/or palmar aluminum, plastic, or carbon fiber bars or metal springs are used to limit excessive range of motion.
- Velcro straps and D-ring closures anchor the braces to the hand, wrist, and forearm, and provide for adjustments in fit.
- Most of the functional braces allow for unrestricted motion of the fingers and thumb.

➠ **Position of the patient:** Sitting on a taping table or bench with the wrist and hand in a neutral position.

➠ **Preparation:** Apply the brace directly to the skin. Loosen all straps.

Application of functional designs should follow manufacturer's instructions that are included with the braces when purchased. The following guidelines pertain to most braces.

➠ **Application:**

**STEP 1:** Apply most of the designs by placing the brace onto the involved hand, wrist, and forearm. Align the dorsal and/or palmar bar(s), wrap the outer shell around the hand, wrist, and forearm, and anchor the strap(s) (Fig. 10–19A). Reposition the bars if necessary.

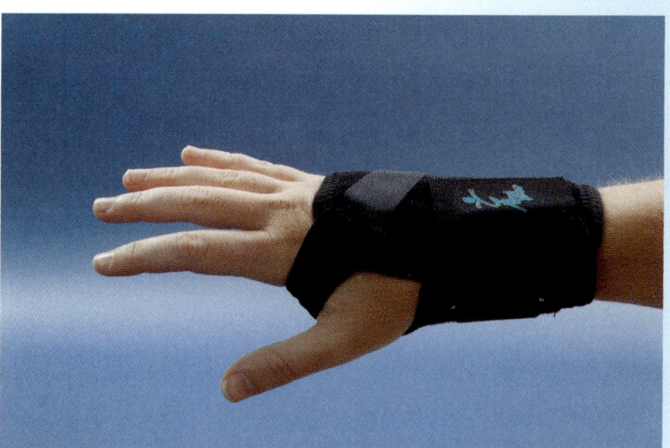

**Fig. 10–19 A**

**STEP 2:** When using other designs, place the neoprene material outer shell over the fingers and pull in a proximal direction until positioned over the wrist (Fig. 10–19B). Anchor the straps.

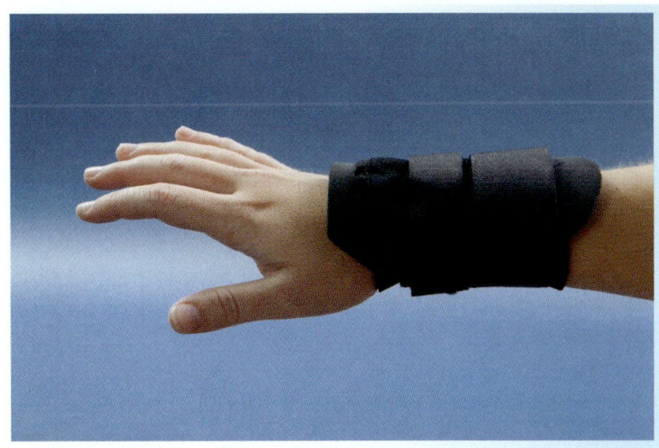

**Fig. 10–19 B**

---

**Clinical Application Question 3**

A nuclear lab technician has been suffering from numbness and tingling in the fingertips of the right thumb, index, and middle fingers for the past month. Two weeks ago, she was seen by a physician and diagnosed with carpal tunnel syndrome. She was fitted with an off-the-shelf brace to immobilize the right wrist in a neutral position. She wore the brace at night only. Ergonomic changes to her office and lab have been made, and in only 2 weeks, she responded well to the treatment. Nonetheless, her symptoms have now returned despite the ergonomic changes and continued night splinting. The lab technician awakens with pain in the right wrist and wonders if any damage occurred to the brace in her luggage during a recent airline trip to a national meeting.

➠ **Question: What can be done in this situation?**

---

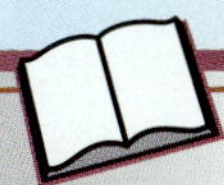

## EVIDENCE SUMMARY

A small study[25] investigated the stiffness characteristics of various wrist brace designs among 20 healthy, right-handed dominant subjects. Twelve circumferential prophylactic, rehabilitative, and functional braces with palmar, dorsal, palmar and dorsal, or no bars were evaluated with a robot driven apparatus that applied a slow torque to the braced wrist in combinations of passive wrist flexion and extension and radial and ulnar deviation range of motion. Researchers[25] found significantly greater stiffness in wrist flexion than extension among braces with a palmar bar and palmar and dorsal bar, significantly greater stiffness in wrist extension than flexion among designs with a dorsal bar, and significantly greater stiffness in wrist radial than ulnar deviation in designs with palmar, dorsal, and palmar and dorsal bars. Among all braces in the study, designs with palmar and dorsal bars demonstrated significantly greater stiffness to passive wrist range of motion compared to palmar bar designs and dorsal bar braces produced significantly greater stiffness in wrist extension than flexion compared to palmar bar and palmar and dorsal bar designs. Palmar, dorsal, and palmar and dorsal bar braces demonstrated significantly greater stiffness in range of motion compared to braces with no bars. Additional research is needed to evaluate different brace designs and their efficacy on the reduction of wrist range of motion in the prevention and treatment of injuries and conditions. Findings from these investigations can assist health care professionals in selecting the most appropriate design based on brace construction and patient preferences and needs such as reductions in specific range(s) of motion.

---

**CUSTOM-MADE**    Figure 10–20

➠ **Purpose:** Construct custom-made braces from thermoplastic material to provide moderate support and to immobilize, limit range of motion, and correct structural abnormalities for a variety of wrist injuries and conditions (Fig. 10–20). Use these braces when preventing and treating sprains, TFCC injury, fractures, dislocations, tendinitis, tenosynovitis, nerve entrapment and compression syndromes, and postoperative procedures. This technique is effective when off-the-shelf brace designs are not available.

**Wrist**

## DETAILS

Custom-made braces can be used during rehabilitative, work, and casual activities. Custom-made braces may be used with the hand and wrist compression wrap technique.

➡ **Materials:**
  • Paper, felt tip pen, thermoplastic material, ⅛ inch or ¼ inch foam or felt or 2 inch or 3 inch moleskin, a heating source, an elastic wrap, taping scissors
➡ **Position of the patient:** Sitting on a taping table or bench with the wrist and hand in a neutral position.
➡ **Preparation:** Design the brace with a paper pattern (see Fig. 1–10) on the dorsal aspect from the MCP joints, across the wrist, and finish at the distal forearm. For the palmar aspect, begin at the MCP joints, continue across the wrist, and finish at the distal forearm. The pattern should cover the entire dorsal or palmar surface of the hand, wrist, and forearm and not cause constriction of finger and thumb motion. Mold and shape the material over the area in the desired range of wrist motion as indicated by a physician.
➡ **Application:**

**STEP 1:** Attach ⅛ inch or ¼ inch foam or felt or 2 inch or 3 inch moleskin to the inside surface of the material (Fig. 10–20) to prevent irritation.

**STEP 2:** Place the brace on the dorsal or palmar hand, wrist, and forearm directly to the skin. Anchor the brace with the figure-of-eight taping or wrapping technique.

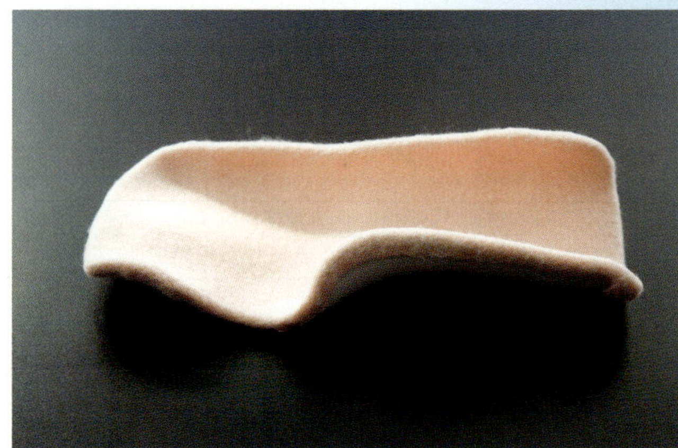

**Fig. 10–20** *Custom-made thermoplastic palmar wrist splint with moleskin lining.*

## EVIDENCE SUMMARY

Among nonsurgical interventions for carpal tunnel syndrome, splinting the wrist in a neutral position may decrease pressure on the median nerve by limiting wrist flexion and extension.[26] Splinting the wrist during sleep—night splinting—is commonly attempted first in the conservative treatment of the condition.[27,28] Full-time splinting may be indicated initially or with unsuccessful night splinting. Evidence-based clinical practice guidelines for the management of carpal tunnel syndrome developed in 2016 by the American Academy of Orthopaedic Surgeons[29] recommends splinting to improve patient reported pain and functional outcomes. A 2012 evidence-based review[30] was conducted to compare splinting, other nonsurgical interventions, and no treatment for the management of carpal tunnel syndrome. The results among 19 studies demonstrated limited evidence to support the efficacy of off-the-shelf and custom-made braces worn at night for 3 months or less in lessening pain levels and improving functional status compared to no treatment. The review[30] also revealed insufficient evidence to determine the most effective brace design and splinting period and the effectiveness of splinting compared to other nonsurgical interventions.

Several small investigations since 2012 have found evidence to support the use of splinting. Researchers[31] showed that a treatment program consisting of full-time splinting and educational sessions for 8 weeks resulted in greater relief of symptoms and improvement in functional status compared with no splinting and education among subjects with chronic carpal tunnel syndrome. Examining splinting and level of symptoms, researchers[32] found night splinting for 90 days resulted in a significant reduction in subjective pain scores among subjects suffering night-only symptoms compared with subjects symptomatic day and night.

Other researchers[33] demonstrated that 1 week of night splinting decreased MRI signal intensity of the median nerve at the inlet of the carpal tunnel in subjects with carpal tunnel syndrome. This decrease in signal intensity among patients with carpal tunnel syndrome has been associated with a reduction in edema in the area.[34,35] Using custom-made night splints for 6 weeks, researchers[36] found a neutral splint and a separate neutral splint that extended distally to immobilize the MCP joints produced a significant reduction in visual analogue scales of pain perception and significant increases in pinch and grip strength and functional status compared to baseline measures. Among the splints, the design with MCP immobilization resulted in significantly lower visual analogue scales of pain perception and significantly greater functional status. No differences were reported between the splints in pinch and grip strength. Other researchers[37] compared night splinting for 4 weeks and a local steroid injection for

the management of chronic carpal tunnel syndrome. Both interventions resulted in significant improvements in subjective measures of symptom severity and functional status compared to baseline measures. The findings also demonstrated no significant differences in symptom severity and functional status between night splinting and steroid injection. However, the injection resulted in significantly greater subjective patient satisfaction and objective hand dexterity.

Bracing techniques are commonly used in the conservative management of carpal tunnel syndrome. The evidence, although limited, suggests splinting is more effective than no treatment. More quality research is needed to investigate the long-term efficacy of bracing and whether other nonsurgical interventions are more effective to lessen symptoms. Selection and use of bracing techniques should be based on the patient's symptoms and compliance with the treatment protocol.

---

**...IF/THEN...**

**IF** off-the-shelf functional braces excessively restrict sport- or work-specific movements, **THEN** consider designing a custom-made brace; mold the brace with the wrist in a functional position while maintaining the necessary support and/or limits in range of motion.

---

## SLINGS

➡ **Purpose:** Slings provide support and immobilization when treating wrist injuries and conditions.
  • Use slings (see Fig. 8–19) when treating sprains, TFCC injury, fractures, dislocations, overuse injuries and conditions, and postoperative procedures.

---

# Padding Techniques

Use foam, felt, and thermoplastic materials to absorb shock, lessen compressive and repetitive stresses, and provide protection to the wrist. The techniques are used when preventing and treating contusions, ganglion cysts, fractures, dislocations, and postoperative procedures.

## CAST PADDING    Figure 10–21

➡ **Purpose:** With approval from a physician, an athlete can return early to activity following a fracture, dislocation, or surgery by placing the hand and wrist in a rigid or semirigid cast. NCAA[38] and NFHS[39] rules require padding casts to protect the injured athlete and her or his competitors from injury (Fig. 10–21).
➡ **Materials:**
  • Paper, felt tip pen, closed-cell, slow-recovery foam or similar material of at least ½ inch thickness, 2 inch or 3 inch width by 5 yard length elastic wrap, 1½ inch or 2 inch elastic tape and pre-wrap, or self-adherent wrap, taping scissors

➡ **Position of the patient:** Sitting on a taping table or bench with the hand and wrist in the casted position.
➡ **Preparation:** Construct a paper pattern of the cast area to be padded. Trace this pattern onto closed-cell, slow-recovery foam or similar material and cut out the pad with taping scissors.
➡ **Application:**

**STEP 1:**   Place the foam over the cast (Fig. 10–21A). Anchor the padding with a 2 inch or 3 inch elastic wrap, 1½ inch or 2 inch elastic tape, or self-adherent wrap with moderate roll tension ◀▬▶ (Fig. 10–21B). When using elastic tape, first apply pre-wrap over the padding to protect the foam from the tape adhesive. The foam may be reused multiple times.

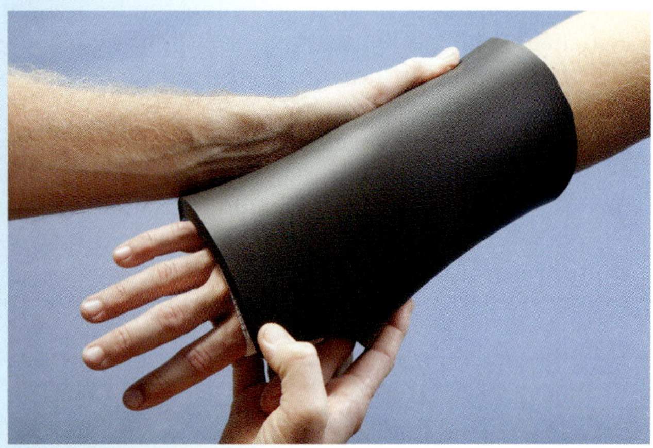
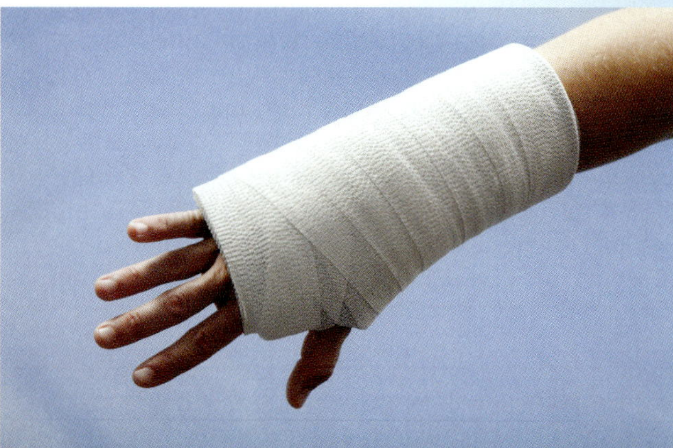

**Fig. 10–21 A**   **Fig. 10–21 B**

## CUSTOM-MADE

➡ **Purpose:** Custom-made pads constructed of thermoplastic material absorb shock and provide protection when preventing and treating wrist contusions. This technique and steps of application can be found at FADavis.com.

## DONUT PADS

➡ **Purpose:** When treating contusions, fractures, and ganglion cysts, use a donut pad to lessen the amount of compression over an area by dispersing the stress outward (see Fig. 3–26).
   • Construct the pads from ⅛ inch or ¼ inch foam or felt or purchase them pre-cut with adhesive backing.
   • Attach the pad directly to the skin over the hook of the hamate with adhesive gauze material (see Fig. 3–15) or with the figure-of-eight taping or wrapping technique.

### Clinical Application Question 4

The offensive center on the football team comes in after practice complaining of pain in the dorsal right wrist. An evaluation reveals a small palpable lump over the area. He sustained a second-degree right wrist sprain last season but has returned to full activities, including his hobby of weightlifting. The team physician examines the athlete and believes a ganglion cyst has formed. At this time, the physician recommends symptomatic treatment and prevention of any known causative factors.

➡ **Question: What techniques are appropriate in this situation?**

### . . . IF/THEN . . .

**IF** padding is required to cover a rigid or semirigid cast, **THEN** consider using thermomoldable foam; after heating and molding, the foam retains the shape of the cast, allowing for easy reapplication.

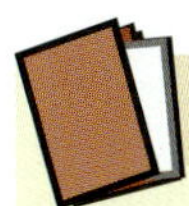

## EVIDENCE-BASED PRACTICE

Tracey Fife agrees to go in-line skating with her office co-workers on Saturday morning. Tracey has never been in-line skating but believes her background in high school sports and motocross will provide for a quick learning curve. She visits an in-line skating store and purchases skates and elbow and knee pads, but she does not feel comfortable wearing wrist guards and decides not to purchase them.

On Saturday morning, Tracey arrives at the park and receives instructions and tips from her co-workers. She immediately begins to skate on the asphalt path. Lacking skate control and the ability to stop, Tracey soon loses control when the front wheel of the right skate strikes a small rock on the path. She falls on her right outstretched arm, forcing her wrist into excessive extension upon contact with the path. Her co-workers help Tracey to her feet and advise her to see a physician. Tracey is able to drive to the local hospital and is seen in the emergency room. The attending physician evaluates Tracey and finds tenderness over the ulnar aspect of the wrist and pain with active extension, flexion, and radial and ulnar deviation. Radiographs are obtained and demonstrate no bony pathology. The physician believes she has sustained a second-degree right wrist sprain. He immobilizes the right wrist and refers her to Lozman Orthopedic Clinic, located next to the hospital.

Three days later, Tracey is seen in the clinic by JoAnn Clark, a PT/AT who worked with Tracey last year for a motocross-related injury. JoAnn and an orthopedic physician are conducting the weekly in-house clinic for the local high school athletes and examine Tracey when they finish. The physician agrees with the earlier diagnosis and decides to immobilize Tracey's right wrist for 2 weeks. Tracey is to avoid in-line skating and motocross activities during this time. Tracey returns to the clinic after 2 weeks of immobilization for her follow-up evaluation. The physician finds a decrease in pain with the available active range of motion and no fractures on follow-up radiographs. The physician allows Tracey to begin a therapeutic exercise program with JoAnn, including 2 additional weeks of night splinting.

The therapeutic exercise program is moving ahead well, and the physician allows Tracey to progress back into her athletic activities if adequate support is provided to her wrist. The physician and JoAnn discuss techniques to provide support during in-line skating and motocross activities. JoAnn is comfortable with searching for a technique to use during in-line skating but is uncertain if the same technique would be effective and safe for motocross. As JoAnn begins to search techniques for in-line skating, she schedules a visit to the local motocross track with Tracey to better understand the sport and equipment. Tracey and JoAnn watch the riders on the course and later examine the protective gear worn by riders and a dirt bike similar to Tracey's model. JoAnn creates a list of unique features she will need to consider in the selection of a technique for Tracey: a lower profile construction with adequate support that allows use with motocross protective gloves and body armor jacket and allows full control of the throttle and brake on the dirt bike handlebars.

1. Develop two clinically relevant questions from the case in the PICO format to generate answers for the selection of a (1) technique for in-line skating and (2) technique for motocross for Tracey. The questions should include the population or problem, the intervention, a comparison intervention (if relevant), and the clinical outcome of interest.

2. Design a search strategy and search to find the best evidence to answer the clinical questions. The strategies should include relevant search terms, electronic databases, online journals, and print journals to use for the search. Discussions with your faculty, preceptor, and other health care professionals can provide evidence from expert opinion.

3. Choose two to three full text studies or reviews from each of your searches or the chapter references. Evaluate and appraise each article to determine its value and usefulness to the case. Ask these questions for each study: (1) Are the results of the study valid? (2) What are the actual results? and (3) Are the findings clinically relevant to my patients? Prepare a summary of the evaluation with answers to the questions and rank the articles based on the evidence hierarchy in Chapter 1.

4. Integrate findings from the evidence, your clinical experience, and Tracey's goals and preferences into the case. Consider which techniques may be appropriate for each situation.

5. Evaluate the EBP process and your experience within the case. Consider these questions in the evaluation.

Were the clinical questions answered?

Did the searches generate quality evidence?

Was the evidence evaluated appropriately?

Was the evidence, your clinical experience, and Tracey's goals and values integrated to make the clinical decision?

Did the interventions produce successful clinical outcomes for Tracey?

Was the EBP experience positive for JoAnn and Tracey?

## WRAP-UP

- Compressive, shear, rotary, and repetitive forces, abnormal ranges of motion, and structural abnormalities can result in acute and chronic injuries and conditions to the wrist.
- The circular wrist and figure-of-eight taping techniques provide support, limit range of motion, and anchor protective padding.
- The fan, strip, "X," and semirigid cast taping techniques support and limit range of motion of the wrist.
- Posterior splints and slings provide immobilization following injury and/or surgery.
- Elastic and self-adherent wraps provide compression and anchor braces and pads.
- Prophylactic, rehabilitative, functional, and custom-made bracing techniques provide compression, protection, stability, and immobilization; limit range of motion; and correct structural abnormalities.
- Cast padding techniques are used to protect the injured athlete and his or her opponents during practices and competitions and are required by NCAA and NFHS rules.
- Custom-made and donut padding techniques absorb shock, lessen stress, and provide protection.

## FADAVIS ONLINE RESOURCES

- Posterior splint technique two
- Custom-made pad

## WEB REFERENCES

**Medscape**
https://emedicine.medscape.com
- This site provides access to information about acute and chronic wrist injuries and conditions.

**American Academy of Family Physicians**
https://www.aafp.org/home.html
- This site allows you access to the *American Family Physician* and online articles about wrist injuries and conditions.

**Sports-health**
https://www.sports-health.com/
- This website allows you access to information about the anatomy and treatment of a variety of wrist injuries and conditions.

**Wheeless' Textbook of Orthopaedics**
http://www.wheelessonline.com/
- This website allows access to anatomy, diagnostic imaging, and management information on a variety of wrist injuries.

## REFERENCES

1. Starkey, C, and Brown, SD: Examination of Orthopedic and Athletic Injuries, ed 4. F.A. Davis, Philadelphia, 2015.
2. Keir, PJ, and Rempel, DM: Pathomechanics of peripheral nerve loading. Evidence in carpal tunnel syndrome. J Hand Ther 18:259–269, 2005.
3. Xiang, H, Kelleher, K, Shields, BJ, Brown, KJ, and Smith, GA: Skiing- and snowboarding-related injuries treated in U.S. emergency departments, 2002. J Trauma 58:112–118, 2005.
4. Flores, AH, Haileyesus, T, and Greenspan, AI: National estimates of outdoor recreational injuries treated in emergency departments, United States, 2004–2005. Wilderness Environ Med 19:91–98, 2008.
5. Jerosch, J, Heidjann, J, Thorwesten, L, and Lepsien, U: Injury pattern and acceptance of passive and active injury prophylaxis for inline skating. Knee Surg Sports Traumatol Arthrosc 6:44–49, 1998.
6. Houshian, S, and Andersen, HM: Comparison between in-line and rollerskating injury. A prospective study. Scand J Med Sci Sports 10:47–50, 2000.
7. Warda, LJ, and Yanchar NL: Canadian Paediatric Society, Injury Prevention Committee. Position Statement: Skiing and snowboarding, 2019. https://www.cps.ca/en/documents/position/skiing-snowboarding-injury
8. Moore, MS, Popovic, NA, Daniel, JN, Boyea, SR, and Polly, DW: The effect of a wrist brace on injury patterns in experimentally produced distal radial fractures in a cadaveric model. Am J Sports Med 25:394–401, 1997.
9. Staebler, MP, Moore, DC, Akelman, E, Weiss, AP, Fadale, PD, and Crisco, JJ III: The effect of wrist guards on bone strain in the distal forearm. Am J Sports Med 27:500–506, 1999.
10. Grant-Ford, M, Sitler, MR, Kozin, SH, Barbe, MF, and Barr, AE: Effect of a prophylactic brace on wrist and ulnocarpal joint biomechanics in a cadaveric model. Am J Sports Med 31:736–743, 2003.
11. Greenwald, RM, Janes, PC, Swanson, SC, and McDonald, TR: Dynamic impact response of human cadaveric forearms using a wrist brace. Am J Sports Med 26:825–830, 1998.
12. Giacobetti, FB, Sharkey, PF, Bos-Giacobetti, MA, Hume, EL, and Taras, JS: Biomechanical analysis of the effectiveness of in-line skating guards for preventing wrist fractures. Am J Sports Med 25:223–225, 1997.
13. Maurel, ML, Fitzgerald, LG, Miles, AW, and Giddins, GE: Biomechanical study of the efficacy of a new design of wrist guard. Clin Biomech 28:509–513, 2013.
14. Russell, K, Hagel, B, and Francescutti, LH: The effect of wrist guards on wrist and arm injuries among snowboarders: A systematic review. Clin J Sport Med 17:145–150, 2007.

15. Hwang, IK, Kim, KJ, Kaufman, KR, Cooney, WP, and An, KN: Biomechanical efficiency of wrist guards as a shock isolator. J Biomech Eng 128:229–234, 2006.

16. Kim, KJ, Alian, AM, Morris, WS, and Lee, YH: Shock attenuation of various protective devices for prevention of fall-related injuries of the forearm/hand complex. Am J Sports Med 34:637–643, 2006.

17. Burkhart, TA, and Andrews, DM: The effectiveness of wrist guards for reducing wrist and elbow accelerations resulting from simulated forward falls. J Appl Biomech 26:281–289, 2010.

18. Cheng, SL, Rajaratnam, K, Raskin, KB, Hu, RW, and Axelrod, TS: Splint-top fracture of the forearm: A description of an in-line skating injury associated with the use of protective wrist splints. J Trauma 39:1194–1197, 1995.

19. Rønning, R, Rønning, I, Gerner, T, and Engebretsen, L: The efficacy of wrist protectors in preventing snowboarding injuries. Am J Sports Med 29:581–585, 2001.

20. Heitkamp, H-C, Horstmann, T, and Schalinski, H: In-line skating: Injuries and prevention. J Sports Med Phys Fitness 40:247–253, 2000.

21. Machold, W, Kwasny, O, Gässler, P, Kolonja, A, Reddy, B, Bauer, E, and Lehr, S: Risk of injury through snowboarding. J Trauma 48:1109–1114, 2000.

22. Machold, W, Kwasny, O, Eisenhardt, P, Kolonja, A, Bauer, E, Lehr, S, Mayr, W, and Fuchs, M: Reduction of severe wrist injuries in snowboarding by an optimized wrist protection device: A prospective randomized trial. J Trauma 52:517–520, 2002.

23. Hagel, B, Pless, IB, and Goulet, C: The effect of wrist guard use on upper-extremity injuries in snowboarders. Am J Epidemiol 162:149–156, 2005.

24. Slaney, GM, Finn, JC, Cook, A, and Weinstein, P: Wrist guards and wrist and elbow injury in snowboarders. Med J Aust 189:412, 2008.

25. Seegmiller, DB, Eggett, DL, and Charles, SK: The effect of common wrist orthoses on the stiffness of wrist rotations. J Rehabil Res Dev 53:1151–1166, 2016.

26. Darowish, M, and Sharma, J: Evaluation and treatment of chronic hand conditions. Med Clin N Am 98:801–815, 2014.

27. Prentice, WE: Rehabilitation Techniques for Sports Medicine and Athletic Training, ed 6. Slack, New Jersey, 2015.

28. Viera, AJ: Management of carpal tunnel syndrome. Am Fam Physician 68:265–272, 279–280, 2003.

29. American Academy of Orthopaedic Surgeons. AAOS Management of Carpal Tunnel Syndrome Evidence-Based Clinical Practice Guideline. https://www.aaos.org/globalassets/quality-and-practice-resources/carpal-tunnel/cts_cpg_4-25-19.pdf, 2019.

30. Page, MJ, Massey-Westropp, N, O'Conner, D, and Pitt, V: Splinting for carpal tunnel syndrome. Cochrane Database Syst Rev (7);CD010003, 2012.

31. Hall, B, Lee, HC, Fitzgerald, H, Byrne, B, Barton, A, and Lee, AH: Investigating the effectiveness of full-time wrist splinting and education in the treatment of carpal tunnel syndrome: A randomized controlled trial. Am J Occup Ther 67:448–459, 2013.

32. Halac, G, Demir, S, Yucel, H, Niftaliyev, E, Kocaman, G, Duruyen, H, Kendirli, T, and Asil, T: Splinting is effective for night-only symptomatic carpal tunnel syndrome patients. J Phys Ther Sci 27:993–996, 2015.

33. Schmid, AB, Elliott, JM, Strudwick, MW, Little, M, and Coppieters, MW: Effect of splinting and exercise on intraneural edema of the median nerve in carpal tunnel syndrome—an MRI study to reveal therapeutic mechanisms. J Orthop Res 30:1343–1350, 2012.

34. Cudlip, SA, Howe, FA, Clifton, A, Schwartz, MS, and Bell, BA: Magnetic resonance neurography studies of the median nerve before and after carpal tunnel decompression. J Neurosurg 96:1046–1051, 2002.

35. Uchiyama, S, Itsubo, T, Yasutomi, T, Nakagawa, H, Kamimura, M, and Kato, H: Quantitative MRI of the wrist and nerve conduction studies in patients with idiopathic carpal tunnel syndrome. J Neurol Neurosurg Psychiatry 76:1103–1108, 2005.

36. Golriz, B, Ahmadi Bani, M, Arazpour, M, Bahramizadeh, M, Curran, S, Madani, SP, and Hutchins, SW: Comparison of the efficacy of a neutral wrist splint and a wrist splint incorporating a lumbrical unit for the treatment of patients with carpal tunnel syndrome. Prosthet Orthot Int 40:617–623, 2016.

37. So, H, Chung, VCH, Cheng, JCK, and Yip, RML: Local steroid injection versus wrist splinting for carpal tunnel syndrome: A randomized clinical trial. Int J Rheum Dis 21:102–107, 2018.

38. National Collegiate Athletic Association: 2014-15 NCAA Sports Medicine Handbook, ed 25. NCAA, Indianapolis, 2014. http://www.ncaapublications.com/productdownloads/MD15.pdf.

39. National Federation of State High School Associations: 2018 Football Rules Book. National Federation of State High School Associations, Indianapolis, 2019.

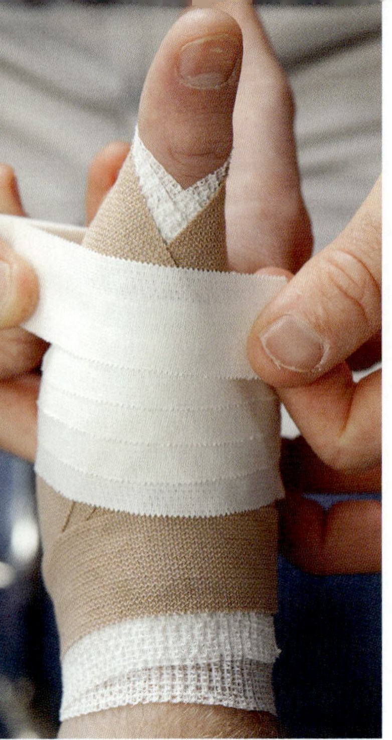

# 11

# Hand, Fingers, and Thumb





## INJURIES AND CONDITIONS

The hand, fingers, and thumb are essential to athletic, work, and casual activities such as catching a basketball, typing, and gardening. Because the hand, fingers, and thumb play a significant role in daily activities, injuries occur frequently. Although gloves do offer protection, shearing forces, compressive forces, and excessive range of motion often result in bony and soft tissue injury. Common injuries to the hand, fingers, and thumb include:

- Contusions
- Sprains
- Dislocations
- Fractures
- Tendon ruptures
- Blisters

## Contusions

Contusions to the hand, fingers, and thumb are frequent in sports because of the minimal protection for the bony structures.[1] Contusions are also common with work activities. Accumulation of edema is more frequently seen in the dorsal rather than the palmar hand because of the differences in the loose and elastic properties of the dorsal skin compared to the inelastic properties of the palmar skin.[2] Mechanisms of injury include shear and compression forces. A contusion can result, for instance, when a diver strikes the diving board with her hand, fingers, and/or thumb while twisting in the air, sustaining a compressive force to the structures.

## Sprains

Sprains typically occur to the fingers and thumb as a result of hyperextension and varus or valgus forces.[3] Finger and thumb sprains involve injury to the collateral ligaments and often to the capsular and tendinous tissues (Fig. 11–1). Sprains may occur at the metacarpophalangeal (MCP), **proximal interphalangeal (PIP), or distal interphalangeal (DIP) joints.** A sprain of the ulnar collateral ligament **(gamekeeper's thumb)** results from forceful abduction and hyperextension of the proximal phalanx.[4] For example, a sprain to the ulnar collateral ligament can happen as a softball player slides headfirst into third base, making initial contact with the thumb, causing abduction and hyperextension (Fig. 11–2).

> **DETAILS**
> The name "gamekeeper's thumb" originates from the gamekeepers who managed the game animals on private lands. These people were subjected to the abduction/hyperextension mechanism during their job-related tasks, which included snapping the necks of fowl with their hands.

## Dislocations

Dislocations can occur at the MCP, PIP, and DIP joints of the fingers and thumb. The causes are extreme flexion, or extension, rotation, or compressive loads to the tip of the fingers or thumb.[5] Only qualified health care professionals should attempt reductions. All patients with dislocations should be referred to a physician for radiographic examination. A dislocation at the PIP joint can result, for instance, when a bare-handed fan at a baseball game catches a line drive foul ball over the first base dugout, causing a compressive load to the distal finger and hyperextension at the PIP joint (Fig. 11–3).

## Fractures

Fractures are seen in the carpals, metacarpals, or phalanges and are caused by compressive, rotational, or axial forces[1] (Fig. 11–4). Compressive forces that may cause a fracture include, for example, dropping a dumbbell on the hand or having an opponent fall on a player's fingers while tackling in football. A fracture of the fourth or fifth metacarpal (**boxer's fracture**) is caused by a direct axial force and may result from an improperly thrown punch[6] (Fig. 11–5).

## Tendon Ruptures

A rupture of the extensor digitorum tendon at its distal attachment (**mallet finger**) often causes an accompanying avulsion fracture of the distal phalanx. The distal phalanx is forced into flexion while being held in extension from a direct blow to the tip of the finger.[7] For example, an extensor digitorum rupture can occur as a basketball player extends the fingers and thumb to receive a pass from a teammate and the ball strikes the tip of the finger, causing violent flexion of the distal phalanx (Fig. 11–6).

## Blisters

Blisters are commonly seen in athletic and work activities that involve the use of the hands on equipment. Shearing forces on the palmar aspect of the fingers and thumb in sports such as baseball, softball, rowing, and weight training can result in the development of blisters.

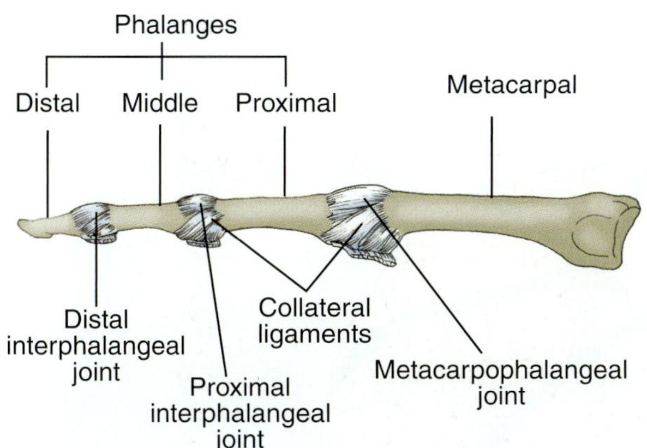


**Fig. 11–1** *Bones and collateral ligaments of the metacarpophalangeal, proximal interphalangeal, and distal interphalangeal joints of the fingers.*

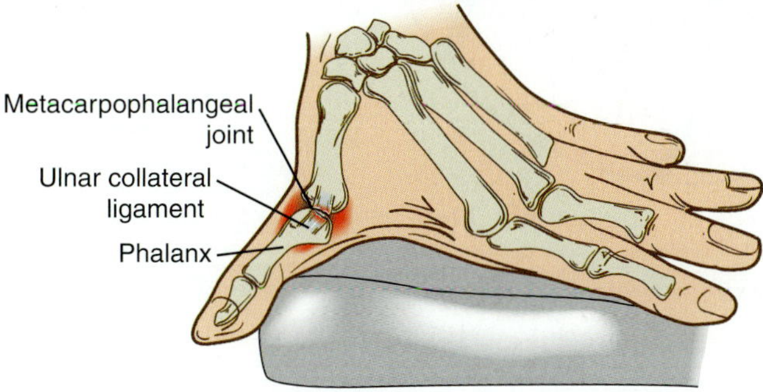


**Fig. 11–2** *Ulnar collateral ligament sprain (gamekeeper's thumb).*

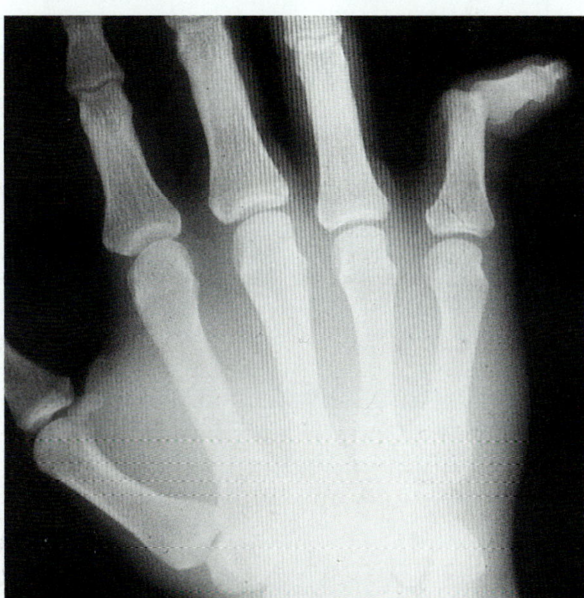

**Fig. 11–3** *Radiograph of a dislocation of the fifth proximal interphalangeal joint (PIP joint). (Courtesy of Starkey, C. and Brown, SD. Examination of Orthopedic & Athletic Injuries. 4th ed. Philadelphia, PA: F.A. Davis Company: 2015.)*

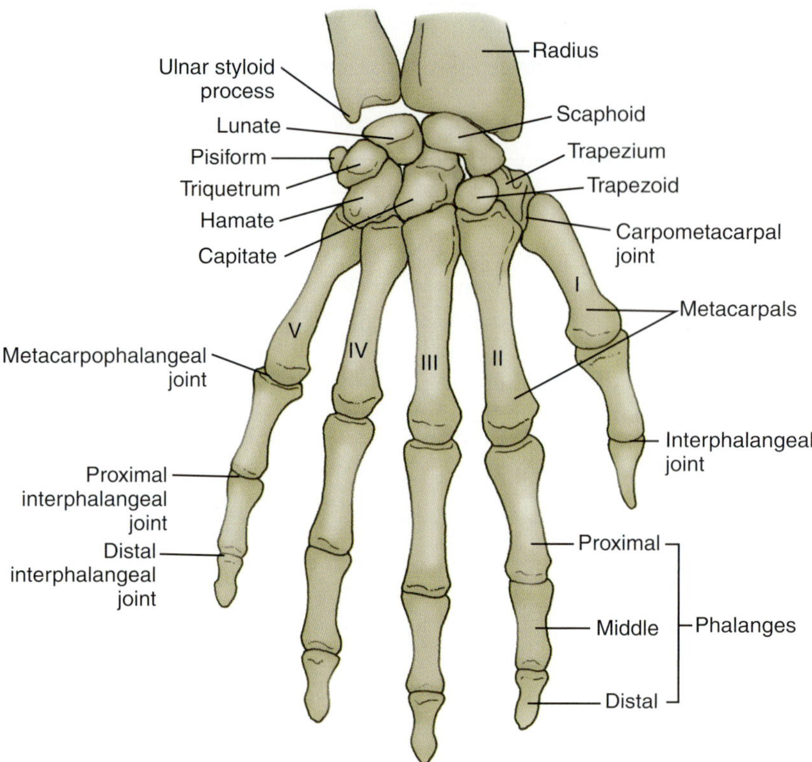


**Fig. 11–4** *Bones and joints of the hand, fingers, and thumb.*

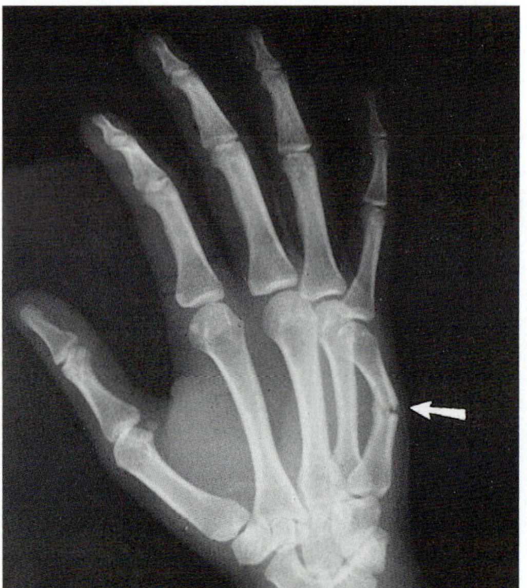

**Fig. 11–5** *Oblique view of the hand demonstrates a midshaft fracture of the fifth metacarpal (arrow), with dorsal angulation at the fracture site. (Courtesy of McKinnis, LN. Fundamentals of Musculoskeletal Imaging, 4th ed. Philadelphia, PA: F.A. Davis Company: 2014.)*

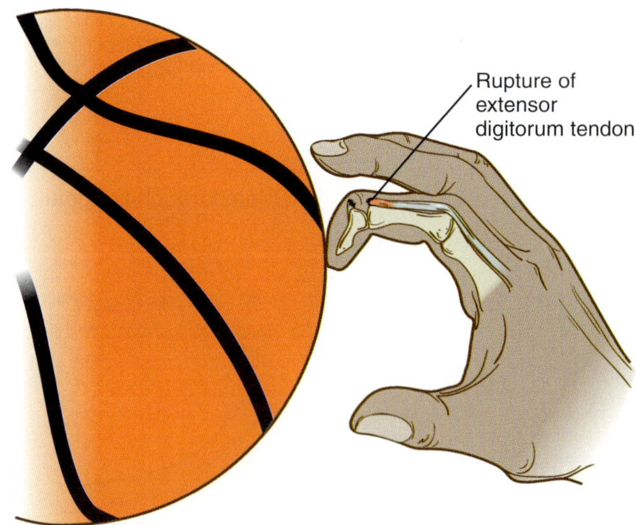


**Fig. 11–6** *Extensor digitorum tendon rupture (mallet finger).*

# Taping Techniques

Taping techniques for the hand, fingers, and thumb can be used for a variety of injuries and conditions. Most techniques are used to provide support and lessen excessive range of motion when preventing and treating sprains and postdislocation and postfracture injuries. Other techniques are used to prevent and treat injuries to the skin.

## BUDDY TAPE    Figure 11–7

➡ **Purpose:** Use the buddy tape technique to provide mild to moderate support to the collateral ligaments of the fingers following sprains and postdislocation and postfracture injuries. As the name implies, the injured finger is taped together with its buddy, the largest adjacent finger, to provide support (Fig. 11–7).

➡ **Materials:**
• ½ inch non-elastic tape, ⅛ inch foam or felt, adherent tape spray, taping scissors
*Option:*
• 1 inch non-elastic or elastic tape

➡ **Position of the patient:** Sitting on a taping table or bench with the hand and fingers in a neutral position.

➡ **Preparation:** Apply adherent tape spray to the fingers. Cut the ⅛ inch foam or felt to the length of the shortest finger to be taped. The buddy tape technique may be applied directly to the skin or over sports-specific gloves.

➡ **Application:**

**STEP 1:**    Apply a strip of ½ inch non-elastic tape around the foam or felt at the proximal end, then place the foam or felt between the fingers to retain anatomical alignment ◀▥▥▶ (Fig. 11–7A).

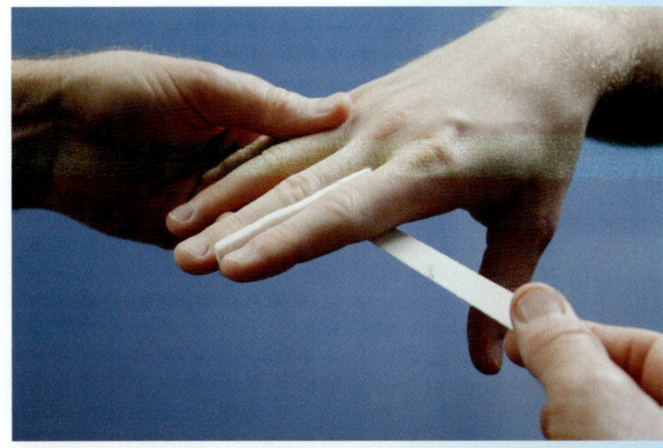

**Fig. 11–7 A**

**STEP 2:**    Encircle the fingers between the MCP and PIP joints with the ½ inch non-elastic tape strip with moderate roll tension ◀▥▥▶ (Fig. 11–7B). This *lock-in* strip will prevent the foam or felt from dislodging and loosening during activity as perspiration and moisture begin to affect the tape adhesive.

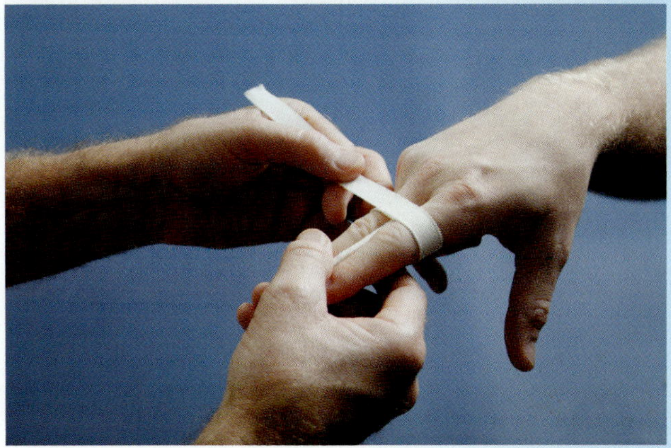

**Fig. 11–7 B**

*Steps Cont.*

**STEP 3:**   Maintaining alignment of the fingers, tape the fingers together with ½ inch non-elastic tape between the MCP and PIP joints, between the PIP and DIP joints, and around the distal phalanx, if necessary, with three to five circular strips with moderate roll tension ◄▬▬► (Fig. 11–7C). End the tape strips on the dorsal aspect of the fingers to prevent unraveling due to contact with equipment during activity. Do not place tape directly over the joints.

*Option:*   *One inch non-elastic or elastic tape may be used for the circular strips on large fingers to provide adequate support or prevent constriction. Note, the use of elastic tape may allow for less support and greater range of motion.*

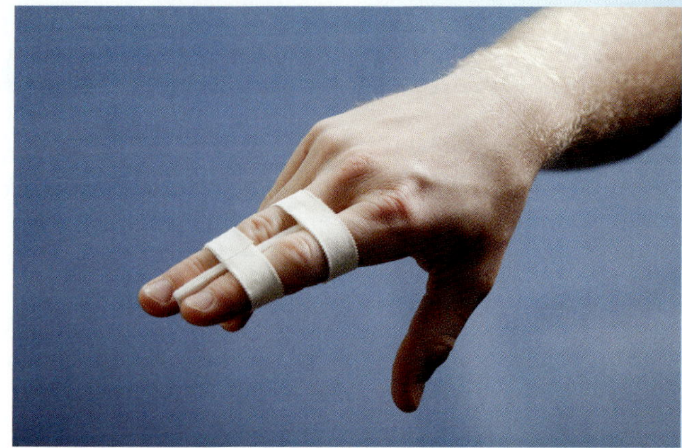

**Fig. 11–7 C**

**STEP 4:**   Apply an additional lock-in strip following completion of these circular strips ◄▬▬►.

**Helpful Hint |**

Begin the additional lock-in technique by anchoring a strip of tape under the proximal circular strip on the dorsal aspect of the finger (Fig. 11–7D). Continue distally over the distal end of the foam or felt with moderate roll tension and finish by anchoring under the proximal circular strip on the palmar aspect of the finger (Fig. 11–7E). Apply an additional proximal circular strip between the MCP and PIP joints with moderate roll tension to serve as an anchor.

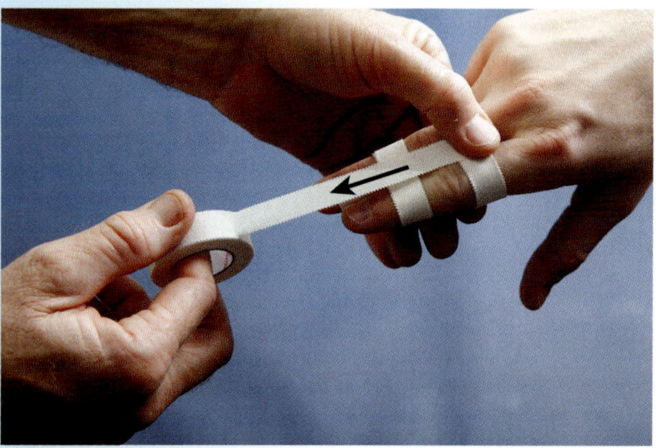
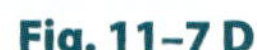

**Fig. 11–7 D**

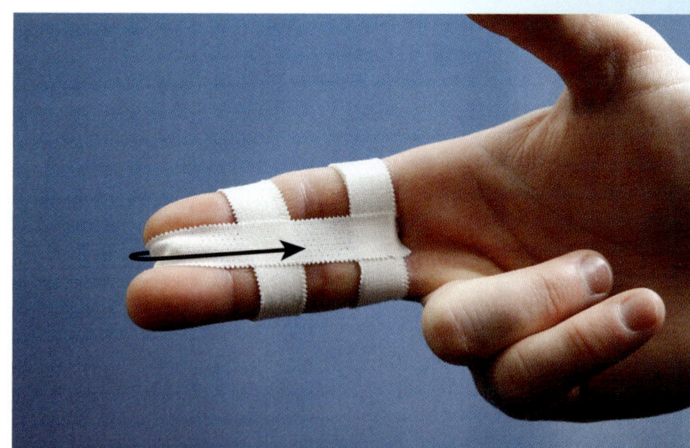

**Fig. 11–7 E**

## EVIDENCE SUMMARY

Several small studies have investigated the efficacy of the buddy tape technique in the management of finger sprains and fractures and complications associated with the technique. Examining PIP joint collateral ligament injuries in fingers two through five, researchers[8] found the buddy tape technique and active finger and hand range of motion exercises for 3 to 4 weeks resulted in satisfactory results in grip strength, active finger range of motion, and physical function at 6 months post-injury compared to the uninjured extremity. The researchers[8] also reported that delayed treatment of these injuries was significantly associated with lower grip strength, active finger range of motion, and physical function perception outcomes. The buddy tape technique has been recommended by several[9–11] and used for the treatment of undisplaced, stable phalangeal fractures of fingers two through five. In a small study among pediatric patients, researchers[12] compared the effects of the buddy tape technique with a forearm palmar hand splint in the treatment of undisplaced and displaced phalangeal fractures. At post-injury day 5, there were no differences in the risk of secondary fracture displacements among the displaced proximal and middle phalangeal fractures between the buddy tape and splint techniques. The buddy tape technique resulted in significantly greater visual analogue scales of comfort perception by parents at day 5 compared to the splint with no differences in comfort perception found at day 21. The researchers[12] reported no significant differences in active finger range of motion between the buddy tape technique and splint in a 21 day period.

Complications associated with the use of the buddy tape technique were examined in two small investigations. Using a questionnaire among 55 orthopedic and hand surgeons, researchers[13] reported that the buddy tape technique was used in the management of PIP and MCP joint injuries and phalangeal and metacarpal fractures. Complications associated with the technique were low patient compliance from patients removing the tape and skin trauma caused by the tape adhesive underneath the tape and between the injured and non-injured finger. However, other researchers[12] found no skin trauma or compliance issues among a pediatric population using the buddy tape technique in the management of undisplaced and displaced phalangeal fractures. While additional research is needed on the efficacy of the buddy tape technique and other immobilization techniques, these findings appear to indicate that the buddy tape technique may provide effective immobilization in the management of finger sprains and fractures. Clinicians should also understand the importance of appropriate follow-up with patients after application of taping, wrapping, bracing, and padding techniques to lessen adverse outcomes.

---

### "X" TAPE    Figure 11–8

➠ **Purpose:** The "X" technique also provides mild to moderate support to the collateral ligaments of the PIP joint of the finger following sprains and postdislocation and postfracture injuries. Use this technique with patients who require support but also desire independent motion of all fingers (Fig. 11–8).

➠ **Materials:**
• ½ inch non-elastic tape, adherent tape spray, taping scissors

➠ **Position of the patient:** Sitting on a taping table or bench with the hand and fingers in a neutral position.

➠ **Preparation:** Apply adherent tape spray to the involved finger.

**Helpful Hint |**
Use a cotton-tipped applicator to apply adherent tape spray to the finger. This method will concentrate adherent on the specific areas and prevent spreading to adjacent fingers. The use of adherent is recommended, especially in warm environments.

➠ **Application:**

**STEP 1:** Using ½ inch non-elastic tape, alternate the application of angled strips directly to the skin over the lateral (Fig. 11–8A) and medial (Fig. 11–8B) joint lines of the PIP joint with moderate roll tension, forming an "X." Each strip should reach proximal and distal to the PIP joint but not over the DIP or MCP joints.

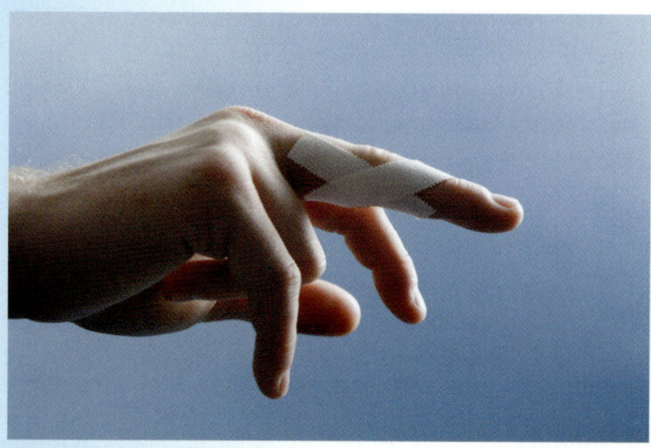

Fig. 11–8 A

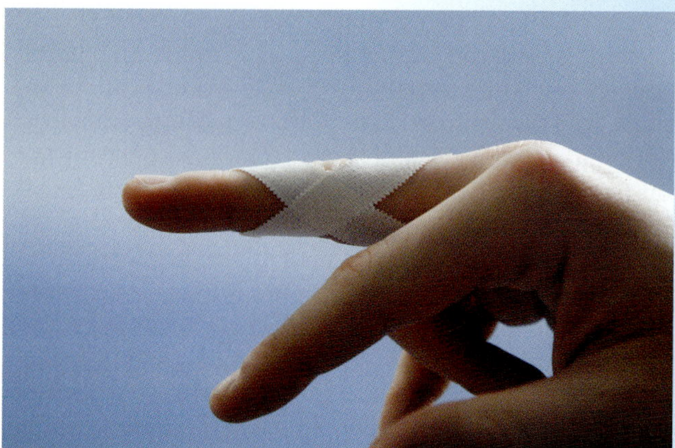

Fig. 11–8 B

**STEP 2:** After applying an "X" on each side of the PIP joint, repeat the procedure, overlapping the tape ⅛–¼ inch (Fig. 11–8C).

**STEP 3:** Place circular anchors at the proximal and distal ends of the "X" strips with moderate roll tension, leaving the ends of the anchors on the dorsal aspect of the finger ◄⫼► (Fig. 11–8D).

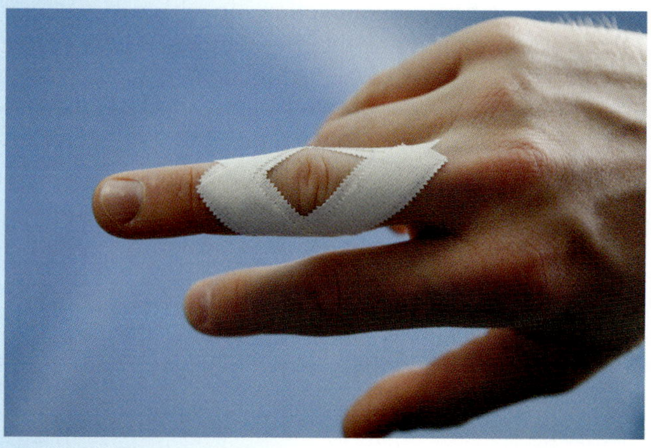

Fig. 11–8 C

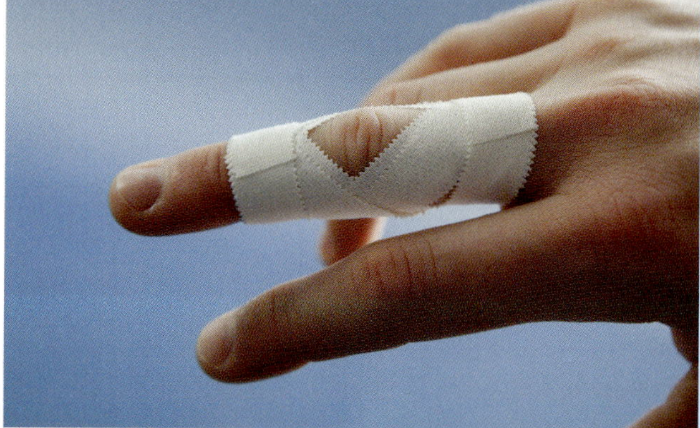

Fig. 11–8 D

## Clinical Application Question 1

While diving for a loose ball during practice, a guard on the women's basketball team dislocates the PIP joint of her left fourth finger. Following a reduction and evaluation by a physician, she is cleared to return to practice. You apply the buddy tape technique to support the injured finger. Soon, she approaches and reports that the technique is uncomfortable.

➠ **Question: What actions can you take in this situation?**

## ELASTIC MATERIAL     Figures 11–9, 11–10, 11–11

➠ **Purpose:** Several methods are available to cover wound dressings and attach pads to the hand, fingers, and thumb when treating wounds, contusions, and blisters. The material should possess elastic properties and great adhesive strength and not impede hand, finger, and thumb motion. Three methods are illustrated in the application of the technique; they differ based on the site of the wound or contusion.

### Elastic Material Technique One

➡ **Materials:**
  • Adhesive gauze material, taping scissors
➡ **Position of the patient:** Sitting on a taping table or bench with the hand and fingers in a neutral position.
➡ **Preparation:** Apply adhesive gauze material directly to the skin and use without adherent tape spray.
➡ **Application:**

**STEP 1:** Cut the piece of material to overlap a sterile wound dressing or pad from ½ inch to 1 inch to provide an effective anchor base to the skin.

**Helpful Hint |**
It is best to round all corners of the material to prevent the edges from being removed by contact with clothing or equipment.

**STEP 2:** After application of sterile materials, donut pad, or friction-reducing lubricant, place the piece of the adhesive gauze material directly on the skin (Fig. 11–9).

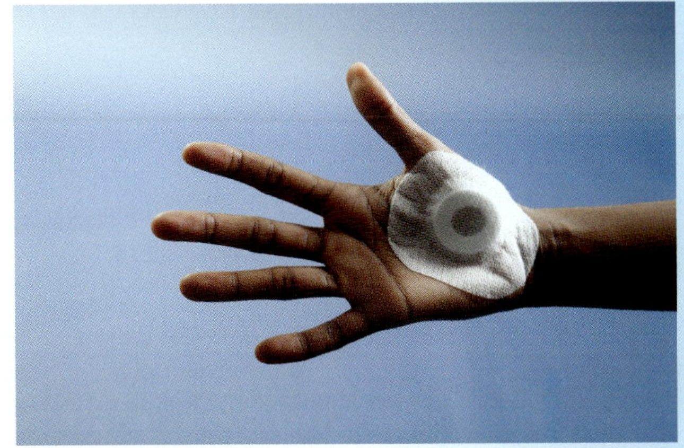

**Fig. 11–9**

### Elastic Material Technique Two

➡ **Materials:**
  • Adhesive gauze material, 1 inch or 1½ inch non-elastic tape, taping scissors
  *Option:*
  • 2 inch or 3 inch lightweight or heavyweight elastic tape
➡ **Position of the patient:** Sitting on a taping table or bench with the hand and fingers in a neutral position.
➡ **Preparation:** Apply sterile materials, donut pad, or friction-reducing lubricant to the palmar hand. Apply technique two directly to the skin.
➡ **Application:**

**STEP 1:** Cut adhesive gauze material into a 12–16 inch strip.

*Option:* *If adhesive gauze material is not available, use 2 inch or 3 inch lightweight or heavyweight elastic tape.*

**STEP 2:** Fold the strip and cut a hole in the middle slightly smaller than the finger.

**STEP 3:** Place the hole in the strip over the fingertip. Pull the strip firmly in a proximal direction to the web space between the fingers (Fig. 11–10A). If necessary, trim the strip to prevent irritation of the web space of adjacent fingers.

**STEP 4:** Smooth the adhesive gauze material to the palmar and dorsal hand.

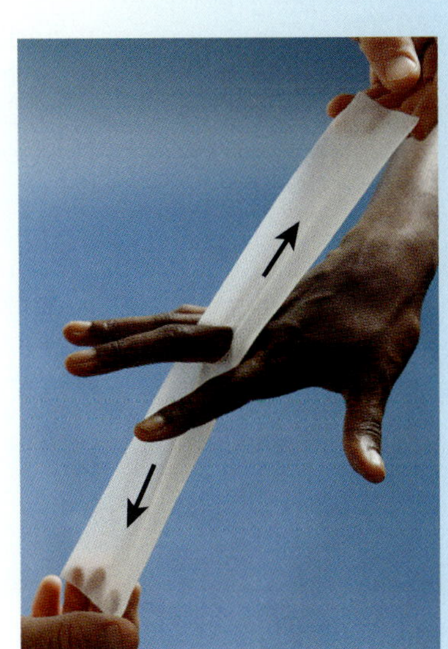

**Fig. 11–10 A**

*Steps Cont.*

**STEP 5:** Finish the strip at the wrist, cutting any excess with taping scissors. Anchor the strip in a circular pattern with 1 inch or 1½ inch non-elastic tape around the wrist with moderate roll tension ⬅▮▮▮▮▮➡ (Fig. 11–10B).

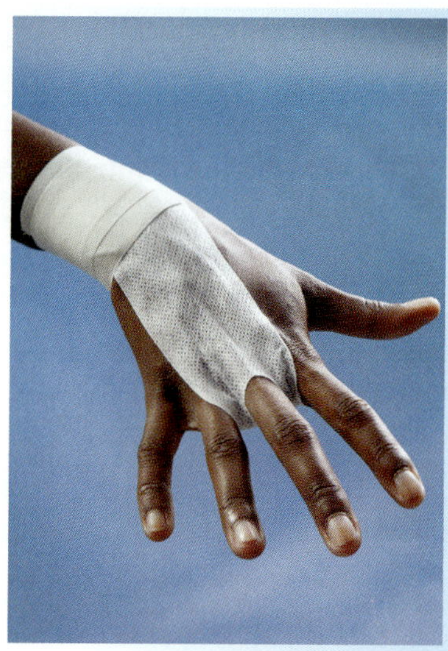

**Fig. 11–10 B**

### Elastic Material Technique Three

**DETAILS**

Use adhesive gauze material or lightweight elastic tape also to manage finger, thumb, and fingertip wounds and blisters. Fingertip bandages often are too large, resulting in excess bandage material, affecting use and sensation of the finger.

➟ **Materials:**
  - Adhesive gauze material, taping scissors
  *Options:*
  - 2 inch or 3 inch lightweight elastic tape
  - ½ inch non-elastic tape
➟ **Position of the patient:** Sitting on a taping table or bench with the hand, fingers, and thumb in a neutral position.
➟ **Preparation:** Apply sterile materials, donut pad, or friction-reducing lubricant to the finger or thumb. Apply technique three directly to the skin.
➟ **Application:**

**STEP 1:** Cut a piece of the adhesive gauze material to cover an area from the fingertip to just proximal to the DIP or PIP joint.

*Option:* *If adhesive gauze is not available, 2 inch or 3 inch lightweight elastic tape may be used.*

**STEP 2:** Place the fingertip in the center of the adhesive gauze material (Fig. 11–11A).

**STEP 3:** Fold the sides over the finger, avoiding wrinkles.

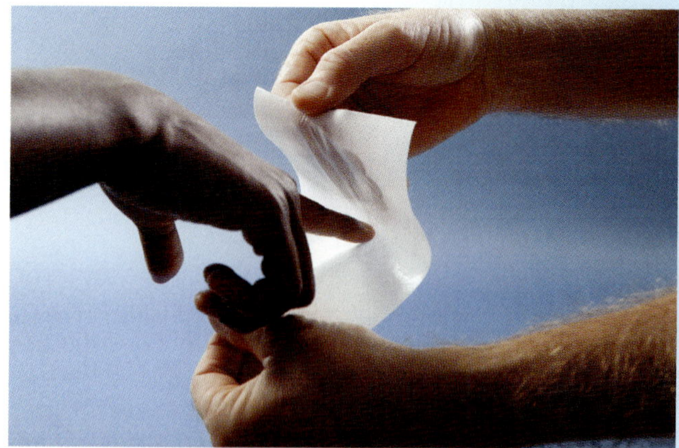

**Fig. 11–11 A

**STEP 4:**   Press the sides of the material firmly together against the finger (Fig. 11–11B).

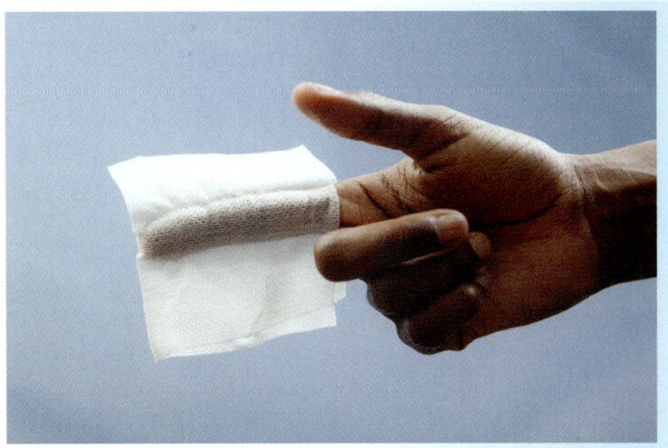

**Fig. 11–11 B**

**STEP 5:**   Cut the excess material away from the sides, leaving enough of the material to maintain adherence (Fig. 11–11C).

*Option:*   *Place circular strips of ½ inch non-elastic tape around the distal, middle, and/or prox-imal phalanx with moderate roll tension to anchor the material or tape* ◀▬▬▶*. End the tape strips on the dorsal finger to prevent unraveling.*

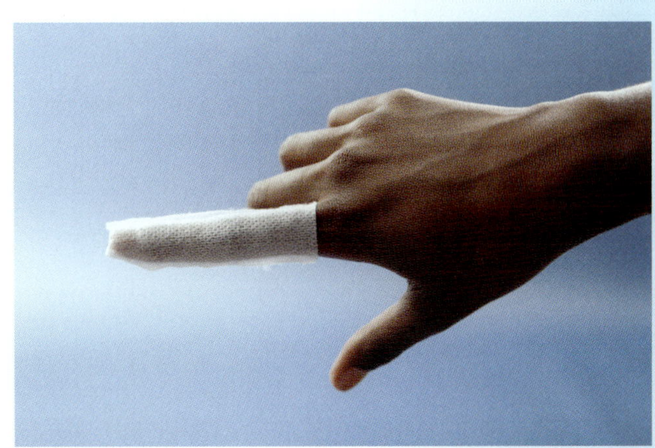

**Fig. 11–11 C**

## THUMB SPICA     Figures 11–12, 11–13, 11–14, 11–15, 11–16

The thumb spica technique is simply a figure-of-eight pattern encircling the wrist and thumb. This technique provides mild to moderate support and limits excessive abduction and extension at the MCP joint. Use the technique when preventing and treating thumb sprains and postdislocation and postfracture injuries. The spica may be applied with varying amounts of support and in combination with sports-specific gloves. This section first illustrates the basic spica, explores several variations, and discusses the addition of other materials for maximum support.

### Basic Thumb Spica

➠ **Purpose:** The basic thumb spica provides mild to moderate support and lessens excessive range of motion of the MCP joint when preventing and treating thumb sprains and postdislocation and postfracture inju-ries (Fig. 11–12).

➠ **Materials:**
   • 1 inch non-elastic or elastic tape, 1½ inch non-elastic tape
   *Option:*
   • Pre-wrap or self-adherent wrap
➠ **Position of the patient:** Sitting on a taping table or bench with the hand and thumb in a neutral position.
➠ **Preparation:** Apply the basic thumb spica directly to the skin.

*Hand, Fingers, and Thumb*

*Option:*  *Apply one to three layers of pre-wrap around the wrist and continue around the thumb, returning to the wrist to lessen irritation ◄▦▦▦►. Self-adherent wrap may be applied in place of pre-wrap. Apply the self-adherent wrap as illustrated in Step 1 below (Fig. 11–12A).*

▦► **Application:**

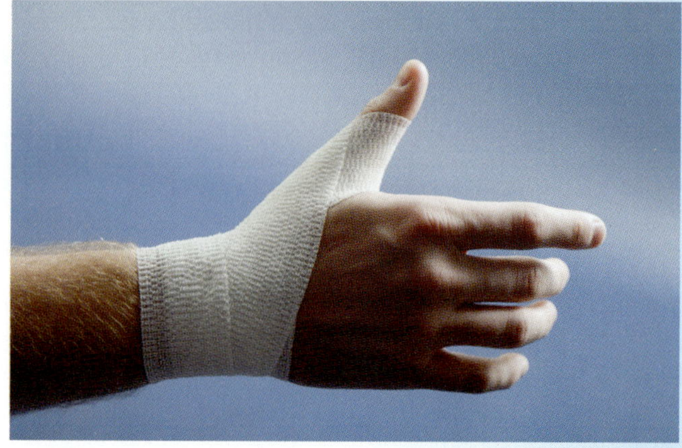

Fig. 11–12 A

**STEP 1:**  Anchor a strip of 1 inch non-elastic or elastic tape to the medial dorsal surface of the wrist and continue in a medial-to-lateral direction around the wrist to the MCP joint of the thumb with moderate roll tension (Fig. 11–12B).

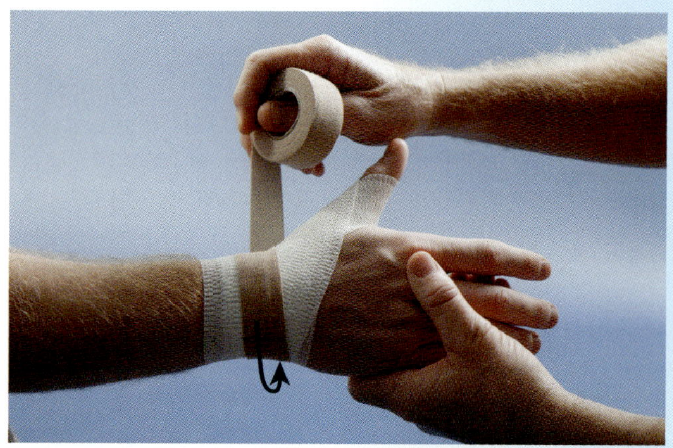

Fig. 11–12 B

**STEP 2:**  Next, cross the MCP joint, encircle the thumb, and anchor on the dorsal surface of the wrist with moderate roll tension (Fig. 11–12C). Slightly adduct and flex the thumb while applying the anchor dorsally to lessen excessive abduction and extension.

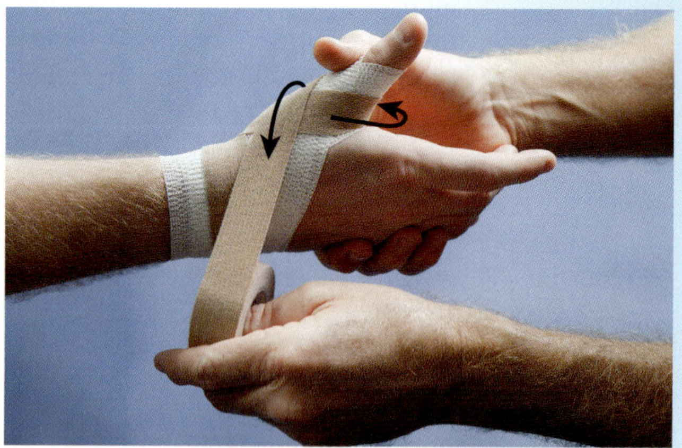

Fig. 11–12 C

**STEP 3:** Apply two to three strips of 1 inch non-elastic or elastic tape in the medial-to-lateral pattern with moderate roll tension, overlapping each by ¼–½ of the tape width in a proximal direction on the thumb (Fig. 11–12D). The tape strips should remain proximal to the **interphalangeal joint (IP)** of the thumb. The strips may be applied in an individual or continuous figure-of-eight pattern around the thumb and wrist.

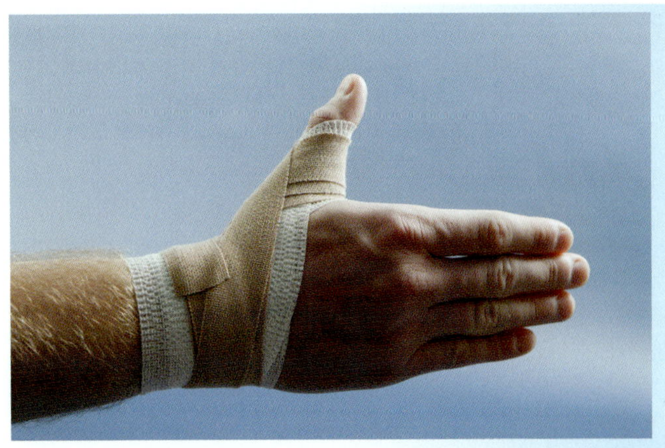

**Fig. 11–12 D**

**STEP 4:** Anchor the strips with moderate roll tension around the wrist with 1 inch or 1½ inch non-elastic tape in a circular pattern ◄━━━► (Fig. 11–12E).

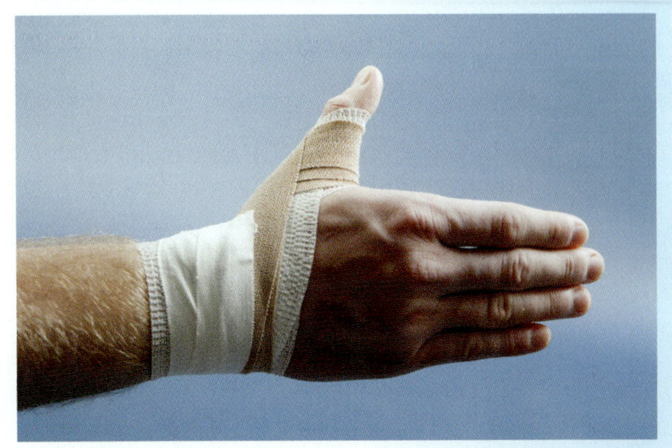

**Fig. 11–12 E**

### *Variation One*

➠ **Purpose:** This variation to the basic thumb spica technique provides mild to moderate support and limits range of motion of the MCP joint without restricting wrist motion (Fig. 11–13).
➠ **Materials:**
  • 1 inch non-elastic or elastic tape
➠ **Position of the patient:** Sitting on a taping table or bench with the hand and thumb in a neutral position.
➠ **Preparation:** Apply variation one directly to the skin or over pre-wrap or self-adherent wrap.
➠ **Application:**

**STEP 1:** Using 1 inch non-elastic or elastic tape, anchor on the medial dorsal aspect of the hand and continue in a medial-to-lateral pattern around the hand with moderate roll tension, remaining distal to the ulnar styloid process (Fig. 11–13A).

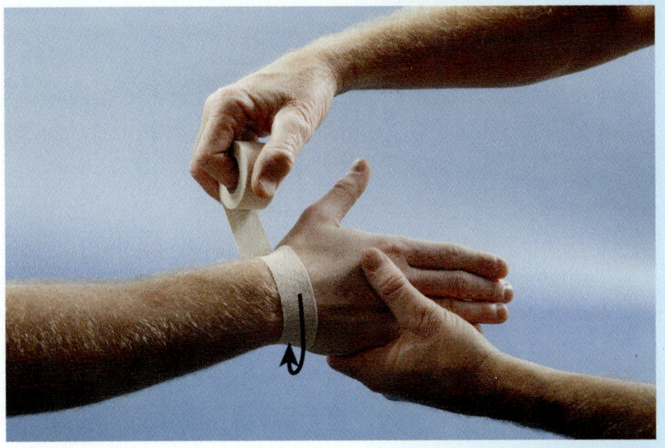

**Fig. 11–13 A**

*Steps Cont.*

**STEP 2:** At the MCP joint, encircle the thumb and finish on the dorsal hand with moderate roll tension (Fig. 11–13B). Slightly adduct and flex the thumb while applying the anchor dorsally.

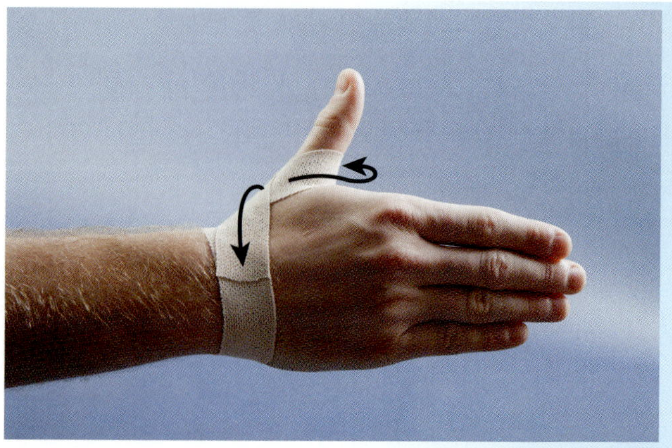

Fig. 11–13 B

**STEP 3:** Apply two to three additional spica strips with 1 inch non-elastic or elastic tape in an individual or continuous medial-to-lateral pattern, overlapping by ¼–½ of the tape width in a proximal direction on the thumb, and anchor on the dorsal hand (Fig. 11–13C). The tape should remain distal to the ulnar styloid process and proximal to the IP joint of the thumb. Do not apply anchor strips around the wrist.

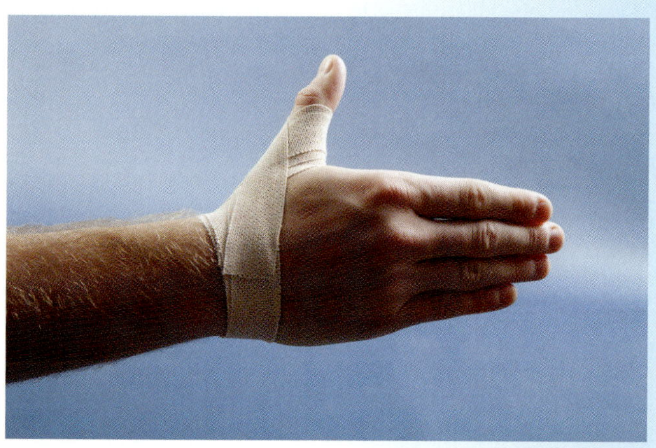

Fig. 11–13 C

**. . . IF/THEN . . .**

**IF** a thumb spica technique is required for a basketball player to support the MCP joint following a sprain, **THEN** consider using variation one, which will provide support and allow for full range of motion at the wrist with minimal effect on wrist flexion and extension during shooting.

### Variation Two

⇒ **Purpose:** When an injury requires greater support and reduction in range of motion of the MCP joint, use the circular wrist taping technique (see Fig. 10–7) or the following additional materials with the thumb spica taping (Fig. 11–14).

⇒ **Materials:**
- 1 inch non-elastic and elastic tape, 1½ inch non-elastic tape, pre-wrap or self-adherent wrap, discarded tape core from 2 inch or 3 inch tape, taping scissors

⇒ **Position of the patient:** Sitting on a taping table or bench with the hand and thumb in a neutral position.

➠ **Preparation:** Apply two to three layers of pre-wrap or self-adherent wrap as shown with the basic spica technique. Cut a discarded tape core to form a tear drop shape slightly larger than the MCP joint (Fig. 11–14A). Round the corners to prevent sharp edges and irritation to the skin.

➠ **Application:**

**STEP 1:** Apply two to three basic spica strips with 1 inch elastic tape in an individual or continuous pattern with moderate roll tension.

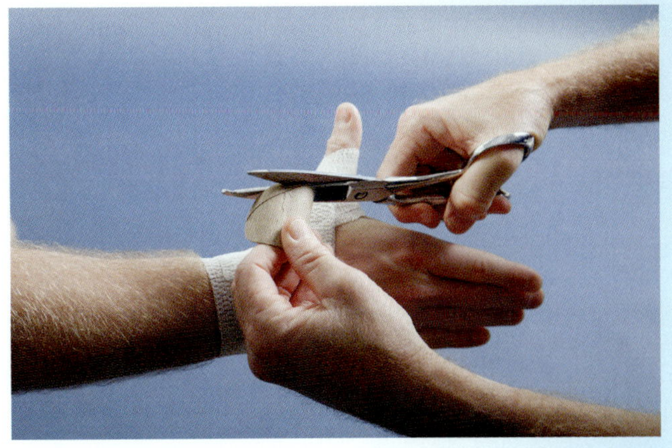

Fig. 11–14 A

**STEP 2:** Place the tape core over the MCP joint (Fig. 11–14B) and apply three to five additional 1 inch elastic tape basic spica strips with moderate roll tension in an overlapping fashion (Fig. 11–14C). The tape should remain proximal to the IP joint of the thumb.

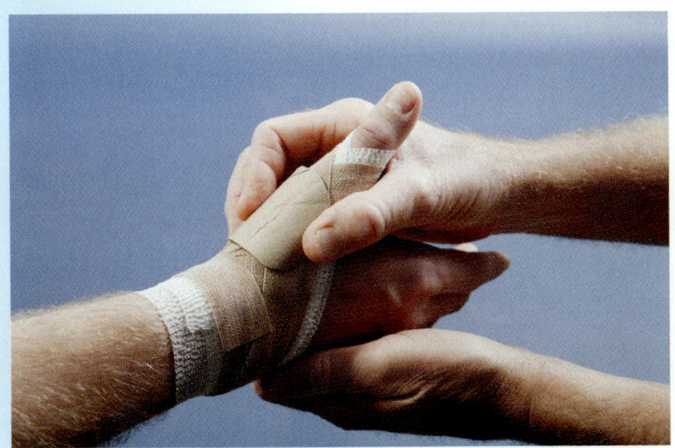

Fig. 11–14 B

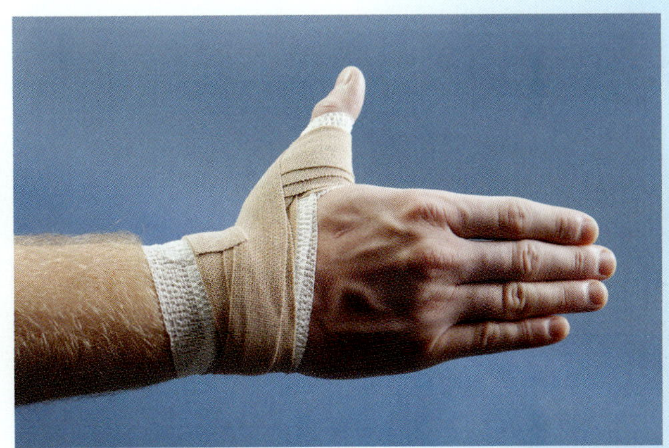

Fig. 11–14 C

**STEP 3:** Apply one to two 1 inch non-elastic tape basic spica strips with moderate roll tension and anchor at the wrist (Fig. 11–14D).

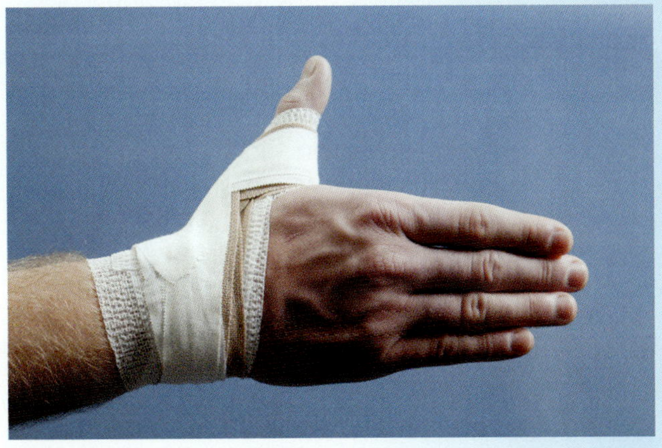

Fig. 11–14 D

*Steps Cont.*

**STEP 4:** Anchor the strips with 1 inch or 1½ inch non-elastic tape around the wrist in a circular pattern with moderate roll tension ◄▬▬► (Fig. 11–14E).

**STEP 5:** Apply the circular wrist taping technique for additional support.

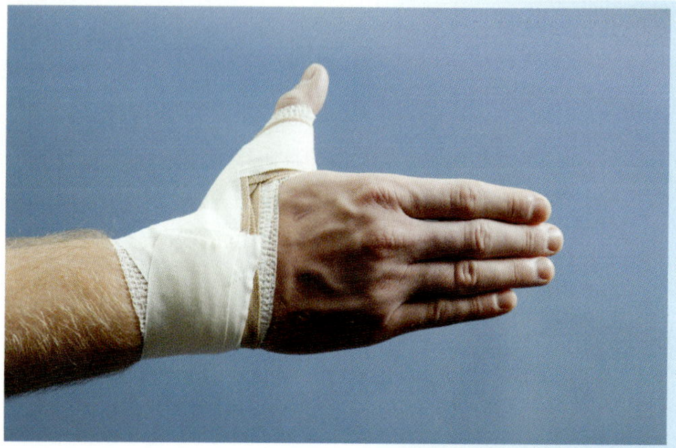

Fig. 11–14 E

### Variation Three

➤ **Purpose:** Mold and apply thermoplastic material to provide additional support to the MCP joint. The size and shape of the material depends on the amount of support needed. Use a small tear drop shape to cover the MCP joint and provide moderate support, or use a custom-made brace to encase the entire thumb for moderate support and immobilization (Fig. 11–15).

➤ **Materials:**
  • Paper, felt tip pen, thermoplastic material, a heating source, 1 inch non-elastic and elastic tape, 1½ inch non-elastic tape, pre-wrap or self-adherent wrap, 2 inch width moleskin, taping scissors

➤ **Position of the patient:** Sitting on a taping table or bench with the hand and thumb in a neutral position.

➤ **Preparation:** Apply two to three layers of pre-wrap or self-adherent wrap as shown with the basic spica technique. Design the tear drop shape with a paper pattern (see Fig. 1–10). Cut, mold, and shape the thermoplastic material on the MCP joint (Fig. 11–15A). Apply 2 inch moleskin to the inside surface of the material to prevent irritation.

➤ **Application:**

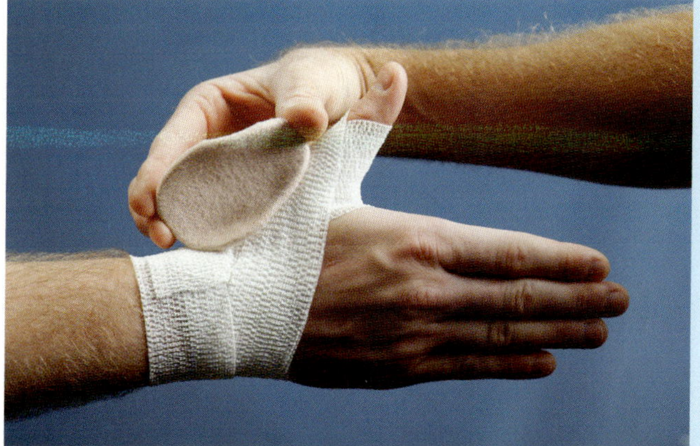

Fig. 11–15 A

**STEP 1:** Apply two to three 1 inch elastic tape basic spica strips with moderate roll tension. Apply the strips in an individual or continuous pattern.

**STEP 2:** Next, place the thermoplastic material over the MCP joint and secure with three to four overlapping 1 inch elastic tape basic spica strips with moderate roll tension (Fig. 11–15B). The tape should remain proximal to the IP joint of the thumb. One to two 1 inch non-elastic tape basic spica strips may be applied to provide additional support.

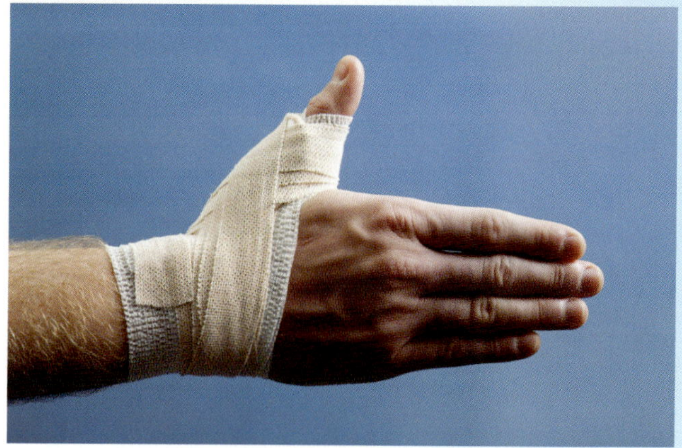

Fig. 11–15 B

**STEP 3:**   Anchor at the wrist in a circular pattern with 1 inch or 1½ inch non-elastic tape with moderate roll tension ◄▦► (Fig. 11–15C).

**STEP 4:**   The circular wrist taping technique may be applied for additional support.

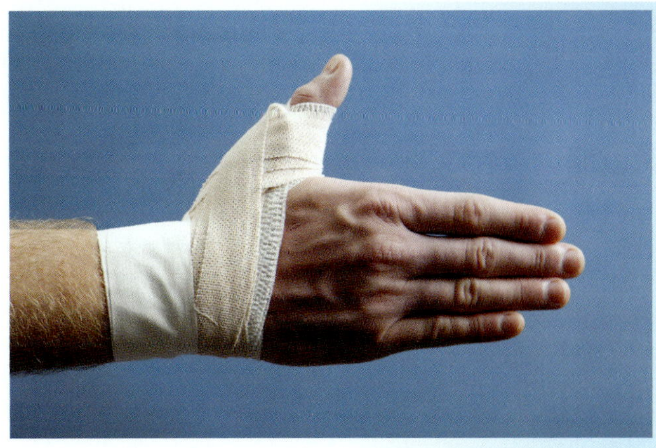

**Fig. 11–15 C**

### Anchor Technique to the Basic Spica and Spica Variations

➡ **Purpose:** Place horizontal strips over the MCP joint following application of the basic spica or spica variations to aid in limiting joint motion (Fig. 11–16). Consider using these strips to provide additional support to the MCP joint when preventing and treating sprains and postdislocation and postfracture injuries.

➡ **Materials:**
  • ½ inch and 1 inch non-elastic tape

➡ **Position of the patient:** Sitting on a taping table or bench with the hand and thumb in a neutral position.

➡ **Preparation:** Apply the basic thumb spica or one of the spica variations.

➡ **Application:**

**STEP 1:**   Begin proximal to the MCP joint and apply individual 1 inch non-elastic tape strips with equal tension inward toward the joint. Anchor each strip on the medial and lateral aspect of the thumb. Continue the strips in a distal direction, overlapping by ½ of the tape width, and finish just distal to the MCP joint (Figs. 11–16A and 11–16B).

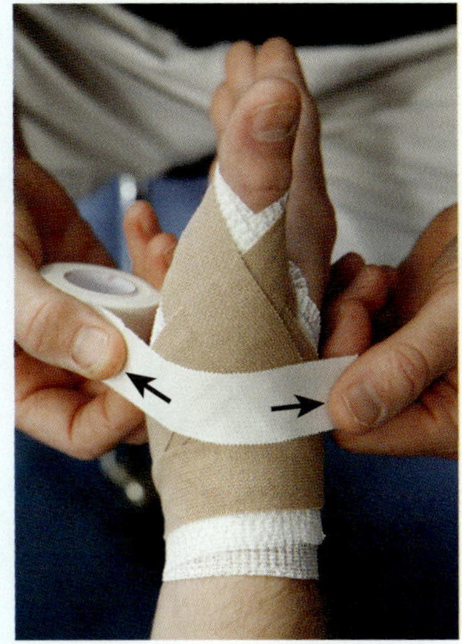

**Fig. 11–16 A**

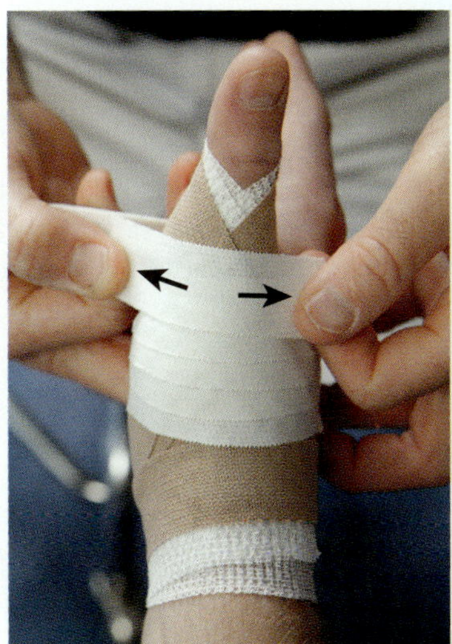

**Fig. 11–16 B**

*Steps Cont.*

**STEP 2:** Anchor the horizontal strips by placing a ½ inch non-elastic tape strip with mild to moderate roll tension from the wrist, under and around the thumb, and finish on the wrist (Fig. 11–16C).

**STEP 3:** Apply a 1 inch non-elastic tape circular anchor around the wrist with moderate roll tension ◀▦▶.

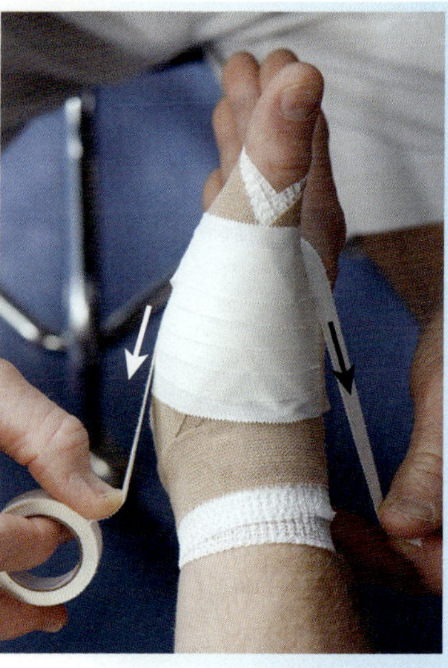

**Fig. 11–16 C**

**. . . IF/THEN . . .**

**IF** applying a thumb spica taping technique for football linemen to prevent and treat MCP injuries, **THEN** consider using variation two, three, and/or the anchor technique; these techniques provide additional support and can be applied under or over gloves.

## THUMB SPICA SEMIRIGID CAST         Figure 11–17

▦ **Purpose:** A semirigid cast provides maximum support and limits MCP joint and wrist range of motion (Fig. 11–17). This cast should be applied only by qualified health care professionals. Use the thumb spica cast when treating sprains and postdislocation and postfracture injuries upon a return to activity. The cast may be reused if removed carefully following athletic or work activities.

▦ **Materials:**
- 2 inch or 3 inch semirigid cast tape, gloves, water, self-adherent wrap, ⅛ inch foam or felt, 2 inch elastic tape, taping scissors

  *Option:*
- Thermoplastic material, a heating source

▦ **Position of the patient:** Sitting on a taping table or bench with the hand, thumb, and wrist in the position to be immobilized (as indicated by a physician) and the fingers in abduction.

▦ **Preparation:** Pad bony prominences with ⅛ inch foam or felt to lessen the occurrence of irritation.

▦ **Application:**

**STEP 1:**   Apply two to three layers of self-adherent wrap to the hand, thumb, and wrist with mild to moderate roll tension with the basic thumb spica and figure-of-eight patterns (see Figs. 10–8 and 11–12).

**STEP 2:**   Using 2 inch or 3 inch semirigid cast tape, anchor on the medial dorsal surface of the wrist and proceed around the wrist and thumb with the basic thumb spica pattern with moderate roll tension (Fig. 11–17A). Depending on the patient's size, the cast tape may need to be cut partially when encircling the thumb (Fig. 11–17B).

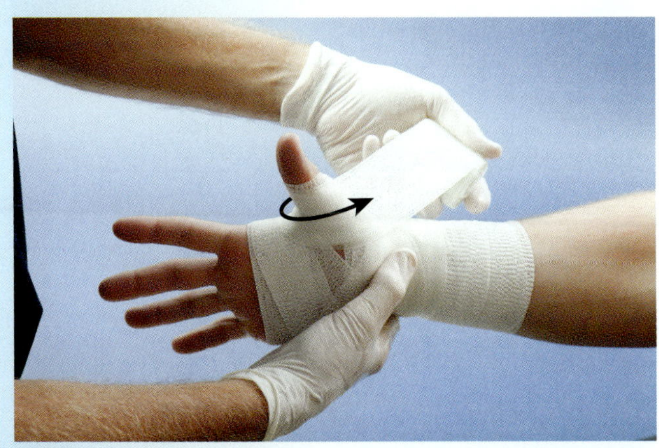

**Fig. 11–17 A**                                                          **Fig. 11–17 B**

**STEP 3:**   Alternate the basic thumb spica pattern with figures-of-eight involving the hand and wrist with moderate roll tension, overlapping the tape by ⅓–⅔ of its width (Fig. 11–17C). The cast tape should remain proximal to the MCP joints of fingers two through five and proximal to the IP joint of the thumb.

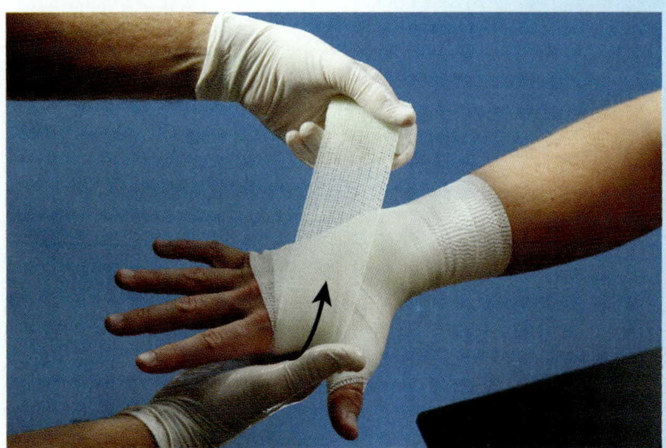

**Fig. 11–17 C**

*Option:*   *Incorporate thermoplastic material over the MCP joint for additional support (Fig. 11–17D).*

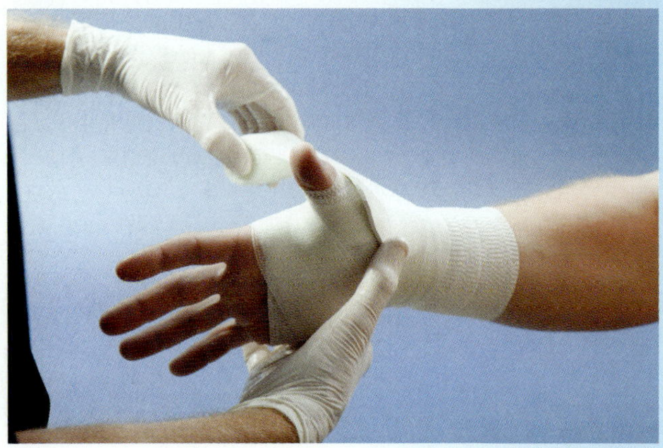

**Fig. 11–17 D**

*Steps Cont.*

**STEP 4:** Finish the tape on the dorsal wrist and smooth and mold the cast with the hands (Fig. 11–17E).

**STEP 5:** Prior to athletic practices and competitions, cover the semirigid cast with closed-cell, slow-recovery foam or similar material of at least ½ inch thickness (see Figs. 11–26A and 11–26B).

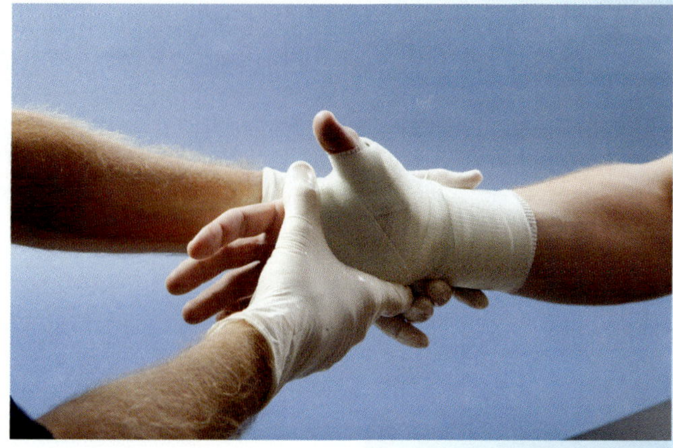

Fig. 11–17 E

**STEP 6:** Following athletic or work activities, remove the cast with taping scissors along the ulnar aspect of the cast (Fig. 11–17F). Allow the inside of the cast to dry overnight by removing the self-adherent wrap and placing the cast in a well-ventilated area.

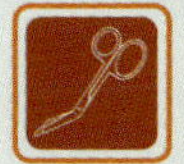

**Helpful Hint |**
Place a tongue depressor inside the cast to spread the edges apart to ensure drying.

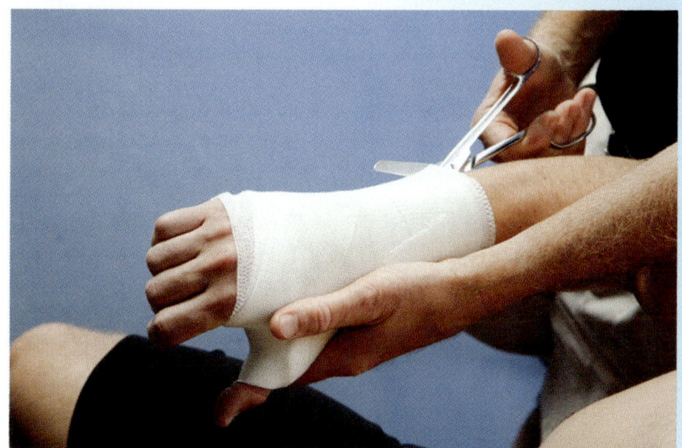

Fig. 11–17 F

**STEP 7:** When reusing, apply two to three layers of self-adherent wrap to the hand, thumb, and wrist with the basic thumb spica and figure-of-eight patterns with moderate roll tension. Replace the cast on the hand, thumb, and wrist, and anchor with 2 inch elastic tape or self-adherent wrap in a circular pattern with moderate roll tension ◀▬▶ (Fig. 11–17G).

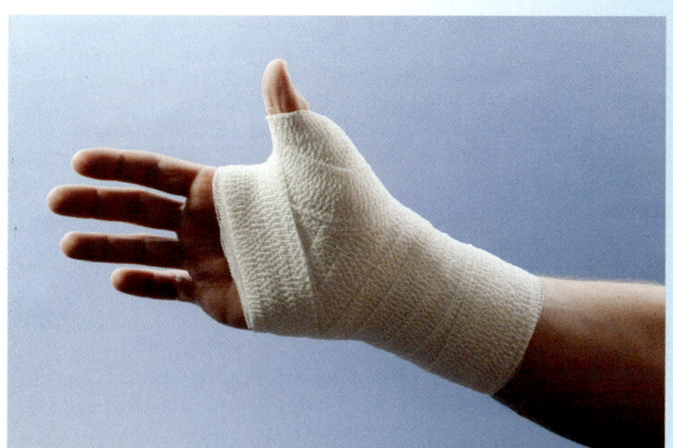

Fig. 11–17 G

## FIGURE-OF-EIGHT TAPE

**Purpose:** The figure-of-eight tape technique is used to anchor padding when preventing and treating hand injuries and conditions.
  • Use the figure-of-eight tape technique (see Fig. 10–8) to attach protective padding when preventing and treating contusions.

### Clinical Application Question 2

During the middle of the season, an offensive tackle on the football team sustains a third-degree right thumb ulnar collateral ligament sprain during practice. After surgery, he is immobilized in a rigid thumb spica cast for 3 weeks. Rehabilitation begins, after which he and the surgeon begin to discuss his return to activity. The surgeon allows a return to activity based on the following guidelines:

Postoperative weeks 3–6: Return to practice and competition at postop week 4 with maximum support: splinting of the right thumb during non-athletic activities.

Postoperative weeks 6–8: Continue athletic participation with moderate support: discontinue non-athletic activity splinting.

**Question: What techniques can be used in this situation?**

# Wrapping Techniques

Wrapping techniques provide compression and support when treating hand, finger, and thumb injuries and conditions. Elastic wraps, tapes, and sleeves, self-adherent wrap, and conforming gauze are used to control swelling following injury. Wraps may be used to anchor protective padding following soft tissue and bone injuries.

## HAND AND WRIST COMPRESSION WRAP         Figure 11–18

**Purpose:** The hand and wrist or finger and thumb compression wrap technique reduces mild, moderate, or severe swelling and inflammation by applying mechanical pressure[14] when treating contusions, sprains, dislocations, and tendon ruptures (Fig. 11–18).

**Materials:**
  • 2 inch, 3 inch, or 4 inch width by 5 yard length elastic wrap, metal clips, 1½ inch non-elastic or 2 inch elastic tape, ⅛ inch or ¼ inch foam or felt, taping scissors
  • 1 inch elastic tape or self-adherent wrap for the fingers or thumb
  *Options:*
  • 2 inch, 3 inch, or 4 inch width self-adherent wrap
  • ¼ inch or ½ inch open-cell foam

**Position of the patient:** Sitting on a taping table or bench with the wrist and hand in a pain-free position and the fingers in abduction.

**Preparation:** Place ⅛ inch or ¼ inch foam or felt over the inflamed area directly on the skin.

**Application:**

**STEP 1:** For the hand, anchor the elastic wrap on the dorsal hand in a circular pattern just distal to the MCP joints of fingers two through five and apply the hand and wrist compression wrap technique (see Figs. 10–15 and 11–18A).

*Options:* *If an elastic wrap is not available, 2 inch, 3 inch, or 4 inch self-adherent wrap may be used. Place a ¼ inch or ½ inch open-cell foam pad over the dorsal hand for additional compression to assist in venous return (see Fig. 11–27A). Apply the pad directly on the skin and cover with the hand and wrist compression wrap.*

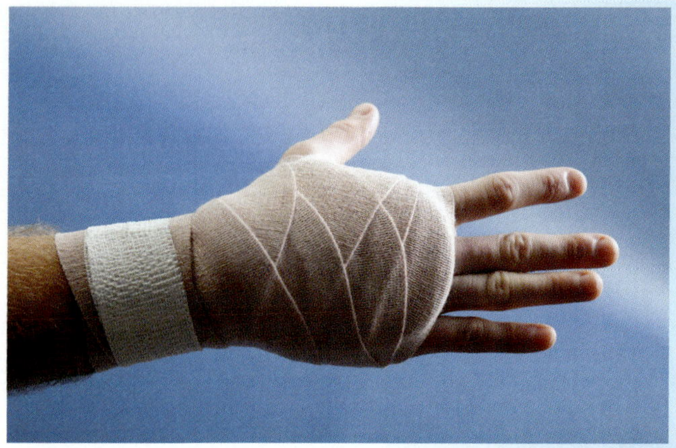

**Fig. 11–18 A**

**STEP 2:** For the fingers or thumb, apply 1 inch elastic tape or self-adherent wrap in a distal-to-proximal circular pattern over the finger or thumb ◄▬▬► (Fig. 11–18B). Apply pressure greatest at the distal end and less toward the proximal end. The tip of the finger or thumb should remain exposed to monitor circulation. No additional anchor is required.

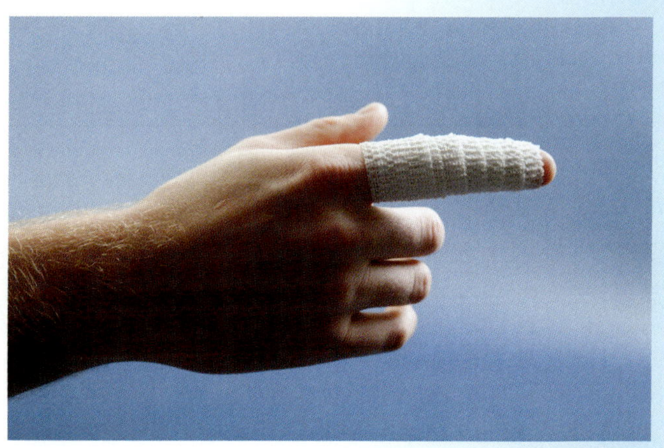

**Fig. 11–18 B**

## FINGER SLEEVES   Figure 11–19

➠ **Purpose:** Use finger sleeves to provide mild to moderate support and compression to the PIP joint to reduce mild, moderate, or severe swelling when treating sprains (Fig. 11–19). The benefit of this technique is that the patient can apply the sleeve without assistance following application instruction.

➠ **Design:**
- The sleeves are available off-the-shelf in predetermined sizes based on finger width measurements.
- Most sleeves are constructed of nylon and elastic or neoprene materials in a single or double finger design.
- The design of the sleeve allows for normal range of motion at the DIP joint.

➠ **Materials:**
- Off-the-shelf single or double finger sleeve

➠ **Position of the patient:** Sitting on a taping table or bench with the hand, fingers, and thumb in a pain-free position.

➠ **Preparation:** Apply the finger sleeve directly to the skin.

➠ **Application:**

**STEP 1:** To apply, pull the sleeve onto the finger(s) in a proximal direction (Fig. 11–19). No anchors are necessary; the sleeves are washable and reusable.

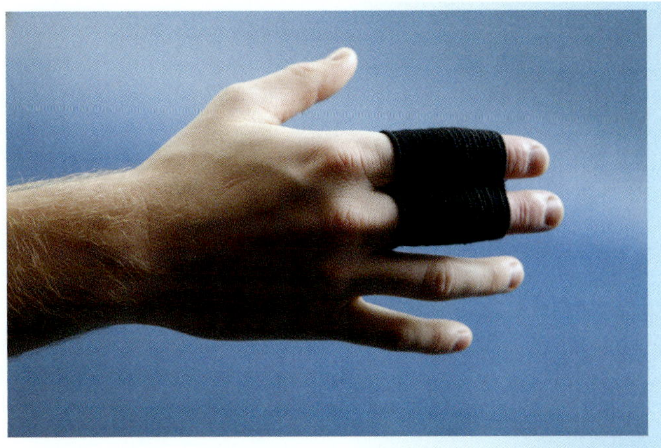

**Fig. 11–19**

## BOXER'S WRAP     Figure 11–20

➡ **Purpose:** The boxer's wrap is similar to the technique used under boxing gloves to pad the hands, but this technique can also be used as a compression wrap for the hand to lessen mild, moderate, or severe swelling following contusions (Fig. 11–20). The boxer's wrap padding technique is discussed later in the chapter.

➡ **Materials:**
  • 1½ inch, 2 inch, or 3 inch conforming gauze or self-adherent wrap, 1½ inch non-elastic tape, ⅛ inch or ¼ inch foam or felt, taping scissors
  ***Option:***
  • ¼ inch or ½ inch open-cell foam

➡ **Position of the patient:** Sitting on a taping table or bench with the hand, fingers, and thumb in a pain-free position and the fingers in abduction.

➡ **Preparation:** Apply the boxer's wrap directly to the skin. Eighth of an inch or ¼ inch foam or felt may be placed over the inflamed area to assist in venous return.

➡ **Application:**

**STEP 1:** Anchor 1½ inch, 2 inch, or 3 inch conforming gauze or self-adherent wrap to the medial dorsal surface of the wrist and continue in a medial-to-lateral direction around the wrist with moderate roll tension (Fig. 11–20A).

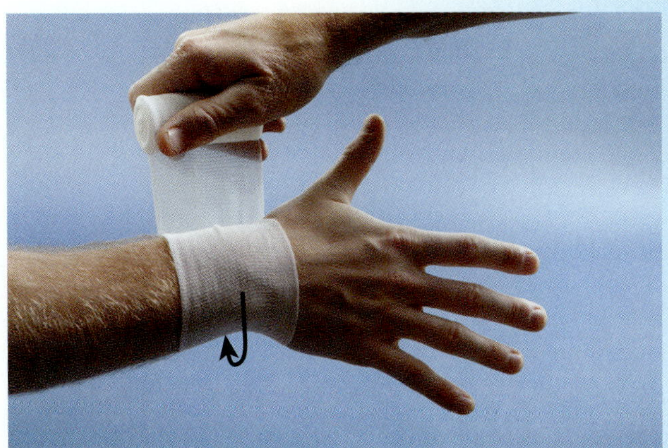

**Fig. 11–20 A**

*Steps Cont.*

**STEP 2:** From the wrist, continue to apply the conforming gauze or wrap across the dorsal aspect of the hand, encircle the second finger at the MCP joint with mild to moderate roll tension, then return and anchor around the wrist in a medial-to-lateral direction (Fig. 11–20B).

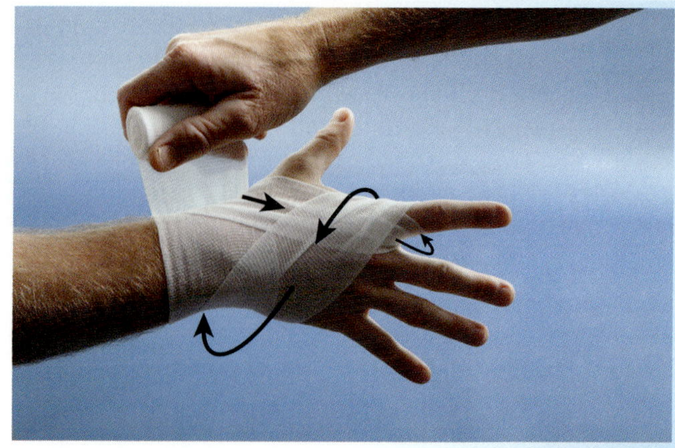

Fig. 11–20 B

**STEP 3:** Continue with this pattern, encircling the third, fourth, and fifth fingers at the MCP joint (Fig. 11–20C). Instruct the patient to flex the fingers actively and make a fist when making each pass around the MCP joint.

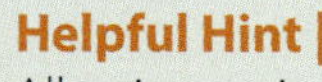

**Helpful Hint |**
Allowing active flexion of the fingers during the technique will prevent the conforming gauze or self-adherent wrap from constricting and abrading the finger web space.

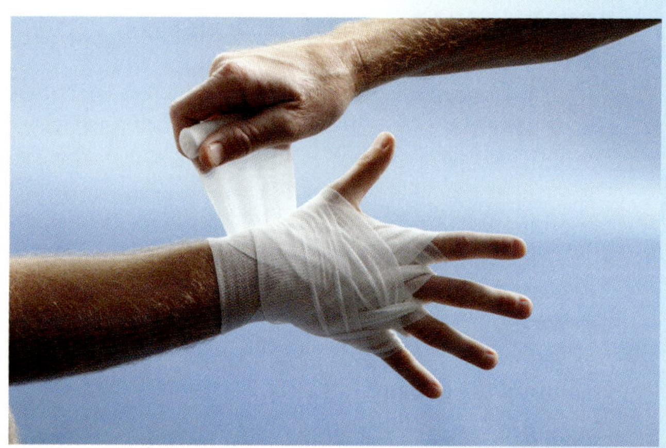

Fig. 11–20 C

**STEP 4:** Next, apply two to three basic thumb spicas with moderate roll tension with the gauze or wrap (Fig. 11–20D).

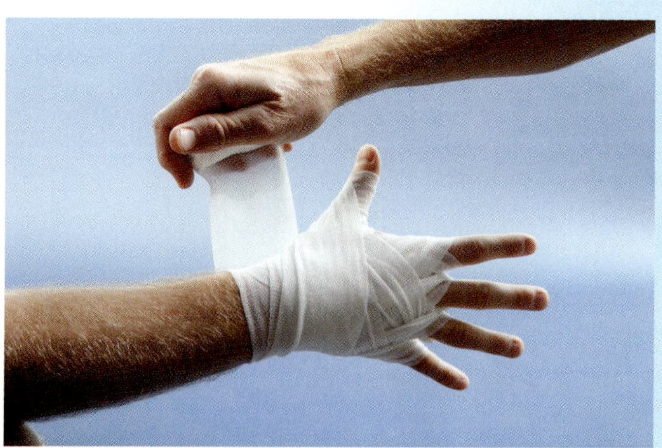

Fig. 11–20 D

**STEP 5:** Cover the remainder of the hand with overlapping figures-of-eight (see Fig. 10–8) with moderate roll tension and anchor loosely around the wrist (Fig. 11–20E).

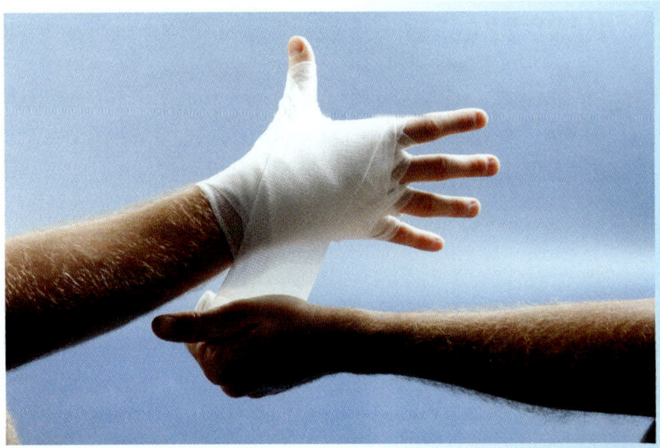

Fig. 11–20 E

**STEP 6:** Apply a loose anchor of 1½ inch non-elastic tape around the wrist ◄▦► (Fig. 11–20F).

*Option:* *Consider using a ¼ inch or ½ inch open-cell foam pad over the dorsal hand for additional compression. Apply the pad directly to the skin and cover with the boxer's wrap.*

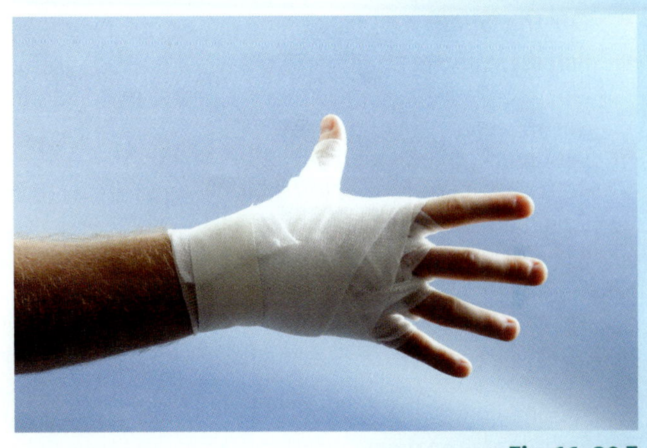

Fig. 11–20 F

## FIGURE-OF-EIGHT WRAP

▦► **Purpose:** The figure-of-eight wrap technique anchors protective padding when preventing and treating hand injuries and conditions.
  • Use the technique illustrated in Chapter 10 (see Fig. 10–16) to attach pads when preventing and treating contusions.

### ...IF/THEN...

**IF** using a finger or thumb brace and swelling and inflammation are present, **THEN** apply a compression wrap technique underneath the brace to control swelling and inflammation; note, a larger size brace may be needed to ensure proper fit, support, and immobilization of the finger and/or thumb.

# Bracing Techniques

Bracing techniques are used to prevent and treat acute and chronic hand, finger, and thumb injuries and conditions. The off-the-shelf and custom-made designs provide compression, support, and immobilization and lessen range of motion. Several other braces used for hand and thumb injuries and conditions were discussed in Chapter 10.

## HAND BRACES   Figure 11–21

**Purpose:** Off-the-shelf and custom-made hand braces provide support and immobilization and limit range of motion when treating fractures of the fourth and fifth metacarpals (Fig. 11–21). These braces are commonly referred to as gutter splints, forming a channel around the fourth and fifth fingers, hand, wrist, and distal forearm. Two methods are illustrated in the application of the technique. Choose a technique according to patient preferences and available supplies.

### DETAILS
The braces are commonly used following acute injury in the conservative management of a boxer's fracture. Off-the-shelf and custom-made designs can also be used in combination with the hand and wrist compression wrapping technique.

### Off-the-Shelf

**Purpose:** Off-the-shelf hand braces are used when treating stable fractures of the fourth and fifth meta-carpals. The braces provide compression, moderate support, and immobilization and reduce range of motion.

**Design:**
- Off-the-shelf right or left style designs are available in predetermined sizes corresponding to wrist cir-cumference measurements.
- The open design braces are constructed of a nylon/polyester material outer shell with a polypropylene felt lining.
- Malleable dorsal and palmar aluminum bars incorporated into the shell are used to limit range of motion of the wrist, hand, and fingers four and five.
- Velcro straps and D-ring closures anchor the braces to the wrist, hand, and fingers and allow for adjust-ments in fit.

**Position of the patient:** Sitting on a taping table or bench with the wrist, hand, and fingers in the position to be immobilized (as indicated by a physician).

**Preparation:** Apply the off-the-shelf braces directly to the skin.

Instructions for the application of hand braces are included with each brace when purchased. The following guidelines pertain to most braces.

**Application:**

**STEP 1:**  Loosen the straps and unfold the brace.

**STEP 2:**  Place the fourth and fifth fingers, hand, and wrist into the brace and continue pulling the brace toward the forearm. Insert the fifth finger through the attached loop (Fig. 11–21A).

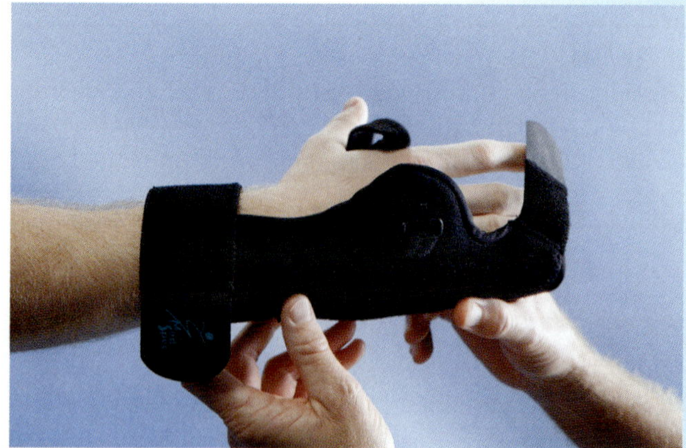

**Fig. 11–21 A**

**STEP 3:** Wrap the outer shell around the fingers, hand, and wrist. The application of straps will depend on the specific brace design. Begin application of most designs by pulling the strap around the wrist and anchoring. Next, pull the strap over the thenar web space, through the D-ring closure, and anchor. Last, anchor the strap around the distal fingers (Fig. 11–21B).

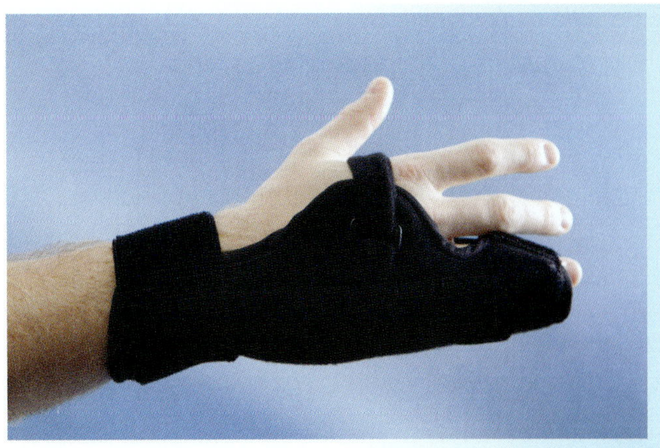

**Fig. 11–21 B**

### Custom-Made

⟹ **Purpose:** Construct custom-made braces from thermoplastic material when off-the-shelf designs are not available. These designs also provide moderate support, compression, and immobilization and limit range of motion in the treatment of stable fractures of the fourth and fifth metacarpals.

⟹ **Materials:**
  • Paper, felt tip pen, thermoplastic material, ⅛ inch foam or 2 inch or 3 inch width moleskin, a heating source, ½ inch or 1 inch non-elastic tape, 1½ inch or 2 inch self-adherent wrap, taping scissors

⟹ **Position of the patient:** Sitting on a taping table or bench with the wrist, hand, and fingers in the position to be immobilized (as indicated by a physician).

⟹ **Preparation:** Design the brace with a paper pattern. Apply this technique directly to the skin.

⟹ **Application:**

**STEP 1:** Using paper, make a pattern from the dorsal and palmar surfaces of the distal ends of the fourth and fifth fingers, continue in a proximal direction across the dorsal and palmar hand, then across the wrist, and finish on the distal forearm. The pattern should conform to the fourth and fifth fingers and the ulnar aspect of the hand, wrist, and forearm similar to a gutter.

**STEP 2:** Apply the buddy tape technique to fingers four and five (see Fig. 11–7).

**STEP 3:** Using the pattern, cut the thermoplastic material, then heat. Mold and shape the material over the area in the desired position as indicated by a physician. Trim the brace if necessary.

**STEP 4:** Attach ⅛ inch foam or 2 inch or 3 inch moleskin to the inside surface of the material to prevent irritation (Fig. 11–21C).

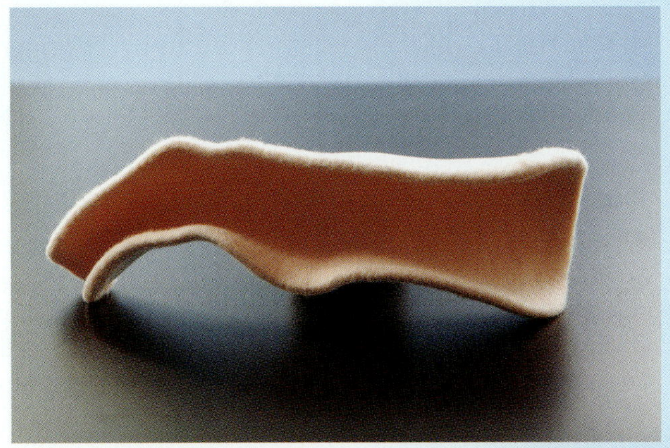

**Fig. 11–21 C**

*Steps Cont.*

**STEP 5:** Place the brace over the fingers, hand, wrist, and forearm. Anchor the brace with the circular wrist taping or figure-of-eight taping or wrapping technique (see Figs. 10–7, 10–8, and 10–16). Apply three to four circular strips around the distal brace with 1½ inch or 2 inch self-adherent wrap with moderate roll tension ◄▬► (Fig. 11–21D). End the wrap on the dorsal aspect of the brace to prevent unraveling.

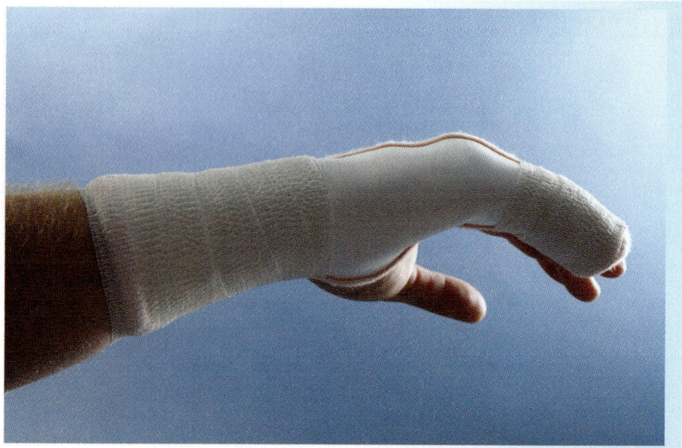

**Fig. 11–21 D**

## EVIDENCE SUMMARY

The efficacy of various interventions for the conservative treatment of boxer's fractures has been examined in three separate evidence-based reviews. A 2016 review of five studies[15] compared reduction of the fracture and cast immobilization with soft wrapping and buddy taping without reduction. The results showed that soft wrapping and buddy taping produced greater metacarpophalangeal range of motion and grip and wrist strength among the subjects. The researchers[15] found no differences in rates of healing, patient-reported satisfaction and pain scores, and time to return to work among the interventions. A separate 2016 meta-analysis[16] of six randomized controlled trials examined complication rates among conservative and surgical interventions for the management of boxer's fractures. Complications in the trials included infection, pain, neurological injury, tendon injury, and postsurgical hardware removal or revision. The findings showed conservative interventions resulted in lower rates of complications when compared to surgical techniques. A 2005 evidence-based review[17] investigated the efficacy of various interventions for the conservative management of boxer's fractures. Five studies were included in the review, but none described the primary outcome measure: function as demonstrated through validated hand function scores. As a result, the authors[17] found no evidence from the data to recommend one best method of treatment among gutter splints, braces, and casts; compression wraps; and functional taping techniques. Further well-designed, high-quality studies among various populations are warranted to determine which intervention produces the greatest clinical and functional outcomes following a fifth metacarpal fracture.

## FINGER BRACES    Figure 11–22

▬► **Purpose:** Use off-the-shelf and custom-made finger braces to provide support and immobilization and to limit range of motion when treating sprains, fractures, and tendon ruptures (Fig. 11–22). Two methods are illustrated in the application of the technique. Choose a technique according to patient preferences and available supplies.

### Off-the-Shelf

▬► **Purpose:** Several off-the-shelf bracing techniques may be used to treat an extensor digitorum tendon rupture and/or distal phalanx fracture. Use these braces to provide moderate support and complete immobilization of the DIP joint. Regardless of which design is used, rotate the brace from the dorsal to the palmar aspect of the finger frequently to prevent maceration of the skin. While the brace is being changed, maintain extension in the DIP joint. Other designs provide mild support and limit range of motion when treating PIP or DIP joint sprains.

**DETAILS**
Finger braces are commonly used to provide support for athletes in a variety of sports but can also be useful with work and casual activities.

➠ **Design:**
  - Off-the-shelf braces are available in predetermined sizes in universal fit designs based on finger length or width measurements.
  - Some designs are constructed of plastic materials and are purchased in kits that include several types of braces in pre-molded sizes.
    - These braces allow for minimal adjustments in fit and are attached to the finger with non-elastic or elastic tape.
  - Other braces are constructed of malleable aluminum with an open-cell foam pad lining.
    - These designs allow for adjustments in fit depending on the injury and condition and are attached with non-elastic or elastic tape.
  - Another design uses a semirigid plastic strip incorporated into adhesive material that wraps over the finger to limit range of motion.

➠ **Materials:**
  - ½ inch non-elastic or 1 inch non-elastic or elastic tape, taping scissors

➠ **Position of the patient:** Sitting on a taping table or bench with the hand, fingers, and thumb in a neutral position. Place the DIP joint of the involved finger or thumb in extension.

➠ **Preparation:** Apply the off-the-shelf braces directly to the skin.

➠ **Application:**

**STEP 1:** Apply some designs by placing the brace over the tip of the finger or thumb. Continue to apply the brace in a distal-to-proximal direction until the tip of the finger or thumb contacts the distal end of the brace. The finger or thumb should fit snugly in the brace (Fig. 11–22A).

**STEP 2:** Anchor with mild to moderate roll tension at the proximal end of the brace with ½ inch non-elastic or 1 inch non-elastic or elastic tape. Apply three to five continuous circular patterns ◀▦▶ (Fig. 11–22B). End the pattern on the dorsal aspect of the finger or thumb to prevent unraveling.

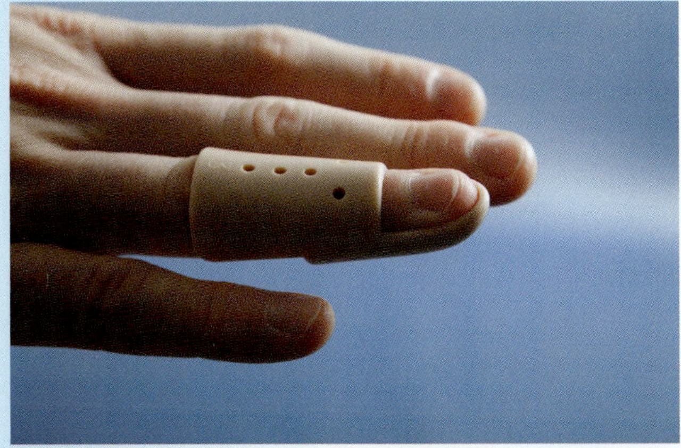

**Fig. 11–22 A**

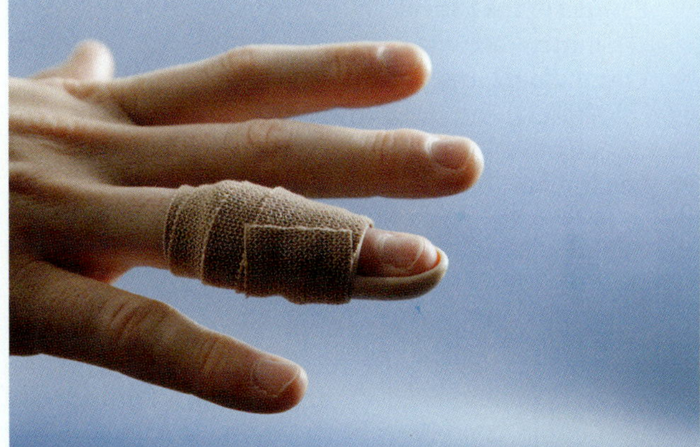

**Fig. 11–22 B**

**STEP 3:** Other designs require cutting and molding to the finger or thumb. Cut a piece of the aluminum material in a length from proximal to the DIP joint to the distal end of the finger or thumb (Fig. 11–22C).

**STEP 4:** Trim any sharp edges of the aluminum to prevent injury and slightly bend the distal end of the brace to maintain full extension in the DIP joint.

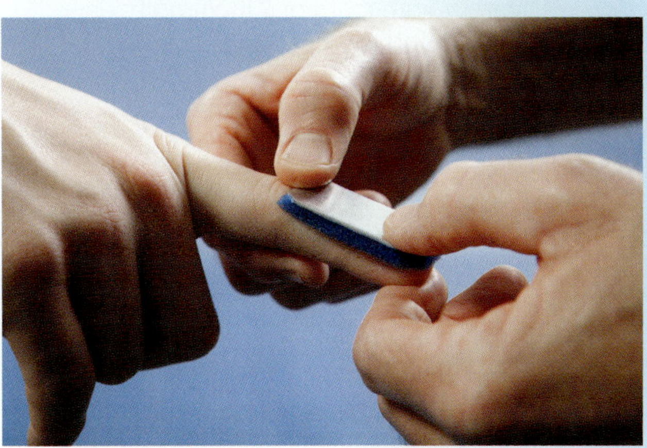

**Fig. 11–22 C**

*Steps Cont.*

**Hand, Fingers, and Thumb**

**STEP 5:**  Apply the brace on the dorsal or palmar aspect of the finger or thumb. Anchor ½ inch or 1 inch non-elastic tape on top of the brace and apply three to five continuous circular patterns around the distal and proximal ends of the brace with moderate roll tension, positioning the DIP joint in full extension ◄▥▥▥► (Fig. 11–22D). End the pattern on the dorsal aspect of the finger or thumb.

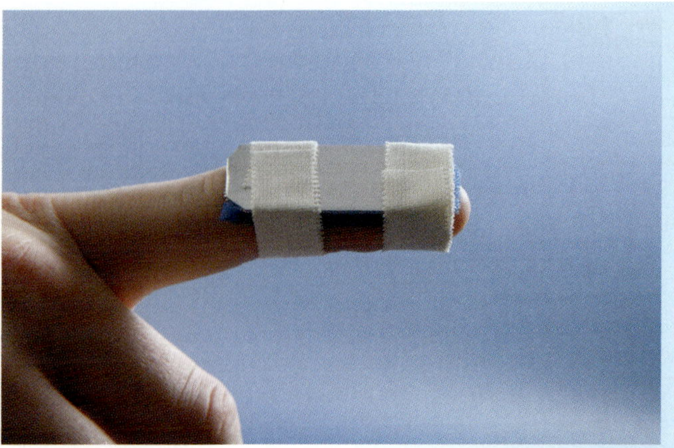

**Fig. 11–22 D**

### Custom-Made

▥▶ **Purpose:** Use thermoplastic material to custom-fit a brace to the finger and thumb when off-the-shelf designs are not available. This technique also provides moderate support and immobilization of the DIP joint when treating an extensor digitorum tendon rupture and/or distal phalanx fracture. Rotate these braces from the dorsal to the palmar aspect of the finger or thumb frequently to prevent maceration of the skin. Maintain extension in the DIP joint while the brace is being changed. Custom-made finger and thumb designs are reusable.

▥▶ **Materials:**
  • Paper, felt tip pen, thermoplastic material, ⅛ inch foam or 2 inch width moleskin, a heating source, ½ inch or 1 inch non-elastic tape, taping scissors

▥▶ **Position of the patient:** Sitting on a taping table or bench with the hand, fingers, and thumb in a neutral position. Place the DIP joint of the involved finger or thumb in extension.

▥▶ **Preparation:** Design the brace with a paper pattern or estimate the width and length from proximal to the DIP joint to the distal end of the finger or thumb. Heat the thermoplastic material. Apply this technique directly to the skin.

▥▶ **Application:**

**STEP 1:**  Fit and mold the material to the dorsal or palmar aspect of the finger or thumb (Fig. 11–22E). Remember to keep the DIP joint in full extension during fitting. Trim the edges of the material to prevent injury and cover the inside surface with ⅛ inch foam or 2 inch moleskin for comfort.

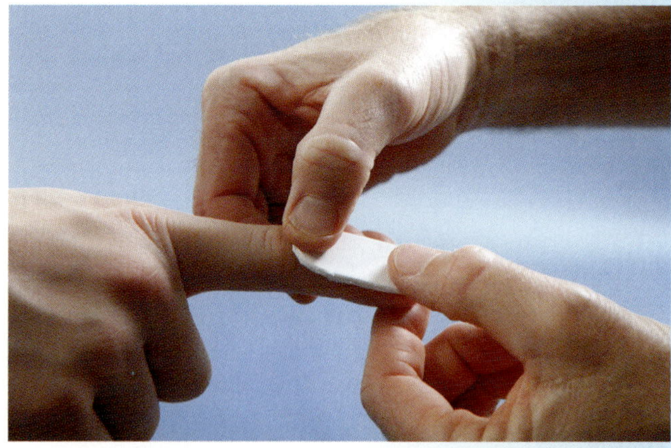

**Fig. 11–22 E**

**STEP 2:** Apply the brace on the dorsal or palmar finger or thumb. Place ½ inch or 1 inch non-elastic tape on top of the brace and anchor with three to five continuous circular patterns around the distal and proximal ends of the brace with moderate roll tension ◀▬▬▶ (Fig. 11–22F). Maintain full extension of the DIP joint. End the pattern on the dorsal aspect of the finger or thumb.

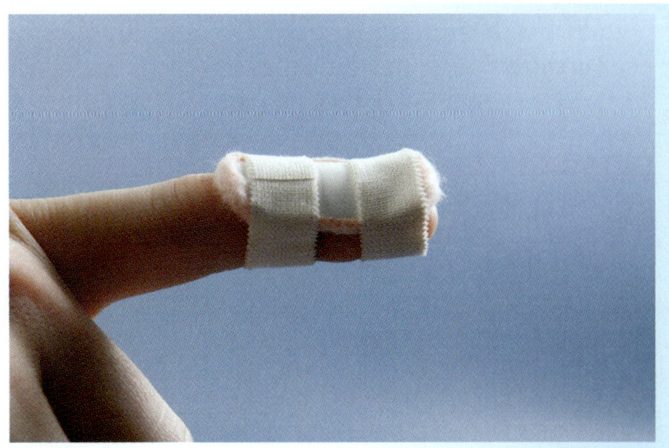

**Fig. 11–22 F**

## EVIDENCE SUMMARY

Several evidence-based reviews have investigated various treatment interventions, immobilization periods, and brace designs for the management of mallet finger. Mallet finger is typically treated with conservative interventions consisting of a period of immobilization using a brace or splint. Examining surgical and conservative treatments, two separate reviews[18,19] found conservative management with brace immobilization was effective for uncomplicated mallet finger injuries. A 2018 systematic review[19] that included five studies revealed a mean extensor lag in the DIP joint of 5.7 degrees following surgical treatment and 7.6 degrees following conservative treatment. However, the researchers[19] suggested that the differences in extensor lag among the interventions were not clinically significant. Most researchers suggest splinting the DIP joint in neutral to slight hyperextension[20–22] for 6 to 8 weeks with additional weeks of splinting indicated if extensor lag in the DIP joint remains after the initial period of immobilization.[20,22] In a 2004

review, researchers[23] found insufficient evidence among four studies of poor quality to determine the effectiveness of off-the-shelf and custom-made braces and which design is more appropriate following injury. However, three more recent reviews[19,22,24] revealed no differences in extensor lag between off-the-shelf and custom-made braces following 6 to 8 weeks of immobilization. One review[24] reported that off-the-shelf braces produced greater occurrences of skin complications (maceration, pain, ulceration) compared with custom-made designs. In a separate review,[19] surgical interventions resulted in greater occurrences of complications compared with off-the-shelf and custom-made braces. The current evidence in the literature supports conservative management for uncomplicated mallet finger injuries. Decisions regarding the type of brace design to implement, off-the-shelf or custom-made, should be guided by clinician expertise and patient preferences, such as needs of athletic and work activities and level of comfort.

**DETAILS**

Whether off-the-shelf or custom-made braces are worn on the dorsal or on the palmar aspect of the fingers and thumb depends on the activities of the patient. Away from sport or work, apply the brace on the palmar aspect. During sport or work activity, **tactile** sensation of the finger and thumb is often required. In these cases, apply the brace to the dorsal aspect of the finger and thumb.

## THUMB BRACES      Figure 11–23

▬▶ **Purpose:** Off-the-shelf and custom-made thumb braces provide compression and support and limit range of motion during athletic and work activities. These braces also provide compression and immobilization when away from these activities. Use these designs when preventing and treating sprains, dislocations, and postfracture injuries of the thumb (Fig. 11–23). Note that some rehabilitative wrist braces, discussed in Chapter 10, can be used to treat thumb sprains, dislocations, and postfracture injuries. Two methods are illustrated in the application of the thumb bracing technique. Choose according to patient preferences and available supplies.

### Off-the-Shelf

▪▶ **Purpose:** Use off-the-shelf thumb braces to provide compression, moderate support, and immobilization and lessen range of motion when preventing and treating sprains, dislocations, and postfracture injuries.

## DETAILS
Thumb braces are commonly used to provide support for athletes in a variety of sports. The braces can also be used with work and casual activities.

▪▶ **Design:**
- Off-the-shelf universal fit and right or left style designs are available in predetermined sizes corresponding to wrist circumference measurements. Some designs are available in universal sizes.
- Most braces are constructed of a neoprene or nylon material outer shell with a Lycra or cotton material lining.
- Most designs have a dorsal thermoplastic bar incorporated into the outer shell to prevent excessive abduction and extension at the MCP joint. Many of these are malleable.
- Several designs use a neoprene strap that wraps around the wrist and thumb to limit excessive range of motion.
- The braces are attached to the thumb and wrist with polyethylene or neoprene straps with Velcro or D-ring closures and allow for adjustments in fit.
- Most of the designs cover the wrist but allow for unrestricted motion of the hand and fingers two through five.

▪▶ **Position of the patient:** Sitting on a taping table or bench with the hand and thumb in a neutral position.

▪▶ **Preparation:** Apply the brace directly to the skin or over sports-specific gloves.
   Follow the manufacturer's application instructions during the application of the braces. The following guidelines apply to most designs.

▪▶ **Application:**

**STEP 1:**   Loosen the straps and unfold the brace.

**STEP 2:**   Place the brace onto the involved thumb (Fig. 11–23A). Wrap the outer shell around the thumb and/or wrist. If a bar is included, align the bar on the dorsal thumb.

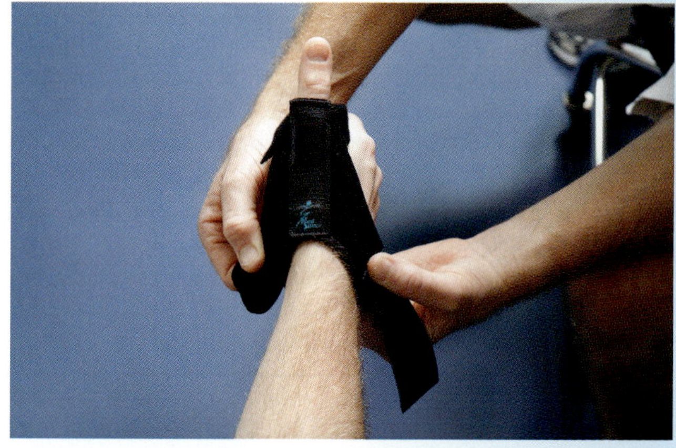

**Fig. 11–23 A**

**STEP 3:**   The application of straps will depend on the specific brace design. Apply most by pulling the strap(s) at the wrist tight and anchoring with Velcro (Fig. 11–23B). When using other designs, wrap the strap around the thumb and/or wrist and anchor.

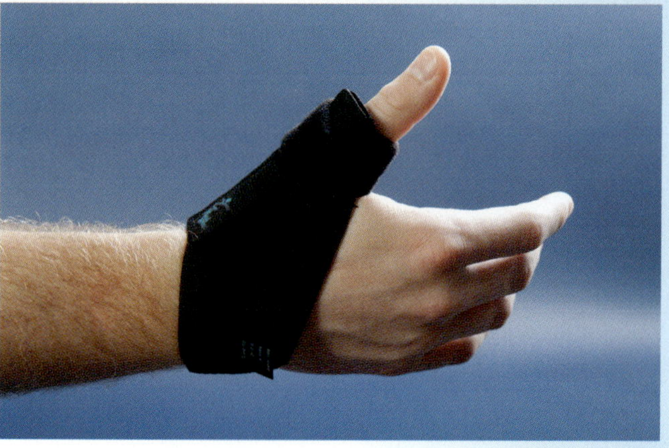

**Fig. 11–23 B**

### Custom-Made

➠ **Purpose:** Construct custom-made designs from thermoplastic material to provide moderate support and immobilization and to limit range of motion to prevent and treat sprains, dislocations, and postfracture injuries. These braces are commonly used when off-the-shelf designs are not available.

➠ **Materials:**
  • Paper, felt tip pen, thermoplastic material, ⅛ inch foam or 2 inch width moleskin, a heating source, an elastic wrap, 2 inch or 3 inch width by 5 yard length elastic wrap, self-adherent wrap, or pre-wrap and 1 inch elastic tape, taping scissors

➠ **Position of the patient:** Sitting on a taping table or bench with the hand and thumb in a neutral position.

➠ **Preparation:** Design the brace with a paper pattern from just distal to the IP joint, over the MCP joint, and partially incorporate the wrist. Mold and shape the material to the thumb and wrist. Apply ⅛ inch foam or 2 inch moleskin to the inside surface of the brace to prevent irritation.

   Apply the brace directly to the skin or over pre-wrap or self-adherent wrap (see Fig. 11–12A). These braces may also be applied over sports-specific gloves.

➠ **Application:**

**STEP 1:**  Position the brace on the thumb (Fig. 11–23C).

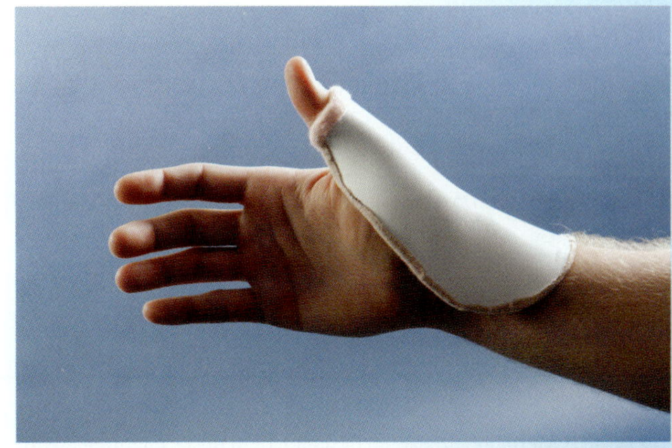

**Fig. 11–23 C**

**STEP 2:**  Anchor the brace with the basic thumb spica pattern with a 2 inch or 3 inch width by 5 yard length elastic wrap, self-adherent wrap, or pre-wrap and 1 inch elastic tape with mild to moderate roll tension (Fig. 11–23D).

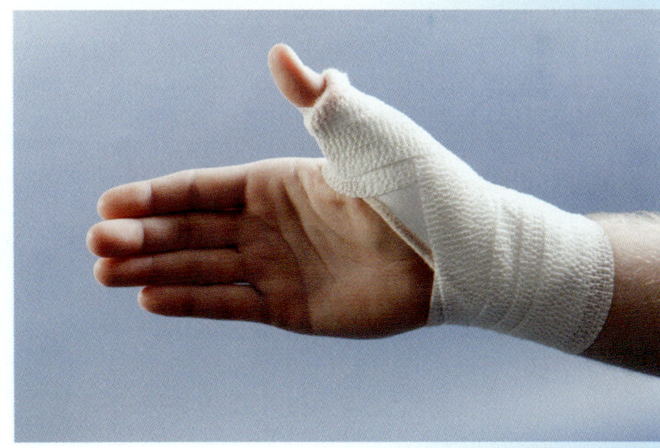

**Fig. 11–23 D**

## EVIDENCE SUMMARY

The use of various immobilization methods for the conservative management of uncomplicated gamekeeper's thumb has been examined in a 2019 evidence-based review.[20] The findings from four studies demonstrated positive functional outcomes with immobilization of the MCP joint for 4 weeks, limiting adduction and abduction range of motion while allowing for controlled flexion and extension.

### Clinical Application Question 3

The center fielder on the baseball team suffers a first-degree left thumb ulnar collateral ligament sprain while sliding into second base. Following an evaluation, your team physician allows the center fielder to return to play if protected from further injury. The athlete bats and throws right handed and is the leading base stealer on the team.

➡ **Question: What techniques are appropriate for practices and competitions?**

### . . . IF/THEN . . .

**IF** a finger brace is required for support in patients participating in athletic and/or work activities, **THEN** consider constructing a custom-made design; these designs are lower-profile, and dorsal application will allow for tactile sensation.

# Padding Techniques

A variety of padding material provides shock absorption, protection, and compression and lessens stress for hand, finger, and thumb injuries and conditions. Felt and foam may prevent and treat contusions, sprains, and blisters. Use thermoplastic material and foam to cover rigid and semirigid casts when returning to activity postoperatively or while treating sprains, dislocations, and fractures.

## BOXER'S WRAP    Figure 11–24

➡ **Purpose:** As previously discussed, padding is the traditional use of the boxer's wrap. The wrap is effective in absorbing shock and preventing contusions and in treating injuries to the hand that require padding (Fig. 11–24).

### DETAILS

The wrap is useful for athletes in baseball, field hockey, football, gymnastics, ice hockey, lacrosse, softball, and boxing activities and can also be used in combination with sports-specific gloves.

➡ **Materials:**
- 1½ inch, 2 inch, or 3 inch conforming gauze or self-adherent wrap, 1½ inch non-elastic tape, 2 inch elastic tape, 1 inch non-elastic or elastic tape, ⅛ inch or ¼ inch foam or felt, taping scissors

➡ **Position of the patient:** Sitting on a taping table or bench with the hand, fingers, and thumb in a neutral position and the fingers in abduction.

➡ **Preparation:** Cut a piece of ⅛ inch or ¼ inch foam or felt to cover the dorsal area of the hand. The pad may be extended to cover the MCP joints of the fingers. Apply the boxer's wrap directly to the skin or over a sports-specific glove.

➡ **Application:**

**STEP 1:**  Place the pad on the dorsal hand directly on the skin (Fig. 11–24A). Anchor 1½ inch, 2 inch, or 3 inch conforming gauze or self-adherent wrap to the medial dorsal surface of the wrist and apply the boxer's wrap with moderate roll tension as illustrated in Figure 11–20.

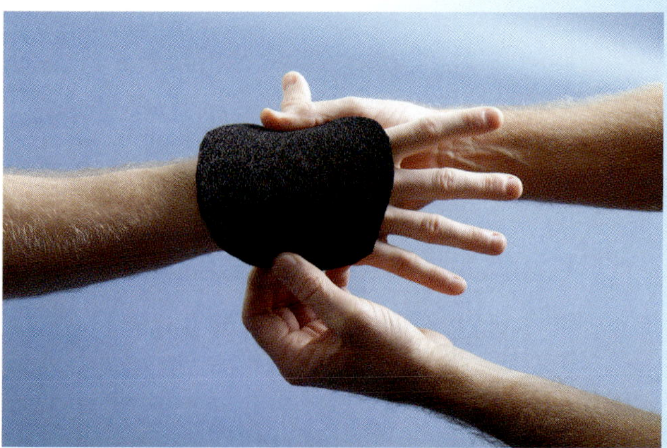

**Fig. 11–24 A**

**STEP 2:** Using 2 inch elastic tape or self-adherent wrap, cover the boxer's wrap with two to four additional figure-of-eight (see Fig. 10–8) patterns with moderate roll tension (Fig. 11–24B).

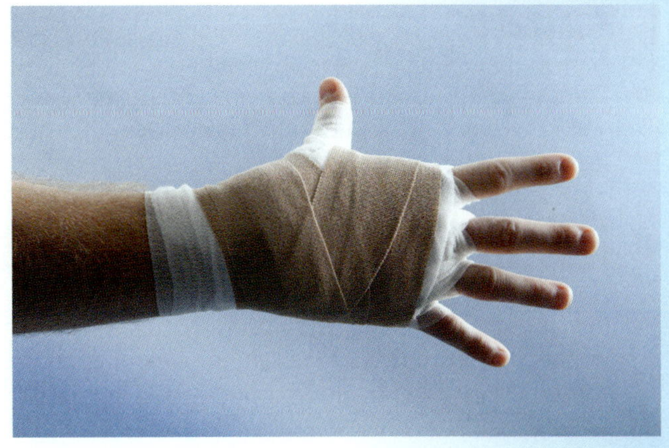

Fig. 11–24 B

**STEP 3:** Apply two to three basic thumb spicas with 1 inch non-elastic or elastic tape with moderate roll tension for additional support (Fig. 11–24C).

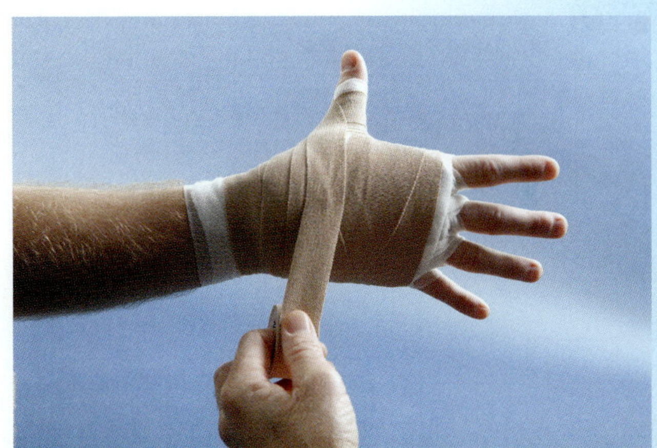

Fig. 11–24 C

**STEP 4:** Finish the figure-of-eight and/or basic thumb spica on the dorsal wrist and anchor with 1½ inch non-elastic tape in a circular pattern with moderate roll tension ◄▬▬► (Fig. 11–24D). Note that the circular wrist taping technique (see Fig. 10–7) may also be applied for additional support.

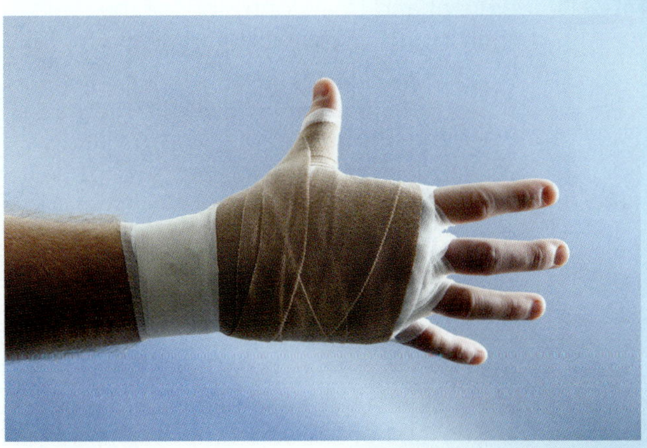

Fig. 11–24 D

## | **FOAM PADS**    Figure 11–25

➠ **Purpose:** Several padding designs constructed of foam absorb shock and lessen friction and pressure when preventing and treating finger and thumb contusions and blisters (Fig. 11–25).

➠ **Materials:**
- Off-the-shelf finger and thumb sleeves in predetermined sizes based on finger width measurements
- Off-the-shelf foam donuts or ¼ inch or ½ inch closed-cell foam, taping scissors

➠ **Position of the patient:** Sitting on a taping table or bench with the hand, fingers, and thumb in a neutral position.

➠ **Preparation:** Cut and fit the appropriate size of the sleeve to overlap the injured area on the fingers and thumb. Quarter inch or ½ inch closed-cell foam may be cut to the appropriate size donut. If the area of the finger or thumb allows, cut the pad to extend in all directions ½ inch to 1 inch beyond the painful area. Mark the painful area on the piece of foam and cut out the area with taping scissors, creating a hole (see Fig. 3–26). This hole protects the painful area from stress and/or impact.

➠ **Application:**

**STEP 1:**  Pull the sleeve onto the finger and thumb directly on the skin, in a distal-to-proximal pattern (Fig. 11–25A). No adherent tape spray or anchor strips are required. The sleeves can be cleaned and reused.

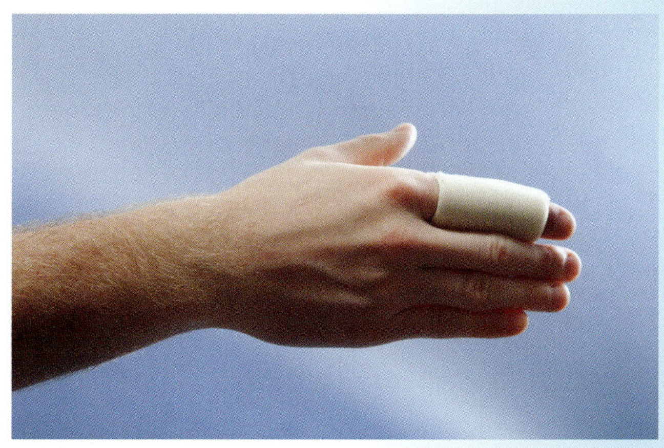

**Fig. 11–25 A**

**STEP 2:**  Prevent and treat contusions of the thumb and palm associated with athletic bat usage by using an off-the-shelf or custom-made closed-cell foam donut. Place the donut over the thumb directly on the skin under a sports-specific glove or use over a glove (Fig. 11–25B). The donut does not require anchors and is reusable.

**STEP 3:**  The off-the-shelf or custom-made pad may be attached to the thumb using the basic thumb spica technique with 1 inch elastic tape or self-adherent wrap with moderate roll tension (see Fig. 11–12).

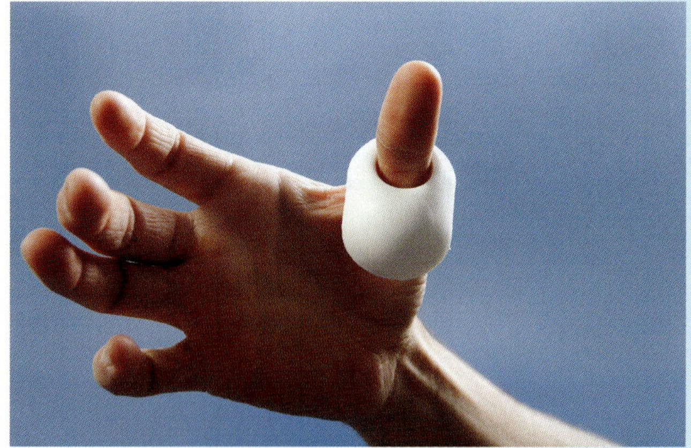

**Fig. 11–25 B**

## CAST PADDING    Figure 11–26

➠ **Purpose:** The cast padding technique protects the injured athlete and her or his competitors from injury and meets NCAA[25] and NFHS[26] rules (Fig. 11–26). Use the technique to cover rigid or semirigid casts when an athlete returns to activity following a fracture, dislocation, or surgery.

➠ **Materials:**
- Paper, felt tip pen, closed-cell, slow-recovery foam or similar material of at least ½ inch thickness, 2 inch or 3 inch width by 5 yard length elastic wrap, 2 inch or 3 inch elastic tape and pre-wrap, or self-adherent wrap, taping scissors

*Option:*
- Thermoplastic material, a heating source

➠ **Position of the patient:** Sitting on a taping table or bench with the hand, fingers, and thumb in the casted position.

➠ **Preparation:** Begin by making a paper pattern of the cast area to be padded. Trace the pattern onto closed-cell, slow-recovery foam or similar material, then cut the pad with taping scissors.

➠ **Application:**

**STEP 1:** Apply the foam over the cast and anchor with a 2 inch or 3 inch elastic wrap, 2 inch or 3 inch elastic tape, or self-adherent wrap with moderate roll tension ◀▬▬▶ (Fig. 11–26A). If using elastic tape, first cover the padding with pre-wrap to protect the foam from the tape adhesive ◀▬▬▶. The foam may be reused.

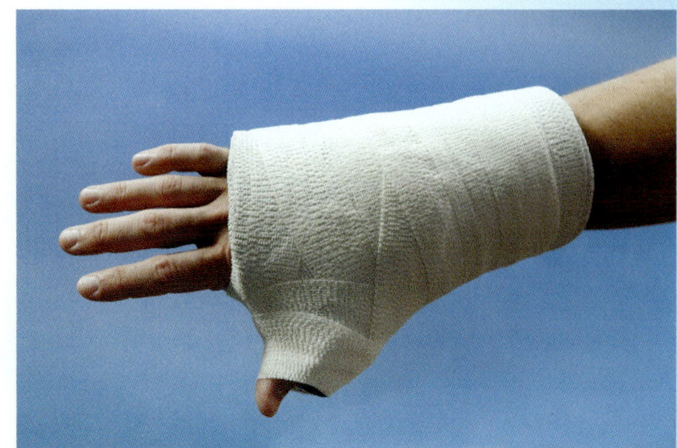

Fig. 11–26 A

*Option:*    *A decision to cover the fingers and/or thumb for additional protection depends on the activity and sport-position of the patient. For example, a semirigid, padded hood of thermoplastic material may be constructed for a football lineman to protect the fingers and thumb from injury (Fig. 11–26B). Because a linebacker or defensive back requires use of his fingers and thumb, a hood may not be advisable. Pad the hood with appropriate material to meet NCAA[25] and NFHS[26] rules (Fig. 11–26C).*

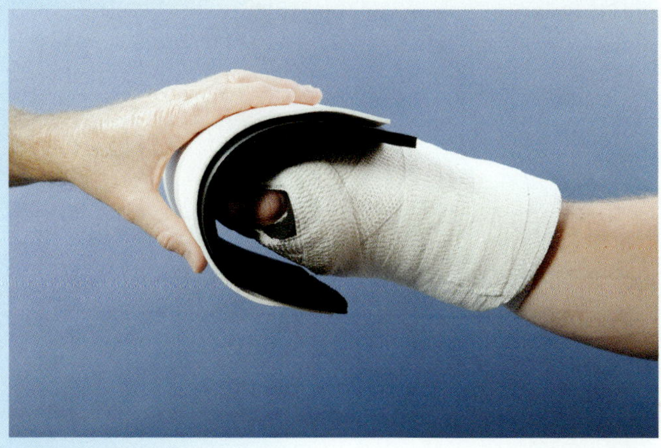

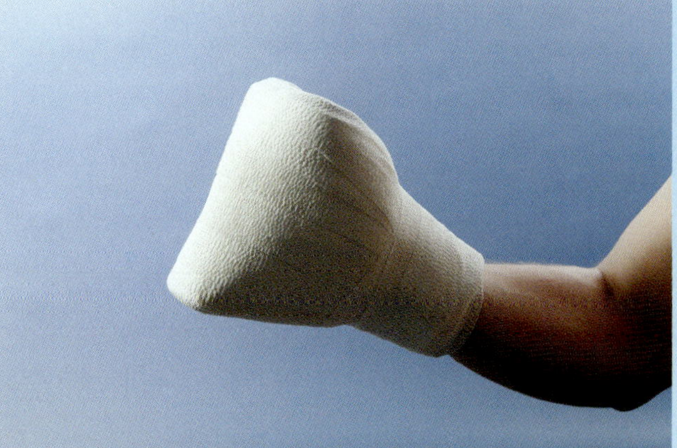

Fig. 11–26 B                              Fig. 11–26 C

## COMPRESSION WRAP PAD          Figure 11–27

➡ **Purpose:** The compression wrap pad assists in reducing mild, moderate, or severe swelling when treating hand contusions and sprains (Fig. 11–27).

➡ **Materials:**
• ¼ inch or ½ inch open-cell foam, taping scissors

➡ **Position of the patient:** Sitting on a taping table or bench with the wrist and hand in a pain-free position and the fingers in abduction.

➡ **Preparation:** Apply the pad directly to the skin.

➡ **Application:**

**STEP 1:**  Extend the pad across the dorsal hand, from the first MCP joint to the fifth MCP joint, and from the MCP joints to the wrist (Fig. 11–27A).

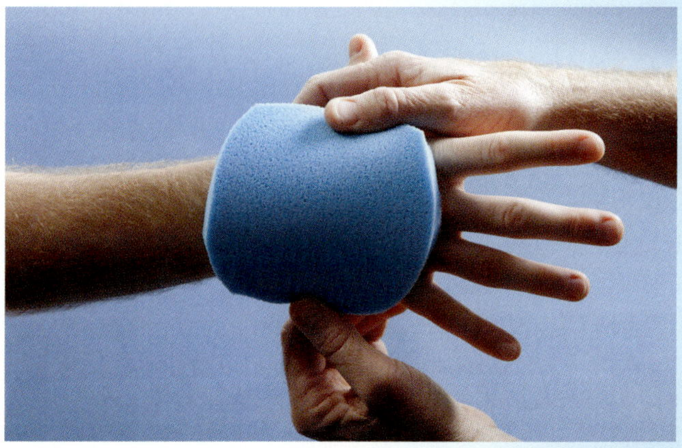

**Fig. 11–27 A**

**STEP 2:**  Place the pad over the dorsal hand and apply the hand and wrist compression (see Fig. 10–15) or boxer's wrap technique (see Fig. 11–20) (Fig. 11–27B).

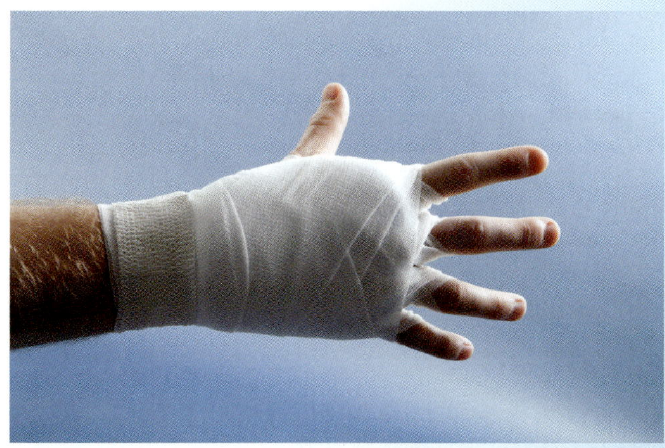

**Fig. 11–27 B**

### Clinical Application Question 4

At the company picnic, the data entry department won the horseshoe tossing contest, but several members sustained blisters to the palmar aspect of the fingertips. On Monday, the members could not use their keyboards because of pain and pressure associated with the blisters.

➡ **Question: How can you manage this situation?**

## MANDATORY PADDING

Protective equipment for the hand, fingers, and thumb is required in several high school and intercollegiate sports. The NCAA[25] and the NFHS[26] require that athletes participating in fencing, field hockey, ice hockey, and lacrosse wear protective padding during all practices and competitions. The majority of these pads are purchased off-the-shelf; the designs are constructed for specific sports and positions. Chapter 13 will provide a more in-depth discussion of these padding techniques.

### ...IF/THEN...

**IF** padding of the dorsal hand and support of the first MCP joint are needed for a field hockey or lacrosse athlete following injury, **THEN** consider applying the boxer's wrap with foam or felt over the dorsal hand and a tape core or thermoplastic material over the first MCP joint for additional padding or support, respectively.

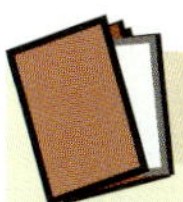

## EVIDENCE-BASED PRACTICE

In the bottom of the seventh inning, Grey Zelda moved to his right to field a line drive hit quickly toward him. Grey is the third baseman on his fastpitch softball team. The team is in the quarterfinals of the men's state championship tournament. Grey immediately raised his gloved hand across his chest and followed the ball as it quickly moved to his right. He placed his right hand on the edge of the glove to help secure the ball. As the ball approached his glove, it struck the tip of his extended right fourth finger. Grey was unable to catch the ball and the batter reached first base. The next batter on the opposing team hit a pop fly to right field and Grey's team won, advancing to the semifinals. After the game, Grey's teammates encouraged him to visit the tournament medical area to have his finger evaluated. Grey refused to go and believed it was just a sprained finger and planned to apply ice when he returned to the hotel.

Grey awoke the next morning with pain and swelling present over the distal fourth finger. He also noticed that he was unable to fully extend the tip of the finger. Grey continued to apply ice and taped fingers three and four together to provide support. Grey and several teammates decided to drive to the softball park and watch the first semifinal game of the day, as their game was in the evening. While in the stands, Grey attempted to retrieve a foul ball. He was unable to grip the ball and decided to walk to the medical area and have his finger evaluated.

Grey entered the medical area and was first seen by Steve Elder, the AT covering the tournament. Steve gathered a complete history from Grey, including information about his occupation as an explosive ordinance disposal expert. Steve observed the distal phalanx resting in 25 to 35 degrees of flexion. Swelling and point tenderness were present in the distal interphalangeal joint. Grey was unable to actively extend the distal phalanx but allowed Steve to passively move it into extension. Steve completed his evaluation and maintained extension of the distal interphalangeal joint. Steve believed Grey sustained a rupture of the extensor digitorum tendon. The tournament physician approached and examined Grey. The evaluation produced the same findings. On-site radiographs demonstrated no bony pathology. The physician agreed with Steve that Grey sustained a rupture of the extensor digitorum tendon in his fourth finger. Grey realized he could not continue play in the tournament and asked what type of treatment was required. The physician and Steve discussed the recommended immobilization time and techniques with Grey. Grey was concerned how the immobilization may interfere with his occupation as an explosive ordinance disposal expert. His work involves packing and pouring of explosives, connecting primers and fuses, laying and attaching Primacord between charges, and disposing of explosive ordnance, requiring the ability to grasp and manipulate small objects. Steve and the physician were uncertain which immobilization technique would be appropriate in this situation to safely return Grey to work and softball activities.

1. Develop a clinically relevant question from the case in the PICO format to generate answers for the selection of an immobilization technique for Grey. The question should include the population or problem, the intervention, a comparison intervention (if relevant), and the clinical outcome of interest.

2. Design a search strategy and search to find the best evidence to answer the clinical question. The strategy should include relevant search

*Continued*

terms, electronic databases, online journals, and print journals to use for the search. Discussions with your faculty, preceptor, and other health care professionals can provide evidence from expert opinion.

3. Choose three to five full text studies or reviews from your search or the chapter references. Evaluate and appraise each article to determine its value and usefulness to the case. Ask these questions for each study: (1) Are the results of the study valid? (2) What are the actual results? and (3) Are the findings clinically relevant to my patients? Prepare a summary of the evaluation with answers to the questions and rank the articles based on the evidence hierarchy in Chapter 1.

4. Integrate findings from the evidence, your clinical experience, and Grey's goals and preferences into the treatment program. Consider which immobilization techniques may be appropriate for Grey.

5. Evaluate the EBP process and your experience within the case. Consider these questions in the evaluation.

Was the clinical question answered?

Did the search generate quality evidence?

Was the evidence evaluated appropriately?

Was the evidence, your clinical experience, and Grey's goals and values integrated to make the clinical decision?

Did the intervention produce successful clinical outcomes for Grey?

Was the EBP experience positive for Steve and Grey?

## WRAP-UP

- Shear, compression, and rotational forces and extreme ranges of motion can cause injury to the hand, fingers, and thumb.
- The buddy and "X" taping techniques support the collateral ligaments of the fingers.
- Elastic material and tape provide protection when treating hand, finger, and thumb wounds.
- The thumb spica taping technique and its variations and the thumb spica semirigid cast technique provide support to the MCP joint when preventing and treating sprains and postdislocation and postfracture injuries.
- The figure-of-eight taping and wrapping techniques are used to attach protective padding to the hand.
- The hand and wrist, finger sleeves, and boxer's wrap compression techniques reduce swelling and inflammation following injury.
- Off-the-shelf and custom-made brace designs support, limit range of motion, and immobilize the hand, fingers, and thumb following sprains, dislocations, fractures, and tendon ruptures.
- The boxer's wrap, foam, and compression wrap padding techniques provide shock absorption, protection, and compression.
- Cast padding techniques provide protection for both injured athletes and opponents and are required by NCAA and NFHS rules.
- The NCAA and NFHS require that protective equipment be used for the hand, fingers, and thumb in several sports.

## WEB REFERENCES

**American Society for Surgery of the Hand**

http://www.assh.org/handcare/

- This site allows you to search for information on hand injuries and conditions.

**OrthoInfo**

https://orthoinfo.aaos.org

- This website allows access to information regarding the anatomy, examination, and treatment of hand, fingers, and thumb injuries and conditions.

**Medline Plus**

https://medlineplus.gov/handinjuriesanddisorders.html

https://medlineplus.gov/fingerinjuriesanddisorders.html

- This site provides general hand, finger, and thumb information on a variety of injuries and treatments.

## REFERENCES

1. Prentice, WE: Principles of Athletic Training: A Guide to Evidence-Based Clinical Practice, ed 16. McGraw-Hill, New York, 2017.

2. Houglum, PA: Therapeutic Exercise for Musculoskeletal Injuries, ed 4. Human Kinetics, Champaign, IL, 2016.

3. Anderson, MK: Foundations of Athletic Training: Prevention, Assessment, and Management, ed 6. Wolters Kluwer, Philadelphia, 2017.

4. Kim, S, Endres, NK, Johnson, RJ, Ettlinger, CF, and Shealy JE: Snowboarding injuries: Trends over time and

comparisons with alpine skiing injuries. Am J Sports Med 40:770–776, 2012.

5. Cahalan, TD, and Cooney, WP: Biomechanics. In Jobe, FW, Pink, MM, Glousman, RE, Kvitne, RS, and Zemel, NP (eds): Operative Techniques in Upper Extremity Sports Injuries. Mosby, St. Louis, 1996.

6. Starkey, C, and Brown, SD: Examination of Orthopedic and Athletic Injuries, ed 4. F.A. Davis, Philadelphia, 2015.

7. Wilson, RL, and Hazen, J: Management of joint injuries and intraarticular fractures of the hand. In Hunter, JM, Mackin, EJ, and Callahan, AD (eds): Rehabilitation of the Hand: Surgery and Therapy, ed 4. Mosby, St. Louis, 1995.

8. Roh, YH, Koh, YD, Go, JY, Noh, JH, Gong, HS, Baek, GH: Factors influencing functional outcome of proximal interphalangeal joint collateral ligament injury when treated with buddy strapping and exercise. J Hand Ther 31:295–300, 2018.

9. Baltera, RM, Hastings, H, Sachar, K, and Jitprapaikulsarn, S: Fractures and dislocations: Hand. In Hammert, WC, Calfee, RP, Bozentka, DJ, and Boyer, MI (eds): ASSH Manual of Hand Surgery. Lippincott Williams & Wilkins, Philadelphia, 2010.

10. Day, CS: Fractures of the metacarpals and phalanges. In Wolfe, SW, Hotchkiss, RN, Pederson, WC, Kozin, SH, and Cohen, MS (eds): Green's Operative Hand Surgery, ed 7. Elsevier, Philadelphia, 2016.

11. Nellans, KW, and Chung, KC: Pediatric hand fractures. Hand Clin 4:569–578, 2013.

12. Weber, DM, Seiler, M, Subotic, U, Kalisch, M, and Weil, R: Buddy taping versus splint immobilization for paediatric finger fractures: A randomized controlled trial. J Hand Surg Eur 1753193418822692. doi: 10.1177/1753193418822692, 2019. [Epub ahead of print]

13. Won, SH, Lee, S, Chung, CY, Lee, KM, Sung, KH, Kim, TG, Choi, Y, Lee, SH, Kwon, DG, Ha, JH, Lee, SY, and Park, MS: Buddy taping: Is it a safe method for treatment of finger and toe injuries. Clin Orthop Surg 6:26–31, 2014.

14. Prentice, WE: Rehabilitation Techniques for Sports Medicine and Athletic Training, ed 6. SLACK, Thorofare, New Jersey, 2015.

15. Dunn, JC, Kusnezov, N, Orr, JD, Pallis, M, and Mitchell, JS: The boxer's fracture: Splint immobilization is not necessary. Orthopedics 39:188–192, 2016.

16. Zong, SL, Zhao, G, Su, LX, Liang, WD, Li, LG, Cheng, G, Wang, AJ, Cao, XQ, Zheng, QT, Li, LD, and Kan, SL: Treatments for the fifth metacarpal neck fractures. Medicine (Baltimore) 95:e3059, 2016.

17. Poolman, RW, Goslings, JC, Lee, J, Statius Muller, M, Steller, EP, and Struijs, PAA: Conservative treatment for closed fifth (small finger) metacarpal neck fractures. Cochrane Database Syst Rev (3);CD003210, 2005.

18. Smit, JM, Beets, MR, Zeebregts, CJ, Rood, A, and Welters, CF: Treatment options for mallet finger: A review. Plast Reconstr Surg 126:1624–1629, 2010.

19. Lin, JS, and Samora, JB: Surgical and nonsurgical management of mallet finger: A systematic review. J Hand Surg Am 43:146–163 e2, 2018.

20. McVeigh, KH, Berger, TG, Cudahy, R, Dekker, TM, Brigham, TJ, and Braxton, JC: An evidence-based approach to casting and orthosis management of the pediatric, adolescent, and young adult population for injuries of the upper extremity: A review article. Clin J Sport Med doi: 10.1097/JSM.0000000000000718, 2019. [Epub ahead of print]

21. Rayan, GM, and Mullins, PT: Skin necrosis complicating mallet finger splinting and vascularity of the distal interphalangeal joint overlying skin. J Hand Surg Am 12:548–552, 1987.

22. Valdes, K, Naughton, N, and Algar, L: Conservative treatment of mallet finger: A systematic review. J Hand Ther 28:237–246, 2015.

23. Handoll, HHG, and Vaghela, MV: Interventions for treating mallet finger injuries. Cochrane Database Syst Rev (3);CD004574, 2004.

24. Witherow, EJ, and Peiris, CL: Custom made finger orthoses have fewer skin complications when compared to prefabricated finger orthoses in management of mallet injury: A systematic review and meta-analysis. Arch Phys Med Rehabil 96:1913–1923, 2015.

25. National Collegiate Athletic Association: 2014–15 Sports Medicine Handbook, ed 25. NCAA, Indianapolis, 2014. http://www.ncaapublications.com/productdownloads/MD15.pdf.

26. National Federation of State High School Associations: 2018 Field Hockey Rules Book. National Federation of State High School Associations, Indianapolis, 2019.

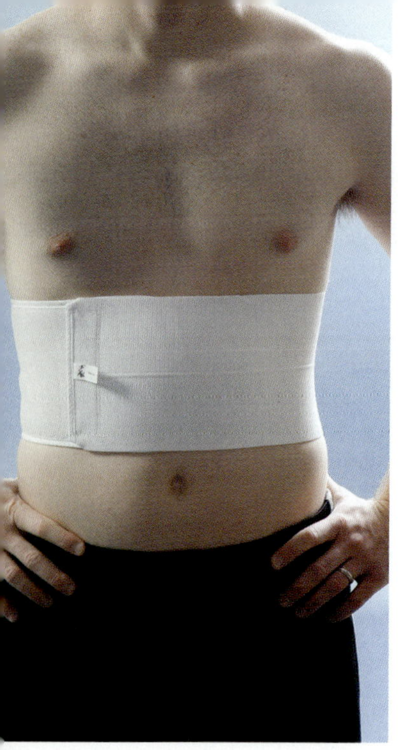

# 12

# Thorax, Abdomen, and Spine

## INJURIES AND CONDITIONS

Injury to the thorax, abdomen, and spine can occur during athletic and work activities as a result of acute and chronic forces, stresses, and movements. Direct and indirect forces can cause a contusion, fracture, and costochondral injury. Sprains can occur from excessive range of motion and strains from violent muscular movements and overload. Participation in collision and contact sports can predispose an athlete to brachial plexus and overuse injuries and conditions of the spine, all of which are caused by excessive range of motion, compression, and repetitive stress. Common injuries to the thorax, abdomen, and spine include:

- Contusions
- Sprains
- Strains
- Fractures
- Costochondral injury
- Brachial plexus injury
- Overuse injuries and conditions

## Contusions

Contusions to the thorax, abdomen, and spine are the result of compressive forces and can involve soft tissue and/or bony structures. A direct blow to the thorax can result in a contusion of the ribs, breasts, and intercostal musculature (Figs. 12–1 and 12–2). Although uncommon in sports, a severe fall on the ground or on rigid sports equipment may cause a **pulmonary contusion.** A pulmonary contusion can result, for example, as a football wide receiver is violently tackled by two defensive backs on the sideline, landing on unattended helmets near the benches. Contusions of the abdominal wall and kidneys are more likely to occur in collision sports and in sport and work activities with high-speed projectiles.[1] Because of external exposure, the male genitalia can be injured by direct forces. These injuries are common in athletic activities as a result of being kicked or struck with equipment. The thoracic and/or lumbar areas are susceptible to contusions in sports that do not require protective padding over these areas, such as basketball, football, and soccer. A contusion to the right lumbar musculature can occur, for instance, when a right-handed football quarterback releases the ball for a pass

396

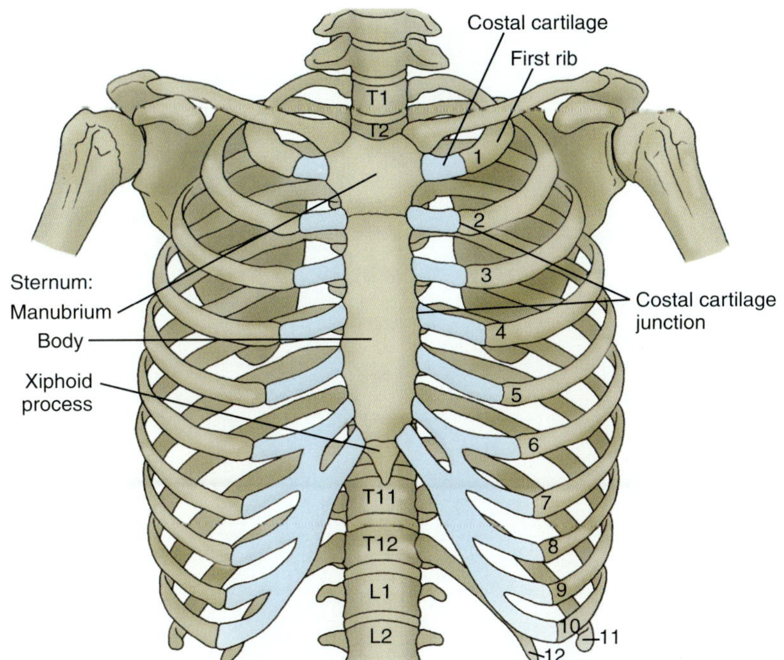



**Fig. 12–1** *Bones of the anterior thorax.*

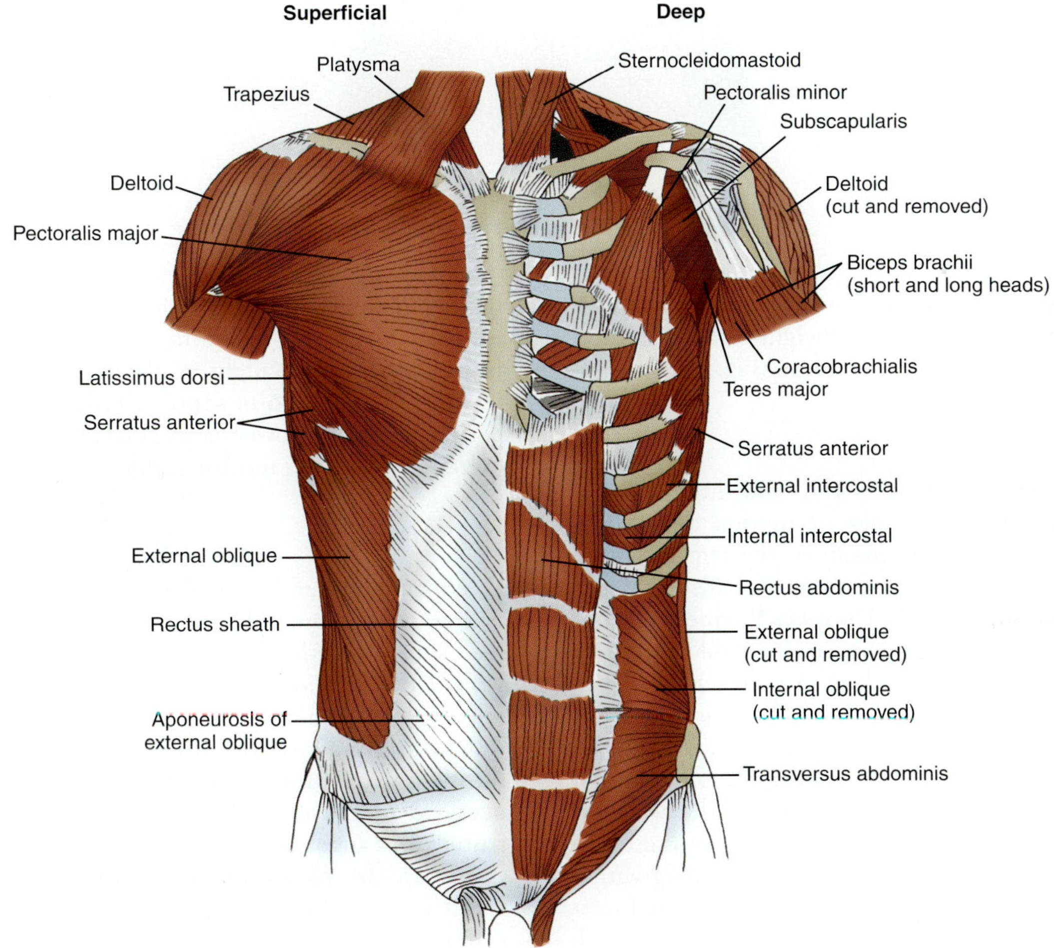



**Fig. 12–2** *Superficial and deep muscles of the anterior thorax and abdomen.*

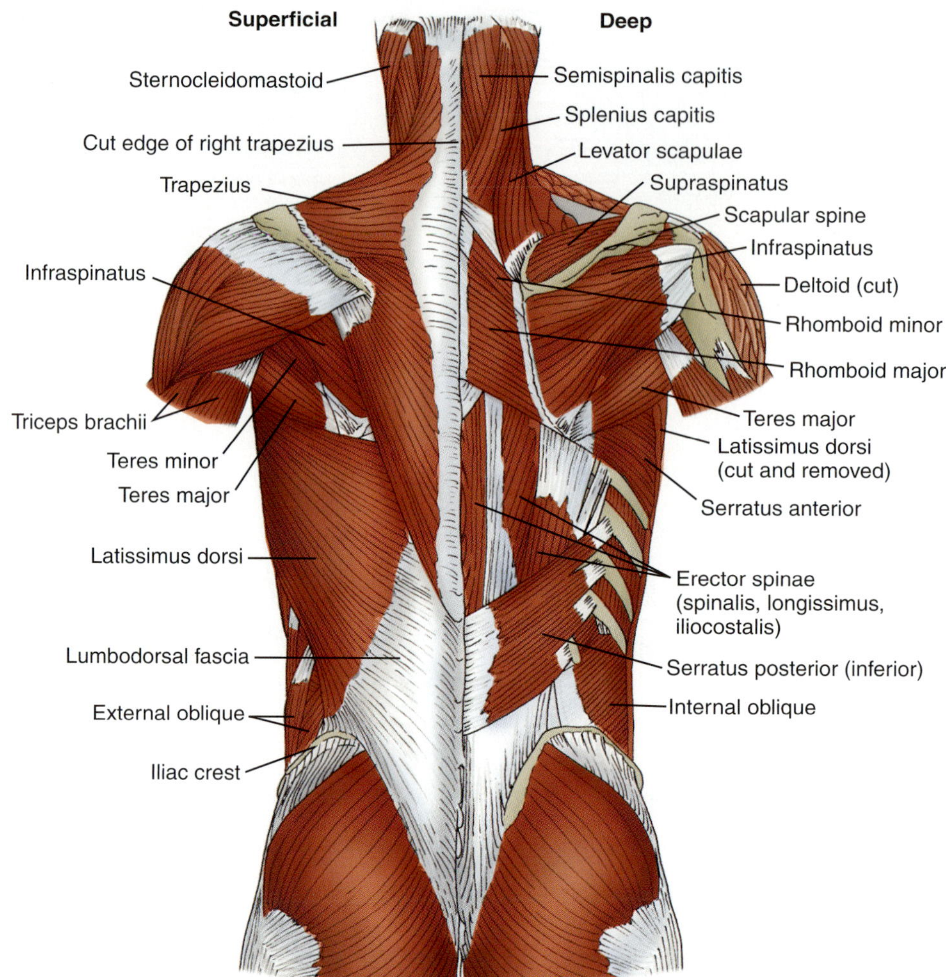



**Fig. 12–3** *Superficial and deep muscles of the posterior thorax and spine.*

downfield and is struck with an opponent's shoulder pads (Fig. 12–3). A fall from a height or a direct blow can lead to a contusion of the coccyx (Fig. 12–4).

## Sprains

Sprains to the thorax, cervical, and lumbar areas are caused by excessive range of motion and repetitive stress. Repetitive movement of the female breasts during athletic activities, as a result of inadequate support, can cause injury to the **Cooper's ligament.** Forced neck flexion, extension, or rotation or sudden contractions of the musculature can lead to a cervical facet joint sprain. A cervical sprain can result, for example, when a wrestler's head and neck are held in a headlock by an opponent during a takedown, causing flexion and rotation of the neck. Abnormal positioning of the head and neck over an extended length of time can also result in a sprain or acute torticollis (**wryneck**). Sleeping with a too-small or too-large pillow and sitting hunched over a desk reading without support for the head and neck can lead to a sprain or acute torticollis. Activities that require maximal trunk flexion and/or extension with rotation can cause injury to the lumbar facet joints. Injury can occur acutely or through repetitive stress. Improper lifting and/or spotting techniques during the performance of a power clean or dead lift strengthening exercise can cause a lumbar sprain.

## Strains

Overload and sudden, violent movements can cause strains to the musculature of the thorax, abdomen, and spine. Overload during active contractions and violent deceleration movements can result in a pectoralis major strain. A strain can occur as a recreational weightlifter increases the amount of weight on the bar during a maximum repetition bench press, resulting in overload of the musculature. Sudden rotation of the trunk can cause injury to the intercostal musculature. Injury to the rectus abdominis can be the result of sudden, violent trunk movements, such as twisting and extension. For example, a strain can occur as a tennis player serves a ball with an overhand motion during

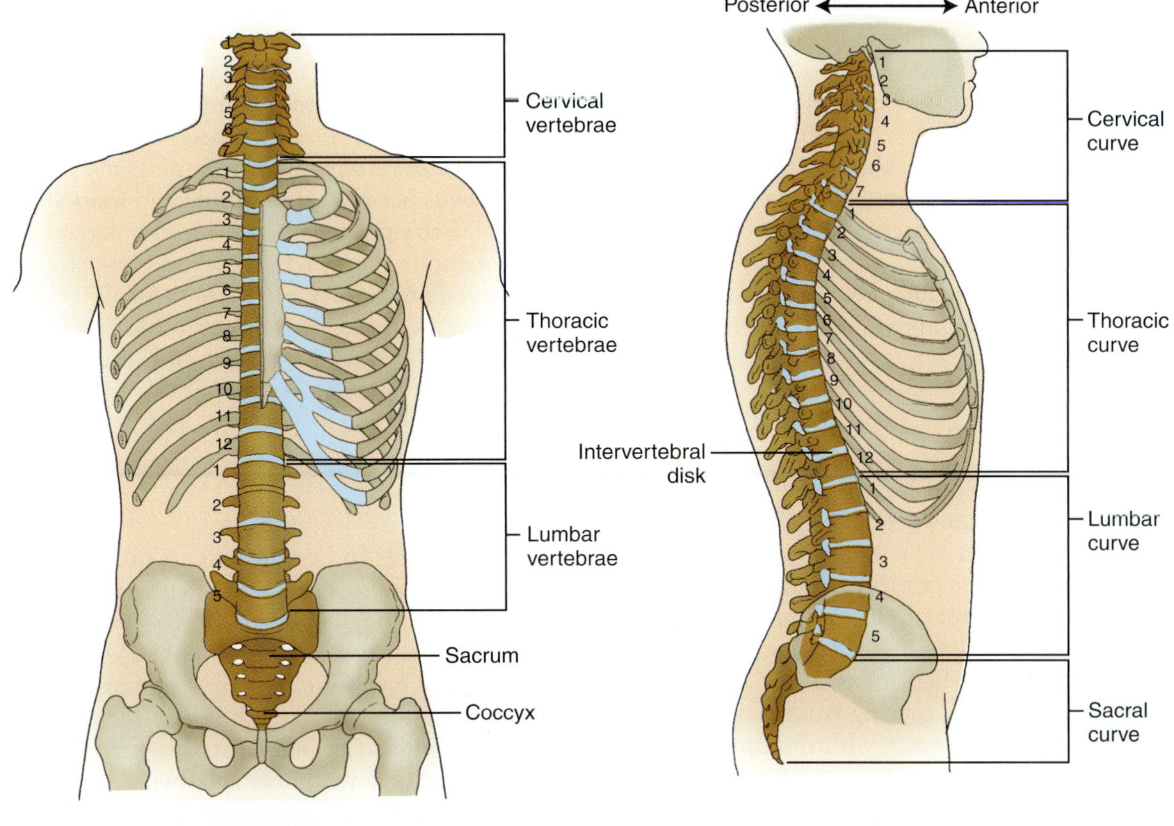



**Fig. 12–4** *Vertebral column demonstrating the normal spinal curves.*

a match, resulting in excessive extension and twisting of the thorax (Fig. 12–5). Cervical strains occur in the same manner as sprains—forced range of motion and sudden muscular contractions; both injuries can occur simultaneously.[2] Trunk extension, in combination with overload stresses and structural abnormalities of the spine, can result in a lumbar strain. Repetitive lifting, **scoliosis,** and **lumbar lordosis** can contribute to a lumbar strain.

## Fractures

Fractures to the thorax, abdomen, and spine may involve the ribs, vertebrae, and coccyx. Rib fractures can result from direct and indirect forces. A direct force to the anterior or posterior thorax severe enough to produce a fracture commonly injures the lateral and anterior portions of the fifth through the ninth ribs.[3] A lateral/anterior fracture to the sixth and seventh ribs can occur, for example, as a baseball base runner attempts to score with the catcher blocking home plate, colliding with the catcher's helmet and face guard. Acute and stress fractures can also be the result of indirect forces, such as violent muscular contractions, repetitive stresses, and training

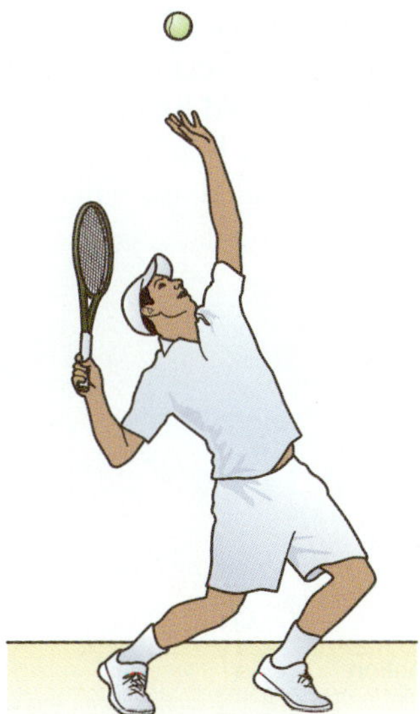

**Fig. 12–5** *Rectus abdominis strain.*

errors. Stress fractures have been reported among athletes participating in crew, golf, volleyball, tennis, gymnastics, and baseball.[4,5] Faulty sport movements and excessive training without appropriate recovery, causing abnormal muscular contractions and overload, can also result in a rib fracture. Forced hyperflexion, hyperextension, and axial loading of the head and neck can cause a cervical vertebral fracture. For example, a fracture can occur as a defensive football player, leading with his head and top of the helmet (spear tackling), tackles a ball carrier, causing hyperflexion and axial loading of the head and neck. A coccygeal fracture can occur through direct forces resulting from a fall from a height. A fracture can result as a gymnast dismounts from the uneven bars and loses her balance, landing violently on the mat in a seated position.

## Costochondral Injury

Separation of the costal cartilage junction at the sternum and/or ribs is commonly referred to as a dislocation or sprain (see Fig. 12–1). Mechanisms of injury include direct compression, violent trunk rotation, and forced flexion and horizontal abduction of the arm. For example, a dislocation or sprain can occur as a basketball guard dives toward a loose ball and is struck and turned to the left by an opponent, causing trunk rotation and direct compression upon contact with the court.

## Brachial Plexus Injury

A stretch/traction or compression brachial plexus injury (**burner** or **stinger**) is most common among athletes participating in football, ice hockey, lacrosse, and wrestling[6–9] (Fig. 12–6). A stretch/traction injury can occur when the shoulder and clavicle are depressed and the neck is forced into lateral flexion in the opposite direction away from the involved brachial plexus. A stretch/traction injury to the left brachial plexus can result as a football fullback is tackled and falls directly onto his left shoulder with his neck forced into lateral flexion to the right. Violent external rotation, abduction, and extension of the arm can also result in a stretch/traction injury. A compression injury to the brachial plexus can be the result of neck extension and rotation to the same side or with impingement of the brachial plexus between the scapula and football shoulder pads at **Erb's point** on the anterior lateral neck. At this location, the brachial plexus is most superficial. A compression injury of the right brachial plexus can occur, for example, as a football linebacker, using his right shoulder, tackles a tight end, causing impingement of the brachial plexus between the scapula and shoulder pads.

## Overuse

Overuse injuries and conditions are caused by excessive, repetitive stress to the spine. Repetitive axial loading and compression, common in collision and contact sports, may result in a herniation of a cervical disk (see Fig. 12–4). Over time, repetitive diving, tackling, and blocking in football, and heading the ball in soccer can contribute to degenerative changes of the cervical disk. Congenital weakness and hyperextension of the trunk associated with gymnastics, weightlifting, blocking in football, and spiking in volleyball can cause a defect in the pars interarticularis[10–12] (Fig. 12–7). This defect, referred to as spondylolysis, typically leads to a unilateral stress fracture of the pars interarticularis (Fig. 12–8). With continued stress, the defect can progress bilaterally. The resulting condition, spondylolisthesis, allows movement of the superior vertebra on the vertebra beneath it. Spondylolysis and spondylolisthesis can occur at any point along the spine, but are most common at the L4–L5 or L5–S1 levels.[13–15]

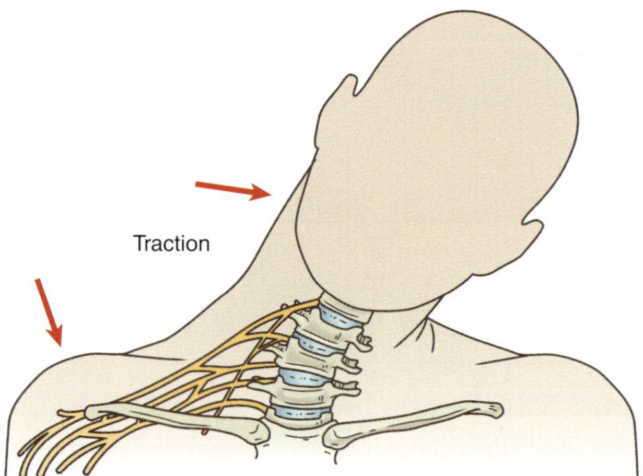


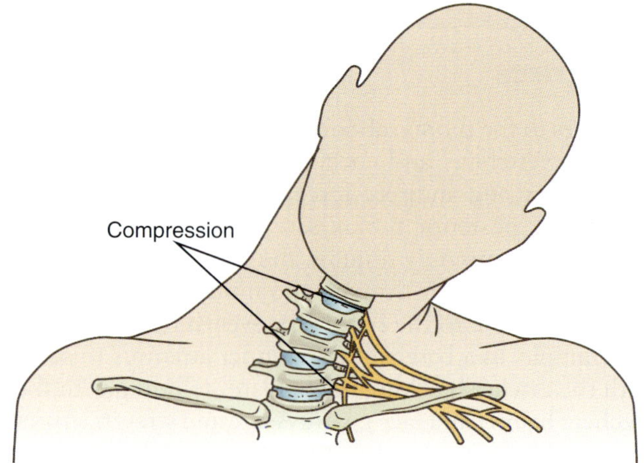


**Fig. 12–6** *Brachial plexus injury.* **A** *Stretch/traction.* **B** *Compression.*

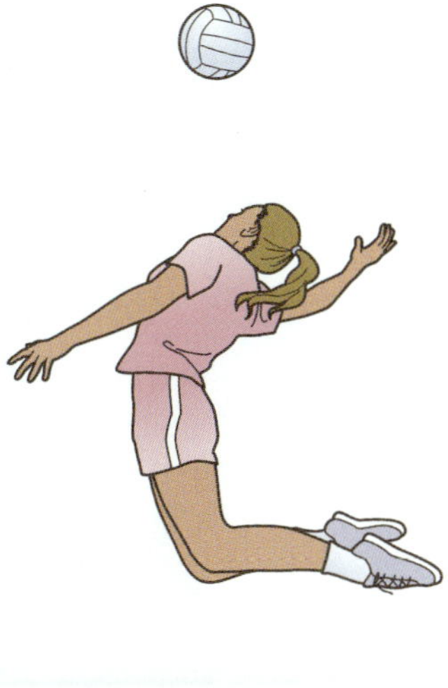

**Fig. 12–7** *Trunk hyperextension with spiking in volleyball.*

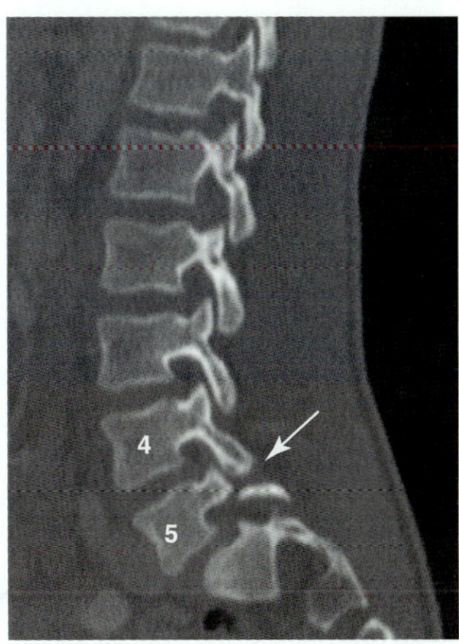

**Fig. 12–8** *Sagittal CT reformat of a 14-year-old boy with a bilateral spondylolysis at L5. Arrow points to the right L5 pars defect. Compare to the normal pars at more superior levels. (Courtesy of McKinnis, LN, and Mulligan, M. Musculoskeletal Imaging Handbook. Philadelphia, PA: F.A. Davis Company: 2014.)*

# Taping Techniques

Taping techniques are used when preventing and treating contusions and fractures of the thorax, abdomen, and spine to anchor off-the-shelf and custom-made protective padding. Padding techniques are illustrated in the Padding section.

## CONTUSION/FRACTURE TAPE     Figure 12–9

➡ **Purpose:** Use the contusion/fracture technique to absorb shock while anchoring off-the-shelf and custom-made pads to the thorax, abdomen, and spine to prevent and treat contusions and fractures (Fig. 12–9).
➡ **Materials:**
  • 2 inch, 3 inch, or 4 inch heavyweight elastic tape, adherent tape spray, taping scissors
➡ **Position of the patient:** Sitting on a taping table or bench or standing with the arms at the side of the body.
➡ **Preparation:** Apply the contusion/fracture technique directly to the skin.
➡ **Application:**

**STEP 1:**  Apply adherent tape spray over the pad area and 4–6 inches beyond, over the thorax, abdomen, and/or spine. Allow the spray to dry.

**STEP 2:**  Cut several strips of 2 inch, 3 inch, or 4 inch heavyweight elastic tape in lengths that will cover the pad and extend 4–6 inches beyond the pad on the two sides. Place the pad over the injured area.

*Steps Cont.*

**STEP 3:**   Next, apply the tape strips with the release-stretch-release sequence illustrated in Chapter 8 (see Fig. 8–10) ◀▥▥▶. Overlap the strips by ½ the width of the tape and apply enough strips to cover the majority of the pad (Fig. 12–9).

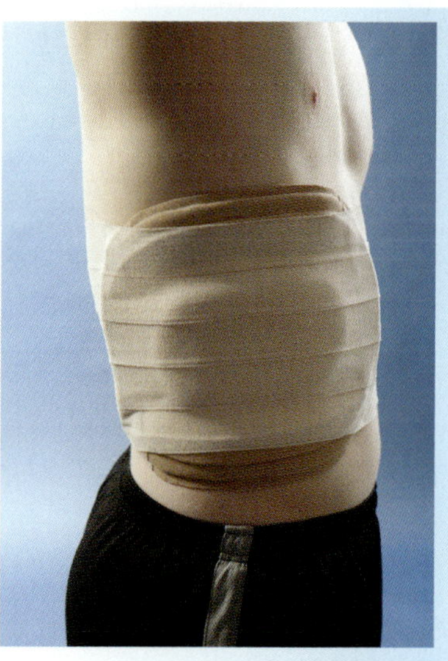

**Fig. 12–9**

# Wrapping Techniques

Use wrapping techniques to provide compression, support, and immobilization and to anchor protective padding to the thorax, abdomen, and spine when preventing and treating soft tissue and bony injuries. Elastic wraps and tapes are used following contusions, strains, and fractures to lessen swelling and to provide immobilization following rib fractures. These materials may also be used to anchor protective padding to prevent and treat contusions, strains, fractures, and costochondral injury.

## DETAILS

Exercise care when applying elastic wraps to the thorax, abdomen, and spine. Follow application guidelines and have the patient inhale during application to prevent restriction of chest movement and normal breathing patterns. Should the patient experience shortness of breath, an increase in pain, and/or have a rapid, weak pulse or low blood pressure,[2] suspect a serious thoracic injury/condition and immediately refer the patient to a physician.

## THORAX AND ABDOMEN COMPRESSION WRAP          Figure 12–10

▥▶ **Purpose:** The thorax and abdomen compression wrap technique is used to control mild, moderate, or severe swelling when treating thorax, abdomen, and spine contusions, strains, and fractures (Fig. 12–10).
▥▶ **Materials:**
 • 6 inch width by 5 yard length or 4 inch or 6 inch width by 10 yard length elastic wrap determined by the size of the patient, metal clips, 2 inch or 3 inch elastic tape, taping scissors
 *Option:*
 • ¼ inch or ½ inch foam or felt
▥▶ **Position of the patient:** Standing on the ground with the arms placed on the lateral hips in a relaxed position.
▥▶ **Preparation:** To lessen migration, apply adherent tape spray, tape strips, or anchors directly to the skin (see Fig. 1–7).
 *Option:*
 • Place a ¼ inch or ½ inch foam or felt pad over the inflamed area directly on the skin to provide additional compression and assist in controlling swelling.
▥▶ **Application:**

**STEP 1:**  Anchor the end of the wrap directly to the skin just inferior to the injured area and encircle the anchor ◄▬► (Fig. 12–10A).

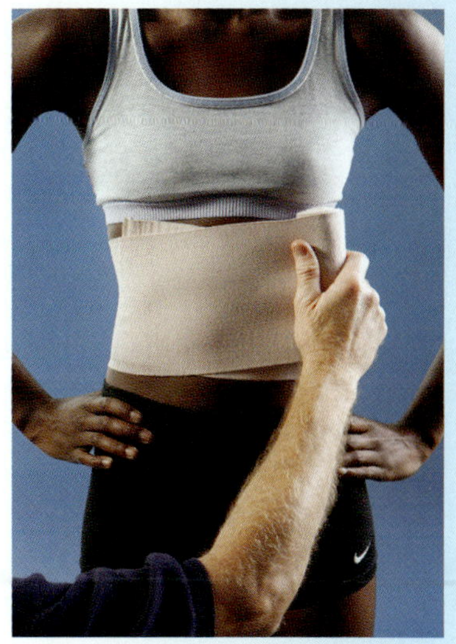

Fig. 12–10 A

**STEP 2:**  Continue to apply the wrap in a spiral pattern in a distal-to-proximal direction, overlapping by ⅓–½ of the wrap width (Fig. 12–10B). Apply the greatest amount of roll tension distally and lessen tension as the wrap continues proximally.

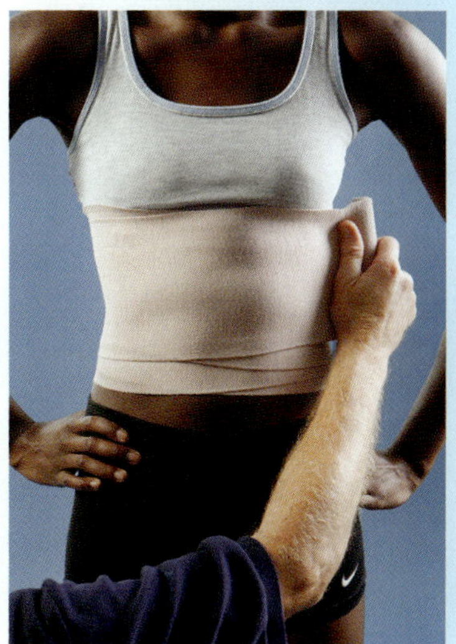

Fig. 12–10 B

**STEP 3:**  Anchor the wrap with Velcro, metal clips, or loosely applied 2 inch or 3 inch elastic tape ◄▬► (Fig. 12–10C). Finish and anchor the tape over the circular tape pattern on the anterior thorax or abdomen to ensure adherence and prevent unraveling and irritation.

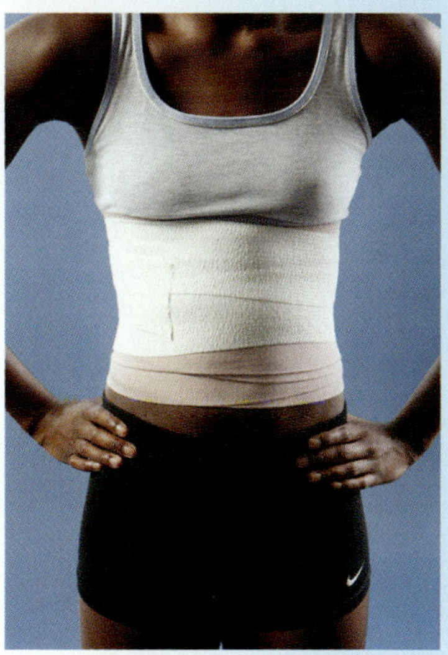

Fig. 12–10 C

## CIRCULAR WRAP    Figure 12–11

➡ **Purpose:** The circular wrap technique is used to provide compression and mild support and to anchor off-the-shelf and custom-made pads to the thorax, abdomen, and spine when preventing and treating contusions, strains, fractures, and costochondral injury (Fig. 12–11).

➡ **Materials:**
- 6 inch width by 5 yard length or 4 inch or 6 inch width by 10 yard length elastic wrap, 2 inch or 3 inch elastic tape, taping scissors

➡ **Position of the patient:** Standing on the ground with the arms placed on the lateral hips in a relaxed position.

➡ **Preparation:** To lessen migration, apply adherent tape spray, tape strips, or anchors directly to the skin.

➡ **Application:**

**STEP 1:**   To provide support, anchor the end of the wrap directly on the skin and encircle the anchor ◄▬▬► (Fig. 12–11A).

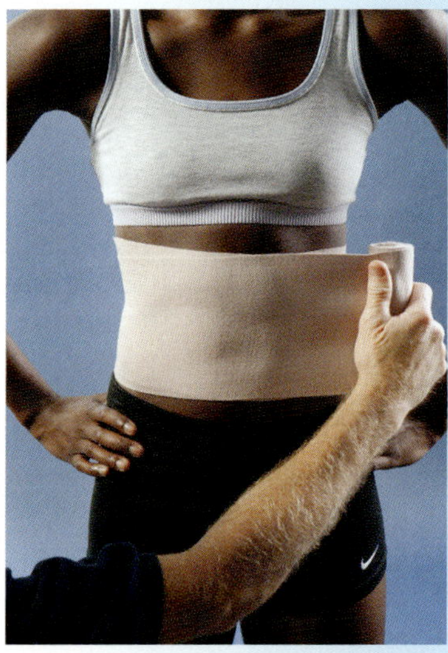

**Fig. 12–11 A**

**STEP 2:**   Continue to apply the wrap in a circular pattern, overlapping by ⅓–½ of its width, with moderate roll tension in a distal-to-proximal or proximal-to-distal direction (Fig. 12–11B).

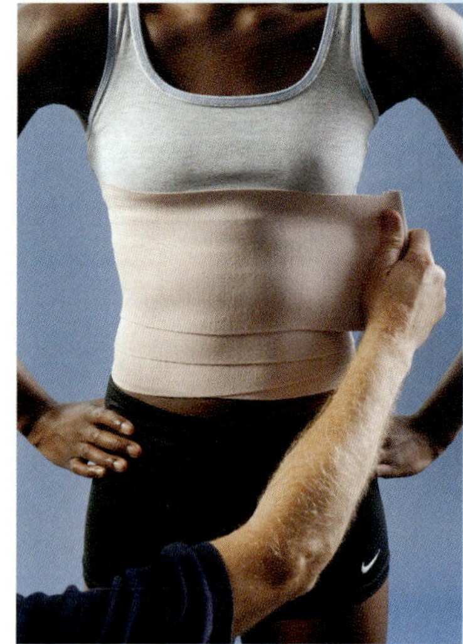

**Fig. 12–11 B**

**STEP 3:**  To attach a pad, place the pad over the injured area directly on the skin (Fig. 12–11C). Apply the circular wrap technique, leaving a small area in the middle of the pad exposed.

**STEP 4:**  Anchor the support wrap with Velcro or 2 inch or 3 inch elastic tape with moderate roll tension with two to three continuous circular patterns. Finish the tape on the circular tape pattern over the anterior thorax or abdomen to prevent unraveling.

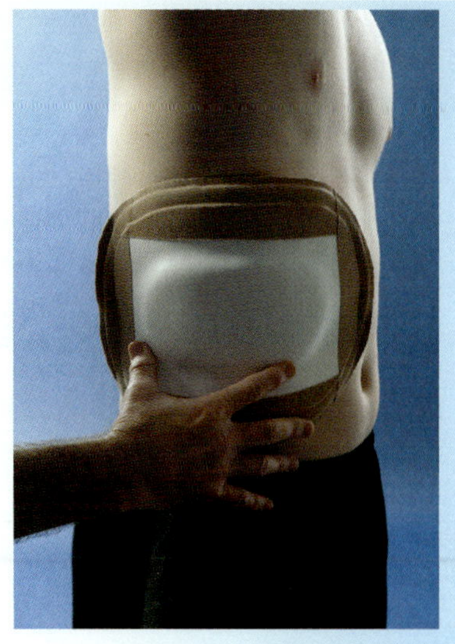

**Fig. 12–11 C**

**STEP 5:**  When using a pad, anchor 2 inch or 3 inch elastic tape directly on the exposed portion of the pad (Fig. 12–11D) and apply one to two continuous circular patterns over the wrap and pad with moderate roll tension ◄▭► (Fig. 12–11E). Anchor the tape over the anterior thorax or abdomen on the circular tape pattern. To prevent migration, a distal circular strip of elastic tape may be applied with distal-to-proximal tension; anchor the loose end on the circular tape pattern. No additional anchors are needed.

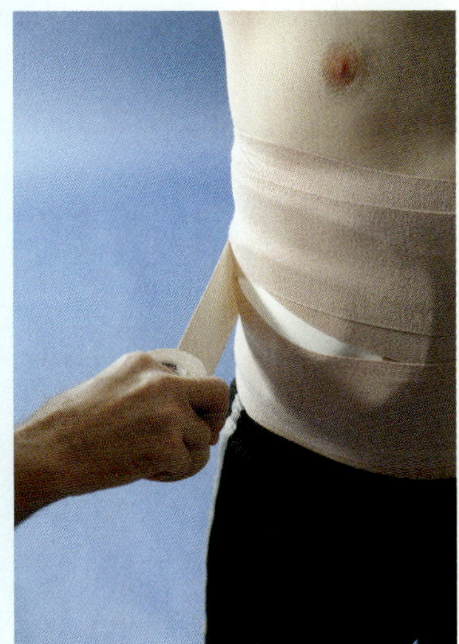

**Fig. 12–11 D**

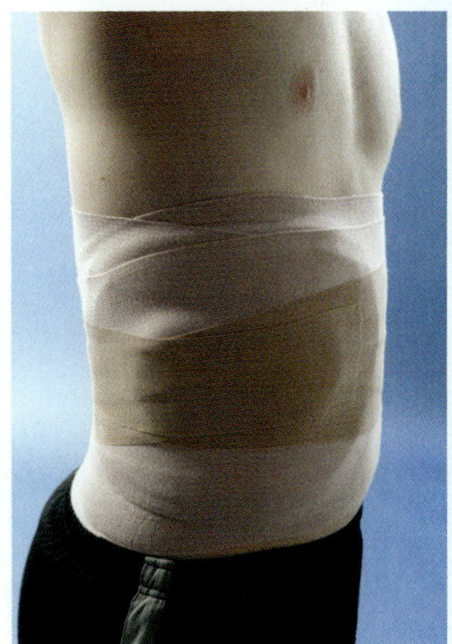

**Fig. 12–11 E**

## ⚕ SWATHE RIB WRAP

◄▭► **Purpose:** Use the swathe rib wrap technique in the immediate treatment of rib fractures to provide mild to moderate support and immobilization to the ribs by anchoring the arm to the involved side of the thorax, immobilizing the shoulder. This technique and steps of application can be found at FADavis.com.

# Bracing Techniques

Bracing techniques for the thorax, abdomen, and spine provide compression and support, lessen range of motion, and correct structural abnormalities. The braces are available in off-the-shelf designs and can be used for a variety of injuries and conditions.

## RIB BELTS    Figure 12–12

➠ **Purpose:** Rib belts are designed to provide compression and mild to moderate support to the thorax following injury (Fig. 12–12). Use these braces to treat rib contusions and fractures, intercostal strains, and costochondral injury.

### DETAILS
Rib belts can be used for athletes in a variety of sports. The braces can also be used with work and casual activities and are reusable.

➠ **Design:**
- Off-the-shelf braces are available in universal fit and male and female designs in predetermined sizes based on circumference measurements of the thorax. Some designs are available in universal sizes.
- Most designs are constructed of elastic materials with a foam/flannel, soft laminated foam, or cotton knit inner lining.
- The braces measure between 4 and 12 inches in width; most female designs are contoured for comfort and fit.
- Some designs have elastic or plastic inserts or stays incorporated into the belt to provide additional support.
- The braces are anchored to the thorax with Velcro closures.

➠ **Position of the patient:** Standing on the ground with the arms placed on the lateral hips in a relaxed position.

➠ **Preparation:** Apply the brace directly to the skin or over a tight-fitting shirt.
Follow the manufacturer's instructions when applying the braces. The following guidelines pertain to most designs.

➠ **Application:**

**STEP 1:**    Loosen the closures and place the belt around the thorax.
Position the foam inner lining over the injured area (Fig. 12–12A).

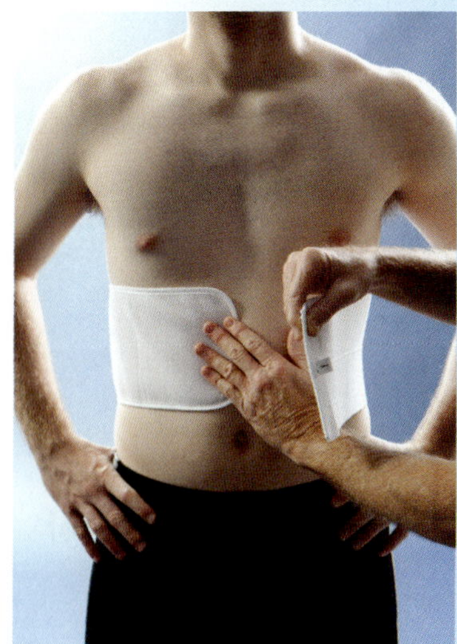

**Fig. 12–12 A**

**STEP 2:**    As the patient inhales, pull the belt with moderate tension and anchor with Velcro closures over the abdomen or back (Fig. 12–12B). Adjust the belt if needed to prevent constriction of chest movement and breathing patterns.

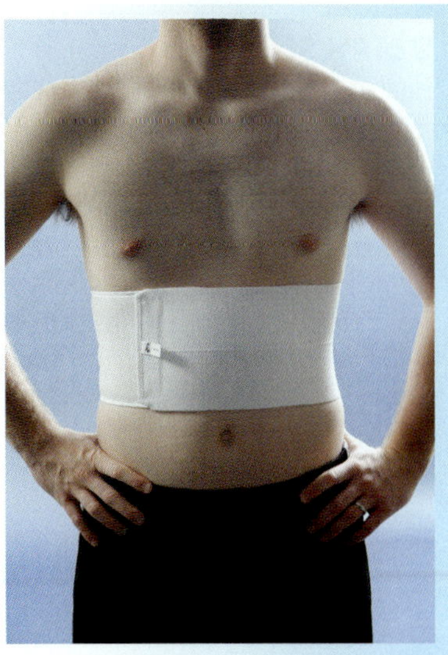

**Fig. 12–12 B**

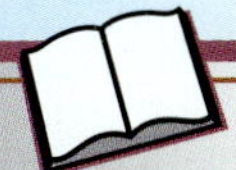

## EVIDENCE SUMMARY

The treatment of rib fractures with compression and support has been questioned. Limited evidence[16,17] has shown that compression and support wraps and/or belts may reduce pain levels in some patients. In contrast, others[4,18] have found no reduction in pain levels and restriction in the already limited ability to inspire among patients with fractures. Mechanical restriction may also increase pain levels further and predispose the patient to **hypostatic pneumonia,** which may occur from hypoventilation due to the pain and mechanical restriction.[16,19,20] Rib belts are designed to provide compression and support to the injured area of the thorax. However, some[20] have suggested that it is difficult to immobilize a specific region of the thorax without immobilizing the entire thorax, as the thorax functions as a single entity during breathing.

### Clinical Application Question 1

During training for an upcoming triathlon, a preschool teacher sustains a costal cartilage separation while performing medicine ball exercises in the gym. She is seen by a physician and allowed to continue training using an off-the-shelf rib belt after several days of rest. She progresses back into training and is symptom-free until reaching pre-injury intensity levels. At this level, she has difficulty with normal breathing patterns and experiences an increase in pain as a result of wearing the belt.

➡ **Question: How can you manage this situation?**

### ...IF/THEN...

**IF** an athlete requires compression and support to the thorax when being treated for a costochondral injury during a return to activity, **THEN** consider using an off-the-shelf rib belt rather than an elastic wrap; with repetitive trunk flexion and extension and perspiration, the elastic wrap and tape may roll and/or bunch distally and become uncomfortable.

## LUMBAR SACRAL BRACE    Figure 12–13

➡ **Purpose:** Use lumbar sacral braces when preventing and treating lumbar sprains, rectus abdominis and lumbar strains, spondylolysis, and spondylolisthesis (Fig. 12–13). These braces provide compression and moderate support, lessen range of motion, and correct structural abnormalities.

## DETAILS
Lumbar sacral braces can be used for athletes participating in a variety of sports. The braces can also be useful with work and casual activities.

➠ **Design:**
  - The braces are available off-the-shelf in universal fit designs in predetermined sizes based on waist circumference measurements. Some braces are available in universal sizes.
  - These braces are constructed of a cotton/polyester, perforated elastic or vinyl, polyester/nylon, or neoprene material outer shell with a soft foam or neoprene inner lining.
  - Most designs have adjustable nylon, elastic, or neoprene strap(s) incorporated in the outer shell to provide additional compression and support. With some braces, these straps may be removed when not in use.
  - The braces measure between 4 and 13 inches in width; some female designs are contoured for comfort and fit.
  - Many designs use rigid or semirigid neoprene, plastic, thermoplastic, foam, air or gel bladder, silicone, or steel spring stays or inserts over the lumbar, sacral, and/or abdominal areas to provide additional compression and support.
  - Most of the stays/inserts can be molded and/or adjusted for individual fit, while others can be removed when not in use.
  - Other designs are constructed of malleable anterior and posterior rigid plastic panels connected with high-tension elastic cords. The cords allow for adjustments in compression and fit.
  - Some designs commonly used in weightlifting are manufactured of leather and are available with a foam inner lining.
  - Several designs are available with detachable shoulder straps to lessen migration.
  - The braces are attached to the trunk through Velcro and/or D-ring closures or buckles and allow for adjustments in fit.

➠ **Position of the patient:** Standing on the ground with the arms placed on the lateral hips in a relaxed position.

➠ **Preparation:** Apply the brace directly to the skin or over a tight-fitting shirt and pant.
  Specific instructions for applying the braces are included with each design. Carefully follow the step-by-step procedures for proper fit and support. The following application guidelines pertain to most braces.

➠ **Application:**

**STEP 1:**  Begin by loosening the straps. Position the brace over the lumbar/sacral area and wrap the ends around the waist (Fig. 12–13A).

**STEP 2:**  When using some braces, position the stays/inserts over the lumbar/sacral and/or abdominal area to achieve the objective of the technique.

**Helpful Hint |**
If plastic or metal stays/inserts are incorporated into rib belts or lumbar sacral braces, monitor the position of the stays/inserts during use; the stays/inserts can migrate superiorly or inferiorly from the outer shell and injure the soft tissue.

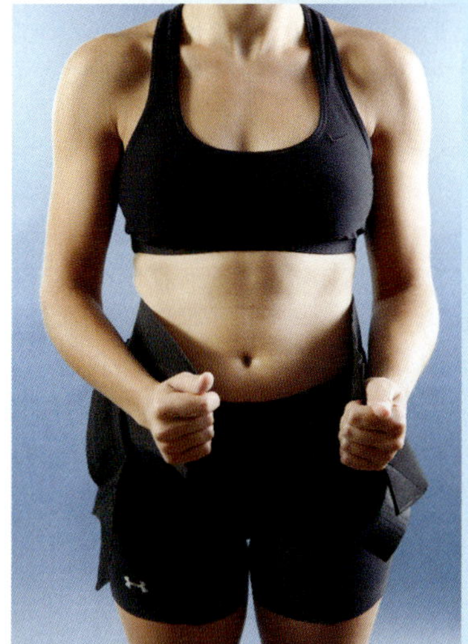

**Fig. 12–13 A**

**STEP 3:** When using most designs, pull the ends with moderate tension as the patient inhales and anchor over the abdomen with Velcro and/or D-ring closures (Fig. 12–13B).

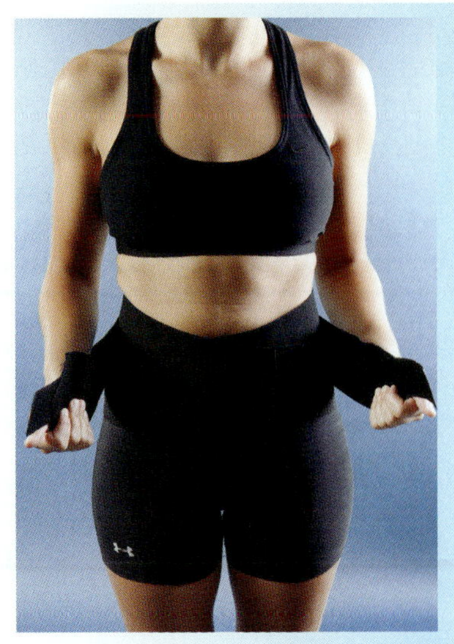

**Fig. 12–13 B**

**STEP 4:** Applying and adjusting straps will depend on the specific brace design. When using many designs, pull the straps incorporated into the outer shell around the waist toward the abdomen and anchor with Velcro closures (Fig. 12–13C). Adjust the brace and/or straps for comfort and fit if necessary.

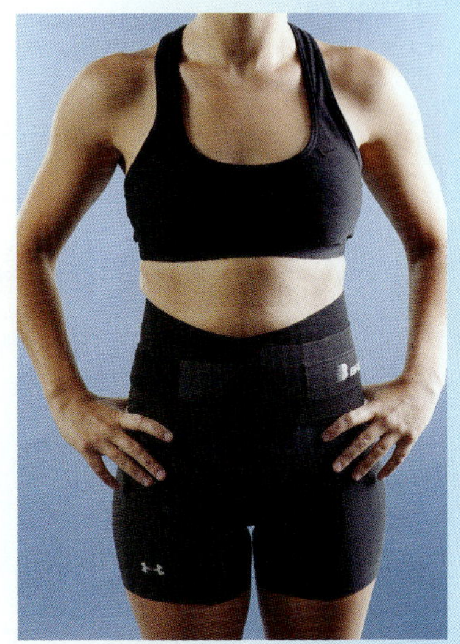

**Fig. 12–13 C**

## EVIDENCE SUMMARY

Lumbar sacral braces are commonly used for the prevention and treatment of various injuries and conditions of the abdomen and spine to provide support, compression, and restriction in range of motion. While many health care professionals continue to utilize these braces in prevention and treatment programs, researchers have demonstrated inconclusive evidence in determining their effectiveness compared with other interventions or no treatment.

A 2008 evidence-based review[21] investigated the effectiveness of lumbar sacral braces in the prevention and treatment of non-specific low back pain. Seven randomized controlled trials (RCTs) among individuals in various work settings examined the prevention of low back pain. The results produced moderate evidence that the braces were no more effective in the prevention of short- or long-term low back pain or time lost from work compared to no treatment. The data also showed no differences between brace use and lifting technique training for the prevention of long-term low back pain and time lost from work. Eight RCTs were included in the review[21] examining the effects of lumbar sacral braces in the treatment of low back pain. The researchers found limited evidence showing no differences with brace use compared to no interventions or other interventions (therapeutic exercise, manipulation, massage) for the reduction of short-term pain and improvement of functional outcomes in patients with acute, subacute, or chronic pain. A 2011 review[22] investigated the effectiveness of physical and rehabilitation interventions (exercise, modalities, education, lumbar sacral braces) for the treatment of non-specific chronic low back pain among adults. Based on the search criteria, no RCTs investigating the efficacy of lumbar sacral braces were identified for inclusion in the review.

The results of these reviews[21,22] provide minimal evidence to support the use of lumbar sacral braces for the prevention and treatment of low back pain. Future RCTs are warranted to examine various interventions used alone or in combination among patients in specific subgroups (acute or chronic pain) to identify successful techniques based on subgroup characteristics.

## CERVICAL COLLAR    Figures 12–14 and 12–15

➤ **Purpose:** Cervical collars are used to provide support and immobilization and to lessen range of motion when preventing and treating sprains, acute torticollis, strains, stable fractures, disk herniation of the cervical spine, and brachial plexus injury. Two cervical collar designs are illustrated below.

### Rehabilitative Technique

➤ **Purpose:** The rehabilitative brace technique is designed to provide moderate to maximal support and complete immobilization of the cervical spine following injury and surgery (Fig. 12–14).

➤ **Design:**
- Rehabilitative braces are available in two basic designs: a rigid and semirigid collar.
- These off-the-shelf braces are available in predetermined sizes based on neck circumference measurements in universal fit designs. Some designs are available in universal sizes.
- The rigid designs consist of an outer shell constructed of polyethylene or thermoplastic materials with a foam inner lining.
- Some of the rigid designs are used for the acute immobilization of the cervical spine following injury (extrication collar) while others are used when complete immobilization is required for extended periods of time.
- Most acute designs allow for adjustments in neck circumference and length measurements during application.
- These braces are typically one piece in design; some can be purchased in various neck lengths.
- The braces are manufactured with openings to allow for pulse checks, airway procedures, and visual inspection.
- Acute braces are attached to the cervical spine through Velcro closures and can be used in most acute injury situations. Most designs are reusable.
- Most rigid, extended wear designs consist of two pieces and are constructed with extra inner padding for comfort. These braces can also be adjusted for comfort and fit and are attached with Velcro closures.
- Semirigid collar designs are manufactured of soft, medium-density foam covered with stockinet.
- The braces are one piece in design, contoured and adjustable for fit, and available in various neck lengths. These braces are anchored with Velcro closures.

### DETAILS
Rigid, extended wear braces can be used during rehabilitative and low intensity work and casual activities. Semirigid designs can be used during rehabilitative and low intensity work and casual activities and are washable and reusable.

**Helpful Hint |**
To lessen soiling and excessive wear, cover the semirigid brace with stockinet. The stockinet can be changed and washed as needed.

➠ **Position of the patient:** Lying, sitting, or standing on the ground with the neck in a pain-free position.
➠ **Preparation:** Apply rehabilitative braces directly to the skin.
   Instructions for application of the braces are included with each design. For proper application, follow the step-by-step procedure. The following general application guidelines apply to most rigid and semi-rigid designs.
➠ **Application:**

**STEP 1:**  When using some rigid acute designs, measure the length from the shoulder to the chin of the patient and adjust the brace to this measurement. Do not adjust the brace while it is on the patient.

**STEP 2:**  Continue application of adjustable and most other acute designs by placing the anterior brace under the chin (Fig. 12–14A).

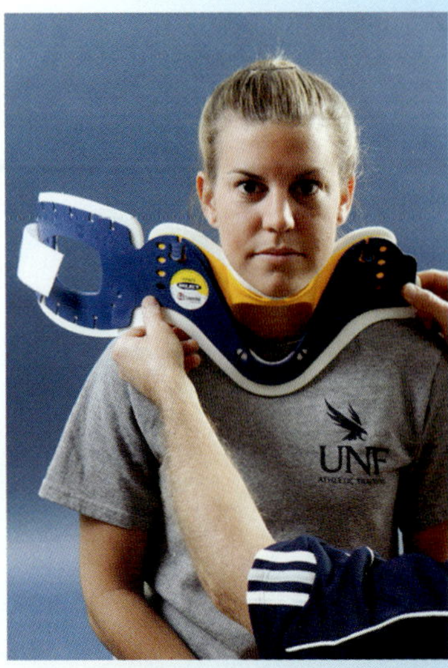

**Fig. 12–14 A**

**STEP 3:**  Next, position and wrap the brace around the neck (Fig. 12–14B). Anchor the brace with Velcro closures with moderate tension (Fig. 12–14C).

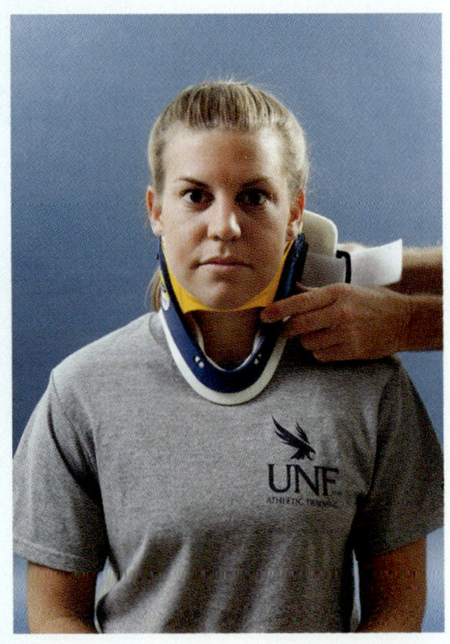

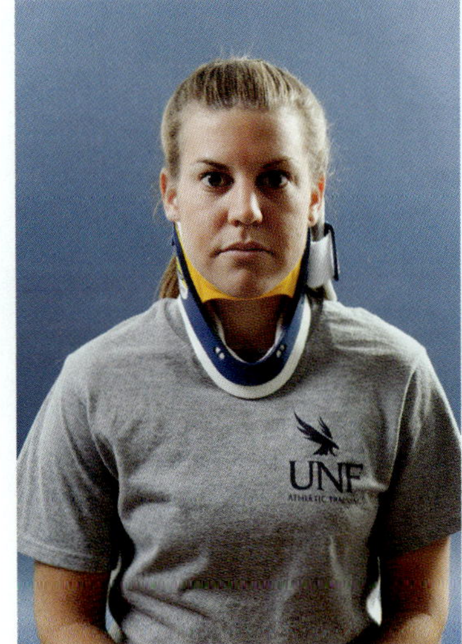

**Fig. 12–14 B**          **Fig. 12–14 C**

**DETAILS**

Note, these are general application guidelines—appropriate care of suspected cervical spine injuries is vital to prevent further trauma. For more complete information, see the Web References.

*Steps Cont.*

**STEP 4:** Begin applying rigid, extended wear designs by placing the anterior piece of the brace under the chin (Fig. 12–14D). When using some designs, wrap the elastic strap around the neck and anchor on the anterior brace.

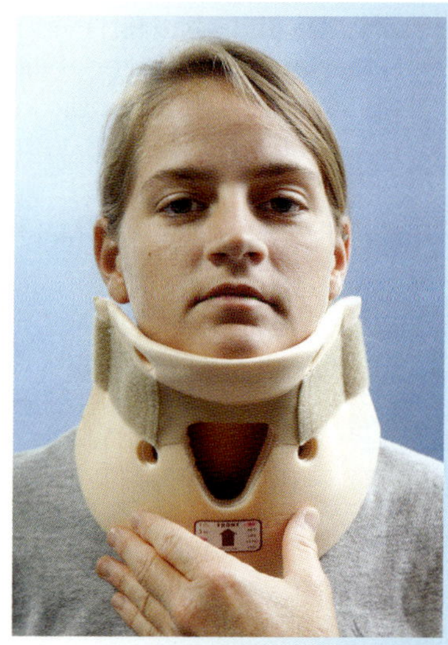

**Fig. 12–14 D**

**STEP 5:** Next, place the posterior piece of the brace around the posterior neck (Fig. 12–14E).

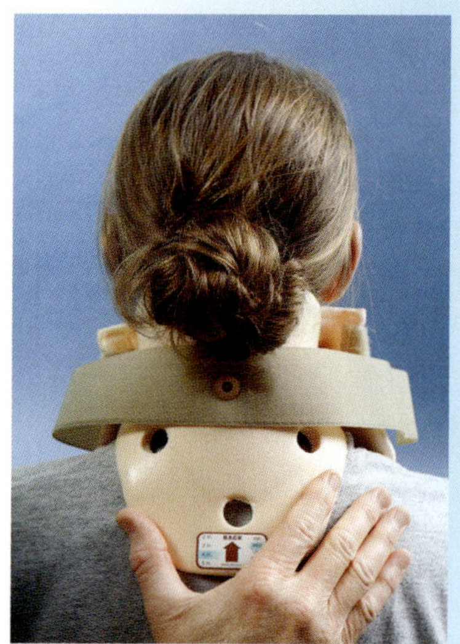

**Fig. 12–14 E**

**STEP 6:** Using moderate tension, anchor the brace with Velcro closures (Fig. 12–14F). Readjust the brace if necessary.

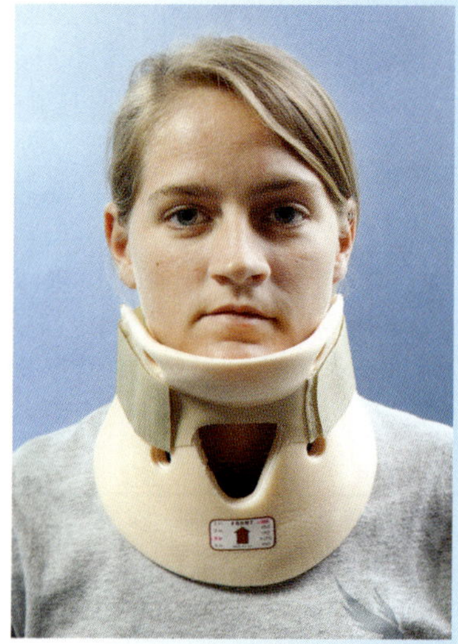

**Fig. 12–14 F**

**STEP 7:** When using semirigid designs, position the contoured area of the brace under the chin and wrap the ends around the neck with moderate tension (Fig. 12–14G). Anchor with Velcro closures. If necessary, readjust the brace.

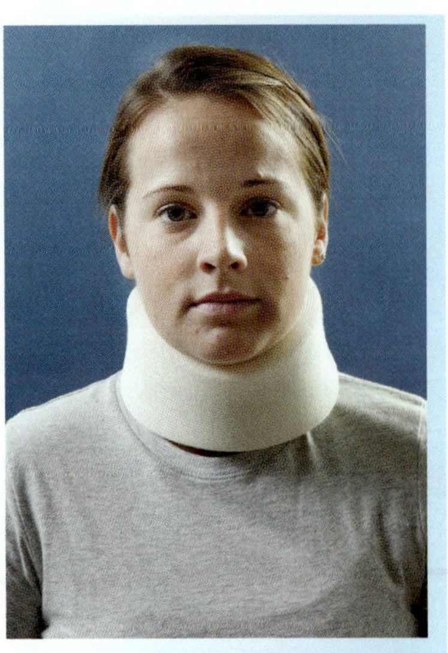

**Fig. 12–14 G**

### Functional Technique

➡ **Purpose:** Functional braces are designed to provide moderate support, absorb shock, and limit range of motion when preventing and treating cervical sprains, strains, disk herniation, and brachial plexus injury for football players (Fig. 12–15). The designs lessen excessive cervical extension and lateral flexion, but allow for normal flexion. Use these functional braces combined with football shoulder pads.

➡ **Design:**
- The braces are available off-the-shelf in predetermined sizes corresponding to neck circumference measurements or the weight of the patient in universal fit designs. Some designs can be purchased in universal sizes.
- Some designs consist of a pre-molded, closed-cell polyethylene foam collar incorporated into a padded foam vest.
- The collar on some vest designs can be adjusted to lessen specific ranges of motion.
- One vest design uses an optional plate manufactured from rigid plastic materials that attaches directly to the collar to provide additional support.
- Vest designs are worn underneath or attached to the neck opening of football shoulder pads and are secured to the pads with laces and/or straps.
- Other functional braces are manufactured of rigid materials and are bolted directly to football shoulder pads.

**Helpful Hint |**
Because some functional collar designs are anchored directly to shoulder pads, the pads must be properly fitted and correctly worn. With contact, braces that attach to the top of shoulder pads may migrate away from the cervical area, allowing for excessive range of motion and/or compression.[23] Belts and/or buckles that anchor shoulder pads to the shoulder and upper torso should always be applied and worn snugly to lessen migration of the pads and collar.

- Some functional designs are constructed of both open- and closed-cell foams and are attached to football shoulder pads with laces and/or bolts.
- These foam braces are available in flat and roll designs in various thicknesses based on the injury and the desired range of motion.

➡ **Position of the patient:** Standing with the arms at the side of the body.

➡ **Preparation:** Attach the functional brace to the shoulder pads. Apply the shoulder pads directly to the skin or over a shirt.

Follow the step-by-step application instructions included with each design. The following general application guidelines pertain to most functional designs.

➡ **Application:**

**STEP 1:** When using vest designs, position the collar through the neck opening of the shoulder pads (Fig. 12–15A). Anchoring of the brace to the pads depends on the design. When using most designs, anchor the vest with laces (Fig. 12–15B).

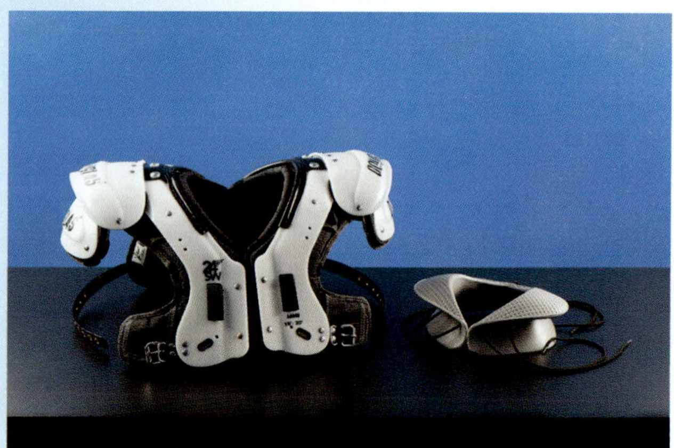

**Fig. 12–15 A** *Functional cervical collar. (Left) Football shoulder pads. (Right) Vest design.*

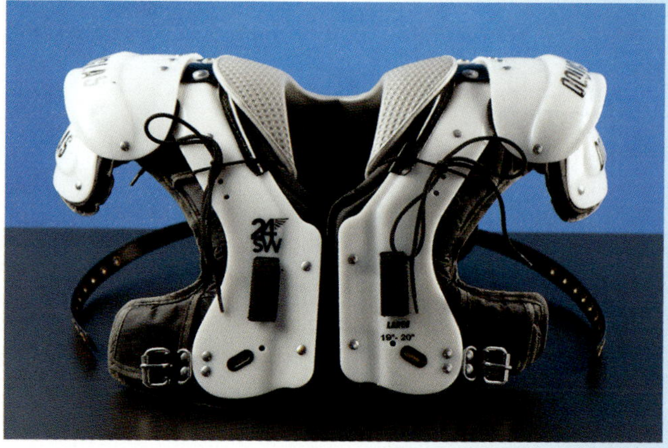

**Fig. 12–15 B** *Vest design attached to football shoulder pads.*

**STEP 2:** Attach other designs directly to the shoulder pads with bolts and/or laces (Fig. 12–15C).

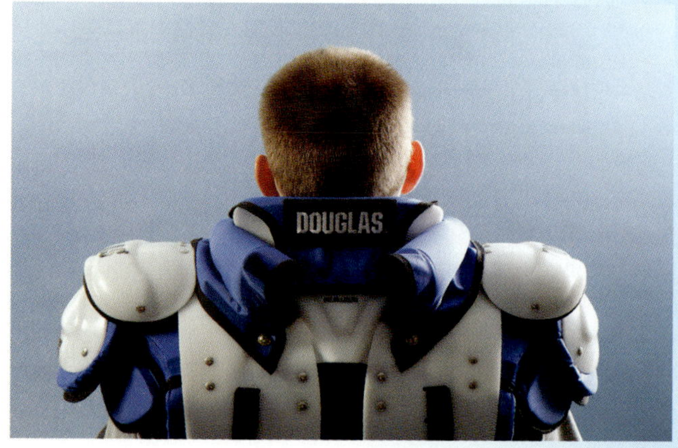


**Fig. 12–15 C**

**. . . IF/THEN . . .**

**IF** a functional cervical collar technique is indicated to treat a compression brachial plexus injury, **THEN** consider using a padded foam vest design; this brace will limit range of motion, and the foam vest may lessen compression/impingement over Erb's point.

## EVIDENCE SUMMARY

Functional cervical collars are designed to reduce cervical hyperextension and lateral flexion in the prevention and treatment of brachial plexus injury. While use of cervical collars is common in football, there is minimal evidence in the literature examining their efficacy. A 2015 evidence-based review[24] that included four studies investigated the effectiveness of functional cervical collars in the reduction of brachial plexus injury among athletes participating in contact sports. Two studies conducted in controlled settings found significant reductions in active and passive cervical hyperextension with vest, nylon strap, foam roll, and custom-made designs compared with shoulder pads alone. However, vest, nylon strap, and foam roll designs allowed for additional hyperextension when a passive overload was applied. The brace designs in the two studies failed to show a restriction in passive lateral flexion. A separate study in the review[24] used dynamic impact testing and demonstrated reductions in head acceleration and force transmission through the neck from top impact with foam and synthetic roll designs; restrictions in cervical hyperextension from front impact with vest and foam and synthetic roll designs; and reductions in lateral flexion from side impact with a synthetic roll brace. A small study in the review[24] examined incidence rates of brachial plexus injury with functional cervical collar use. The findings revealed a reduction in the incidence and severity of symptoms among tackle football athletes during a 1-year period.

Several recommendations have been made toward the prevention of brachial plexus injury and the use of functional cervical collars. Some researchers[6,25–27] have suggested that the braces should be mandatory to lessen the frequency of injury for athletes who experience recurrent episodes or have experienced an isolated severe injury or a single injury in a high-risk playing position. Based on the mechanism of injury and the data from the limited studies, prevention of injury may involve more than just functional bracing techniques. Some researchers[28–30] recommend a comprehensive rehabilitation program consisting of strength, flexibility, and neuromuscular exercises for the neck and shoulder girdle. Others suggest instruction of proper tackling and hitting techniques[7,30,31] and use of properly fitted shoulder pads and helmets.[7,9,30] While this limited evidence appears to provide some support for the benefit of functional cervical collars, additional research is needed with current designs to determine the effectiveness of functional cervical collars in the prevention and treatment of injury. These investigations could compare the effects of different collar and shoulder pad designs on the restriction of cervical range of motion and the effects of various neck and shoulder strengthening and flexibility programs and player education, used individually or in combination, on rates of injury to determine the most effective intervention(s).

### Clinical Application Question 2

A freshman defensive back on the intercollegiate football team suffers a grade one brachial plexus injury during a tackling drill in preseason practice. His medical history reveals chronic episodes of the injury in high school. He used a foam roll functional brace in high school and is currently wearing a similar design. An evaluation with the team physician concludes with a discussion of preventive bracing techniques.

➡ **Question: What bracing techniques are appropriate for the player's return to activity?**

## SLINGS

➡ **Purpose:** Slings provide support and immobilization when treating thorax and spine injuries and conditions.
- Use slings (see Fig. 8–19) to treat pectoralis major strains and brachial plexus injury.

# Padding Techniques

A variety of off-the-shelf padding techniques can be used to prevent and treat injuries and conditions of the thorax, abdomen, and spine. Custom-made pads may also be constructed from thermoplastic material and foam. Padding of the thorax, abdomen, and spine is required in several interscholastic and intercollegiate sports. These padding techniques will be discussed further in Chapter 13.

## OFF-THE-SHELF    Figures 12–16 and 12–17

➠ **Purpose:** Off-the-shelf padding techniques are available in a variety of designs to provide shock absorption and protection. Use these techniques when preventing and treating rib, abdominal, kidney, pulmonary, genital, breast, and coccygeal contusions; Cooper's ligament sprains; rib, coccygeal, and stable cervical fractures; and costochondral and brachial plexus injury. Following is a description of two basic designs.

### Soft, Low-Density

### DETAILS

Soft, low-density pads are commonly used to provide shock absorption to the thorax, abdomen, and spine of athletes participating in a variety of sports. The pads can be used in combination with mandatory protective equipment, among different sports, or worn alone. Use the pads with work and casual activities. These pads may be washed and reused.

➠ **Design:**
- These universal fit designs are available in predetermined sizes based on chest or waist circumference measurements or age of the patient.
- Shirt designs are manufactured of polyester/spandex materials with thermal foam pads incorporated in the inner lining over the ribs, kidney, and spine to provide shock absorption.
- Padded shorts are constructed of nylon/spandex materials with a mesh covering.
- These designs contain ethylene vinyl acetate (EVA) foam incorporated in the inner lining over the coccyx and spine area.
- The shorts extend from the mid thigh area to the waist; most have an elastic waistband.
- Bra and top designs are manufactured of nylon/spandex materials with additional foam incorporated to support and protect the breast.
- Individual pad designs are constructed of varying thicknesses of low-density open- and closed-cell foams; viscoelastic polymer or gel materials are available in a variety of sizes to provide shock absorption of the thorax, abdomen, spine, and coccyx.

➠ **Position of the patient:** Standing with the arms at the side of the body.

➠ **Preparation:** Apply shirts, shorts, bras, tops, and individual pads directly to the skin. Individual pads may also be applied under tight-fitting clothing or within athletic clothing.

➠ **Application:**

**STEP 1:**    To apply a padded shirt, place the shirt over the head and insert the arms through the sleeves. Pull the shirt and pads onto the thorax, abdomen, and spine (Fig. 12–16A). Adjust the pads if needed.

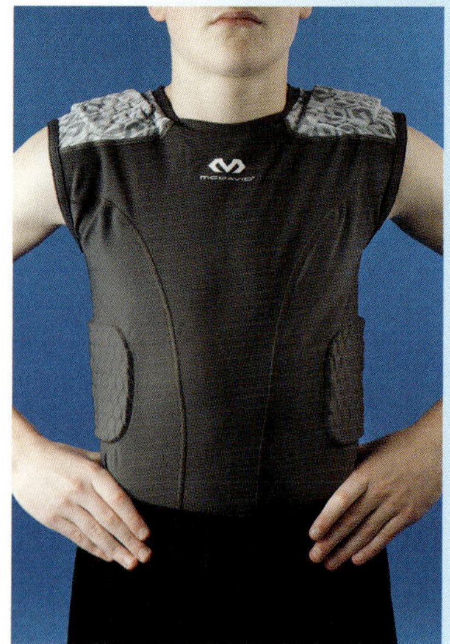

**Fig. 12–16 A**

**STEP 2:**  When using short designs, place the feet into the shorts and pull in a proximal direction until positioned on the waist (Fig. 12–16B). Adjust the pads over the coccyx and spine.

**STEP 3:**  Apply the bra and top designs by placing them over the head and arms. Position the pads over the breasts.

**STEP 4:**  Attach an individual, closed-cell foam pad to the spine and/or coccyx by placing the pad underneath tight-fitting clothing or within athletic girdles (see Fig. 7–22F).

**STEP 5:**  Apply other closed-cell foam designs over the head and shoulders and anchor under the axillae with elastic straps or around the chest with Velcro straps (see Fig. 8–23G).

**STEP 6:**  Attach viscoelastic polymer or gel material pads to the inner lining of football shoulder pads (see Fig. 8–23F). The pads may also be anchored with the contusion/fracture taping technique or circular wrapping technique.

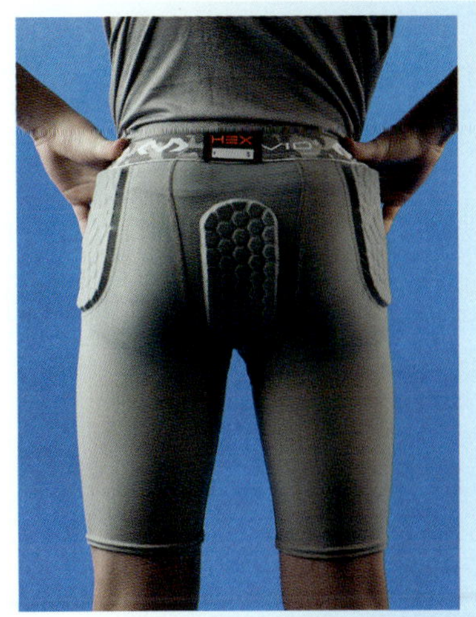

**Fig. 12–16 B**

## EVIDENCE SUMMARY

Soft, low-density padding has been used to prevent brachial plexus injury. Skeleton, viscoelastic polymer, or gel pads attached underneath football shoulder pads may reduce the incidence of injury.[6,32] Use these pads to improve shoulder pad fit, lessen pressure on the cervical spine, and provide additional shock absorption.[33] Some suggest the additional padding may lift the shoulder pads off the shoulders, reducing the amount of lateral flexion of the neck.[7]

### Hard, High-Density

**DETAILS**

Hard, high-density pads are commonly used to provide shock absorption to the thorax, abdomen, and spine of athletes participating in a variety of sports. Use the pads in combination with mandatory sports equipment or wear the pads alone. The pads may be used in work and casual activities and reused.

**DETAILS**

Football shoulder pads can provide protection of the anterior and posterior upper thoracic and cervical areas. However, these pads do not protect the lower rib cage and abdominal areas from injury.[34]

➡ **Design:**
- Universal fit designs are available in prede-termined sizes based on chest circumference measurements or age of the patient (Fig. 12–17A).
- Rib vests or jackets (flak jacket) are con-structed of a high-density plastic material outer shell pre-molded to the contours of the thorax and abdomen. The outer shell is lined with open-cell foam.

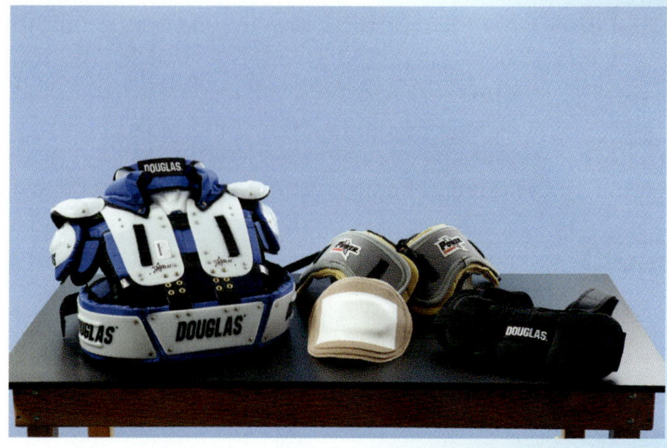

**Fig. 12–17 A** *Variety of hard, high-density pads.*

---

## DETAILS

The term "flak" is an abbreviation for *Flugzeugabwehrkanone*—aircraft attack gun. "Flak" was used to describe German antiaircraft fire during World War II.[35] The name "flak jacket" originates from an armored jacket worn by Allied troops and air crews for protection against bullets and shell fragments.

---

- The pads are available in various lengths and widths depending on the size of the patient and the area to be protected.
- Some designs are attached directly to football shoulder pads with zippers, bolts, and/or nylon straps.
- Other pads are incorporated and attached to the thorax and abdomen with adjustable elastic suspenders.
- Most rib vest/jacket designs are anchored over the anterior thorax/abdomen with laces or Velcro closures.

---

## DETAILS

Vests/jackets designed as mandatory equipment for one sport may be used for another sport. For example, use lacrosse rib pads for an athlete participating in baseball or basketball.

---

- Another pad design uses a high-density plastic plate lined with open-cell foam.
  - These plates are attached directly to football shoulder pads with zippers, bolts, and/or nylon straps over the anterior and/or posterior thorax, abdomen, and spine.
- Athletic cups are constructed of high-density, flexible plastic or carbon laminate materials pre-molded to the contours of the genital area. The edges of these designs are covered with closed-cell foam or viscoelastic polymers to prevent irritation.
  - Designs are available for males and females and are typically used in combination with an elastic supporter.
  - Another cup design is manufactured of low-density polyethylene plastic materials. This cup is designed for female breasts and is used in combination with bras and tops.

➡ **Position of the patient:** Standing with the arms at the side of the body.

➡ **Preparation:** Apply these designs directly to the skin, over or under tight-fitting clothing, or within athletic clothing.

➡ **Application:**

**STEP 1:** Begin application of some rib vests/jackets and plates by attaching the designs to football shoulder pads (Fig. 12–17B). Apply and anchor the shoulder pads.

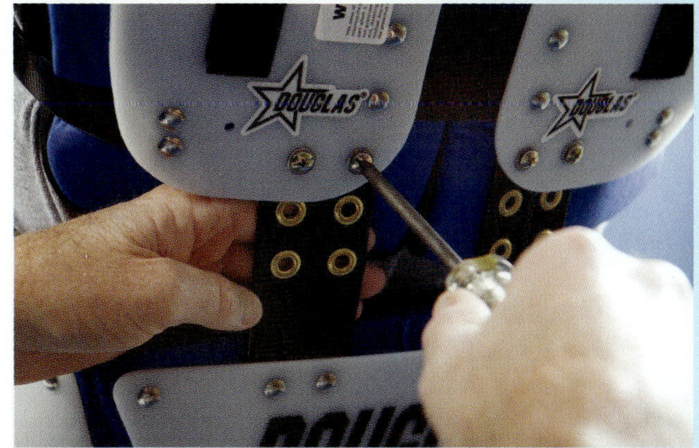

**Fig. 12–17 B**

**STEP 2:** Next, position the vest/jacket or plate over the thorax, abdomen, and/or spine. With most designs, anchor the pads snugly over the anterior thorax/abdomen with laces or Velcro closures (Fig. 12–17C). Adjust the laces or closures if needed to prevent constriction of chest movement and breathing patterns.

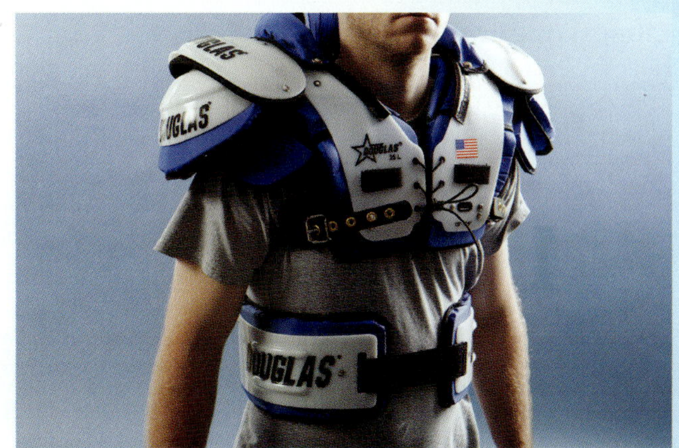

**Fig. 12–17 C**

**STEP 3:** Apply other vests/jackets by placing the suspenders over the shoulders. Position the pads around the thorax, abdomen, and/or spine, and anchor (Fig. 12–17D).

**STEP 4:** When using athletic cup designs, place the feet into an athletic supporter and pull in a proximal direction until the supporter is positioned around the waist. Place the head and arms into a bra or top and position over the breasts.

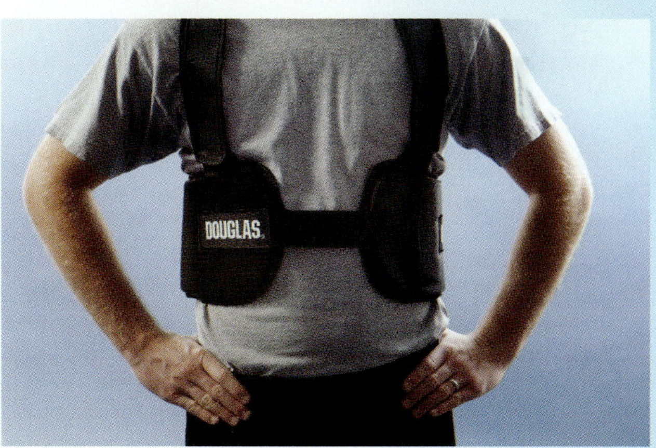

**Fig. 12–17 D**

*Steps Cont.*

**STEP 5:**   Place most cups in a pocket that is incorporated into the supporter or bra/top (Fig. 12–17E). Cups may also be used under tight-fitting clothing.

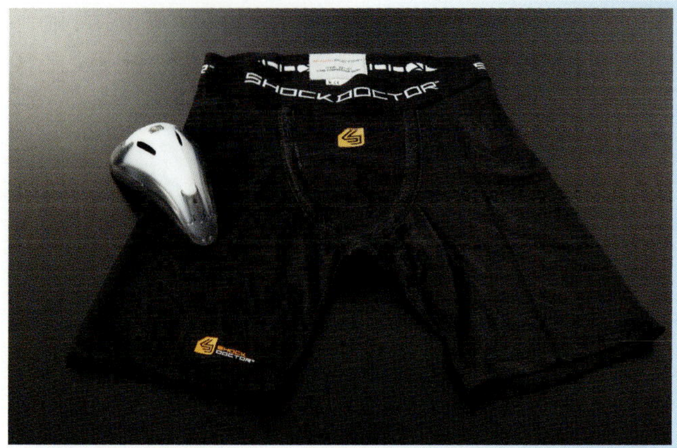

**Fig. 12–17 E**

---

### Clinical Application Question 3

Near the end of the soccer match, an 8-year-old goalie is struck in the mid to low back area by an opponent's elbow during a shot on goal. His team is participating in a state youth tournament out of town. He is unable to continue play and is taken to a local out-patient medical clinic for evaluation. The physician evaluates the goalie and suspects a first-degree kidney contusion. The physician allows a return to play if the area is protected with padding. The team has three matches remaining in the tournament; the goalie's parents will allow him to participate as tolerated. The goalie's parents search the local sporting goods stores for padded rib/thorax vests and jackets, but all the designs are too large for the goalie. Another parent is the coach of the youth football team and commonly carries some protective football equipment in the back of his SUV.

➡ **Question: What padding techniques can you apply in this situation?**

---

## CUSTOM-MADE

➡ **Purpose:** Absorb shock and provide protection when preventing and treating rib, abdominal, kidney, pulmonary, genital, breast, and coccygeal contusions; rib and coccygeal fractures; and costochondral injury with thermoplastic material and foam. Use these pads when off-the-shelf designs are not available.

➡ **Materials:**
  • Paper, felt tip pen, thermoplastic material, ⅛ inch or ¼ inch foam or felt, a heating source, 2 inch or 3 inch elastic tape, an elastic wrap, soft, low-density foam, rubber cement, taping scissors

➡ **Position of the patient:** Standing with the arms at the side of the body.

➡ **Preparation:** Design the pad with a paper pattern. Cut, mold, and shape the thermoplastic material on the thorax, abdomen, and/or spine over the injured area. Attach soft, low-density foam to the inside surface of the material.

➡ **Application:**

**STEP 1:**   Place the pad over the injured area and attach with the contusion/fracture taping or circular wrapping technique. Pad all nonpliable materials to meet NCAA[36] and NFHS[37] rules.

**STEP 2:**   Another option is to attach the custom-made pad to the thorax, abdomen, and/or spine underneath tight-fitting clothing or within athletic clothing.

> **Helpful Hint |**
> If off-the-shelf or custom-made padding techniques irritate the nipples, apply a skin lubricant over the area and cover with a wound dressing or adhesive gauze material.

## | MANDATORY PADDING

Protective equipment is required in several high school and intercollegiate sports. The NCAA[36] and NFHS[37] require that athletes participating in baseball, fencing, field hockey, football, ice hockey, lacrosse, and softball wear protective padding on the thorax, abdomen, and/or spine during all practices and competitions. These pads are typically purchased off-the-shelf; many sport-specific designs are available. A further discussion of these padding techniques can be found in Chapter 13.

### Clinical Application Question 4

A batsman sends a forceful shot to the off side, and a gully is struck in the left anterior ribs with the cricket ball. The gully immediately falls to the ground in pain and is removed from the pitch. An evaluation by a physician, including radiographs, reveals anterior fractures to the sixth and seventh ribs. After several weeks of inactivity, the gully is allowed to return to play.

➡ **Question: What padding techniques can you use to protect the area during play?**

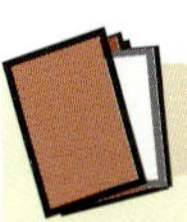

## EVIDENCE-BASED PRACTICE

During the second quarter of the opening game of the season, John Mariani, a junior wide receiver at Round Top College, jumps to catch a pass. As the ball arrives, the safety collides with John, turning him to a semihorizontal position. John maintains possession of the ball, holding it against his right thorax, and falls toward the ground. Upon landing, John's right shoulder strikes the ground, followed by his thorax on top of the ball, then his lower body. The safety simultaneously falls on John, forcing John's head and neck to the left. John remains on the field; Bernadette Chamberlain, AT, immediately comes out to the field. John complains of a burning pain and numbness radiating distally in the right arm and pain in the right lateral thorax. Bernadette begins an initial evaluation as the team physician arrives. Following this evaluation, Bernadette and the team physician help John to the sidelines, where they perform further testing. The evaluation reveals pain and paresthesia in the right shoulder and arm, muscle weakness in the right rotator cuff, point tenderness over the lateral aspect of ribs six through nine, and pain with deep inhalation and coughing. John is taken to the locker room for radiographs. The radiographs are negative; the team physician believes John has sustained a grade two right brachial plexus injury, along with a moderate rib contusion. The team physician requests that support, compression, and immobilization be applied for the shoulder and ribs. Bernadette applies a sling to support and immobilize the right shoulder and the thorax and abdomen wrapping technique to provide compression and support to the thorax and ribs.

John is seen by the team physician in the athletic training facility the next day. An evaluation that includes strength, range of motion, nerve root, myotome, and special tests confirms the original diagnosis. John is placed in a therapeutic exercise program with Bernadette and closely followed by the team physician. After many weeks of treatment and rehabilitation, John achieves pre-injury strength and range of motion and is free of neurological symptoms. The team physician allows John to progress back into football activities and discusses with Bernadette protective options for the cervical and thoracic areas. Bernadette goes to the storage room and returns with multiple sizes and designs of protective techniques. Bernadette and the team physician choose a functional cervical collar and hard, high-density rib pad to limit range of motion of the cervical spine and absorb shock over the thorax.

The return to football activities progresses well, and John enters his first drill since the injury at full speed. While running deep routes, John notices he is unable to rotate his head completely to the right or left to see the ball, so he drops several passes. He then runs several short, turn-in patterns and easily catches the ball, but cannot secure the ball in his arm against the thorax when running. John becomes frustrated and talks with Bernadette about the possibility of removing the brace and pad. Bernadette has experienced positive clinical outcomes with the bracing and padding techniques John is wearing, but realizes this is a unique situation she hasn't seen before. She consults with the team physician and decides to search

*Continued*

for a bracing and padding technique to allow John improved vision and ball control while providing the necessary protection to allow him to continue football activities.

1. Develop two clinically relevant questions from the case in the PICO format to generate answers for the selection of a (1) bracing technique to limit range of motion of the cervical spine and (2) padding technique to absorb shock over the thorax for John. The questions should include the population or problem, the intervention, a comparison intervention (if relevant), and the clinical outcome of interest.

2. Design a search strategy and search to find the best evidence to answer the clinical questions. The strategies should include relevant search terms, electronic databases, online journals, and print journals to use for the search. Discussions with your faculty, preceptor, and other health care professionals can provide evidence from expert opinion.

3. Choose two to three full text studies or reviews from each of your searches or the chapter references. Evaluate and appraise each article to determine its value and usefulness to the case. Ask these questions for each study: (1) Are the results of the study valid? (2) What are the actual results? and (3) Are the findings clinically relevant to my patients? Prepare a summary of the evaluation with answers to the questions and rank the articles based on the evidence hierarchy in Chapter 1.

4. Integrate findings from the evidence, your clinical experience, and John's goals and preferences into the case. Consider which bracing and padding techniques may be appropriate for each situation.

5. Evaluate the EBP process and your experience within the case. Consider these questions in the evaluation.

Were the clinical questions answered?
Did the searches generate quality evidence?
Was the evidence evaluated appropriately?
Was the evidence, your clinical experience, and John's goals and values integrated to make the clinical decisions?
Did the interventions produce successful clinical outcomes for John?
Was the EBP experience positive for Bernadette and John?

## WRAP-UP

- Acute and chronic injuries and conditions to the thorax, abdomen, and spine can be the result of compressive and repetitive forces, excessive range of motion, and overload and violent muscular contractions.
- The contusion/fracture taping and circular wrapping techniques anchor protective padding to the thorax, abdomen, and spine.
- Compression wrap techniques are used to control mild, moderate, and severe swelling following injury.
- The swathe wrapping and sling bracing techniques provide support and immobilization.
- Rib belts and lumbar sacral bracing techniques can be used to provide compression and support, lessen range of motion, and correct structural abnormalities.
- Rehabilitative and functional cervical collar bracing techniques provide support and immobilization, absorb shock, and limit range of motion following injury and surgery.
- Off-the-shelf and custom-made padding techniques constructed of soft, low-density and hard, high-density materials absorb shock and provide protection when preventing and treating injuries and conditions.
- Mandatory protective padding is required by the NCAA and NFHS for the thorax, abdomen, and/or spine in several sports.

## FADAVIS ONLINE RESOURCES

- Swathe rib wrapping technique

## WEB REFERENCES

**National Athletic Trainers' Association**
**National Athletic Trainers' Association Position Statement: Preventing Sudden Death in Sports**
http://natajournals.org/doi/pdf/10.4085/1062-6050-47.1.96?code=nata-site
- This website allows access to recommendations on the prevention and treatment and management of the injured patient.

**National Athletic Trainers' Association Position Statement: Acute Management of the Cervical Spine-Injured Athlete**
http://natajournals.org/doi/pdf/10.4085/1062-6050-44.3.306
- This site allows access to recommendations on the management of catastrophic cervical spine injury in the athlete.

**The Inter-Association Task Force for Preventing Sudden Death in Secondary School Athletics Programs: Best-Practice Recommendations**
https://meridian.allenpress.com/jat/article/48/4/546/191277/The-Inter-Association-Task-Force-for-Preventing
- This website allows access to recommendations on the prevention of injury and use of appropriate equipment.

**National Athletic Trainers' Association: Consensus Recommendations on the Prehospital Care of the Injured Athlete With a Suspected Catastrophic Cervical Spine Injury**
https://meridian.allenpress.com/jat/article/55/6/563/438476/Consensus-Recommendations-on-the-Prehospital-Care
- This website allows access to recommendations on the prehospital management of cervical spine injury in the athlete.

**The Miami Project to Cure Paralysis**
https://www.themiamiproject.org/
- This website allows access to the research center for information about spinal cord injury and ongoing research to find more effective treatments.

## REFERENCES


1. Prentice, WE: Principles of Athletic Training: A Guide to Evidence-Based Clinical Practice, ed 16. McGraw-Hill, New York, 2017.
2. Anderson, MK: Foundations of Athletic Training: Prevention, Assessment, and Management, ed 6. Wolters Kluwer, Philadelphia, 2017.
3. Starkey, C, and Brown, SD: Examination of Orthopedic and Athletic Injuries, ed 4. F.A. Davis, Philadelphia, 2015.
4. Grod, JP: Diagnosis and evaluation of rib fracture. Top Clin Chiropractic 6:49–61, 1999.
5. Gurtler, R, Pavlov, H, and Torg, JS: Stress fracture of the ipsilateral first rib in a pitcher. Am J Sports Med 13:277–279, 1985.
6. Markey, KL, Di Benedetto, M, and Curl, WW: Upper trunk brachial plexopathy: The stinger syndrome. Am J Sports Med 21:650–655, 1993.
7. Feinberg, JH: Burners and stingers. Phys Med Rehab Clin North Am 11:771–784, 2000.
8. Kelly, JD IV: Brachial plexus injuries: Evaluating and treating "burners." J Musculoskel Med 14:70–80, 1997.
9. Chao, S, Pacella, MJ, and Torg, JS: The pathomechanics, pathophysiology and prevention of cervical spinal cord and brachial plexus injuries in athletics. Sports Med 40:59–75, 2010.
10. Granhed, H, and Morelli, B: Low back pain among retired wrestlers and heavyweight lifters. Am J Sports Med 16:530–533, 1988.
11. Micheli, LJ: Back injuries in gymnastics. Clin Sports Med 4:85–93, 1985.
12. Soler, T, and Calderon, C: The prevalence of spondylolysis in the Spanish elite athlete. Am J Sports Med 28:57–62, 2000.
13. Motley, G, Nyland, J, Jacobs, J, and Caborn, D: The pars interarticularis stress reaction, spondylolysis, and spondylolisthesis progression. J Athl Train 33:351–358, 1998.
14. Pezzullo, DJ: Spondylolisthesis and spondylolysis in athletes. Ath Ther Today 4:36–40, 1999.
15. Iwamoto, J, Takeda, T, and Wakano, K: Returning athletes with severe low back pain and spondylolysis to original sporting activities with conservative treatment. Scand J Med Sci Sports 14:346–351, 2004.
16. O'Kane, J, O'Kane, E, and Marquet, J: Delayed complication of a rib fracture. Phys Sportsmed 26:69–77, 1998.
17. Quick, G: A randomized clinical trial of rib belts for simple fractures. Am J Emerg Med 8:277–281, 1990.
18. Lazcano, A, Dougherty, JM, and Kruger, M: Use of rib belts in acute rib fractures. Am J Emerg Med 7:97–100, 1989.
19. Mayberry, JC, and Trunkey, DD: The fractured rib in chest wall trauma. Chest Surg Clin N Am 7:239–261, 1997.
20. Kerr-Valentic, MA, Arthur, M, Mullins, RJ, Pearson, TE, and Mayberry, JC: Rib fracture pain and disability: Can we do better? J Trauma 54:1058–1064, 2003.
21. van Duijvenbode, I, Jellema, P, van Poppel, M, and van Tulder, MW: Lumbar supports for prevention and treatment of low back pain. Cochrane Database Syst Rev (2);CD001823, 2008.
22. van Middelkoop, M, Rubinstein, SM, Kuijpers, T, Verhagen, AP, Ostelo, R, Koes, BW, and van Tulder, MW: A systematic review on the effectiveness of physical and rehabilitation interventions for chronic non-specific low back pain. Eur Spine J 20:19–39, 2011.
23. Archambault, JL: Brachial plexus stretch injury. J Am Coll Health 31:256–260, 1983.
24. Stowers, MDJ, Lemanu, DP, Hill, AG, and Fulcher, ML: Cervical orthoses in preventing brachial plexus and spinal cord injury: A systematic review. New Zeal J Sport Med 42:18–23, 2015.
25. Hovis, WD, and Limbird, TJ: An evaluation of cervical orthoses in limiting hyperextension and lateral flexion in football. Med Sci Sports Exerc 26:872–876, 1994.
26. Koffler, KM, and Kelly, JD 4th: Neurovascular trauma in athletes. Orthop Clin North Am 33:523–534, 2002.
27. Weinstein, SM: Assessment and rehabilitation of the athlete with a "stinger": A model for the management of noncatastrophic athletic cervical spine injury. Clin Sports Med 17:127–135, 1998.
28. Gorden, JA, Straub, SJ, Swanik, CB, and Swanik, KA: Effects of football collars on cervical hyperextension and lateral flexion. J Athl Train 38:209–215, 2003.

29. Cramer, CR: A reconditioning program to lower the recurrence rate of brachial plexus neurapraxia in collegiate football players. J Athl Train 34:390–396, 1999.

30. Cross, KM, and Serenelli, C: Training and equipment to prevent athletic head and neck injuries. Clin Sports Med 22:639–667, 2003.

31. Safran, MR: Nerve injury about the shoulder in athletes, part 2: Long thoracic nerve, spinal accessory nerve, burners/stingers, thoracic outlet syndrome. Am J Sports Med 32:1063–1076, 2004.

32. Di Benedetto, M, and Markey, K: Electrodiagnostic localization of traumatic upper trunk brachial plexopathy. Arch Phys Med Rehabil 65:15–17, 1984.

33. Watkins, RG: Neck injuries in football players. Clin Sports Med 5:215–246, 1986.

34. Levy, AS, Bassett, F, Lintner, S, and Speer, K: Pulmonary barotraumas: Diagnosis in American football players. Am J Sports Med 24:227–228, 1996.

35. Wikipedia: Flak jacket. https://en.wikipedia.org/wiki/Flak_jacket

36. National Collegiate Athletic Association: 2014–15 NCAA Sports Medicine Handbook, ed 25. NCAA, Indianapolis, 2014. http://www.ncaapublications.com/productdownloads/MD15.pdf.

37. National Federation of State High School Associations: 2018 Football Rules Book. National Federation of State High School Associations, Indianapolis, 2019.

# Part Four

# Protective Equipment

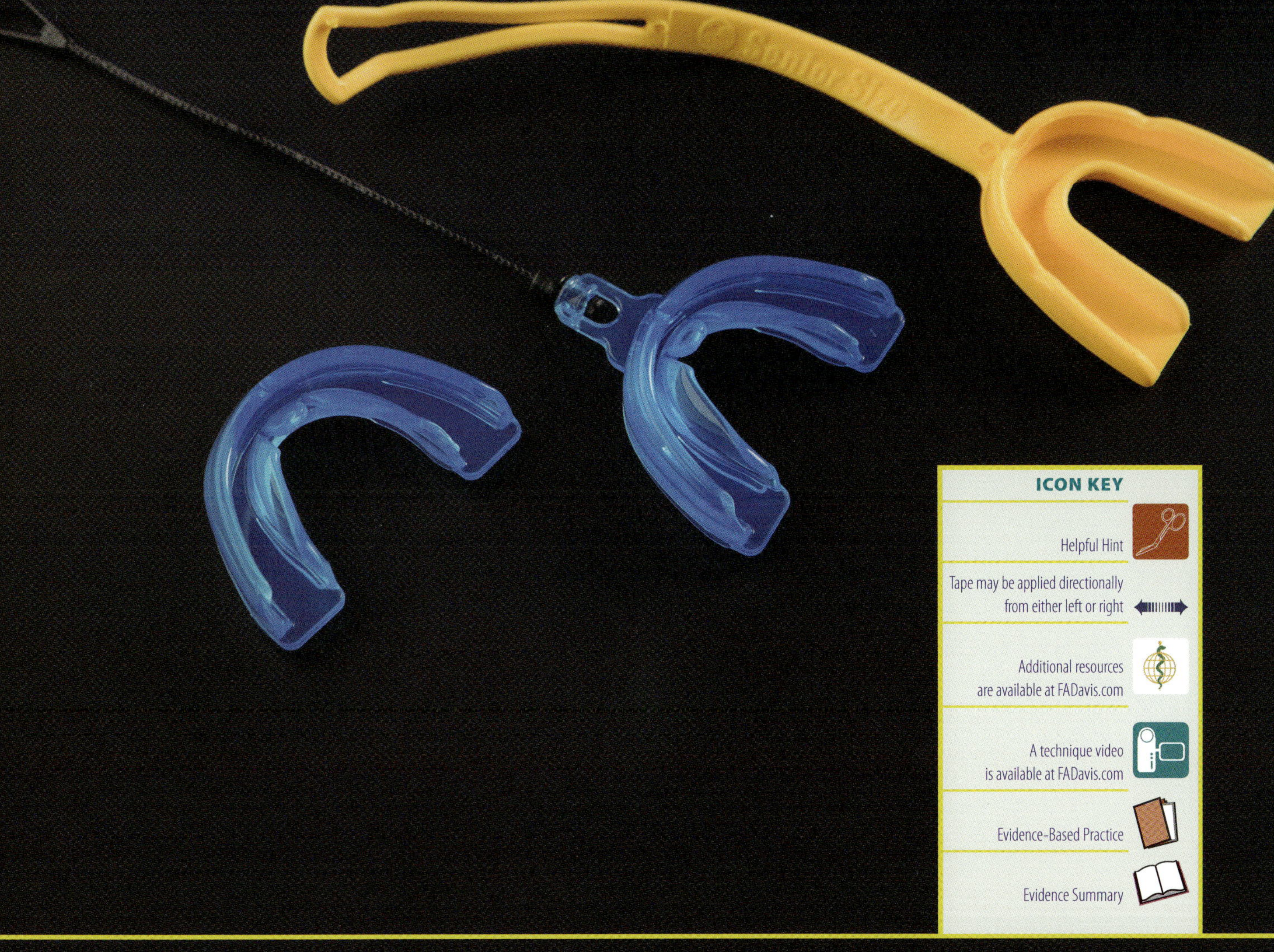

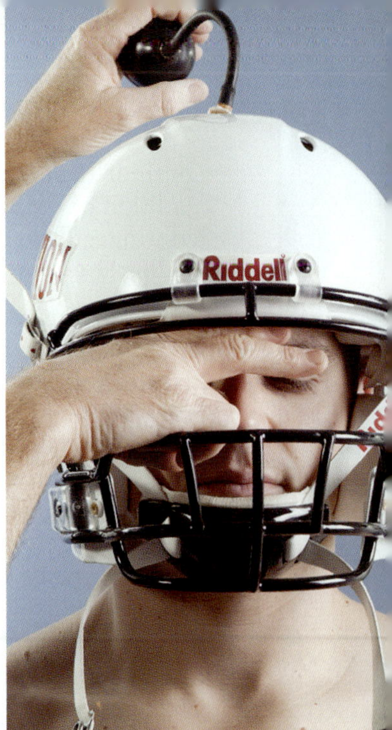

13

# Protective Equipment and Padding





## LIABILITY ISSUES SURROUNDING PROTECTIVE EQUIPMENT

Legal issues surround the design, manufacture, fit, application, and use of protective equipment and padding. The responsibility to ensure appropriate design and use is shared by the individuals who manufacture, purchase, fit, apply, and use the equipment and padding. Manufacturers may be found liable if an individual is injured while using their products or if the products are found to be defective or unfit for their designed purpose. Manufacturers may also be found liable if **foreseeable,** or anticipated, risks associated with the use of the products were not lessened or eliminated.[1] Health care professionals have a duty to fit and apply the protective equipment according to manufacturers' guidelines and intended uses. Modifications to or use of equipment or padding in ways other than the intended purpose can place the liability on the health care professional and/or individual using the equipment and padding. Modifications that result in injury to the individual may lead to liability for the health care provider.

Health care professionals and others involved with protective equipment and padding can use the following recommendations to mitigate vulnerability to liability:

- Select and purchase only high-quality equipment and padding from reputable manufacturers.
- Become familiar with the warning labels and intended purposes for all equipment and padding purchased.
- Read and follow the manufacturer's instructions when fitting the equipment and padding to the individual. Do not attempt to modify and/or alter any equipment and padding.
- Instruct the individual on the use, application, and care of the equipment and padding.
- Ensure that individuals read the warning labels and understand the use and care of the equipment or padding. Have individuals sign a form stating they understand the warning labels and risks involved with the sport or activity.

- Continually monitor the use of and inspect the condition of the equipment and padding.
- Perform regular maintenance on the equipment and padding as recommended by the manufacturer.

Legal issues surrounding protective equipment leave some questions for the health care professional. Can health care professionals be held liable if they don't monitor the equipment regularly or schedule regular reconditioning? Are they liable if they don't fully instruct the individual on the uses of the equipment? A full discussion of these liability issues is outside the scope of this book and can be found elsewhere. For more complete information, see the Web References.

---

**Clinical Application Question 1**

During batting practice prior to a weekend intercollegiate baseball series, the center fielder picks up his batter's helmet and notices that the open- and closed-cell foam inner lining is partially missing. He brings you the helmet and asks if you can replace the padding. The team is away from home this weekend, and no one on the team wears the same size helmet.

➠ **Question: What can you do in this situation to provide protection for the center fielder and avoid legal problems?**

---

# STANDARDS AND TESTING

Many national and international agencies and organizations have been established to protect the individual from ineffective and poorly designed and constructed protective equipment and padding.[2] In response to the high incidence of various acute injuries in sport, recreational, and work activities, these agencies and organizations have developed standards and testing procedures for the manufacturing, maintenance, and use of equipment and padding. The National Operating Committee on Standards for Athletic Equipment (NOCSAE), the Hockey Equipment Certification Council (HECC), ASTM International, the Canadian Standards Association (CSA), the Safety Equipment Institute (SEI), the American National Standards Institute (ANSI), and the U.S. Consumer Product Safety Commission (CPSC) currently set standards and conduct testing and research for protective equipment and padding.

**NOCSAE** was formed in 1969 with the purpose "to commission research directed toward injury reduction."[3] Consisting of representatives from medical associations and societies, interscholastic and intercollegiate athletic associations, and the sports industry, NOCSAE strives to improve the quality of protective equipment

and lessen the occurrence of injury associated with participation in athletic activity through the development of voluntary testing standards.

---

**DETAILS**

The NOCSAE member associations include the American Academy of Pediatrics, American College of Sports Medicine, American College Health Association, American Medical Society for Sports Medicine, American Orthopaedic Society for Sports Medicine, American Football Coaches Association, Athletic Equipment Managers' Association, National Athletic Trainers' Association, National Athletic Equipment Reconditioners' Association, National Collegiate Athletic Association, National Federation of State High School Associations, and the Sports & Fitness Industry Association.

---

At the request of USA Hockey in 1978, **HECC** was formed. HECC currently evaluates the needs and recommendations of amateur hockey–governing bodies in relation to protective equipment and safety.[4] HECC promotes and sponsors research focusing on the prevention and reduction of injuries associated with participation in ice hockey. Equipment certification testing serves to validate manufacturers' certifications and is based on standards developed by other organizations such as ASTM and CSA.

Originally known as the American Society for Testing and Materials, **ASTM International** is a voluntary standards development organization consisting of members from the government, academia, consumers, and manufacturers.[5] Formed in 1898, ASTM International strives to develop standards to direct the production of safer, more efficient and cost-effective products and services. The organization has developed standards directly related to protective equipment, specifically the certification of athletic helmets and eye guards.

**CSA** develops standards to address the needs of business, industry, government, and consumers.[6] The organization serves as a neutral third party to provide a structure and forum for standards development, including safety and prevention. CSA has developed standards for the design and manufacture of ice hockey helmets, face guards, and visors, and lacrosse face guards.

**SEI** administers a voluntary certification program to test occupational and recreational safety and protective equipment.[7] The third-party organization certifies equipment from manufacturers in accordance with organizational standards such as ASTM International and NOCSAE. SEI currently certifies athletic eye guards, helmets, face guards, chest protectors, and shin guards.

Currently, there are published NOCSAE, HECC, ASTM, and CSA Standards for several types of equipment: football, baseball and softball batter's and catcher's, lacrosse, field and ice hockey, and polo helmets and appropriate face guards; ice hockey face protectors and visors; soccer shin guards; baseball, softball, and lacrosse chest protectors; football gloves; and mouth and eye guards. The following provides a brief summary of testing methods for a sample of required helmet and face guard designs.

## Football Helmets

Football helmets are tested with the NOCSAE drop and ram tests to meet NOCSAE Standards.[3] In the drop test, the helmet, excluding face guards and face guard hardware, is placed on a headform (model head) and dropped onto a cylindrical rubber pad with impact on seven different areas of the helmet. During the ram test, the helmet, with attached face guard and face guard hardware, is placed on a headform mounted to a sliding table top. A pneumatic ram is propelled at the helmet, impacting the helmet on six different areas. Football helmets that meet the NOCSAE Standards must be permanently and legibly marked with the manufacturer's name, model, and size. On the exterior of the shell, there should be an easily readable warning label and a SEI/NOCSAE seal.[3]

NOCSAE does not perform surveillance to determine adherence to the football helmet standard. The responsibility to ensure the condition of the helmet falls on the purchaser and wearer. NOCSAE does recommend the implementation of a reconditioning and recertification program for all helmets originally certified when manufactured. The frequency of reconditioning and recertification of helmets is established by the manufacturer and should be based on the age and size of the athlete, amount and intensity of usage, and age of the helmet.[3] Reconditioning and recertification involves the repairing, cleaning, and retesting of helmets with the drop test. At high competition levels, such as intercollegiate and professional football, for example, helmets are reconditioned and recertified at the conclusion of each season. The NOCSAE Standard is not a warranty against injury and resulting liability, but most helmet manufacturers provide a separate 3–5 year warranty on the helmet shell.

---

**DETAILS**

NOCSAE Standards were initiated in response to football injuries. In 1970, NOCSAE developed a helmet standard, which was published in 1973 and implemented in 1974 with new helmet models. The standard has resulted in shell size changes, softer construction materials, and improved quality control during manufacturing.[3]

---

## Baseball and Softball Batter's Helmets

Newly manufactured baseball and softball batter's helmets undergo a projectile impact test to meet the NOCSAE Standard.[3] The helmet is fit on a headform attached to a sliding table top; the test involves an air cannon assembly launching a baseball or softball at the helmet, striking the helmet on six different areas. Baseball and softball batter's helmets meeting the NOCSAE Standard must be permanently and legibly labeled with the manufacturer's name, model, and size. A SEI/NOCSAE seal and the warning label,[3] similar to the football helmet label, must be placed on the exterior shell. A reconditioning and recertification program, as recommended by the manufacturer, should also be used with SEI/NOCSAE-certified baseball and softball batter's helmets.

## Baseball and Softball Catcher's Helmets with Face Guards

NOCSAE Standards for new baseball and softball catcher's helmets with attached face guards consist of the drop test method and projectile impact tests.[3] The face guard must be attached to the helmet during all testing. Baseball and softball catcher's helmets that meet the standard must be marked with a SEI/NOCSAE seal and a warning label[3] in the same manner as batter's helmets. Catcher's helmets, sold by manufacturers without a face guard, must also have a warning statement permanently placed on the exterior shell. Face guards with stand-alone padding must be sold with manufacturer's guidelines indicating which helmet should be used with the guard. A warning statement[3] must be affixed to the mask.

## Lacrosse Helmets with Face Guards

Test standards for new lacrosse helmets with compatible face guards include helmet stability and retention and drop method tests.[3] During all tests, face guards certified by SEI/NOCSAE must be attached to the helmets. In the stability and retention test, the helmet is placed on a headform connected to a stability stand with the retention system fastened. During the test, the headform is canted downward; to pass, the helmet must remain on the headform throughout the test. Drop tests are performed with impacts occurring on a cylindrical rubber pad. Lacrosse helmets with face guards meeting the NOCSAE Standard must be permanently marked with the manufacturer's information.

*Protective Equipment and Padding*

A SEI/NOCSAE seal and a warning statement[3] must be placed on the exterior shell.

## Ice Hockey Helmets

Newly manufactured ice hockey helmets are subjected to retention, stability, drop method, and projectile impact tests to determine certification according to the NOCSAE Standard.[3] During all tests, helmet face guards and face guard hardware are removed. The retention test evaluates the dynamic strength of the chin strap(s) and is conducted by placing the helmet on a head-shaped platform attached to a strength and extension apparatus.[3] First, a weight is dropped, elongating the retention system. Next, the weight is dropped to release the system, allowing removal of the helmet. The stability and drop method tests for ice hockey helmets are similar to the lacrosse helmet tests. Projectile impact tests are conducted with the helmet using an International Ice Hockey Federation puck as a projectile. Ice hockey helmets meeting the NOCSAE Standard are permanently marked with the manufacturer's information, a SEI/NOCSAE seal, and a warning label.[3] HECC[4] and CSA[6] also evaluate new ice hockey player helmets with retention, penetration, and drop method tests. Helmets that meet the standards are marked on the exterior shell with a HECC and/or CSA label.

---

### DETAILS

The governing bodies of interscholastic, intercollegiate, and amateur athletics may require different testing standards for approved protective equipment used in practices and competitions. For example, the National Collegiate Athletic Association (NCAA) and the National Federation of State High School Associations (NFHS) require the use of HECC and/or ASTM Standards for ice hockey helmets and face guards, although NOCSAE performs testing on ice hockey helmets. To ensure compliance, read and follow the governing bodies' regulations prior to purchasing and using protective equipment.

---

### Clinical Application Question 2

You are performing outreach services through the hospital to a local senior league ice hockey team. During a practice, the coach asks if you could replace a face guard on a helmet so he can continue to work with the team on the ice. The coach provides you with the helmet, a new face guard, and tools.

➡ **Question: Can the face guard be replaced without jeopardizing NOCSAE and/or HECC certification?**

---

### ...IF/THEN...

**IF** a helmet is worn incorrectly or the individual uses it for purposes other than those designed or intended, **THEN** a manufacturer or health care professional most likely will not be held liable for injuries sustained while wearing the helmet.

---

# PROTECTIVE EQUIPMENT AND PADDING

Protective equipment and padding are available in many designs, based on the sport, the playing position, the activity, the individual, or the objective of the technique. The designs are constructed from a variety of materials. Some pads are manufactured from soft, low-density materials such as open- and closed-cell foams, while others are made of hard, high-density polycarbonate, Kevlar, or acrylonitrile butadiene styrene (ABS) plastic materials. Several designs are constructed from both soft, low-density and hard, high-density materials. For example, football shoulder pads have a high-density outer shell lined with open- and closed-cell foams. Proper fitting and application of the equipment and padding are critical; carefully follow manufacturers' instructions to prevent injury to the individual and to avoid liability. The following general fitting guidelines apply to most designs.

- Baseball, lacrosse, softball, and soccer shin guards and field hockey shin and leg guards and kickers are manufactured in individual and universal fit designs in predetermined sizes corresponding to lower leg length measurements or age of the individual.
- Ice hockey and lacrosse shoulder pads are available in individual fit designs in predetermined sizes based on chest circumference measurements.
- Baseball, field hockey, football, and softball glove designs are constructed in individual fit, with right- and left-handed designs in predetermined sizes corresponding to tip of the third finger to the wrist length measurements.
- Baseball, field hockey, and softball chest (body) protectors are manufactured in predetermined sizes based on chest circumference and length measurements.
- Baseball and softball batter's and catcher's, field hockey, football, ice hockey, and lacrosse helmets and wrestling ear guards are constructed in individual fit designs in predetermined sizes corresponding to head circumference measurements. For most designs, circumference measurements are taken 1 inch above the eyebrows.
- Baseball, field hockey, lacrosse, and softball throat guards are available in universal fit designs in predetermined sizes.

The governing bodies of interscholastic, intercollegiate, and amateur athletics have established rules that govern the use of mandatory equipment and padding. The NCAA, the National Association of Intercollegiate Athletics (NAIA), the NFHS, the United States Olympic Committee (USOC), and individual state high school athletic associations require equipment/padding in several sports. For our purposes, we will focus on protective equipment and padding required by the NCAA[8] and NFHS.[9–17]

Regardless of the requirements, many athletes wear equipment and padding that are not required. For example, the NCAA does not require baseball catchers to wear a chest protector or shin guards. Catchers nonetheless voluntarily wear the equipment because participation without the padding increases the risk of injury. This section discusses mandatory protective equipment and other standard equipment commonly worn by athletes during participation in practices and competitions. Eye and mouth guards are discussed at the end of the section.

---

### DETAILS

Commotio cordis is a life-threatening condition caused by a blunt, non-penetrating blow to the chest.[18] Although more research is needed, the National Athletic Trainers' Association[19] recommends the use of sport-specific chest protectors during practices and competitions to reduce the risk of injury. A NOCSAE Standard[3] has been developed to test baseball, softball, and lacrosse chest protectors to lessen the risk of injury in sports. All protective equipment should meet appropriate standards and be properly fitted and used by the individual. For more complete information, see the Web References.

---

# Baseball

### *Mandatory Equipment*

On deck, batting, and base running (NCAA and NFHS), retired runners, players/students in coach's boxes, nonadult bat/ball shaggers (NFHS)

- Helmet with double ear-flap design, NOCSAE Standards (NCAA and NFHS), risk of injury warning label (NFHS), non-glare surface (NFHS)

### Catcher

- Helmet, NOCSAE Standards (NCAA)
- Helmet and face mask with dual ear-flap design, NOCSAE Standards (NFHS)
- Throat guard (NCAA and NFHS)
- Chest (body) protector, SEI/NOCSAE Standards (NFHS)
- Shin guards, protective cup (male catcher) (NFHS)

- Helmet and face mask, throat guard, protective cup (male catcher), nonadult while warming up pitcher (NFHS)

### *Standard Equipment*

### Batting

- Gloves

**Batter's helmets** are manufactured of a pre-molded ABS, polycarbonate, carbon fiber/resin, or polyethylene plastic material outer shell with a front bill and double ear flaps and dual-density and/or open- and closed-cell foam inner lining. Several designs are available with a mechanism that allows for adjustments in fit; other designs are manufactured with hardware to attach a chin strap or cup and/or metal face guard (Fig. 13–1).

**Catcher's helmets** and **face guards** are available in a one- or two-piece style. One-piece designs are constructed of a pre-molded fiberglass resin, polymer nylon, Kevlar, or ABS plastic material outer shell lined with open- and closed-cell foam. The face guard is attached to the outer shell; most face guards are manufactured of metal and/or steel compound materials (Fig. 13–2). Several designs are available with adjustable posterior plates and chin straps for adjustments in fit. Two-piece designs consist of an individual helmet and face guard that are used in combination with one another. The helmets are manufactured similarly to batting helmets, with or without a bill and ear flaps. Face guards are constructed of a tubular steel or hollow wire frame. Removable soft padding covered with polyurethane, leather, and/or synthetic leather materials is attached to the wire frame with metal snaps or Velcro closures. Most face guards are anchored over a helmet by a three-way, adjustable elastic harness (Fig. 13–3).

**Throat guards** are manufactured of rigid plastic materials; most throat guards attach to the distal

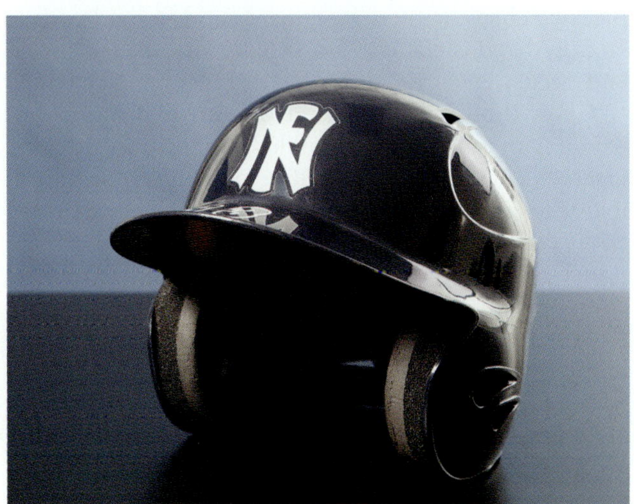

**Fig. 13–1** *Double ear-flap batter's helmet.*

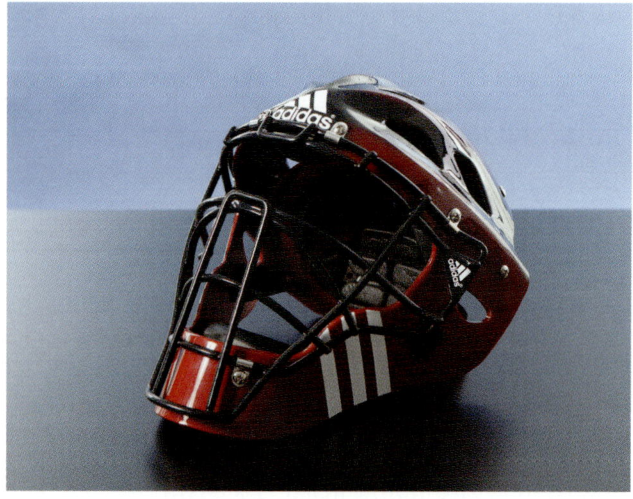
**Fig. 13–2** *One-piece catcher's helmet.*

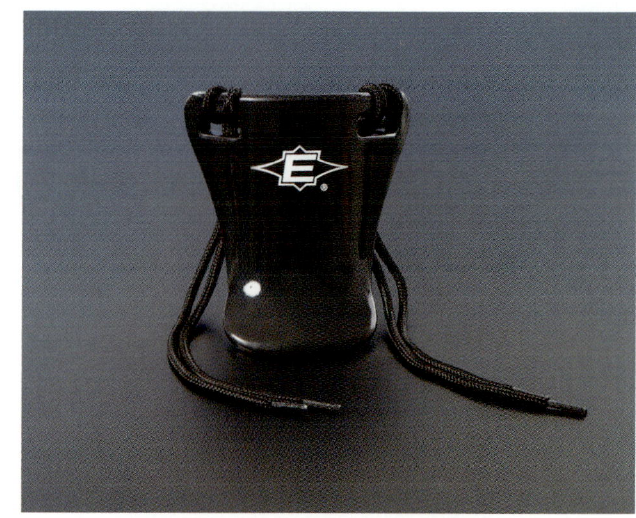
**Fig. 13–4** *Throat guard.*

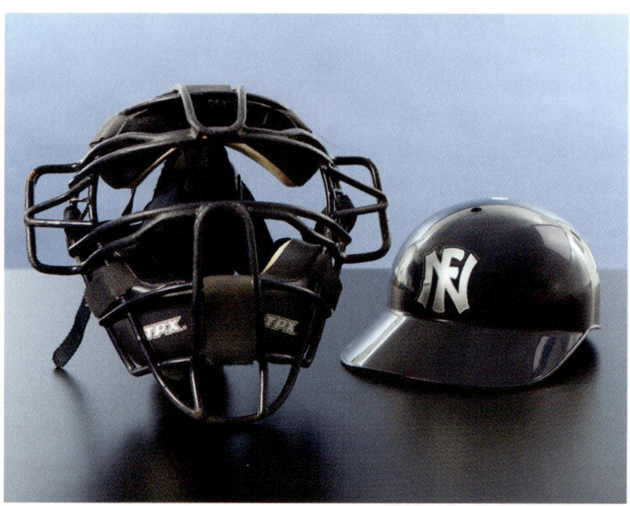
**Fig. 13–3** *Two-piece catcher's helmet.*

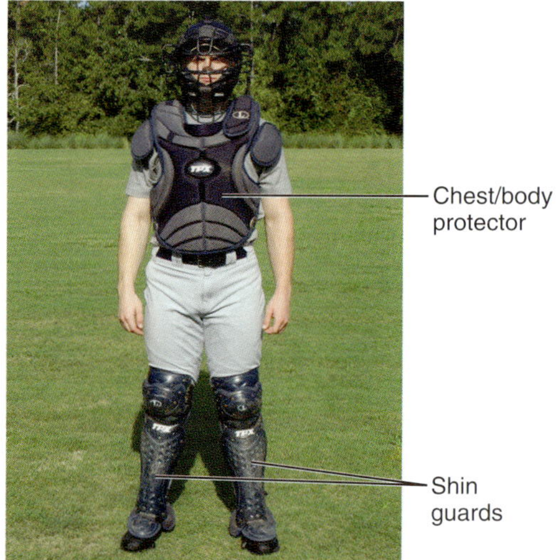

**Fig. 13–5** *Catcher in protective equipment. Chest (body) protector and shin guards.*

face guard with laces or ties (Fig. 13–4). Many one-piece catcher's helmets/face guards and individual face guards are constructed with extensions over the throat and neck.

**Chest (body) protectors** are constructed in individual fit, with right- and left-handed designs, and are manufactured of dual-density and/or open- and closed-cell foam, covered with a nylon mesh material outer lining. Some designs are available with wings or extensions that protect the upper arm and genitalia. The protectors are contoured to allow for unrestricted shoulder and arm range of motion and are attached with an adjustable harness and straps with Velcro and/or D-ring closures (Fig. 13–5).

**Shin guards** are constructed of multiple polycarbonate or other rigid material outer shells incorporated in an inner shell of synthetic leather or nylon material lined with open- and closed-cell or ethylene-vinyl acetate (EVA) foam, air bladder, or rubber padding materials. Shin guards are attached with adjustable nylon straps with metal closures (see Fig. 13–5).

**Protective athletic cups** used in baseball and softball were discussed in Chapter 12 in the Padding section (see Fig. 12–17).

# Field Hockey

## *Mandatory Equipment*

### Goalkeeper

- Helmet with full-face design (NCAA and NFHS), no protruding visor (NFHS)
- Throat guard (NCAA and NFHS)
- Chest protector (NCAA and NFHS)
- Elbow pads (NCAA)
- Gloves (NCAA and NFHS)

- Leg guards (NFHS)
- Kickers (NCAA and NFHS)

### Kicking back (NCAA)

- Helmet
- Throat guard
- Chest protector

### Field athletes (NFHS)

- Eye guard, ASTM 2713 Field Hockey Standards (NFHS)
- Shin guards

### All athletes (NCAA and NFHS)

- Mouth guard, intraoral design covering all upper or lower teeth (NFHS), readily visible color (not white or transparent) (NFHS)

### *Standard Equipment*

### Goalkeeper

- Pants

**Helmets** are manufactured of a pre-molded fiberglass resin, carbon fiber, polyethylene, or polycarbonate plastic material outer shell with an open- and closed-cell foam inner lining. Many designs extend over the throat. A carbon steel wire face guard is attached to the outer shell. The helmets are anchored with an adjustable strap (Fig. 13–6).

**Throat guards** are manufactured of a rigid plastic material inner lining with a pre-molded foam outer shell covered with cotton and/or nylon materials. These guards wrap around the neck and are anchored with Velcro closures (see Fig. 13–6). Some designs extend over the thorax.

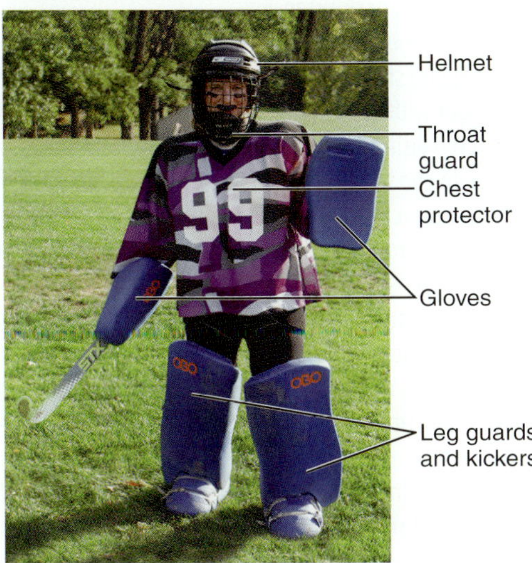


**Fig. 13–6** *Goalkeeper in protective equipment. Helmet, throat guard, chest protector, gloves, and leg guards and kickers.*

**Chest protectors** are manufactured in individual and universal fit designs and are constructed of open- and closed-cell and/or EVA foam with a nylon mesh outer lining. Most wraparound designs have a nylon mesh back. Some designs have additional padding over the thorax; many have detachable pads around the shoulder and arms. Chest protectors are anchored with an adjustable harness and straps with Velcro and/or D-ring closures (see Fig. 13–6).

**Arm** and **elbow pads** are constructed in individual fit designs in predetermined sizes corresponding to mid upper arm to mid forearm length measurements. These pads are manufactured of a spandex and/or nylon material outer shell with a neoprene and/or EVA foam inner lining. Pre-molded polycarbonate or rigid plastic materials are incorporated in the outer shell over the elbow and forearm. Arm and elbow pads are attached with adjustable nylon straps with Velcro closures.

**Gloves** are manufactured of leather materials with spandex or Lycra material finger, thumb, and knuckle gussets with foam and/or gel padding material incorporated throughout the glove. Several designs are available for athletes, excluding the goalkeeper, to protect the nondominant stick hand with foam and/or gel padding material incorporated in the dorsal hand. The gloves are anchored with elastic nylon straps with Velcro closures (see Fig. 13–6).

**Leg guards** and **kickers** are constructed of pre-molded laminate foams and are attached with nylon straps and plastic closures (see Fig. 13–6).

**Mouth guards** are discussed at the end of this section (see Figs. 13–26, 13–27, and 13–28).

**Shin guards** consist of a pre-molded rigid plastic material outer shell with a soft foam inner lining. Some designs are manufactured of thermoplastic or fiberglass materials that allow for custom-fitting. Other guards extend over the medial and lateral malleoli to provide additional protection. Most shin guards are attached with Velcro straps (Fig. 13–7). Some guards have nylon foot stirrups to lessen migration during activity.

# Football

## *Mandatory Equipment*

### All athletes

- Helmet, NOCSAE Standards, risk of injury warning label, attached face mask (NCAA and NFHS), four-point (NCAA and NFHS) or six-point chin strap (NCAA)
- Shoulder pads (NCAA and NFHS)
- Hip, thigh, and coccyx pads (NCAA and NFHS)
- Knee pads (NCAA and NFHS), at least ½ inch (NCAA and NFHS) or ⅜ inch thick (NFHS)

**Protective Equipment and Padding**

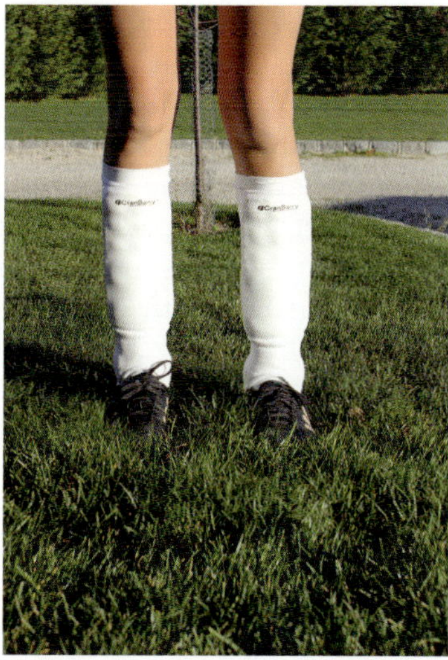

**Fig. 13–7** *Shin guards.*

• Mouth guard, intraoral design covering all upper teeth (NCAA and NFHS) or lower teeth (NFHS), readily visible color (not white or transparent) (NCAA and NFHS) with FDA-approved base materials (FDCS) (NCAA)

## *Standard Equipment*

### All athletes

• Gloves

**Helmets** are manufactured of a polycarbonate alloy or ABS plastic material outer shell. Some designs use one or two crown air bladder(s) and dual-density foam as an inner liner. Other designs use multiple individual pads constructed of an air bladder and dual-density foam. Inflation ports located on the outer shell allow for adjustments of air pressure within the bladders. The foam is available in varying thickness and firmness for adjustments in fit. The air bladders and/or foam padding of most designs are removable for replacement and maintenance. Some designs have sensors incorporated into the inner liner to record head acceleration data resulting from impacts during practices and competitions. Other designs use a scanning process to custom-fit the outer shell and inner liner to the individual.

Helmets are anchored with chin straps in a variety of designs. Chin straps are available in two-, four-, and six-point or snap designs. The straps are constructed of cotton materials with a vinyl coating and are anchored to the helmet with plastic or metal snaps. Other strap designs anchor to the helmet with an adjustable mechanism to allow quick adjustments in tension and fit. Some designs consist of a soft chin cup, while others have a polycarbonate or ABS plastic material cup. Many designs are available with a foam inner lining.

---

**DETAILS**

Removal of athletic equipment such as the helmet, face guard, and shoulder pads in an emergency situation should be performed by well-trained health care professionals. For more complete information, see the Chapter 12 Web References.

---

**DETAILS**

### General Football Helmet Fitting Guidelines[20]

• Place the athlete in a standing position, with the hair at a length worn during the season. Wet the hair to simulate perspiration.
• Use a helmet manufacturer's caliper or measuring tape and measure the circumference of the head above the ears to determine helmet shell size (Fig. 13–8A).
• Select the appropriate helmet shell size. Remove the jaw pads and deflate all air bladders.
• Have the athlete place the helmet on the head.
• Inspect the jaw area to determine what size pads are needed. Select and fit the proper jaw pads (see Fig. 13–8B). The pads should feel firm against the face. When using some designs, inflate the jaw pads with air.
• Inflate crown air bladder(s) through holes in the exterior shell so that the helmet rises to the proper position just above the eyebrows, approximately one to two finger widths or 1 inch (see Fig. 13–8C).
• Center the chin strap cup over the chin. Adjust the chin straps on the side of the helmet to provide equal tension in each strap and anchor (see Fig. 13–8D).
• The chin strap(s) should be positioned underneath the face guard.
• If air bladders are present, inflate side and back air bladders.

• Check for proper fit. The helmet should be fit to snugness rather than comfort or too tight over the crown, front, back, and sides.
• The helmet should cover the base of the skull but not prevent normal range of neck extension.
• The helmet ear holes should align with the ears.
• The face guard should be positioned approximately two to three finger widths from the nose and forehead and allow for unrestricted vision (see Fig. 13–8E).
• Continue to check for proper fit by having the athlete maintain a rigid head and neck position.
• Apply downward pressure on the crown of the helmet with the hands (see Fig. 13–8F). The helmet should not move.
• Grasp the face guard and pull downward (see Fig. 13–8G). The helmet should not move.
• Place the hands on the sides of the helmet, then on the front and back, and attempt to rotate the helmet (see Fig. 13–8H). The helmet should not rotate.
• Remove the helmet, apply shoulder pads, then reapply the helmet. Have the athlete move through several position-specific movements to check for proper fit. The helmet should not move at any time and allow for upper body range of motion.

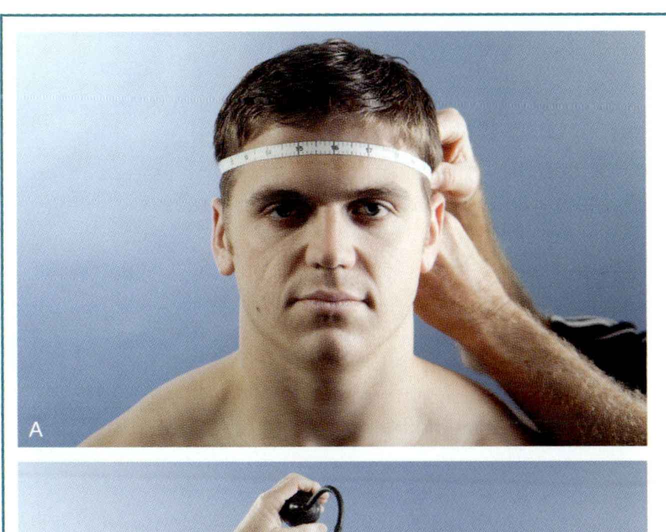
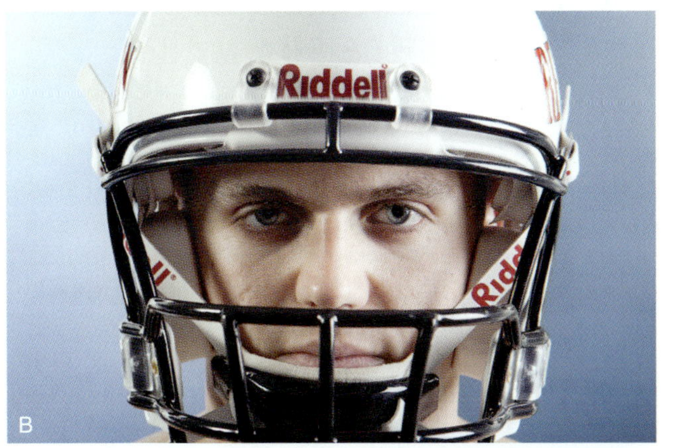
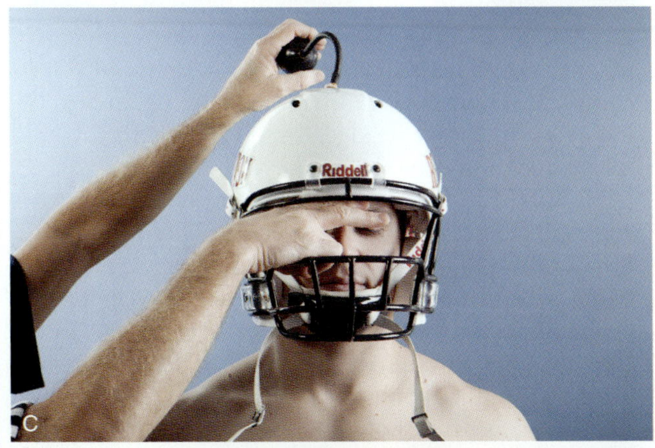
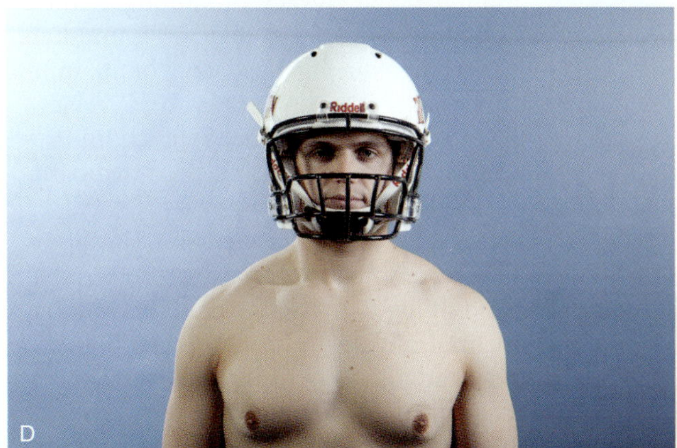
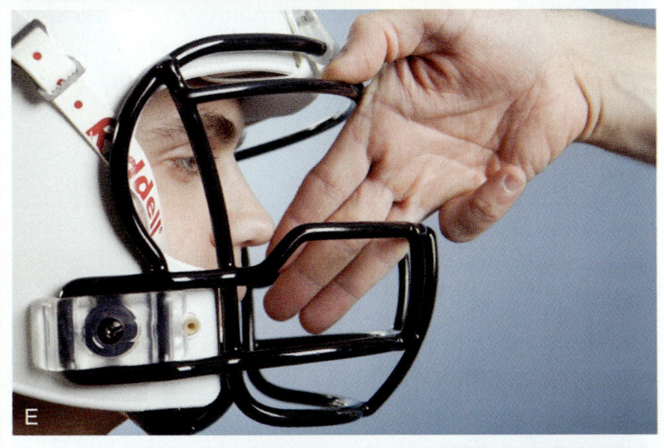
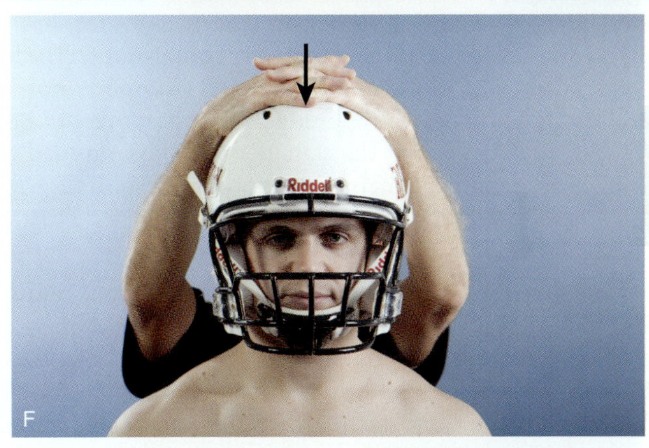
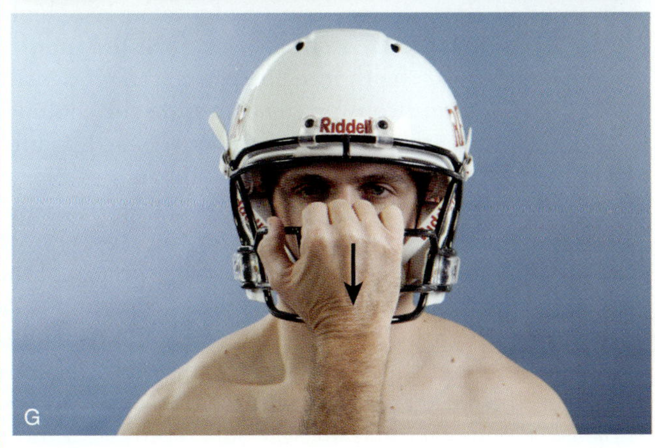
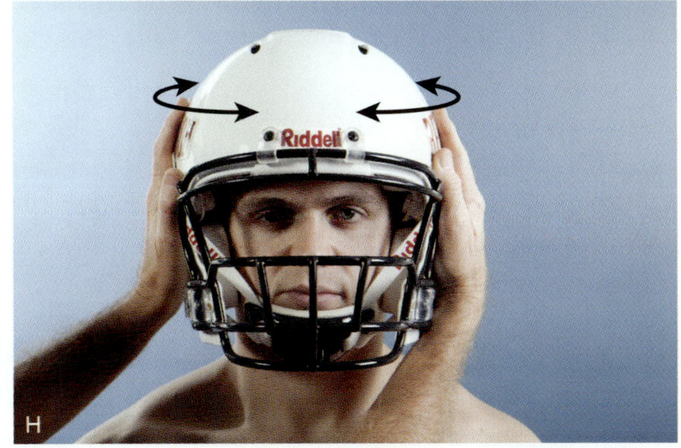

**Fig. 13–8 A–H**

## EVIDENCE SUMMARY

Helmets are mandatory in several NCAA and NFHS sports; these designs are certified according to NOCSAE, HECC, ASTM, SEI, and/or CSA Standards. Although these helmets have met current testing methods, any athlete participating in any sport can sustain a head injury even with the best head protection.[21] Regardless, the use of certified helmets should be enforced to protect the athlete against injury.

What type of protection does a certified helmet provide for the athlete? Helmets are designed primarily to prevent catastrophic injuries. Several evidence-based reviews have examined the efficacy of various helmets in the prevention of injury. A 2016 review[22] found helmets were effective in reducing head and brain injuries among individuals in cycling. In a 2017 review, researchers[23] revealed helmets reduced head injuries among youth and adults participating in snowboarding and skiing activities. Based on this evidence, a 2017 consensus statement from the Concussion in Sport Group[24] strongly recommends the use of helmets in snowboarding and skiing to prevent overall head injury. Position statements from the National Athletic Trainers' Association[25] and the American Medical Society for Sports Medicine[26] provided guidelines for the management and prevention of concussions in sports. The guidelines[25,26] found insufficient evidence to recommend the use of helmets to prevent concussions. The limited evidence in a statement[25] neither supports nor refutes the use of protective headgear in soccer to reduce the risk of concussion. The statements[25,26] recommend the use of certified helmets with appropriate sports.

NOCSAE, HECC, ASTM, SEI, and CSA Standards and testing evaluate the protective value of equipment for the prevention of injury. Helmet standards and testing are designed to evaluate the helmet's ability to prevent catastrophic head injury.[27,28] Other assessment systems[21,27,28] have been developed to test previously certified football, ice hockey, and cycling helmets and soccer headgear. These systems are implemented in combination with NOCSAE, HECC, SEI, and CSA Standards and testing methods to evaluate the protective capabilities of the helmet for the reduction of concussions, provide consumers with performance ratings to guide purchasing decisions, and perhaps drive manufacturers to advance future helmet designs.[27,28] For the complete rankings of football, ice hockey, and cycling helmets and soccer headgear, see Virginia Tech Center for Injury Biomechanics in the Web References.

NOCSAE-, HECC-, ASTM-, SEI-, and/or CSA-certified helmets are not designed to prevent all head injuries but are recommended for athletes when appropriate.[25,26] Helmets should be maintained in their original form and constantly monitored for wear. Use a certified reconditioner to evaluate and repair helmets at regular intervals, and adhere to manufacturer recommendations. Last, athletes should be educated about the proper use of the helmet, safe sport techniques such as blocking and tackling, and the signs and symptoms of acute and chronic trauma to the head and neck. Although significant advancements have been made in helmet designs, additional research and development among all sport helmets is needed to reduce the risk of head injury.

**Face guards** are available in a variety of designs and sizes based on playing position and desired level of protection. Most face guards are constructed of carbon, stainless, or tubular steel or titanium with a vinyl coating. The guards are attached directly on the helmet using plastic grommets and screws. Some designs are available with a quick release mechanism to allow faster removal of the guard.

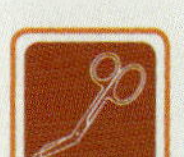

**Helpful Hint |**

When the face guard hardware of a football helmet becomes rusted as a result of environmental conditions and/or perspiration, replace the hardware with parts that meet or exceed original manufacturer specifications. NOCSAE has published a standard to test the corrosion characteristics of face guard hardware.[3] Regular maintenance increases protection and allows for removal of the face guard in an emergency situation.

**Shoulder pads** are constructed in individual fit designs in predetermined sizes based on chest circumference, AC joint to AC joint, or lateral shoulder to lateral shoulder length measurements. The pads are available for each playing position in two basic designs: cantilever and flat. Both designs consist of a two-piece, high-density plastic material arch or outer shell pre-molded to the contours of the thorax. Pre-formed, high-density plastic epaulets and caps or cups covering the shoulder and upper arm are attached to the outer shell. Cantilever designs have a high-density plastic arch or bridge located underneath the outer shell over the AC joint. Cantilevers are used to disperse impact forces away from the shoulder and AC joint to the thoracic surfaces of the pads. Cantilever pads provide the greatest amount of protection but are bulky and restrict glenohumeral joint range of motion. These designs are commonly used by linemen, linebackers, and running backs. Flat pads do not use a cantilever and are less bulky, provide a more contoured fit, and allow greater glenohumeral joint range of motion, but they provide less protection. These designs are commonly worn by quarterbacks, receivers, and defensive backs but can be used with any position.

Construction of the inner lining depends on the specific pad design. Most designs use a combination of open- and closed-cell and/or EVA foams covered with a moisture-resistant nylon material in various individual patterns and sizes. The individual inner lining pads are attached to the outer shell with Velcro or zippers; most designs allow for adjustments in fit. The inner lining forms a channel over the shoulder and AC joint to disperse forces to the thoracic padding. One design uses a system incorporated in the shoulder pad to allow separation and/or removal of the pads in an emergency situation. Shoulder pads are anchored with adjustable anterior and/or posterior laces, elastic straps with T-hook closures, and/or polyurethane belts with buckle closures.

---

## DETAILS

### General Football Shoulder Pad Fitting Guidelines[29]

- Place the athlete in a standing position without a shirt or only wearing a T-shirt. Perform an assessment of the athlete that includes body weight and height, medical history, playing position, and chest circumference and/or shoulder length measurements.
- Match the body type, past injury concerns (AC joint sprain, upper arm contusions, etc.), playing position, and chest/shoulder measurements with a corresponding shoulder pad design. Refer to the manufacturer's sizing chart.
- Place the shoulder pads on the athlete and anchor the laces, straps, and/or belts to achieve a snug fit.
- Next, conduct an anterior, lateral, and posterior visual assessment.
- Anterior: The pads should fully cover the clavicles, AC joints, and pectoralis and trapezius muscles and should extend ½ inch over the deltoid. The collar should provide a comfortable range of motion to the neck, and arms raised overhead should not cause pinching of the neck. The caps/cups should fit snugly over the deltoid muscle. The outer shell should meet evenly with no overlap, and the laces should be tight and centered over the anterior thorax (Fig. 13–9A).
- Lateral: The inner lining should form a channel over the AC joint and not make contact with the AC joint. The caps/cups should cover the deltoid muscle (see Fig. 13–9B).
- Posterior: The outer shell should extend below the inferior angle of the scapula, covering the scapula and trapezius, rhomboids, and latissimus dorsi muscles. If present, the laces should be tight and centered over the posterior thorax. The collar should not cause pinching of the neck (see Fig. 13–9C).
- The last assessment is conducted following application of a helmet and jersey. Have the athlete assume several different upper and lower body movements required by the playing position.
- A properly fitted shoulder pad should be snug over the entire thorax and shoulder but still allow for upper body range of motion.
- The pads should return to the thorax and shoulder after movement.
- A properly worn jersey and sleeves should assist in anchoring the pads to the shoulder, thorax, and upper arm.

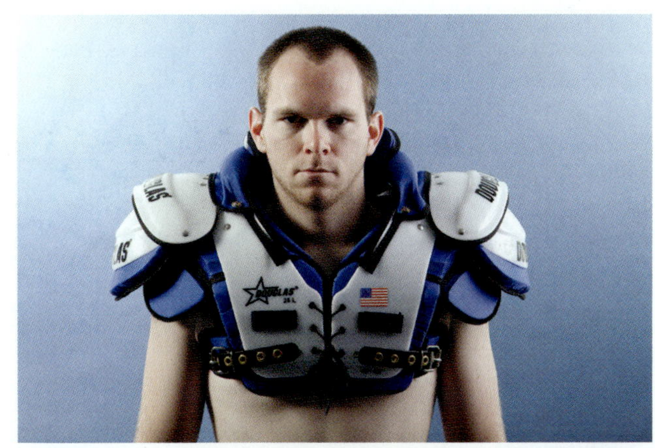

**Fig. 13–9 A**

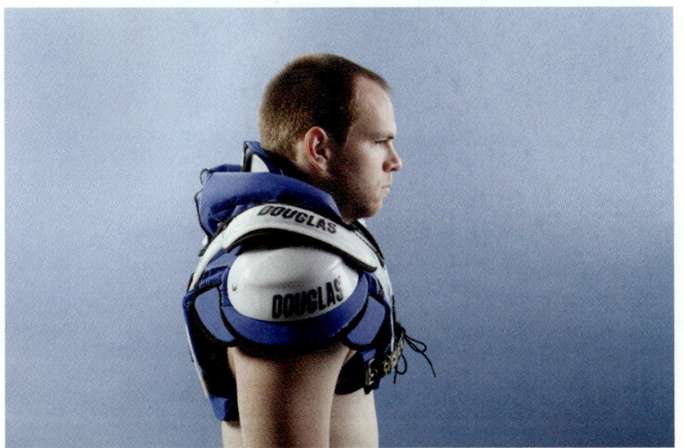

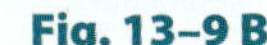

**Fig. 13–9 B**

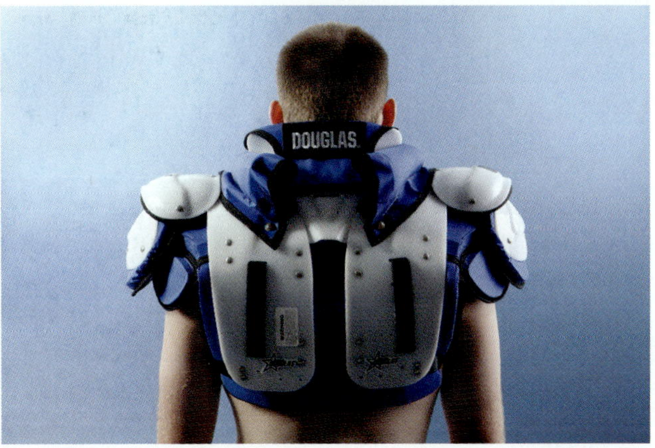

**Fig. 13–9 C**

**Knee, hip, thigh,** and **coccyx pads** are manufactured in individual and universal fit designs in predetermined sizes based on circumference measurements of the thigh or waist or on the age of the individual. Universal fit pads are constructed of varying thicknesses of high-impact or high-density, open- and closed-cell, and EVA foams (see Fig. 7–22A). Some designs are coated with vinyl. Most thigh pads are manufactured with a rigid plastic insert. The individual fit hip and thigh pads are larger in size, with additional padding, than the mandatory designs and are commonly used following injury to provide additional protection (see Figs. 7–22B–C). Mandatory knee, hip, thigh, and coccyx pads are available from most manufacturers in a complete set. These pads are attached in pad pockets of nylon/polyester/ Lycra girdles (see Fig. 7–22F). Some pads are placed into pad pockets of football pants.

**Mouth guard** designs for use in football are illustrated in Figures 13–26, 13–27, and 13–28.

# Ice Hockey

## *Mandatory Equipment*

### All athletes

- Helmet attached with chin strap, HECC Standards (NCAA), HECC-ASTM Standards (NFHS)
- Face mask, HECC-ASTM F 513-89 Eye and Face Protective Equipment for Hockey Players Standard (NCAA), HECC-ASTM Standard (NFHS)
- Mouth guard, intraoral design (NCAA and NFHS), covering all upper teeth (NCAA and NFHS) or lower teeth (NFHS), readily visible color (not transparent) (NFHS)
- Pants, hip pads (NFHS)
- Shin guards (NFHS)
- Protective cup (NFHS)
- Elbow pads (NFHS)
- Shoulder pads (NFHS)
- Gloves (NFHS)

### Goalkeeper

- Leg guards, not to exceed 11 inches in width and 38 inches in length (NFHS)
- Gloves, not to exceed 8 inches in width and 15 inches in length (blocker) (NFHS), maximum circumference of 45 inches (catcher) (NFHS)
- Chest and arm protector (NFHS)
- Throat guard, separate, commercially manufactured (NFHS)

**Helmets** are manufactured of a pre-molded polycarbonate or polyethylene plastic material outer shell and multi-density and/or EVA foam or air bladder inner lining. Many designs are constructed of a two-piece outer shell allowing for adjustments in fit. The helmets

are available with or without face guards. Most face guards are manufactured of a carbon or stainless steel or titanium wire pattern extending over the jaw, permanently attached to the superior outer shell. These helmets are anchored with an adjustable two- or four-point cotton or nylon chin strap (Fig. 13–10). Many designs have a soft chin cup.

**Goalkeeper's helmets** and **face guards** are available in a two-piece style constructed of a pre-molded Kevlar, carbon, fiberglass resin, or polymer nylon material outer shell. An adjustable plate incorporated in the posterior outer shell allows for adjustments in fit. Multi-density foam and gel materials are used for the inner lining. Face guards constructed of carbon or stainless steel wire or titanium are attached to the outer shell. Goalkeeper's helmets are attached with an adjustable elastic or nylon chin strap and/or chin cup (Fig. 13–11).

**Leg guards** or **pads** for goalkeepers are manufactured in individual fit designs in predetermined sizes based on the sum of instep to knee and patella to distal thigh length and the skate size measurements. The designs are

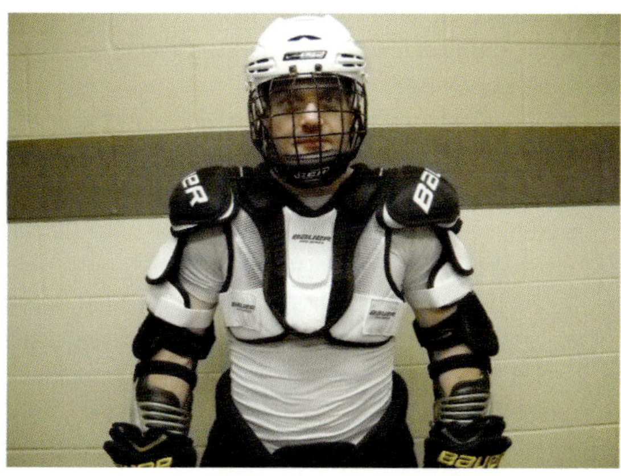

**Fig. 13–10** *Helmet with attached face guard.*

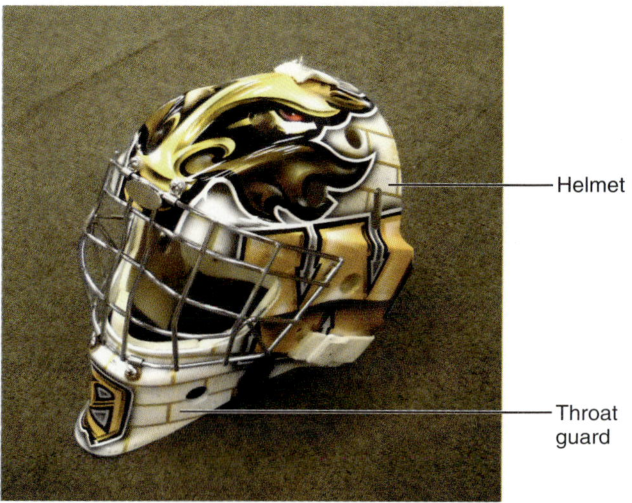



**Fig. 13–11** *Goalkeeper's helmet with attached throat guard.*

constructed of a thick, laminated foam material outer shell covered with synthetic leather and nylon materials. The outer shell is incorporated in a laminated foam inner lining consisting of vertical rolls and wings that extend around the knee, lower leg, ankle, and foot. Most designs are anchored with leather and/or nylon straps with plastic, metal, or Velcro closures (Fig. 13–12).

**Player's gloves** are manufactured in individual fit and right- and left-handed designs, in predetermined sizes in various lengths corresponding to fingertip to mid forearm length measurements or from the fingertips to the distal edge of the elbow pad. The gloves are constructed of a multiple-piece leather, synthetic leather, polyester, or nylon outer shell lined with a moisture-resistant mesh material. Most designs have leather incorporated in the palmar hand, finger, and thumb gussets. Multi-density foam or air bladder padding and polyethylene or Kevlar inserts incorporated throughout the dorsal fingers, thumb, and hand and around the wrist absorb shock and provide protection. These gloves are constructed with two- or three-piece flared or winged cuffs to provide additional protection. Most gloves are anchored with leather straps with Velcro closures (Fig. 13–13).

**Goalkeeper's gloves** consist of a catcher and blocker design. Catchers and blockers are available in individual fit, right- and left-handed designs in predetermined sizes identical to player's gloves. Catchers are worn on the nonstick hand and are manufactured of a multiple-piece leather, synthetic leather, and/or nylon outer shell with a moisture-resistant mesh material inner lining with individual finger and thumb stalls. A leather or synthetic leather mesh pocket is incorporated in the

outer shell. Contoured, high-density foam and/or air and polyethylene inserts are incorporated throughout the glove for protection and improved fit. Catchers are anchored with multiple Velcro straps (Fig. 13–14). Blockers are worn on the stick hand and are constructed

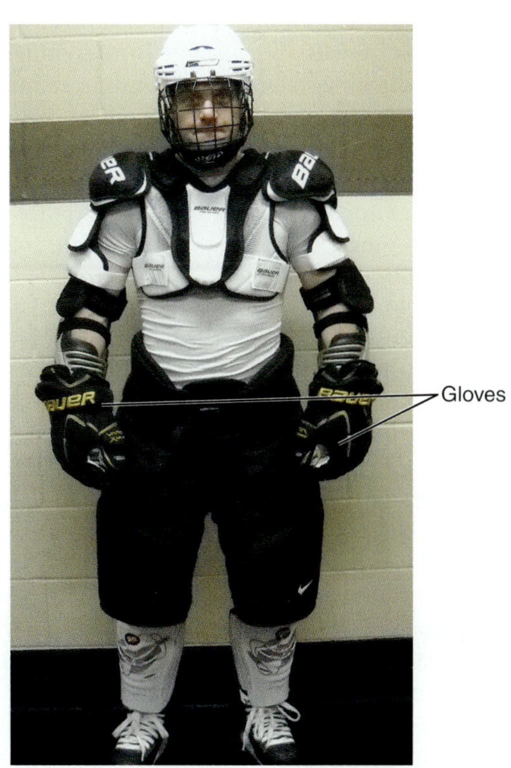


**Fig. 13–13** *Player's gloves.*

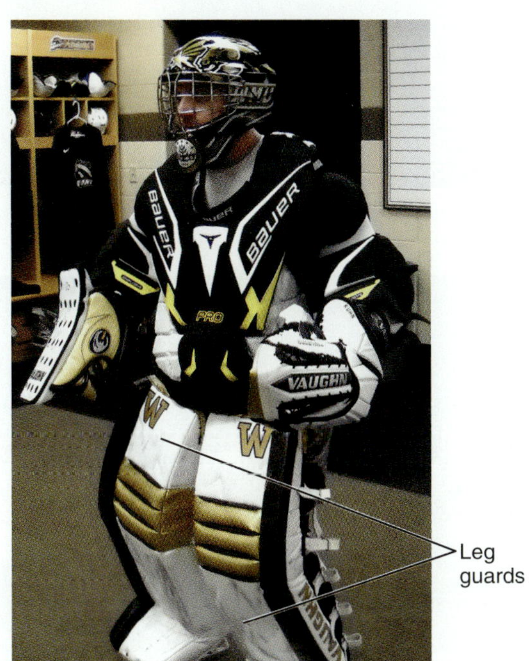


**Fig. 13–12** *Goalkeeper's leg guards.*

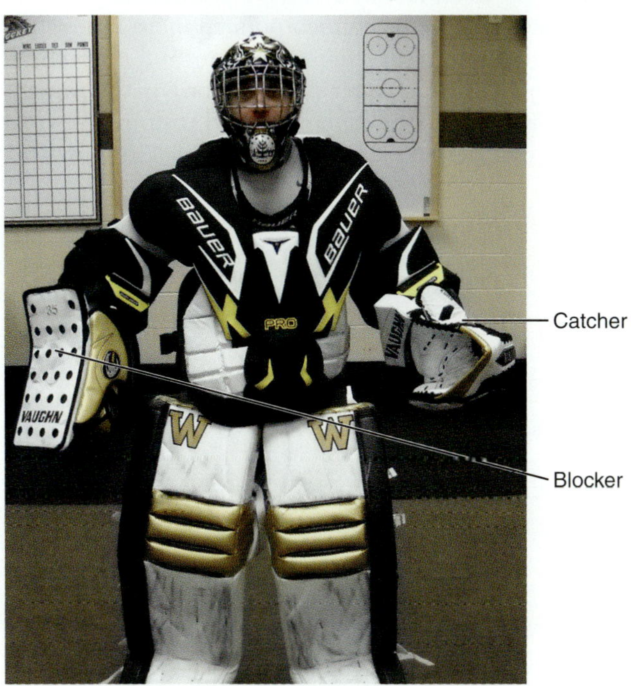


**Fig. 13–14** *Goalkeeper's gloves. Blocker and catcher.*

of dual-density foam with a leather, synthetic leather, or nylon outer shell. A foam padded glove is incorporated in the inner surface of the blocker. Pre-molded, high-density foam and polyethylene inserts provide protection for the first finger, thumb, and wrist. Most designs have finger, thumb, and palmar hand gussets and a strap to anchor the glove. Blockers are attached through various straps with webbing or lace closures.

**Throat guards** are available in individual fit designs in predetermined sizes corresponding to neck circumference measurements. Most guards are constructed of a pre-molded, high-density foam material collar and bib with a ballistic nylon material covering. These throat guards are anchored with adjustable elastic straps with Velcro closures. Other throat guards are manufactured of rigid plastic materials and attach to the distal helmet and face guard with laces or ties (see Fig. 13–11).

**Mouth guards** are discussed in Figures 13–26, 13–27, and 13–28.

**Arm** and **elbow pads** are manufactured in universal and right- and left-handed styles in predetermined sizes based on mid upper arm to mid forearm length measurements or from the distal edge of the shoulder pads to the proximal glove. Most pads are constructed of a polycarbonate or plastic outer shell incorporated in a vinyl, nylon, or woven fabric material inner shell with open- and closed-cell foam padding. The pads are anchored with adjustable nylon straps with Velcro or buckle closures (Fig. 13–15).

**Shin guards** are available in individual and universal fit designs in predetermined sizes based on superior patella to top of the skate length measurements. The designs are manufactured of a polycarbonate or other rigid material outer shell incorporated in an inner shell constructed of various foams. The outer and inner shells are covered with polyester mesh, nylon, or thermoregulatory materials. The inner shell and padding of some designs can be removed and/or adjusted to allow for additional protection and custom-fitting. Most designs are anchored with adjustable nylon straps with Velcro closures (Fig. 13–16).

**Shoulder pads** are manufactured with an outer shell constructed of varying thicknesses of open- and closed-cell and EVA foams covered with a nylon/polyester material. Most designs have a moisture-resistant inner lining. These pads have rigid carbon or polyethylene plastic plates and rounded caps or high-density foam incorporated in the outer shell over the spine, thorax, shoulder, and upper arm. Some designs have a carbon or polyethylene plate over the clavicle; other designs have a detachable abdominal pad. Shoulder pads are anchored with adjustable nylon straps with Velcro closures (Fig. 13–17).

**Chest and arm protectors** are available in individual fit designs in predetermined sizes corresponding to chest circumference measurements. The designs are manufactured of open- and closed-cell block foam pads arranged in various patterns covered with nylon materials. The chest pads have pre-molded carbon or polyethylene plastic plates and caps or high-density foam incorporated over the thorax, abdomen, shoulder,

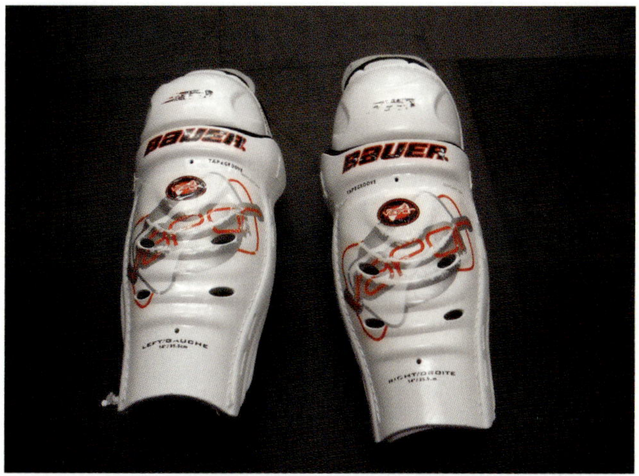

**Fig. 13–16** *Shin guards.*

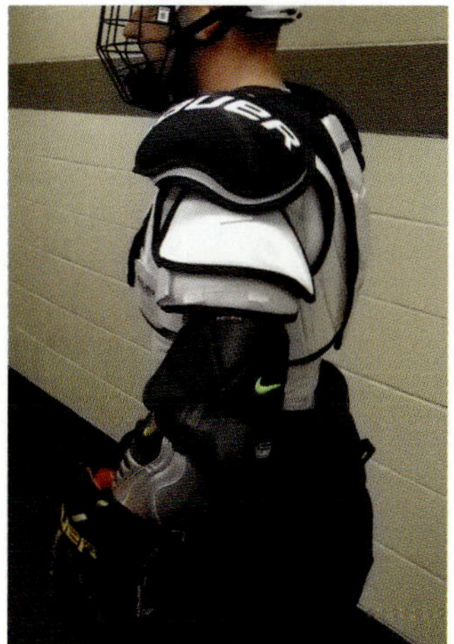

**Fig. 13–15** *Arm and elbow pad.*

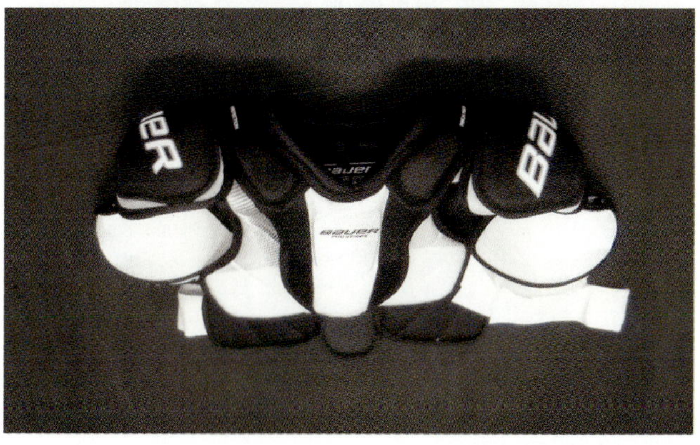

**Fig. 13–17** *Shoulder pads.*

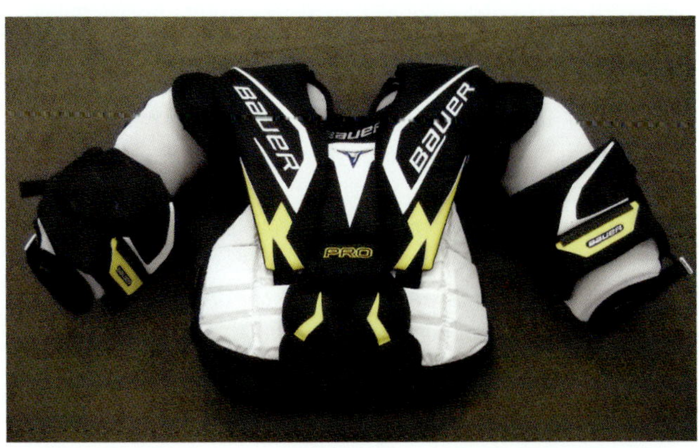

**Fig. 13–18** *Goalkeeper's chest and arm protector.*

upper arm, and elbow. Chest pads are anchored with an adjustable harness and straps with Velcro and/or D-ring closures (Fig. 13–18).

**Protective athletic cups** used in ice hockey were discussed in Chapter 12 in the Padding section (see Fig. 12–17).

# Lacrosse

## Women's and Girls' Lacrosse

### *Mandatory Equipment*

### All athletes

- Eye guard, ASTM Lacrosse Standards (NCAA), ASTM Standard 3077 (NFHS), SEI Standard (NFHS)
- Mouth guard (NCAA and NFHS), intraoral design covering all upper teeth (NCAA and NFHS) or lower teeth (NFHS), any readily visible color (not white or transparent) (NFHS)

### Goalkeeper

- Helmet with attached face mask (NCAA and NFHS), NOCSAE Standards (NFHS), chin strap (NFHS)
- Chest protector (NCAA and NFHS)
- Throat protector (NCAA and NFHS)
- Gloves (NFHS)
- Shin guards (NFHS)
- Thigh pads (NFHS)

## Men's and Boys' Lacrosse

### *Mandatory Equipment*

### All athletes

- Helmet with attached face mask, NOCSAE Standards (NCAA and NFHS), risk of injury warning label (NFHS), chin strap and chin pad (NFHS),

cupped four-point chin strap with high-point hookup, chin pad (NCAA)
- Gloves (NCAA and NFHS)
- Mouth guard, intraoral design covering all upper teeth (NCAA and NFHS) or lower teeth (NFHS), yellow or any other highly visible color (NCAA), any readily visible color (not white or transparent) (NFHS)
- Shoulder pads (NCAA and NFHS), optional for goalkeeper (NFHS)
- Arm pads (NFHS), optional for goalkeeper (NFHS)

### Goalkeeper

- Chest protector (NCAA and NFHS)
- Throat protector (NCAA and NFHS)

**Helmet designs** are constructed of a polyethylene or polycarbonate plastic material outer shell with an inner lining of air bladders and/or dual-density or EVA foam. A visor is incorporated in the outer shell. The face guard is manufactured of carbon steel and is anchored to the outer shell. A rigid plastic chin guard is attached to the distal face guard and extends downward. Most helmets and face guards are anchored with a four-point adjustable chin strap with a chin cup (Fig. 13–19).

**Shoulder pads** can serve as a chest protector and are manufactured of an open- and closed-cell and EVA foams or viscoelastic gel material outer shell covered with a mesh material lining. Most pads have an inner lining of moisture-resistant material. In most designs, polyethylene plastic plates and caps are incorporated in the outer shell over the thorax, shoulder, and upper arm. Some designs use a wire mesh material incorporated in the outer shell over the shoulder to provide additional protection. Shoulder pads are attached with adjustable nylon straps with Velcro closures (see Figs. 13–19 and 13–20).

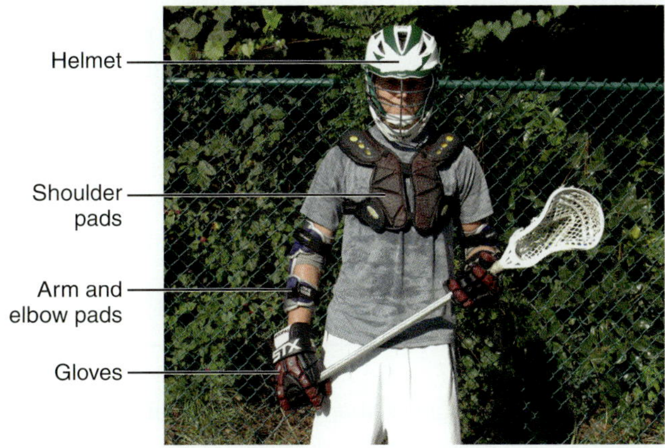


**Fig. 13–19** *Field player in protective equipment. Helmet, shoulder pads, arm and elbow pads, and gloves.*

Protective Equipment and Padding

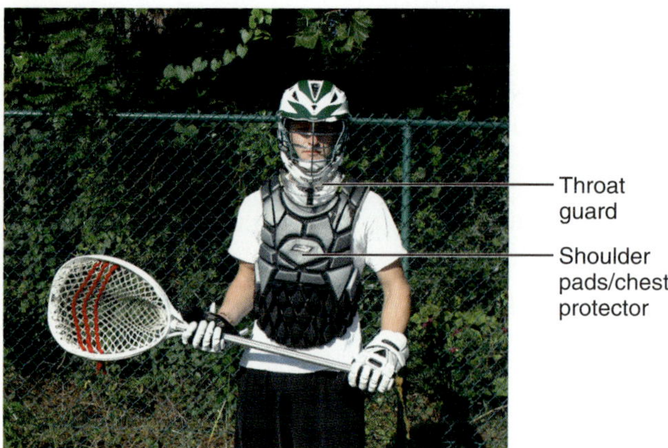


**Fig. 13–20** *Goalkeeper in protective equipment. Shoulder pads/chest protector and throat guard.*

**Arm** and **elbow pads** are manufactured, fit, and attached in the same manner as ice hockey designs (see Fig. 13–19).

**Gloves** are available in individual fit and right- and left-handed designs in various lengths and predetermined sizes based on length measurements similar to ice hockey designs. The multi-piece designs consist of a contoured leather, synthetic leather, and/or vinyl outer shell; moisture-resistant inner lining; finger and thumb gussets; leather or mesh surface on the palmar hand; and flared or winged wrist cuffs. The gloves have multi-density foam and polyethylene inserts incorporated throughout the dorsal finger and hand surface for protection and stability. Most gloves are attached with laces, Velcro closures, or a magnetic closure mechanism (see Fig. 13–19).

**Throat guards** are constructed of rigid plastic material or high-density foam. The guards attach to the distal face guard with laces or nylon straps with metal snaps (see Fig. 13–20).

**Shin guards** are manufactured, fit, and attached in the same manner as field hockey designs (see Fig. 13–7).

**Thigh pads** for goalkeepers are incorporated into nylon/polyester/Lycra pants and are available in individual fit designs in predetermined sizes corresponding to waist circumference measurements. The pant designs have multiple closed-cell foam pads arranged in various patterns over the thigh and hip. The designs are anchored with an elastic waistband.

**Eye guards** for use in lacrosse are discussed at the end of this section (see Fig. 13–25).

**Mouth guard** designs for lacrosse are illustrated in Figures 13–26, 13–27, and 13–28.

---

**DETAILS**

For more complete information on lacrosse helmet fitting, eye protection, and approved protective equipment lists, see the Web References.

---

**Clinical Application Question 3**

During the second half of a soccer match, a forward is tackled and falls to the ground on her left posterior elbow, sustaining a moderate contusion. Following an evaluation by the team physician and several days of treatment, she is allowed to return to play if properly protected.

➡ **Question: What padding technique can you use to provide adequate protection?**

# Soccer

## *Mandatory Equipment*

### All athletes

- Shin guards, NOCSAE Standards, professionally manufactured, age and size appropriate, no alterations (NCAA and NFHS), bottom edge no higher than 2 inches above the ankle (NFHS)

## *Standard Equipment*

### Goalkeeper

- Gloves

**Shin guards** are manufactured of a pre-molded resin, polypropylene, and/or polyurethane material outer shell. Some designs use thermoplastic materials for a custom-fit. The outer shell of the guards is lined with soft, EVA, or closed-cell foam. Many designs are manufactured with padding over the medial and lateral malleoli. Some guards are covered with a nylon mesh material and others with a cotton sock or elastic sleeve. Most shin guards are attached with adjustable nylon straps with Velcro closures (Fig. 13–21). Some designs have nylon foot stirrups.

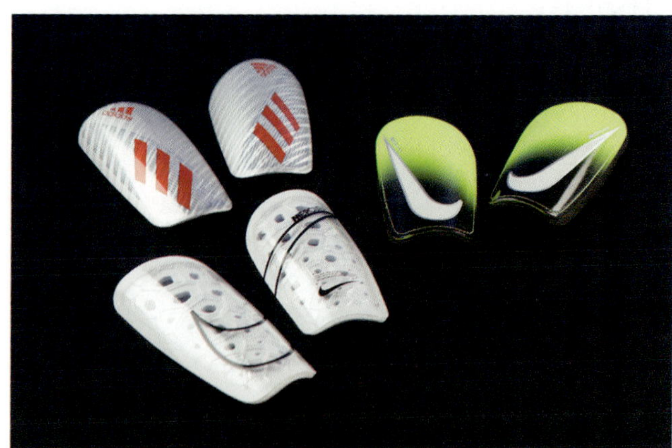

**Fig. 13–21** *Shin guards.*

## EVIDENCE SUMMARY

The majority of injuries sustained during participation in soccer occur to the lower extremities and include minor trauma, such as contusions and high-impact trauma such as fractures.[30] Off-the-shelf shin guards are designed to absorb shock and provide protection in the prevention and treatment of lower leg injuries and conditions. Despite the mandatory use of shin guards in NCAA soccer and softball and NFHS baseball, field hockey, ice hockey, girls' lacrosse, soccer, and softball, limited investigations have been conducted to examine their effectiveness in reducing trauma to the lower leg.

Some researchers have suggested that shin guards may lessen the occurrence of minor trauma,[31,32] while others have demonstrated that guards may protect against lower leg fractures. Among recreational, intercollegiate, amateur, and professional soccer athletes, using shin guards was shown to prevent lower leg fractures.[33–35] This decline in fractures has been attributed to design improvements and mandatory use of shin guards. Other investigations[36] have shown a significant decrease in the rates of lower leg contusions and fractures after implementation of rules for mandatory guard use among recreational and amateur soccer athletes in the Netherlands. Using fiberglass[37] and metal rod[38] lower leg models, other researchers found reductions in peak forces at the proximal and distal ends of the models during controlled impact-loading testing at drop heights of 20, 30, 40, and 50 cm. Other studies[39] examined the effectiveness of custom-made carbon fiber and off-the-shelf polypropylene shin guards among artificial carbon fiber lower leg models. The results demonstrated that the custom-made designs significantly reduced the maximum force and impact duration on the anterior aspect of the model during controlled low- and high-impact forces compared to off-the-shelf designs.[39] Examining off-the-shelf field hockey guards, other researchers[40] found a greater reduction of impact forces on the anterior aspect of an artificial lower leg model during single and repeated drop tests at 60 and 75 mm with a sock normally worn during play and guard compared to a guard only.

The results of these limited investigations provide some evidence to support the use of shin guards to prevent lower leg injuries. However, the level of protection may depend on the size and construction of the guard. Although heavier, thicker, and longer guards most likely provide greater protection, soccer participants prefer lower profile and lighter designs for fit and comfort.[37] Thinner designs constructed from quality materials such as carbon fiber may provide greater protection[39] and comfort, perhaps increasing compliance among wearers. Newly manufactured shin guards undergo impact and retention tests to determine certification according to the NOCSAE Standards.[3] Guards meeting the standard must be permanently marked with the manufacturer's information, intended body size of wearer, and SEI/NOCSAE seal.[3] Based on the evidence and rules governing the mandatory use of shin guards, research is needed to design the optimal shin guard that provides maximal protection and comfort for soccer, field hockey, lacrosse, baseball, softball, and ice hockey participants among all levels.

---

### ...IF/THEN...

**IF** soccer shin guards do not provide adequate protection of the anterior lower leg, **THEN** consider purchasing a larger size or a thermoplastic design; the larger size should extend coverage over the area, and thermoplastic designs can be custom-fit.

## Softball

### *Mandatory Equipment*

On deck, batting, and base running (NCAA and NFHS)
Retired runners, players/students in coach's boxes, non-adult bat/ball shaggers (NFHS)

- Helmet with double ear-flap design, NOCSAE Standards (NCAA and NFHS), risk of injury warning label (NFHS), non-glare surface (NFHS)

### Batting Fast-Pitch (NFHS)

- Helmet and face mask with double ear-flap design, NOCSAE Standards

### Catcher

- Helmet, NOCSAE Standards (NCAA and NFHS), non-glare surface (NFHS)
- Face mask, NOCSAE Standards (NCAA and NFHS)
- Throat guard (NCAA and NFHS)
- Chest (body) protector (NCAA)
- Shin guards, foot to knee (NCAA)
- Body protector, shin guards (NFHS)
- Protective cup (male catcher) while warming up pitcher (NFHS)

### *Standard Equipment*

### Batting

- Gloves

Protective Equipment and Padding

**Helmet, face mask, throat guard, chest and chest (body) protector, shin guard,** and **protective cup designs** are identical to baseball equipment (see Figs. 13–1, 13–2, 13–3, 13–4, and 13–5).

# Wrestling

## Mandatory Equipment

### All athletes

- Ear guard (NCAA and NFHS)
- Mouth guard, intraoral design covering all upper and/or lower teeth, athletes with braces or special orthodontic device (NFHS)

**Ear guards** are available with an outer shell constructed of various nylon and/or neoprene straps with a polypropylene, polycarbonate, and/or air bladder guard incorporated in the straps over the ears. Most ear guards are lined with EVA foam and/or neoprene materials. Some designs use a padded nylon guard that attaches to the outer shell to protect the forehead. Other designs are constructed to limit restriction of hearing. Ear guards are anchored with adjustable nylon and/or neoprene straps with Velcro or metal closures (Fig. 13–22). Some designs are available with a chin cup.

**Mouth guard** designs for wrestling are illustrated in Figures 13–26, 13–27, and 13–28.

# Eye Guards

Eye guards are available in individual fit designs in predetermined sizes corresponding to head circumference measurements and helmet and face guard style. The guards are manufactured in three designs: glasses, shields, and goggles. Eye guards are mandatory in NCAA and NFHS women's and girls' lacrosse and NFHS field hockey but can provide protection for athletes participating in baseball, basketball, fencing, football, ice hockey, rifle, skiing, softball, swimming, volleyball, and water polo. Baseball, fencing, field hockey, football, ice hockey, lacrosse, and softball helmets, face guards, and masks, by design, also provide some protection of the eyes.

**Glasses** are used for protection in baseball, basketball, field hockey, football, ice hockey, lacrosse, and softball. Most designs are manufactured of polycarbonate or Trivex material lenses and are available with ultraviolet (UV) protection, anti-fog, anti-glare, and anti-scratch coatings, as well as prescription vision corrections. The lenses are incorporated in one- or three-piece polycarbonate, synthetic, or other plastic material frames that extend across the eyes and lateral face. The nose piece is padded with foam, rubber, or viscoelastic materials; some frames are lined with these materials for additional protection. Glasses are attached with temples behind the ears and/or adjustable elastic nylon straps (Fig. 13–23).

> **Helpful Hint |**
> Protective eye guards should fit snugly. To test for proper fit, lightly run a finger around the outside perimeter of the eye guard. No gaps large enough to allow a finger to lightly touch the eye should be present.[41]

**Shields** are designed to be used in combination with baseball and softball catcher's, field hockey, football, ice hockey, and lacrosse helmets and face guards to provide protection. These shields are manufactured from polycarbonate, synthetic, or other plastic materials and are coated to provide UV and scratch protection and resist fogging and glare. The shields extend the width of the face guard; most shields are attached on the inside surface of face guards with plastic grommets or wire or plastic ties (Fig. 13–24).

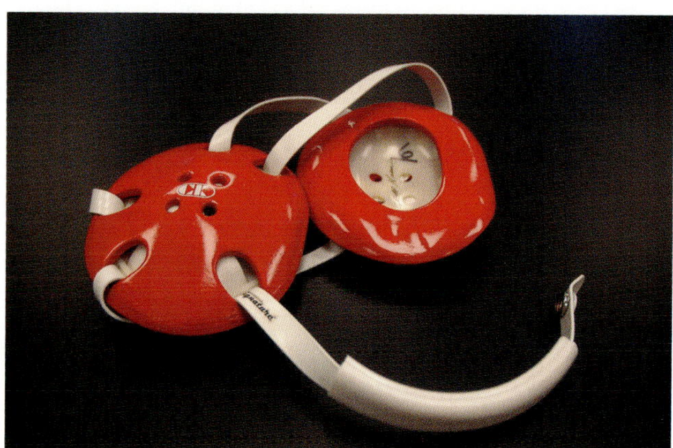

**Fig. 13–22** *Ear guards.*

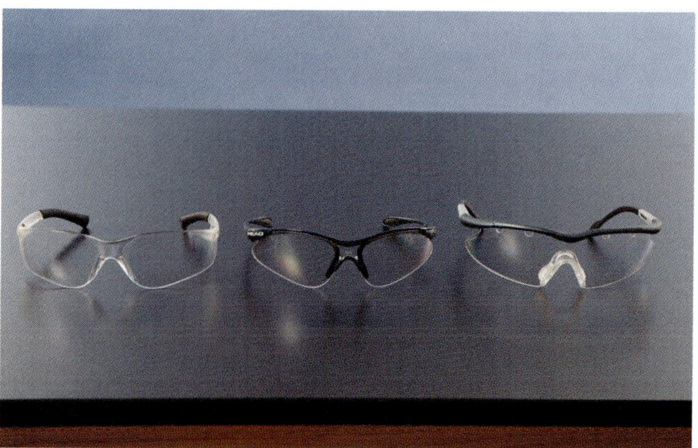

**Fig. 13–23** *Glasses.*

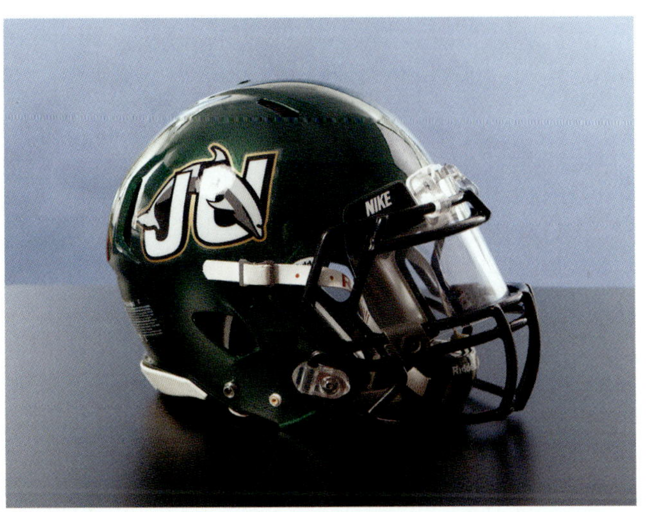

**Fig. 13–24** *Shield attached to a football helmet.*

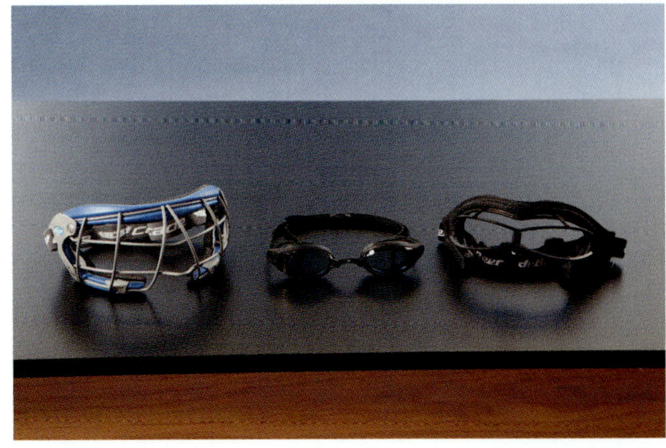

**Fig. 13–25** *Goggles.*

**Goggles** are used to provide protection in field hockey, lacrosse, skiing, swimming, and water polo (Fig. 13–25). Most designs are constructed of polycarbonate or Trivex lenses with UV, anti-scratch, anti-fog, and anti-glare protection. Prescription goggles are also available. Some lacrosse and field hockey designs are constructed of a foam- or silicone-lined, light wire or titanium frame with adjustable elastic straps. Skiing goggles are used in combination with helmets and are attached over the helmet with adjustable nylon straps. Swimming and water polo designs are manufactured in a cup style that fits snugly over the eye socket with water-tight silicone, neoprene, or closed-cell foam gaskets and a flexible nose bridge. Most designs are anchored with adjustable silicon straps.

## EVIDENCE SUMMARY

A risk of injury to the eye is present in any sport that involves a stick or racquet, a ball or other projectile, or body contact. The risk of eye injury does not correlate with the common classifications of collision, contact, and noncontact sports, in which collision and contact sports typically possess the highest risk of injury. With eye injuries, the risk is proportional to the chance of receiving a blow significant enough to result in injury.[42] Sports with a high risk of eye injury include baseball, basketball, boxing, fencing, field hockey, ice hockey, lacrosse, martial arts, paintball, racquetball, softball, and squash.[42] However, at least 90% of eye injuries can be prevented by using off-the-shelf eye guards.[43]

Several investigations have examined incidence rates of eye injury in athletic activities. Researchers[44] have examined incidence rates among different competition levels and sports utilizing data from surveillance systems. Among interscholastic athletes, an incidence rate of 0.68 injury per 100,000 practice and competition sessions was found during the 2005 to 2015 academic years. The highest rates of injury occurred in baseball, boys' basketball, field hockey, and wrestling, respectively. During the 2004 to 2015 academic years, an incidence rate of 1.84 injury per 100,000 practice and competition sessions was found among intercollegiate athletes. Wrestling, women's basketball, field hockey, and men's basketball produced the highest rates of injury, respectively. The researchers[44] revealed rates of injury were significantly higher in competition when compared to practice sessions at the interscholastic and intercollegiate levels. Although categorized as high-risk sports, the study reported no injuries during the periods in interscholastic and intercollegiate ice hockey and intercollegiate women's lacrosse. Over a 23-year period from 1990 to 2012, researchers[45] examined rates of injury caused by sport and recreation activities among U.S. children ≤17 years of age. The researchers reported an incidence rate of 26.9 injury per 100,000 children annually, with basketball, baseball, softball, non-powder gun (paintball, BB, pellet), swimming, and football activities associated with the highest rates. The findings also showed the overall rates of injury decreased slightly during the period.

Rule changes from governing bodies of interscholastic and professional athletics requiring the mandatory use of eye guards have reduced the incidence of injury to the eye. Researchers have examined injury rates before and after implementation of rules for eye guard use and found significant reductions in eye/

orbital injuries during practice and competition sessions among interscholastic field hockey[46] and girls' lacrosse.[47] Others[44] found a reduction in eye injuries following the eye guard mandate in interscholastic field hockey. Based on the small injury counts before and after the mandate, the findings were not significant. During the 2009 to 2015 academic years in which eye guards were mandatory, researchers[48] found no eye injuries in practice and competition sessions among intercollegiate women's lacrosse athletes. Eye guard use also produced reductions in head/face injuries in interscholastic field hockey[46] and girls' lacrosse[47] and face injuries in lacrosse among females 5 to 18 years of age.[49] However, researchers[46,47] found an increase in concussion incidence rates with eye guards among these sports, perhaps as a result of increased awareness and diagnosis of concussions. Others[50] examining the incidence of eye injury in professional ice hockey over a 10 season period found a significant increase in the risk of eye injury when no face half shields were worn. The use of half shields among professional ice hockey athletes has increased from 32% in 2002–2003 to 73% in 2012–2013 seasons.[50] Following a 2013 mandate regarding visor use for all rookie players, the overall use of visors has increased to 87.1% among all professional ice hockey players and 81.7% among all non-rookie players.[51]

In a 2009 systematic review, the use of ice hockey face shields for the prevention of concussions was examined.[52] The findings from three studies among junior, intercollegiate, and professional athletes revealed no differences in concussion rates between the use of full, half, and no face shields. In one study, less practice and competition time loss per concussion was found with the use of full shields compared to half shield designs with intercollegiate athletes. Another study among professional athletes demonstrated no differences in time loss following concussions between the use of face shields and no shield. Using laboratory headforms to examine peak acceleration, one study found that full face guards produced lower measures than half face shields, demonstrating more protection with the guards. A 2017 review[53] found no evidence for the efficacy of ice hockey face shields in the prevention of concussions. A 2013 policy statement[42] from the American Academy of Pediatrics and the American Academy of Ophthalmology recommends the use of eye guards for all individuals participating in sports that have a risk of eye injury and mandatory use of eye guards for functionally one-eyed athletes and athletes recovering from eye surgery or trauma upon recommendation from an ophthalmologist.

Choosing the correct eye guard to lessen the risk of injury involves three steps. First, conduct an eye medical history, examination, and vision screening to identify potential concerns.[54] Second, select and use only those eye guards that meet ASTM, ANSI, NOCSAE, and SEI Standards.[42] Last, have an experienced ophthalmologist, optometrist, optician, or other health care professional select and fit the guards.[42] Glasses should consist of polycarbonate or Trivex lenses and polycarbonate or other thermoplastic material frames with or without foam liners.[43,55] Contact lenses alone do not provide protection; wearers should use glasses, shields, or goggles for protection.[42]

The high risk of eye injury in sports, and the high success in injury prevention when using eye guards, indicates that athletic associations and organizations should consider mandating the use of certified eye guards in high-risk sports. Additional research is needed to evaluate the effectiveness of eye guard use and their effects on visual acuity and overall athletic performance to determine the most effective design to prevent injuries to the eye.

---

### Clinical Application Question 4

The fullback on the football team requires the use of contact lenses during all practices and competitions. Several times during preseason practices, dirt and grass were thrown through the face guard into his eyes, damaging the lenses but fortunately not his eyes. A polycarbonate shield was attached to his helmet and face guard to provide protection. Although the shield protected against large objects entering through the face guard, the debris continued to reach his contact lenses and eyes.

➡ **Question: What techniques can you use to prevent debris from entering the face guard and eyes?**

# Mouth Guards

The ASTM[56] has categorized mouth guards based on the fitting process and the level of comfort and protection provided. The categories include Type I custom-fabricated, Type II mouth-formed, and Type III stock. Custom-fabricated, mouth-formed, or stock mouth guards are mandatory in NCAA and NFHS field hockey, football, ice hockey, and lacrosse and NFHS wrestling, but they can be used in any sport.

**Custom-fabricated** guards are manufactured in individual fit designs corresponding to an upper or lower arch model (Fig. 13–26). Some guards are constructed of thermoplastic materials using a vacuum

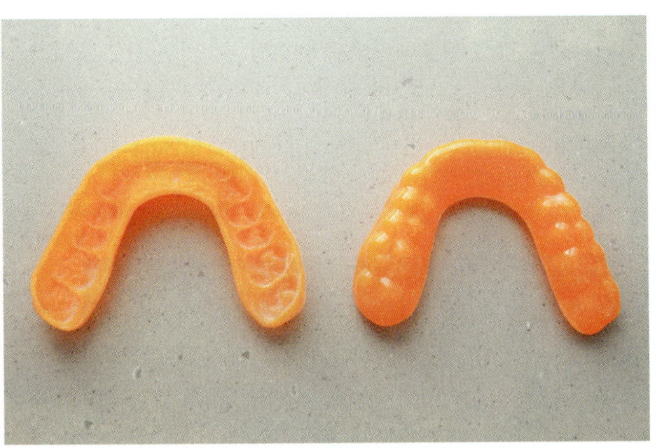

**Fig. 13–26** *Custom-fabricated mouth guards.*

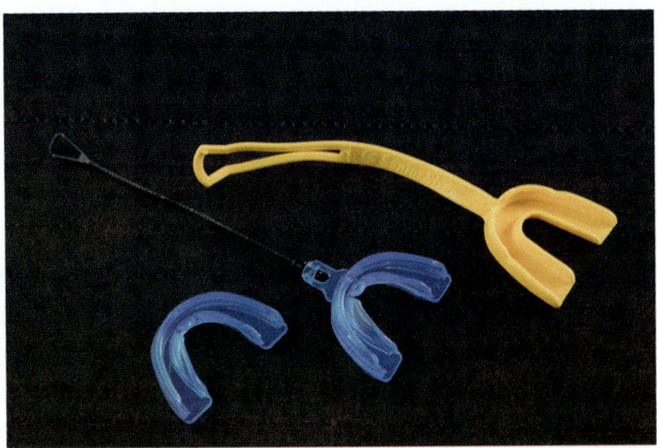

**Fig. 13–27 A** *Mouth-formed mouth guards. (Left) Without loop strap. (Middle and Right) With loop straps.*

process. Other designs are manufactured of thermoplastic or laminated resin materials using a pressure-formed lamination process. These guards are typically manufactured in a dental office or laboratory but can be constructed in-house. Although rarely needed because of the custom-fit, a face guard strap can be incorporated in these designs. A custom-fabrication positive pressure process can be found at FADavis.com ⚫.

**Mouth-formed** designs are manufactured in predetermined sizes corresponding to mouth circumference measurements (Fig. 13–27A). This design is the most commonly used guard. Some designs, referred to as boil and bite guards, are constructed of a thermoplastic material shell, while other designs consist of a rigid material outer shell and an ethyl methacrylate material or gel inner lining. These guards are heated in boiling water and intraorally shaped to the contours of the mouth and teeth, preferably by a dentist. Improper molding by the user can cause inconsistent thickness, fit, and retention of the guard.[57] Mouth-formed guards are anchored to the teeth if properly fit; most are available with a face guard strap.

---

### DETAILS
#### Mouth-Formed Fitting Process
- Hold the mouth guard by the face guard strap and insert the guard into boiling water until the guard becomes pliable (Fig. 13–27B). For many designs, 20–30 seconds is recommended.
- Remove the guard from the water and allow the excess water to drain for approximately 5 seconds.
- Place the guard directly into the mouth. For most designs, position the guard over the upper arch (see Fig. 13–27C). Center the guard over the teeth using the strap as a guide.
- Press the lips together to create a tight seal and aggressively suck the guard against the upper arch to obtain a contoured

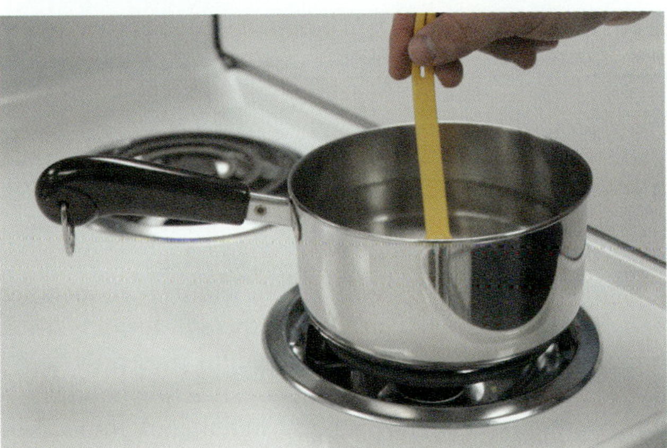

**Fig. 13–27 B**

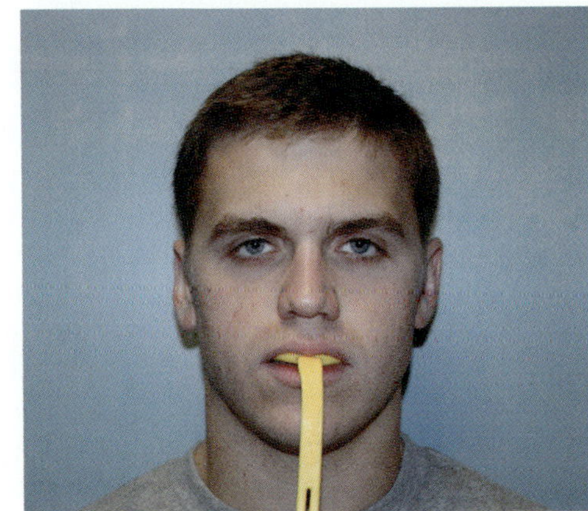

**Fig. 13–27 C**

fit (see Fig. 13–27D). For most designs, 15–30 seconds is recommended.
- During the forming process, do not bring the upper and lower jaw together or bite into the guard.
- Remove the guard from the mouth and rinse in cold water.

- Cutting the posterior ends or trimming the edges next to the gums may lessen the protective properties and increase the risk of injury (see Fig. 13–27E).
- If the guard requires reforming, begin the fitting process with a new guard.

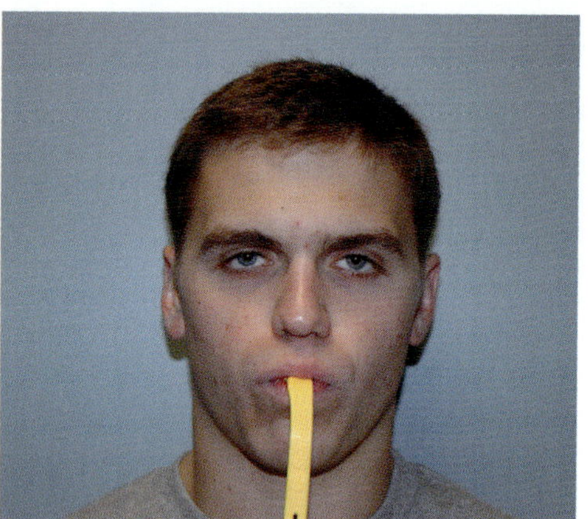

Fig. 13–27 D

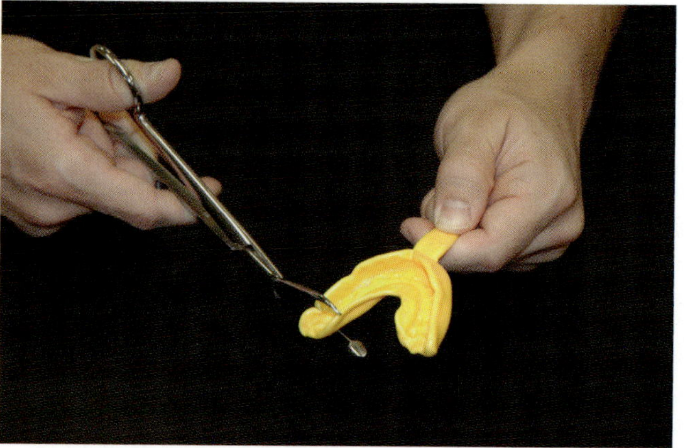

Fig. 13–27 E

**Stock** mouth guards are available in predetermined sizes based on mouth circumference measurements (Fig. 13–28). These guards are constructed of pre-molded rubber, silicone, or polyvinyl materials, are ready to be used upon purchase, and do not allow for customization. Stock mouth guards are anchored by clenching the teeth together and may interfere with speech and breathing. Some designs are available with loop straps to attach the guard to a face guard.

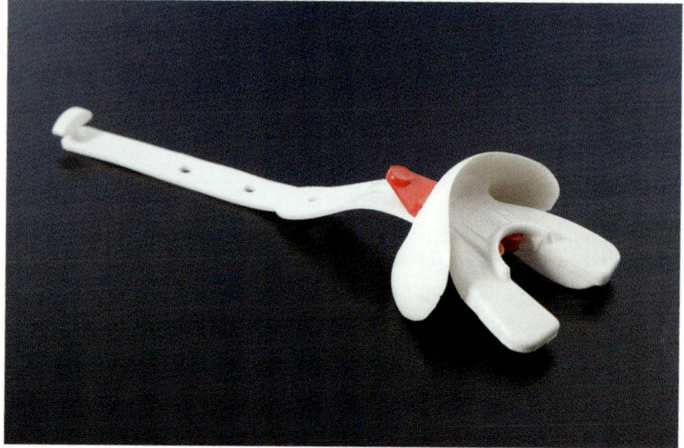

**Fig. 13–28** *Stock mouth guard with loop strap.*

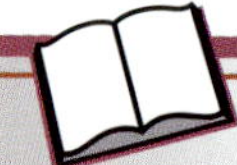

## EVIDENCE SUMMARY

Participation with mouth guards in athletic activities is mandatory for several sports, but the type of design used is often the choice of the institution and/or athlete. A 2010 Academy for Sports Dentistry position statement[58] adopted replacement of the term "mouth guard" with "a properly fitted mouth guard" to promote optimal safety and well-being of athletes. Several characteristics of a properly fitted mouth guard include custom-fabrication from a stone model; guard material meets U.S. Food and Drug Administration approval; adequate coverage and protection of the teeth and surrounding tissues in labial, occlusal, and palatal areas; limited effect on speech; retentive fit and not dislodged on impact; and routine inspection directed by a dentist.[58]

A 2016 National Athletic Trainers' Association position statement[57] examined the efficacy of guards on the prevention of dental injury and presented recommendations for mouth guard construction and care. A 2007 systematic review[59] in the statement demonstrated that the overall risk of orofacial injury was 1.6–1.9 times greater for individuals participating in athletic activities without the use of a mouth guard compared to guard use. Other researchers[60,61] have shown a reduction in the incidence and severity of dental injury with the use of mouth guards. Recommendations from the National Athletic Trainers' Association (NATA)[25,57] and the American Medical Society for Sports Medicine[26] position statements revealed a lack of evidence that mouth guards reduce the risk of concussion among athletes in various sports. The American Dental Association,[62] the American Academy of Pediatric Dentistry,[63] the NATA position statement,[57] and the Academy for Sports Dentistry[58] recommend the use of a properly fitted mouth guard for all individuals participating in recreational or athletic activities that have a risk of dental injury.

The effectiveness of a mouth guard is dependent on the material used, fabrication process, and regular care. NATA position statement recommendations[57] suggest guard construction with thermoplastic materials with labial thickness of 2–3 mm, occlusal 3 mm, and palatal 2 mm. Although more expensive than off-the-shelf designs, custom-fabricated guards meet the properties of a "properly fitted" guard and offer better fit and comfort for the wearer. General recommendations[57] for care of a guard include daily washing in cold or lukewarm water with an oral antimicrobial solution; daily evaluation to confirm fit and damage; storage in a clean, rigid, ventilated container between use; and avoidance of prolonged exposure to direct sunlight or sources of heat.

The choice and use of mouth guard designs appear to be based on general beliefs and perceptions rather than clinical effectiveness.[64] Although recommendations suggest the use of custom-fabricated designs, stock and mouth-formed guards are the most common among athletic populations.[57] Many athletes believe that mouth guards are bulky, uncomfortable, and affect speech and breathing and avoid their use during practices and competitions. Several studies have investigated the effects of mouth guards on functional performance and showed mouth-formed and custom-fabricated designs had overall no negative impact on aerobic,[65–69] strength,[68] and agility[66] performance among athletes.

The evidence supports the use of properly fitted mouth guards for the prevention of dental injury. Health care professionals should educate athletes, parents, and coaches on the effectiveness and use of "a properly fitted mouth guard" for the prevention of injury.[57] Efforts should continue toward the implementation of rule changes in other interscholastic, intercollegiate, amateur, and professional sports to mandate the use of properly fitted mouth guards for all athletes. Additional research is needed to develop an appropriate guard design that provides maximal protection, ease of wear, and cost-effectiveness to encourage usage among individuals in recreational and athletic activities.

---

### DETAILS

For more complete information on the protective mechanisms and recommendations for fabrication of properly fitted mouth guards, see the Web References.

---

### ...IF/THEN...

**IF** an athlete continually bites through a boil and bite mouth guard during use, **THEN** consider replacing the guard with a rigid outer shell mouth-formed or custom-fabricated design.

---

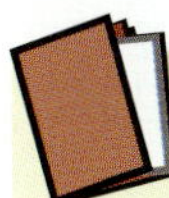

### EVIDENCE-BASED PRACTICE

Tillman University will begin women's lacrosse next year, and Mike McCallum is working to finalize the coordination of medical services for the program. Mike is the Head Athletic Trainer at Tillman University, with over 30 years of experience as an AT but a limited background in lacrosse. He has projected the impact of women's lacrosse throughout the athletic training budget and set aside limited funds for the purchase of mouth guards for the athletes. Mouth guards are not typically purchased through the budget as Tillman University does not have any sports that require their use. Mike has previous experience with several off-the-shelf mouth guard designs used in football and field hockey but begins to question whether these designs are the most effective for lacrosse athletes. He creates a list of relevant details that will be considered in the selection of a mouth guard technique. The list includes:

- The governing sport body requires that all lacrosse athletes must wear an intraoral mouth guard of a readily visible color that covers all upper teeth.
- Based on athlete preferences, the design must be correctly fitted, comfortable to wear, tasteless,

*Continued*

possess retention, and not restrict breathing and speech.

- The design must be cost-effective as the remaining athletic training budget is limited.
- The team dentist will continue to see referred athletes from Tillman University but does not have the equipment to fabricate custom mouth guards in her office.
- A large dental clinic, located 200 miles away, has expressed interest in developing a relationship with Tillman University to fabricate mouth guards for the athletes.
- A retired dentist and supporter of Tillman University's athletic program has begun conversations with Mike about donating the necessary funding to purchase mouth-formed designs for the lacrosse team.

Using this list, Mike searches for a mouth guard design that would result in high compliance with wear and would prevent and lessen the severity of injury among the lacrosse athletes.

1. Develop a clinically relevant question from the case in the PICO format to generate answers for the selection of a mouth guard design for the lacrosse athletes. The question should include the population or problem, the intervention, a comparison intervention (if relevant), and the clinical outcome of interest.
2. Design a search strategy and search to find the best evidence to answer the clinical question. The strategy should include relevant search terms, electronic databases, online journals, and print journals to use for the search. Discussions with your faculty, preceptor, and other health care professionals can provide evidence from expert opinion.
3. Choose three to five full text studies or reviews from your search or the chapter references. Evaluate and appraise each article to determine its value and usefulness to the case. Ask these questions for each study: (1) Are the results of the study valid? (2) What are the actual results? and (3) Are the findings clinically relevant to my patients? Prepare a summary of the evaluation with answers to the questions and rank the articles based on the evidence hierarchy in Chapter 1.
4. Integrate findings from the evidence, your clinical experience, and the patient's goals and preferences into the case. Consider which mouth guard designs may be appropriate for the lacrosse athletes.
5. Evaluate the EBP process and your experience within the case. Consider these questions in the evaluation.

Was the clinical question answered?
Did the search generate quality evidence?
Was the evidence evaluated appropriately?
Was the evidence, your clinical experience, and the lacrosse athletes' goals and values integrated to make the clinical decision?
Did the intervention produce successful clinical outcomes for the lacrosse athletes?
Was the EBP experience positive for Mike and the lacrosse athletes?

## WRAP-UP

- Individuals who design, manufacture, purchase, fit, and use protective equipment and padding share a legal responsibility to ensure safety.
- Purchase only high-quality equipment and padding, follow manufacturer's instructions, do not make modifications, and monitor and perform regular maintenance.
- NOCSAE, HECC, SEI, ASTM, and CSA have established safety standards and testing procedures for the manufacture, maintenance, and use of protective equipment and padding.
- Baseball, football, lacrosse, ice hockey, and softball helmets and face guards and soccer shin guards that meet NOCSAE, SEI, HECC, ASTM, and/or CSA testing standards are permanently branded or stamped with a seal or label.

- The NCAA and NFHS require mandatory protective equipment and padding for athletes participating in many sports.
- Athletes voluntarily wear many protective equipment and padding designs that are not required during practices and competitions.
- Off-the-shelf equipment and padding techniques are available in a variety of universal and custom-fit designs to absorb shock and provide protection.
- Although protective equipment and padding are not designed to prevent all injuries, using such equipment and padding is recommended when appropriate.

## FADAVIS ONLINE RESOURCES

- Custom-fabrication positive pressure process

## WEB REFERENCES

**National Athletic Trainers' Association**
**National Athletic Trainers' Association Position Statement: Preventing and Managing Sport-Related Dental and Oral Injuries**
http://natajournals.org/doi/pdf/10.4085/1062-6050-51.8.01?code=nata-site
- This website allows access to recommendations on the prevention and management of sport-related dental injuries and fabrication of mouth guards.

**National Athletic Trainers' Association Position Statement: Management of Sport Concussion**
http://natajournals.org/doi/pdf/10.4085/1062-6050-49.1.07
- This site allows access to recommendations on the management of sport-related concussions, including the use of helmets in various sports.

**National Athletic Trainers' Association Position Statement: Preventing Sudden Death in Sports**
http://natajournals.org/doi/pdf/10.4085/1062-6050-47.1.96
- This website allows access to recommendations on the prevention and treatment and management of the injured patient.

**Academy for Sports Dentistry**
https://www.academyforsportsdentistry.org/
- This site provides access to information regarding the prevention and treatment of dental injuries in sport, including position statements and resources for health care professionals.

**American Academy of Ophthalmology**
https://www.aao.org
- This site provides you recommendations about appropriate eye guards to prevent sport-related eye injuries.

**American Association of Oral and Maxillofacial Surgeons**
https://www.aaoms.org
- This website allows you access to information about the prevention and treatment of oral sport injuries.

**American Dental Association**
https://www.ada.org/en
- This site allows you access to information on types, standards, and care of mouth guards.

**Canadian Standards Association**
https://www.csagroup.org
- This website allows you to search and purchase standards developed for protective athletic equipment.

**Virginia Tech Center for Injury Biomechanics**
https://beam.vt.edu/research/Center-for-Injury-Biomechanics.html
- This site provides access to interdisciplinary research examining human tolerance to impact loading and helmet ratings for football, ice hockey, and soccer.

**Cornell Law School Legal Information Institute**
https://www.law.cornell.edu
- This website allows access to information about sports law and product liability.

**Douglas**
https://www.douglaspads.com/
- This website is an online catalog for the manufacturer and provides sizing and ordering information for football, baseball, and softball equipment.

**Great Lakes Orthodontics, Ltd.**
https://www.greatlakesdentaltech.com/
- This website provides information about equipment for the custom-fabrication of mouth guards.

**National Collegiate Athletic Association**
https://www.ncaapublications.com
- This website allows access to online rules and guidelines for each sponsored sport in regard to mandatory and recommended protective equipment.

**National Federation of State High School Associations**
https://www.nfhs.org
- This site provides you information about ordering sponsored sport rules and guidelines, which include mandatory and recommended protective equipment.

**National Operating Committee on Standards for Athletic Equipment**
https://www.nocsae.org/
- This site provides access to standards, certifications, and testing procedures for protective equipment.

**Pro-Gear Sports**
http://www.footballshoulderpads.com
- This site allows access to information about protective equipment for football. Additionally, this site provides information about the reconditioning of football shoulder pads.

**Riddell**
https://www.riddell.com
- This site is an online catalog for the protective equipment manufacturer and provides technical, fitting, reconditioning, and ordering information.

**Safety Equipment Institute**
https://www.seinet.org/
- This website allows access to information on the testing of protective equipment and provides a certified product list of equipment with manufacturer name and model.

**Schutt Sports**

https://www.schuttsports.com
- This site provides access to sport-specific catalogs containing protective equipment.

**The Hockey Equipment Certification Council Inc.**

http://www.hecc.net
- This website provides information about the testing and certification of ice hockey equipment.

**USLacrosse**

https://www.uslacrosse.org/safety/sports-science-and-safety-committee
- This site provides access to the Sports Science and Safety Committee and position statements on helmets, mouth guards, and eye guards.

## REFERENCES


1. Konin, JG, and Ray, R: Management Strategies in Athletic Training, ed 5. Human Kinetics, Champaign, IL, 2019.

2. Anderson, MK. Foundations of Athletic Training: Prevention, Assessment, and Management, ed 6. Wolters Kluwer, Philadelphia, 2017.

3. National Operating Committee on Standards for Athletic Equipment. https://nocsae.org/, 2019.

4. The Hockey Equipment Certification Council, Inc. Introduction. http://www.hecc.net/index.html, 2019.

5. ASTM International. Detailed Overview. https://www.astm.org/, 2019.

6. Canadian Standards Association. Codes & Standards. https://www.csagroup.org/codes-standards/, 2019.

7. Safety Equipment Institute. Company Overview. https://www.seinet.org/, 2019.

8. National Collegiate Athletic Association: 2014–15 Sports Medicine Handbook, ed 25. NCAA, Indianapolis, 2014. http://www.ncaapublications.com/productdownloads/MD15.pdf.

9. National Federation of State High School Associations: 2019 Baseball Rules Book. National Federation of State High School Associations, Indianapolis, 2019.

10. National Federation of State High School Associations: 2018 Field Hockey Rules Book. National Federation of State High School Associations, Indianapolis, 2019.

11. National Federation of State High School Associations: 2018 Football Rules Book. National Federation of State High School Associations, Indianapolis, 2019.

12. National Federation of State High School Associations: 2018–19 Ice Hockey Rules Book. National Federation of State High School Associations, Indianapolis, 2019.

13. National Federation of State High School Associations: 2018 Boys Lacrosse Rules Book. National Federation of State High School Associations, Indianapolis, 2019.

14. National Federation of State High School Associations: 2018–19 Soccer Rules Book. National Federation of State High School Associations, Indianapolis, 2019.

15. National Federation of State High School Associations: 2018 Softball Rules Book. National Federation of State High School Associations, Indianapolis, 2019.

16. National Federation of State High School Associations: 2018-19 Wrestling Rules Book. National Federation of State High School Associations, Indianapolis, 2019.

17. National Federation of State High School Associations: 2018 Girls Lacrosse Rules Book. National Federation of State High School Associations, Indianapolis, 2019.

18. Maron, BJ, Gohman, TE, Kyle, SB, Estes, NAM, and Link, MS: Clinical profile and spectrum of commotio cordis. JAMA 287:1142–1146, 2002.

19. National Athletic Trainers' Association. NATA Official Statement on Commotio Cordis. http://www.nata.org/sites/default/files/CommotioCordis.pdf, 2019.

20. Davidson, M: Helmets. Annual Athletic Equipment Managers Association Convention, Kansas City, MO, June 9, 2004.

21. Virginia Tech Department of Biomedical Engineering and Mechanics. Virginia Tech helmet ratings. https://www.helmet.beam.vt.edu/, 2019.

22. Schneider, DK, Grandhi, RK, Bansal, P, Kuntz, GE IV, Webster, KE, Logan, K, Barber Foss, KD, and Myer, GD: Current state of concussion prevention strategies: A systematic review and meta-analysis of prospective, controlled studies. Br J Sports Med 51:1473–1482, 2017.

23. Emery, CA, Black, AM, Kolstad, A, Martinez, G, Nettel-Aguirre, A, Engebretsen, L, Johnston, K, Kissick, J, Maddocks, D, Tator, C, Aubry, M, Dvorák, J, Nagahiro, S, and Schneider, K: What strategies can be used to effectively reduce the risk of concussion in sport? A systematic review. Br J Sports Med 51:978–984, 2017.

24. McCrory, P, Meeuwisse, W, Dvorák, J, Aubry, M, Bailes, J, Broglio, S, Cantu, RC, and et al: Consensus statement on concussion in sport—the 5th international conference on concussion in sport held in Berlin, October 2016. Br J Sports Med 51:838–847, 2017.

25. Broglio, SP, Cantu, RC, Gioia, GA, Guskiewicz, KM, Kutcher, J, Palm, M, and Valovich McLeod, TC: National Athletic Trainers' Association position statement: Management of sport concussion. J Athl Train 49:245–265, 2014.

26. Harmon, KG, Drezner, JA, Gammons, M, and et al: American Medical Society for Sports Medicine position statement: Concussion in sport. Br J Sports Med 47:15–26, 2013.

27. Rowson, S, and Duma, SM: Development of the STAR evaluation system for football helmets: Integrating player head impact exposure and risk of concussion. Ann Biomed Eng 39:2130–2140, 2011.

28. Rowson, B, Rowson, S, and Duma, SM: Hockey STAR: Methodology for assessing the biomechanical performance of hockey helmets. Ann Biomed Eng 43:2429–2442, 2015.

29. Davidson, M: Shoulder pads. Annual Athletic Equipment Managers Association Convention, Kansas City, MO, June 9, 2004.

30. Esquivel, AO, Bruder, A, Ratkowiak, K, and Lemos, SE: Soccer-related injuries in children and adults aged 5 to 49 years in US emergency departments from 2000 to 2012. Sports Health 7:366–370, 2015.

31. Kujala, UM, Taimela, S, Antti-Poika, I, Orava, S, Tuominen, R, and Myllynen, P: Acute injuries in soccer, ice hockey, volleyball, basketball, judo, and karate: Analysis of national registry data. BMJ 311:1465–1468, 1995.

32. Tenvergert, EM, Ton Duis, HJ, and Klasen, HJ: Trends in sports injuries, 1982–1988: An in-depth study on four types of sport. J Sports Med Phys Fitness 32:214–220, 1992.

33. Boden, BP, and Garrett, WE: Tibia and fibula fractures in soccer players. Knee Surg Sports Traumatol Arthrosc 7:262–266, 1999.

34. Cattermole, HR, Hardy, JRW, and Gregg, PJ: The footballer's fracture. Br J Sports Med 30:171–175, 1996.

35. Chang, WR, Kapasi, Z, Daisley, S, and Leach, WJ: Tibial shaft fractures in football players. J Orthop Surg Res 2:11, 2007.

36. Vriend, I, Valkenberg, H, Schoots, W, Goudswaard, GJ, van der Meulen, WJ, and Backx, FJ: Shinguards effective in preventing lower leg injuries in football: Population-based trend analyses over 25 years. J Sci Med Sport 18:518–522, 2015.

37. Francisco, AC, Nightingale, RW, Guilak, F, Glisson, RR, and Garrett, WE, Jr: Comparison of soccer shin guards in preventing tibia fracture. Am J Sports Med 28:227–233, 2000.

38. Bir, CA, Cassatta, SJ, and Janda, DH: An analysis and comparison of soccer shin guards. Clin J Sport Med 5:95–99, 1995.

39. Tatar, Y, Ramazanoglu, N, Camliguney, AF, Saygi, EK, and Cotuk, HB: The effectiveness of shin guards used by football players. J Sports Sci Med 13:120–127, 2014.

40. Ruznan, WS, Laing, RM, Lowe, BJ, and Wilson, CA: Impact attenuation provided by shin guards for field hockey. Sports Eng 21:161–175, 2018.

41. Vinger, P: The mechanisms and prevention of sports eye injuries. https://www.astm.org/COMMIT/The-Mech-and-Prev-of-Sports-Eye-Injuries.pdf, 2019.

42. American Academy of Ophthalmology. Joint Policy Statement: Protective Eyewear for Young Athletes-2013. AAO, San Francisco. https://www.aao.org/clinical-statement/protective-eyewear-young-athletes, 2019.

43. Vinger, PF, Parver, L, Alfaro, DV, III, Woods, T, and Abrams, BS: Shatter resistance of spectacle lenses. JAMA 277:142–144, 1997.

44. Boden, BP, Pierpoint, LA, Boden, RG, Comstock, RD, and Kerr, ZY: Eye injuries in high school and collegiate athletes. Sports Health 9:444–449, 2017.

45. Miller, KN, Collins, CL, Chounthirath, T, and Smith, GA: Pediatric sports- and recreation-related eye injuries treated in US emergency departments. http://pediatrics.aappublications.org/content/pediatrics/141/2/e20173083.full.pdf, 2019.

46. Kriz, PK, Zurakowski, RD, Almquist, JL, Reynolds, J, Ruggieri, D, Collins, CL, d'Hemecourt, PA, and Comstock, RD: Eye protection and risk of eye injuries in high school field hockey. Pediatrics 136:521–527, 2015.

47. Lincoln, AE, Caswell, SV, Almquist, JL, Dunn, RE, Clough, MV, Dick, RW, and Hinton, RY: Effectiveness of the women's lacrosse protective eyewear mandate in the reduction of eye injuries. Am J Sports Med 40:611–614, 2012.

48. Kerr, ZY, Lincoln, AE, Caswell, SV, Klossner, DA, Walker, N, and Dompier, TP: Epidemiology of National Collegiate Athletic Association women's lacrosse injuries, 2009-10 through 2014-15. J Sport Rehabil 27:118–125, 2018.

49. Walls, A, Kasle, D, Aaronson, N, Harley, E, and Waldman, E: A population based analysis of the implementation of pediatric facemasks in girls youth lacrosse. Int J Pediatr Otorhinolaryngol 93:141–144, 2017.

50. Micieli, JA, Zurakowski, D, and Ahmed, II: Impact of visors on eye and orbital injuries in the National Hockey League. Can J Ophthalmol 49:243–248, 2014.

51. Micieli, R, and Micieli, JA: Visor use among National Hockey League players and its relationship to on-ice performance. Inj Prev 22:392–395, 2016.

52. Benson, BW, Hamilton, GM, Meeuwisse, WH, McCrory, P, and Dvorak, J: Is protective equipment useful in preventing concussion? A systematic review of the literature. Br J Sports Med 43:i56–i67, 2009.

53. Schneider, DK, Grandhi, RK, Bansal, P, Kuntz, GE IV, Webster, KE, Logan, K, Barber Foss, KD, and Myer, GD: Current state of concussion prevention strategies: A systematic review and meta-analysis of prospective, controlled studies. Br J Sports Med 51:1473–1482, 2017.

54. Conley, KM, Bolin, DJ, Carek, PJ, Konin, JG, Neal, TL, and Violette, D: National Athletic Trainers' Association position statement: Preparticipation physical examinations and disqualifying conditions. J Athl Train 49:102–120, 2014.

55. Hoskin, AK, Philip, S, Dain, SJ, and Mackley, DA: Spectacle-related eye injuries, spectacle-impact performance and eye protection. Clin Exp Optom 98:203–209, 2015.

56. American Society for Testing and Materials. Standard Practice for Care and Use of Athletic Mouth Protectors. Designation: F697-16. https://www.astm.org/Standards/F697.htm, 2019.

57. Gould, TE, Piland, SG, Caswell, SV, Ranalli, D, Mills, S, Ferrara, MS, and Courson, R: National Athletic Trainers' Association position statement: Preventing and

managing sport-related dental and oral injuries. J Athl Train 51:821–839, 2016.

58. Academy for Sports Dentistry. Position statements. https://www.academyforsportsdentistry.org/index.php?option=com_content&view=article&id=51:position-statements&catid=20:site-content&Itemid=111, 2019.

59. Knapik, JJ, Marshall, SW, Lee, RB, Darakjy, SS, Jones, SB, Mitchener, TA, delaCruz, GG, and Jones, BH: Mouthguards in sport activities: History, physical properties and injury prevention effectiveness. Sports Med 37:117–144, 2007.

60. Glendor, U: Aetiology and risk factors related to traumatic dental injuries: A review of the literature. Dent Traumatol 25:19–31, 2009.

61. Maeda, Y, Kumamoto, D, Yagi, K, and Ikebe, K: Effectiveness and fabrication of mouthguards. Dent Traumatol 25:556–564, 2009.

62. American Dental Association. Oral Health Topics, Mouthguards. https://www.ada.org/en/member-center/oral-health-topics/mouthguards, 2019.

63. American Academy of Pediatric Dentistry. Policy on prevention of sports-related orofacial injuries. AAPD, Chicago, IL. http://www.aapd.org/media/Policies_Guidelines/P_Sports.pdf, 2019.

64. Westerman, B, Stringfellow, PM, and Eccleston, JA: Forces transmitted through EVA mouthguard materials of different types and thickness. Aust Dent J 40:389–391, 1995.

65. Piero, M, Simone, U, Jonathan, M, and et al: Influence of a custom-made maxillary mouthguard on gas exchange parameters during incremental exercise in amateur road cyclists. J Strength Cond Res 29:672–677, 2015.

66. Bailey, SP, Willauer, TJ, Balilionis, G, Wilson, LE, Salley, JT, Bailey, EK, and Strickland, TL: Effects of an over-the-counter vented mouthguard on cardiorespiratory responses to exercise and physical agility. J Strength Cond Res 29:678–684, 2015.

67. Collares, K, Correa, MB, Mohnsam da Silva, IC, Hallal, PC, and Demarco, FF: Effect of wearing mouthguards on the physical performance of soccer and futsal players: A randomized cross-over study. Dent Traumatol 30:55–59, 2014.

68. Duddy, FA, Weissman, J, Lee, RA Sr, Paranjpe, A, Johnson, JD, and Cohenca, N: Influence of different types of mouthguards on strength and performance of collegiate athletes: A controlled-randomized trial. Dent Traumatol 28:263–267, 2012.

69. Gebauer, DP, Williamson, RA, Wallman, KE, and Dawson, BT: The effect of mouthguard design on respiratory function in athletes. Clin J Sport Med 21:95–100, 2011.

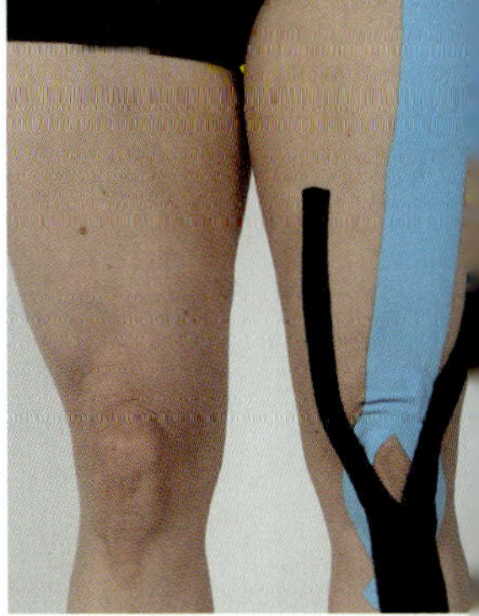

# Kinesio® Taping

Developed in 1973, Kinesio® Taping can be used with patients of any age and condition and during any stage of injury and prevention for 3 to 5 days per application.[1] Kinesio tape is latex free, water resistant, and said to mimic the qualities of the skin. The method can be used alongside many other treatment and modality options.[1] When applied, the tape has the ability to re-educate the neuromuscular system, reduce pain, enhance performance, prevent injury, and promote good circulation and healing while allowing for normal range of motion.[1]

## Physiological Effects

There are five main physiological effects of Kinesio tape: skin, circulatory/lymphatic, fascia, muscle, and joint.[1]

1. Skin. Application of the tape may reduce pain by easing pressure on pain receptors and decrease swelling by increasing fluid movement.[1]
2. Circulatory/lymphatic. Application may speed lymphatic drainage and flow by increasing the amount of space under the skin.[1] It is suggested that improved lymph drainage can cause a decrease in pressure on neural receptors under the skin, with a subsequent reduction in pain.[1]
3. Fascia. Because all layers of the body are interconnected, application of Kinesio tape on the surface of the skin may affect change in deeper tissue groups.[1]
4. Muscle. Application of the tape may have several effects on muscle health and function, such as reduced pain and muscle fatigue, increased range of motion, potential to normalize length/tension ratios, and assistance with tissue recovery.[1]
5. Joint. Kinesio tape may assist with improving joint biomechanics and alignment, reducing protective muscle guarding and pain, facilitating ligament and tendon function, and enhancing kinesthetic awareness.[1]

## Strip Types

Kinesio tape is applied with strips in several different shapes. Scissors are used to cut strips in "X," "I," "Y," fan, donut, and web shapes. Strips are also available in pre-cut shapes. The appropriate shape to select is based on the findings of a clinical assessment, what technique will be applied and the subsequent desired effect, and the length and shape of the body area to be treated.

## Application Instructions

Kinesio Taping techniques involve three steps: (1) assessment/screening of the individual and injury/condition, (2) application of the tape, and (3) reassessment of the individual.[1] Each strip of Kinesio tape contains three zones: a beginning anchor, the therapeutic zone (target tissue), and the base.[1] The anchor and base zones are applied to the skin with no additional stretch on the tape, resulting in 0% tension.[1] Tension should occur in the therapeutic zone when placed over the target tissue. Tension in the tape is created by applying a stretch or pull to both anchors.

Tension guidelines for the application of Kinesio tape are as follows: super light, 0% to 10%; paper off, 10% to 15%; light, 15% to 25%; moderate, 25% to 35%; severe, 50% to 75%; and full, 75% to 100%. Paper off tension, or 10% to 15% tension, occurs when the tape is applied to the skin directly from the paper substrate.

When taping for lymphatic function, 15% to 50% of available tension should be used.[1] The tape should be stretched ≥50% for joint, ligaments, and joint positioning.[1] Following application, lightly rub the tape to activate the adhesive.

There are six general categories of Kinesio Taping corrective techniques. The techniques include mechanical, fascia, space, ligament/tendon, functional, and circulatory/lymphatic.[1] The "X," "I," "Y," fan, donut, and web strips can be used within these categories except when noted.

1. Mechanical. Also known as "positional hold," tape is applied with 50% to 75% tension with downward/inward pressure.[1] This application can provide a positional stimulus to influence a resting desired position, maintain range of motion, maintain circulation, or inhibit pathological movement.[1]
2. Fascia. Referred to as "oscillating tissue," tape is applied with 15% to 50% tension using an oscillating motion to maintain the fascial position by creating or directing movement of the fascia.[1] There are two oscillating techniques that can be applied: side to side and long and short.[1] Tension can be applied at either the tails or in the base of the tape strips.[1]
3. Space. Known as the "lifting" technique, 10% to 50% tension is applied in the middle of the strip.[1] The goal is to decrease pressure on the target tissue by creating recoil and lift over the tissue.[1] The "I,"

strip, donut hole, and web strips are used with this technique.

4. Ligament/tendon. Referred to as the "proprioceptive" technique, tape is applied with 50% to 75% tension with tendon correction and 75% to 100% tension with ligament correction.[1] This technique may decrease stress on the tendon and ligament and generate a signal through the skin to the brain for perception of normal tension on target tissues.[1]

5. Functional. Also termed "spring assist or limit," 50% to 75% tension is used with tape application.[1] This technique provides sensory stimulation to either assist or limit a motion.[1] Tension to the tape is applied through movement and helps with prevention of tissue overstretch, joint hypermobility, and reinjury.

6. Circulatory/lymphatic. Known as "channeling," tape is applied with 0% to 20% tension.[1] The directional pull of the tape may guide exudate to less congested areas through superficial lymphatic pathways.[1] The anchor is often applied proximally, where the exudate flow is desired, and the fan tails are applied over the congested area.[1]

## Contraindications and Precautions

Several contraindications and precautions for the application of Kinesio Taping are mentioned in the literature.[1] Kinesio Taping should not be used over active malignancy sites, cellulitis or skin infection, open wounds, or deep vein thrombosis. Precautions for application include diabetes, kidney disease, congestive heart failure, coronary artery disease or bruits in the carotid artery, and fragile or healing skin. Following application, do not blow dry the tape to activate the adhesive.

## EVIDENCE SUMMARY

The use of Kinesio Taping for the treatment of injuries and conditions has become popular among health care professionals in many clinical settings. The techniques are used alone or in combination with therapeutic modalities and/or rehabilitation programs to lessen levels of pain and increase functional outcomes. Past investigations have produced conflicting evidence to support the efficacy of Kinesio Taping to improve functional performance, strength, range of motion, proprioception, and decrease levels of pain. Based on the methodology in these studies, the findings represent lower levels of evidence limiting application to clinical practice. However, since 2012, 14 separate evidence-based reviews have been published examining the efficacy of Kinesio Taping in the treatment of various injuries and conditions.

Among the more recent reviews, five investigated the use of Kinesio Taping in the treatment of musculoskeletal injuries and conditions. Two separate reviews examined the effects of Kinesio Taping on muscle strength and sports performance outcomes. A 2014 systematic review[2] that included 12 trials revealed no overall clinically significant differences in pain, disability, and quality of life scores between Kinesio Taping and sham taping/placebo, exercises, manual therapy, electrotherapy, and no treatment in the management of patellofemoral pain (PFP), shoulder impingement, plantar fasciitis, and low back and neck pain. A 2014 meta-analysis[3] of eight trials found reductions in levels of pain with Kinesio Taping used alone and in combination with rehabilitation. However, the reductions in pain were not clinically significant when compared with placebo tape, electrotherapy and rehabilitation, McConnell taping technique, and manual therapy for the treatment of PFP and low back and neck pain.

Findings from a 2015 meta-analysis[4] included 17 trials and produced minimal evidence to support the use of Kinesio Taping in the treatment of PFP; de Quervain's tenosynovitis; plantar fasciitis; shoulder impingement; and low back, neck, and myofascial pain. The findings showed Kinesio Taping was superior to no taping, sham taping, and minimal stretching and strengthening exercises for reductions in levels of pain lasting longer than 4 weeks. However, no significant differences in pain were found between Kinesio Taping and various modalities and manual therapy. Examining disability scores, the review[4] revealed no evidence to support that Kinesio Taping decreased scores. Two trials in the review[4] that investigated the effects of Kinesio Taping used in combination with rehabilitation found significant reductions in pain and disability scores compared with rehabilitation alone. A 2016 systematic review[5] that included five trials examined the efficacy of Kinesio Taping on chronic low back pain. Overall, Kinesio Taping was not superior to various modalities, rehabilitation, and sham taping for improving pain and disability scores. Limited evidence showed Kinesio Taping in combination with rehabilitation improved range of motion and motor control outcomes compared with rehabilitation alone. Other trials in the review[5] found limited evidence that Kinesio Taping was superior to sham taping for the improvement of range of motion and muscular endurance. In a 2017 systematic review,[6] five trials among individuals with PFP revealed no significant differences in pain scores with the use of Kinesio Taping, McConnell taping technique, placebo taping, or no taping when used alone. However, significant reductions in pain were demonstrated with Kinesio Taping and McConnell and placebo taping when used in combination with rehabilitation. A separate

2015 meta-analysis[7] of 19 trials examined the effects of Kinesio Taping on increasing muscle strength among healthy adults. Kinesio Taping was shown to have a negligible effect on producing increases in knee extension and flexion, grip, ankle plantar flexion and dorsiflexion, finger extension and flexion, elbow flexion, and trunk flexion muscle strength among healthy individuals. In a 2018 systematic review,[8] 15 trials among healthy subjects examined the effects of Kinesio Taping on various sports performance outcomes. The findings revealed limited evidence to support the use of Kinesio Taping to enhance throwing and kicking ball accuracy, lower extremity muscular power, cycling anaerobic power and capacity, dynamic balance, horizontal and vertical jumping, agility, and sprint and distance running outcome measures. A 2018 clinical practice guideline[9] for the diagnosis, treatment, and prevention of lateral ankle sprains found insufficient evidence that Kinesio Taping provided mechanical support to patients with a history of ankle injury. Kinesio Taping was shown to have a positive effect on postural control and may be beneficial in the prevention of injury among patients with a history of ankle injury.

The available evidence in the literature provides minimal support for the use of Kinesio Taping, alone or in combination with rehabilitation, to lessen levels of pain associated with musculoskeletal injuries and conditions. Overall, it appears Kinesio Taping is no more effective than other commonly used interventions to reduce levels of pain.

Despite the findings reviewed above, health care professionals continue to utilize multiple Kinesio Taping techniques in the treatment of various injuries and conditions. Compared with other interventions, Kinesio Taping may be cost- and time-effective and used as an adjunct within rehabilitation programs. Although support for Kinesio Taping is minimal, clinical decisions should be based on the available evidence, clinician experience and expertise with Kinesio Taping, and patient preferences. Additional research is warranted with well-designed randomized controlled trials using standardized technique applications (tape tension, direction, duration of wear) and outcome measures (pain, range of motion, strength) among various populations to provide stronger evidence for the use of Kinesio Taping in clinical practice.

# Kinesio Taping Techniques

## LATERAL ANKLE SPRAIN LYMPHATIC CORRECTION

⟹ **Purpose:** The lymphatic correction technique is used in the acute treatment of inversion and eversion ankle sprains to reduce mild, moderate, or severe swelling.

⟹ **Materials:**
 • 2 inch or 3 inch Kinesio tape and taping scissors

⟹ **Position of the patient:** Sitting on a taping table or bench with the leg extended off the edge and the foot in a pain-free position.

⟹ **Preparation:** Clean and dry the skin of the patient. Shaving may be necessary for effective application. Apply the tape directly to the skin. Two fan strips of tape are needed for the technique. Cut the fan strips with four to six separate tails.

⟹ **Application:**

**STEP 1:**  Anchor the base of the first fan on the distal aspect of the Achilles tendon with no tension (Fig. A–1A). Activate the adhesive of the strip.

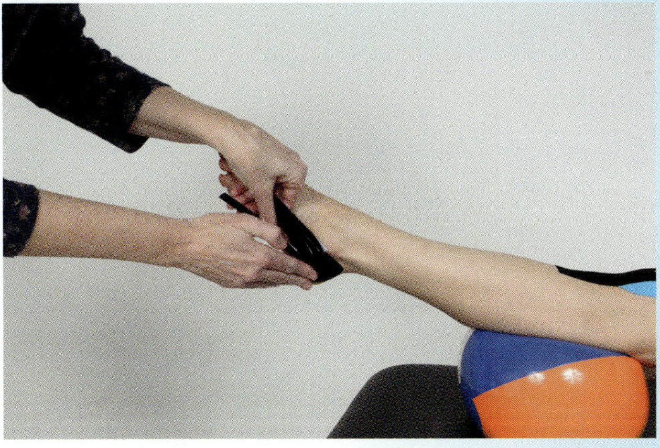

**Fig. A–1 A**

*Steps Cont.*

**STEP 2:** Apply the fan tails over the area of edema on the lateral aspect of the ankle with light tension (15% to 25%). Have the patient actively position the foot in maximum, pain-free plantar flexion and inversion. Continue across the dorsum of the foot and anchor each tail with no tension (Fig. A–1B). Activate the adhesive of the tails prior to further movement by the patient.

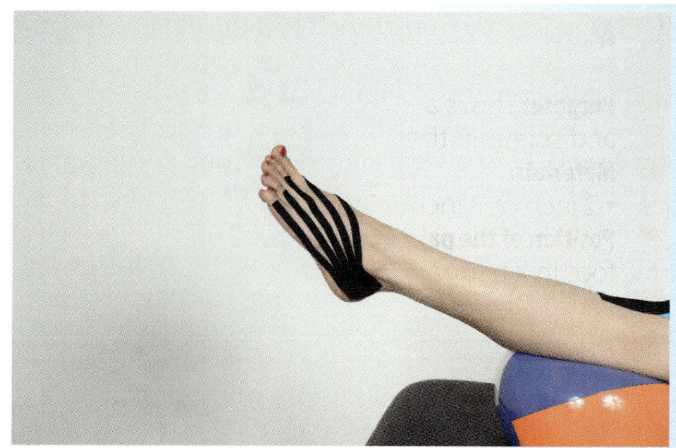

Fig. A–1 B

**STEP 3:** Anchor the base of the second fan on the distal Achilles tendon with no tension (Fig. A–1C).

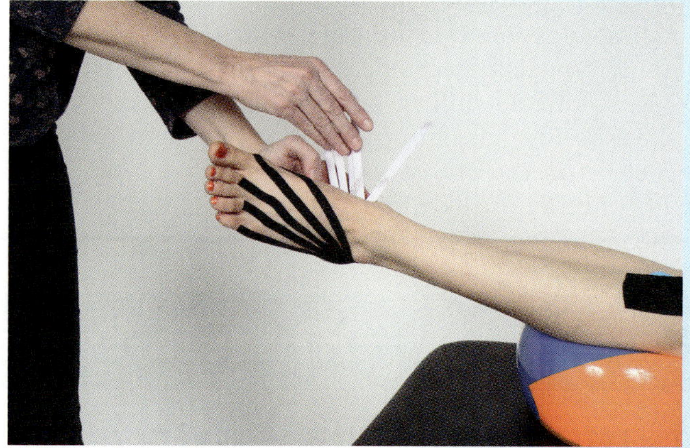

Fig. A–1 C

**STEP 4:** Apply the fan tails over the area of edema on the medial aspect of the ankle with light tension (15% to 25%) (Fig. A–1D). Continue across the dorsum of the foot overlapping the first fan. Anchor each tail with no tension (Fig. A–1E). Activate the adhesive.

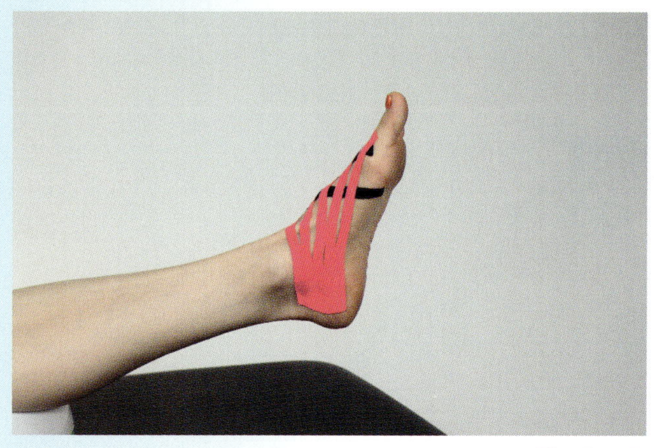

Fig. A–1 D

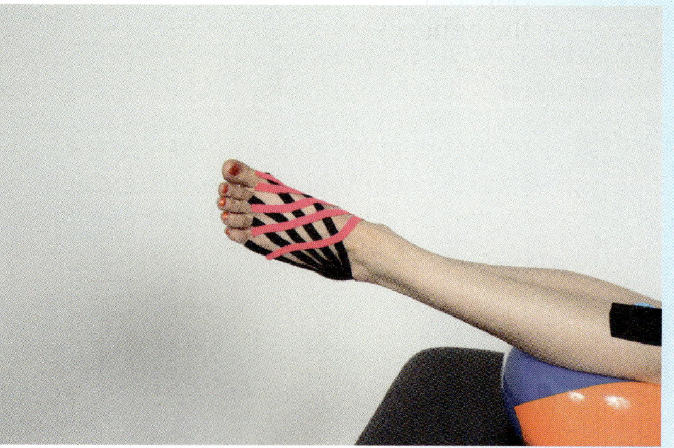

Fig. A–1 E

## ACHILLES TENDON CORRECTION AND INHIBITION

➡ **Purpose:** This is a combination technique used to provide tendon correction and inhibit the gastrocnemius and soleus in the treatment of Achilles tendinitis.

➡ **Materials:**
  • 2 inch or 3 inch Kinesio tape and taping scissors

➡ **Position of the patient:** Prone on a taping table or bench with the lower leg extended off the edge and the foot in a neutral position.

➡ **Preparation:** Clean and dry the skin of the patient. Shaving may be necessary for effective application. Apply the tape directly to the skin. "I" and "Y" strips of tape are needed for the technique.

➡ **Application:**

**STEP 1:** Anchor the base of the "I" strip on the calcaneus with no tension (Fig. A–2A). Activate the adhesive of the strip.

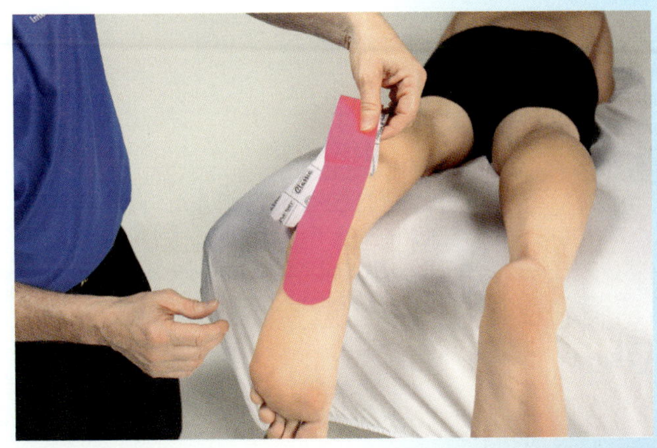

**Fig. A–2 A**

**STEP 2:** Apply the strip with 50% to 75% tension over the Achilles tendon to the musculotendinous junction. Activate the adhesive.

**STEP 3:** Apply the next section of the strip over the posterior lower leg with paper off to light tension (10% to 25%) (Fig. A–2B). Anchor the strip with no tension. Activate the adhesive of the strip.

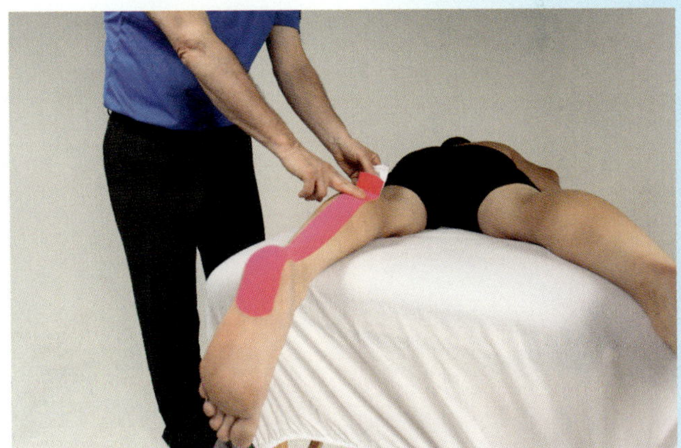

**Fig. A–2 B**

*Steps Cont.*

**STEP 4:** Anchor the base of the "Y" strip on the calcaneus just distal to the "I" strip with no tension (Fig. A–2C). Activate the adhesive. Position the foot into dorsiflexion.

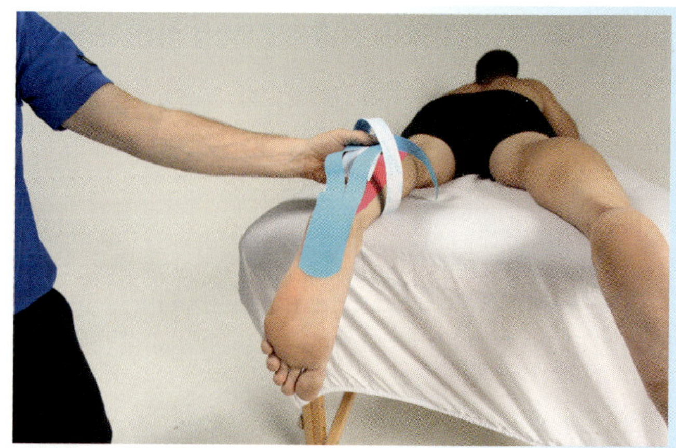

**Fig. A–2 C**

**STEP 5:** Apply the medial tail with paper off to light tension (10% to 25%) along the medial border of the gastrocnemius (Fig. A–2D). Anchor the tail with no tension. Activate the adhesive.

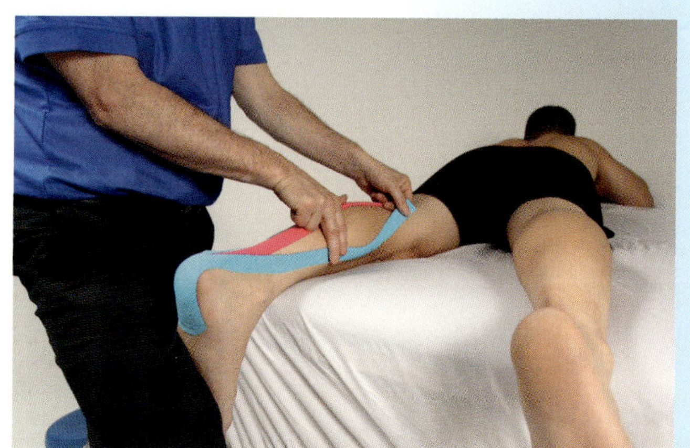

**Fig. A–2 D**

**STEP 6:** Apply the lateral tail with paper off to light tension (10% to 25%) along the lateral border of the gastrocnemius. Anchor the tail with no tension. Activate the adhesive (Fig. A–2E).

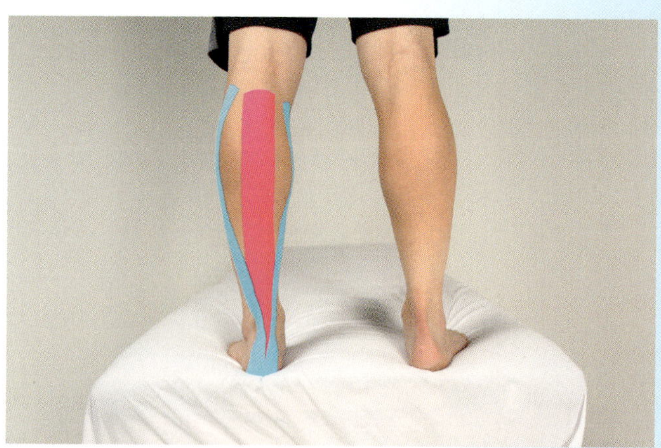

**Fig. A–2 E**

**STEP 7:**  A strip may be applied across the plantar foot to anchor the "I" and "Y" strips, but this is not required (Fig. A–2F).

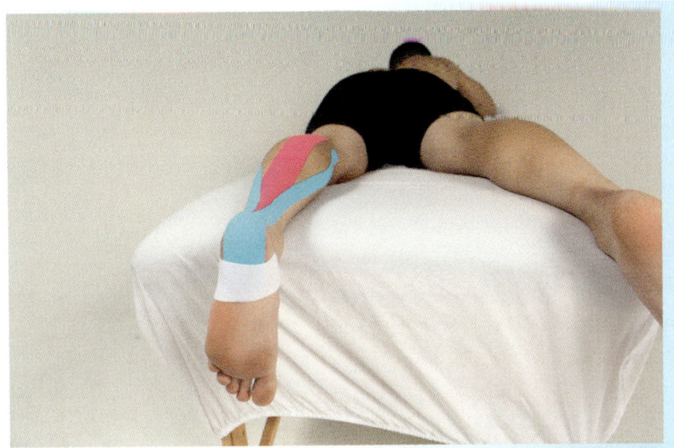

**Fig. A–2 F**

## MEDIAL TIBIAL STRESS SYNDROME INHIBITION AND CORRECTION

➠ **Purpose:** This combination technique is used to inhibit the tibialis anterior and provide mechanical and space correction to the tibia and surrounding tissues in the treatment of medial tibial stress syndrome.
➠ **Materials:**
• 2 inch or 3 inch Kinesio tape and taping scissors
➠ **Position of the patient:** Sitting on a taping table or bench with the leg extended off the edge and the foot in a pain-free position.
➠ **Preparation:** Clean and dry the skin of the patient. Shaving may be necessary for effective application. Apply the tape directly to the skin. "I" and "Y" strips of tape are needed for the technique.
➠ **Application:**

**STEP 1:**  Anchor the base of the "I" strip to the plantar foot over the medial cuneiforms with no tension (Fig. A–3A). Activate the adhesive of the strip. Have the patient actively position the foot into plantar flexion.

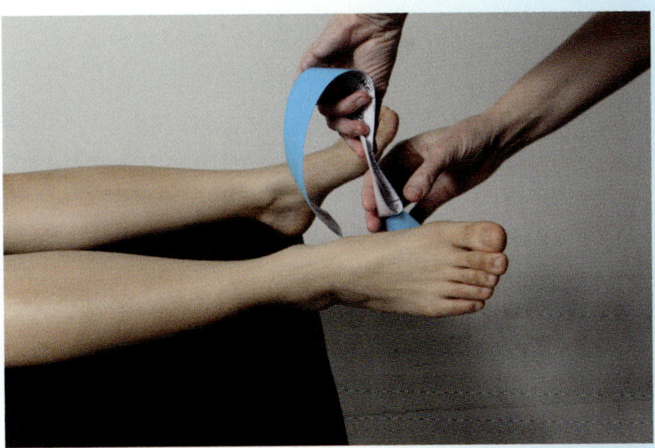

**Fig. A–3 A**

*Steps Cont.*

**STEP 2:**  Apply the "I" strip with light tension (15% to 25%) across the dorsum of the foot and continue over the anterolateral aspect of the lower leg (Fig. A–3B). Anchor the strip with no tension. Activate the adhesive of the strip (Fig. A–3C).

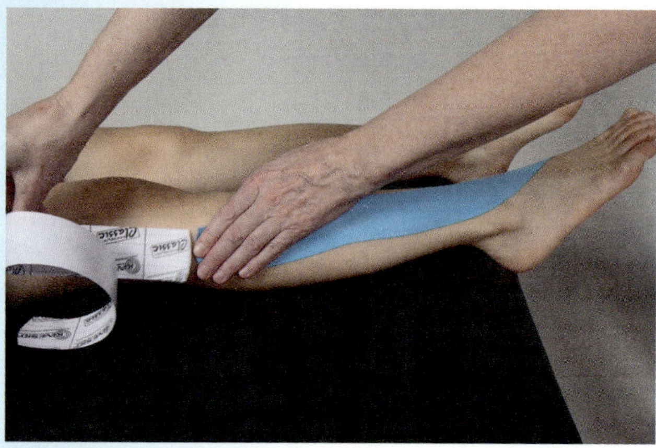

**Fig. A–3 B**

**Fig. A–3 C**

**STEP 3:**  Anchor the base of the "Y" strip on the medial aspect of the tibia inferior to the area of pain with no tension (Fig. A–3D). Activate the adhesive of the strip.

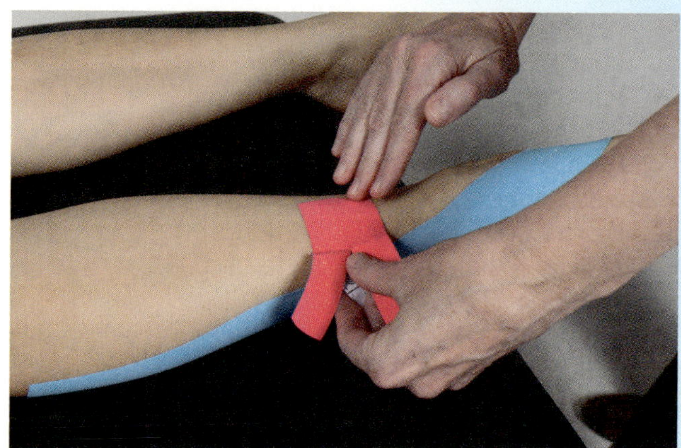

**Fig. A–3 D**

**STEP 4:**  Hold the base of the "Y" strip, then compress and roll the tissue toward the medial border of the tibia. Continue to apply the strip with 50% to 75% tension and inward pressure to the split in the "Y" strip. Activate the adhesive.

**STEP 5:**  Apply the superior tail with paper off to light tension (10% to 25%) across the "I" strip (Fig. A–3E). Anchor the tail with no tension. Activate the adhesive.

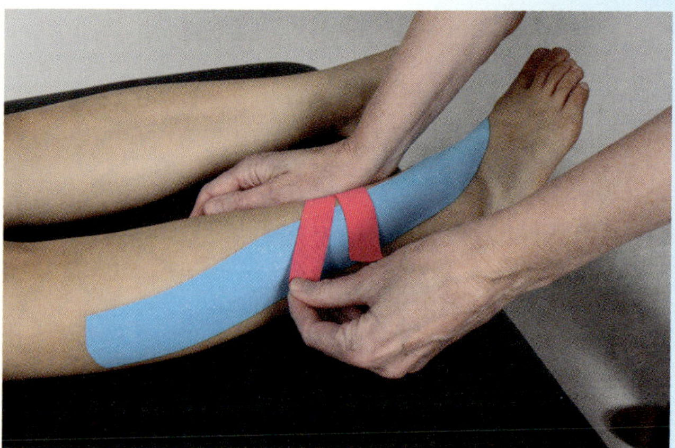

**Fig. A–3 E**

**STEP 6:** Apply the interior tail with 10% to 25% tension across the "I" strip and anchor the tail with no tension. Activate the adhesive (Fig. A–3F).

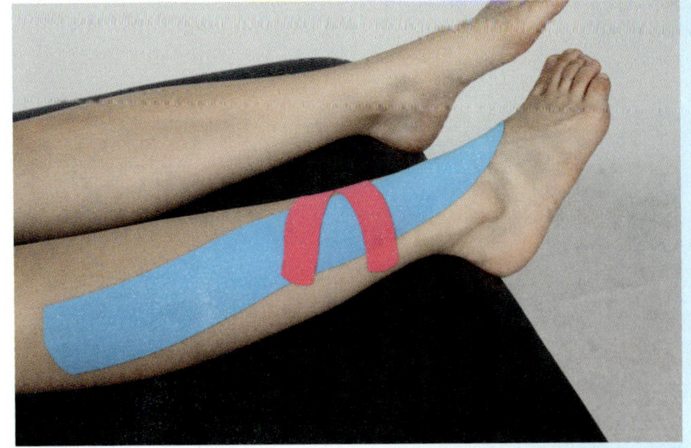

**Fig. A–3 F**

## PATELLAR TENDINITIS FACILITATION

➡ **Purpose:** The facilitation technique is used to treat patellar tendinitis to provide relief of pain and proprioceptive stimulation to the area.
➡ **Materials:**
  • 2 inch or 3 inch Kinesio tape and taping scissors
➡ **Position of the patient:** Sitting on a taping table or bench with the leg extended off the edge.
➡ **Preparation:** Clean and dry the skin of the patient. Shaving may be necessary for effective application. Apply the tape directly to the skin. Two "Y" strips of tape are needed for the technique.
➡ **Application:**

**STEP 1:** Anchor the base of the first "Y" strip at the proximal rectus femoris with no tension (Fig. A–4A). Activate the adhesive of the strip. Have the patient actively position the hip into extension and the knee into flexion.

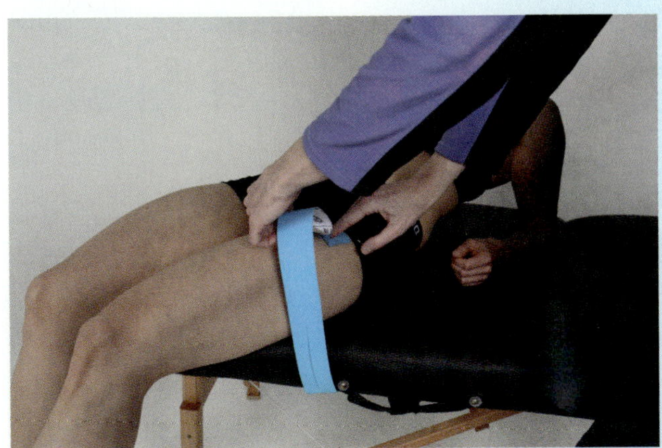

**Fig. A–4 A**

**STEP 2:** Apply the strip with light to moderate tension (15% to 35%) in a distal direction over the rectus femoris until the "Y" reaches the superior pole of the patella. Activate the adhesive.

*Steps Cont.*

**STEP 3:** Apply the medial tail with paper off to light tension (10% to 25%) along the medial border of the patella. Anchor the distal end of the tail near the tibial tubercle with no tension. Activate the adhesive (Fig. A–4B).

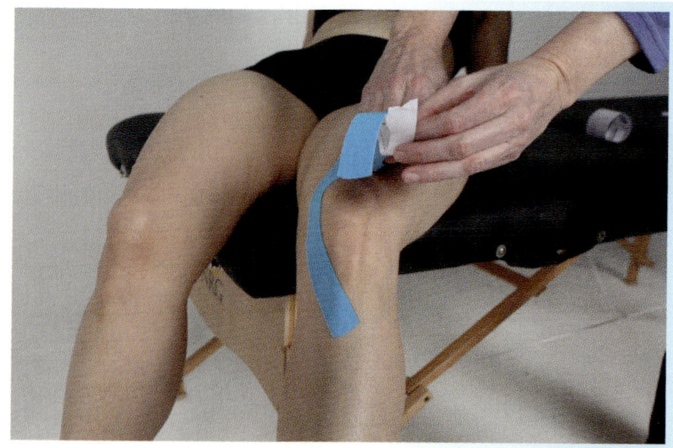

**Fig. A–4 B**

**STEP 4:** Apply the lateral tail with paper off to light tension (10% to 25%) along the lateral border of the patella (Fig. A–4C). Anchor the distal end of the tail near the tibial tubercle with no tension. Activate the adhesive (Fig. A–4D).

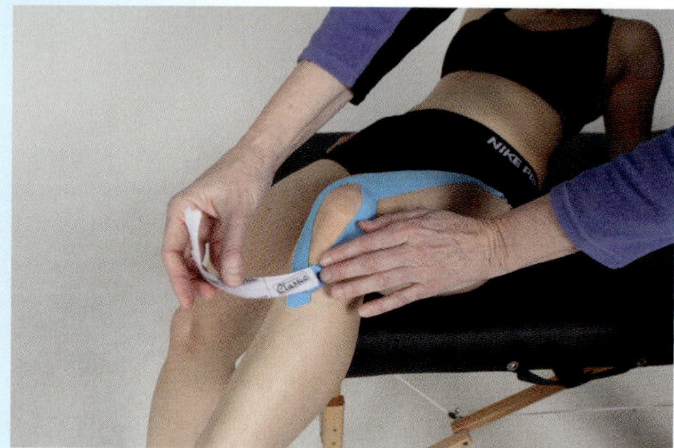

**Fig. A–4 C**

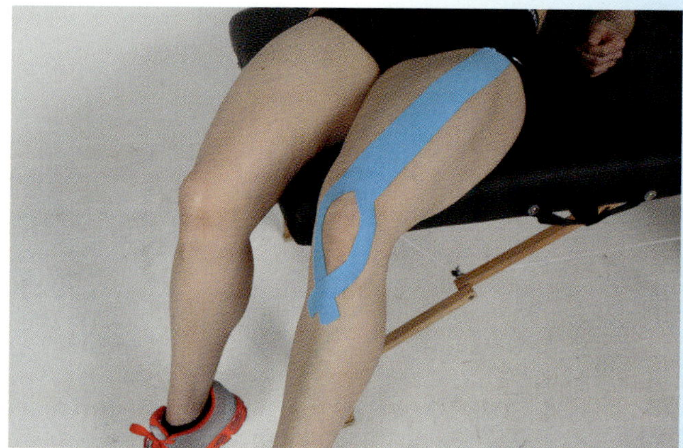

**Fig. A–4 D**

**STEP 5:** With the patient standing, anchor the base of the second "Y" strip 2–3 inches inferior to the tibial tubercle (Fig. A–4E). Activate the adhesive.

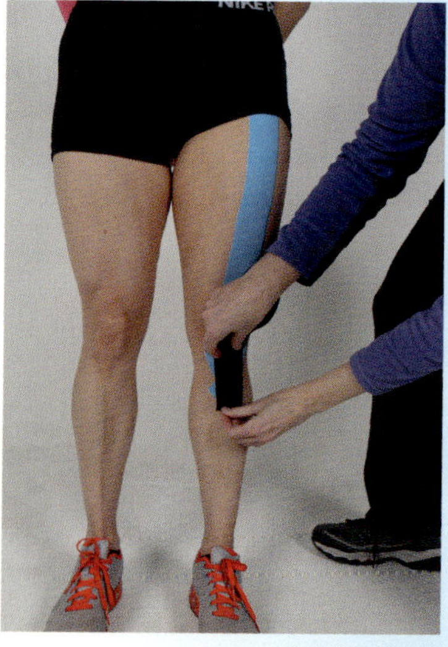

**Fig. A–4 E**

**STEP 6:** Have the patient actively position the knee in slight flexion. Place one hand over the base to ensure no tension is added. Apply the strip with 50% to 75% tension and inward pressure in a proximal direction until the "Y" reaches the inferior pole of the patella. Activate the adhesive.

**STEP 7:** Apply the lateral tail with paper off to light tension (10% to 25%) along the lateral border of the patella. Anchor the distal end over the vastus lateralis with no tension. Activate the adhesive.

**STEP 8:** Apply the medial tail with paper off to light tension (10% to 25%) along the medial border of the patella (Fig. A–4F). Anchor the distal end over the vastus medialis with no tension. Activate the adhesive (Fig. A–4G).

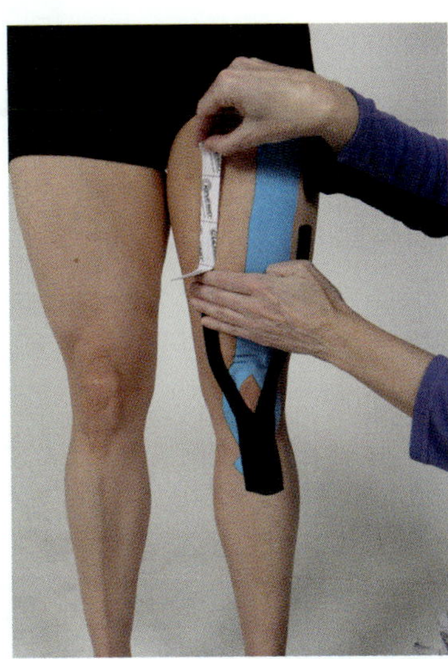 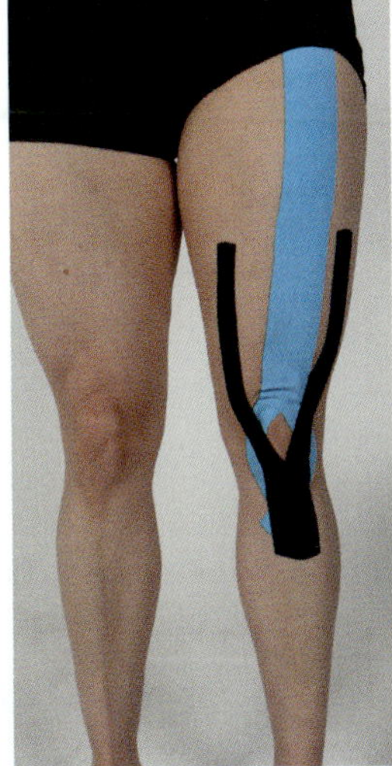

**Fig. A–4 F**                **Fig. A–4 G**

## LATERAL EPICONDYLITIS INHIBITION AND CORRECTION

➭ **Purpose:** This is a combination technique used in the treatment of lateral epicondylitis to reduce edema and pain and provide a fascia and space correction to the painful lateral forearm.
➭ **Materials:**
  • 2 inch or 3 inch Kinesio tape and taping scissors
➭ **Position of the patient:** Standing with the involved arm placed at the side of the body.
➭ **Preparation:** Clean and dry the skin of the patient. Shaving may be necessary for effective application. Apply the tape directly to the skin. Two "Y" strips of tape are needed for the technique.
➭ **Application:**

**STEP 1:** Anchor the base of the first "Y" strip near the base of the second and third metacarpals on the dorsal hand with no tension (Fig. A–5A). Activate the adhesive of the strip.

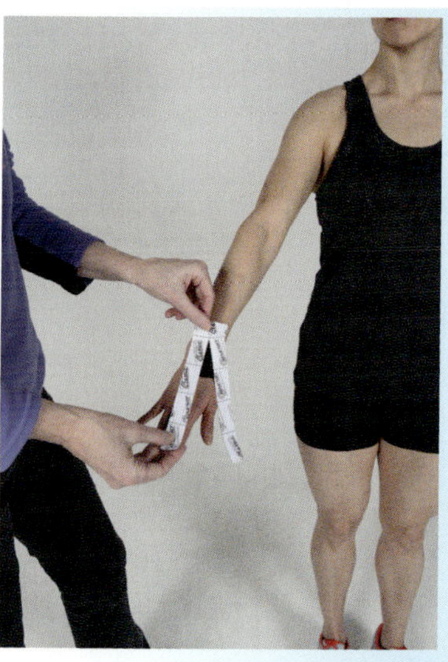

**Fig. A–5 A**

**STEP 2:** Have the patient actively position the wrist in ulnar deviation. Apply the medial tail with paper off to light tension (10% to 25%) along the common extensor muscle group. Anchor the distal end of the tail near the lateral epicondyle with no tension. Activate the adhesive.

**STEP 3:** Apply the lateral tail with paper off to light tension (10% to 25%) along the common extensor muscle group. Anchor the distal end of the tail near the lateral epicondyle with no tension. Activate the adhesive (Fig. A–5B).

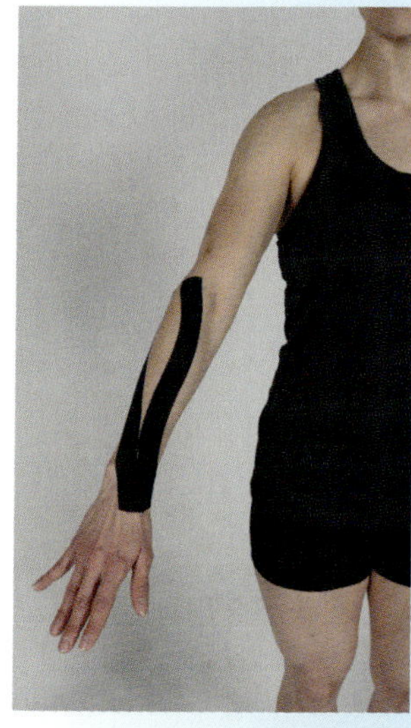

**Fig. A–5 B**

**STEP 4:** Have the patient actively position the elbow in flexion. Anchor the base of the second "Y" strip on the lateral forearm ½–1 inch inferior to the area of pain with no tension (Fig. A–5C). Activate the adhesive.

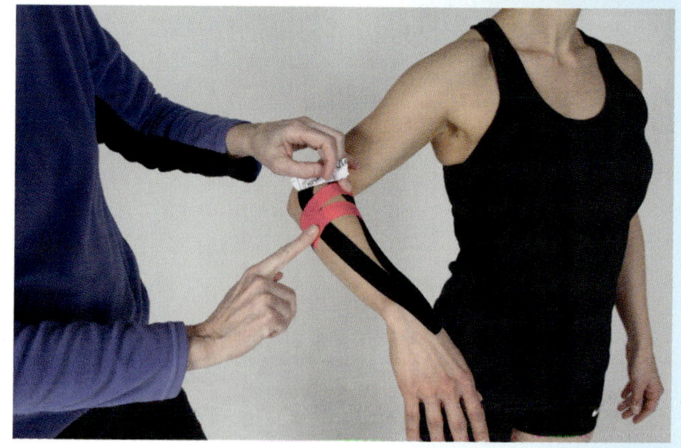

**Fig. A–5 C

**STEP 5:**  Place one hand over the base to ensure no tension is added. Apply 10% to 50% tension to each tail. Move the hand from the base to the area of pain. Release tension in the tails and anchor over the first "Y" strip with no tension (Fig. A–5D). Activate the adhesive.

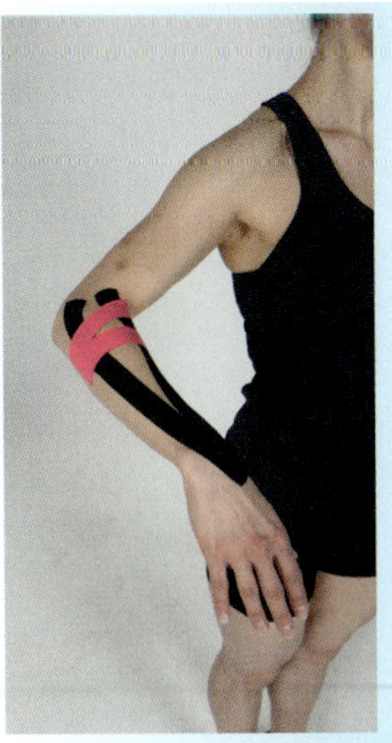

**Fig. A–5 D**

## CARPAL TUNNEL SYNDROME BUTTON HOLE AND CORRECTION

➥ **Purpose:** This combination technique is used in the treatment of carpal tunnel syndrome to provide relief of pain and increase space over the palmar wrist.

➥ **Materials:**
  • 2 inch or 3 inch Kinesio tape and taping scissors

➥ **Position of the patient:** Standing with the involved arm placed at the side of the body.

➥ **Preparation:** Clean and dry the skin of the patient. Shaving may be necessary for effective application. Apply the tape directly to the skin. Two "I" strips of tape are needed for the technique. Cut two holes (button holes) in the middle of one "I" strip, about a palm length into the strip. Do not make the holes too large as this may cause the tape to tear.

➥ **Application:**

**STEP 1:**  Apply the two button holes with no tension over the third and fourth fingers. Anchor the base of the first "I" strip on the dorsal hand with no tension. Activate the adhesive of the strip (Fig. A–6A).

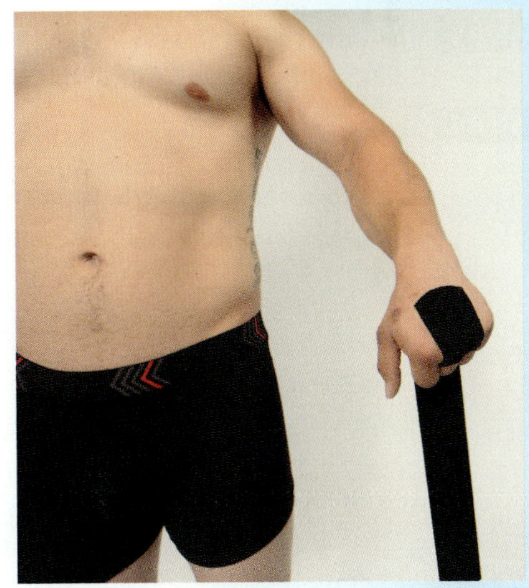

**Fig. A–6 A**

*Steps Cont.*

**STEP 2:** Have the patient actively position the wrist into extension with radial deviation. Apply the strip with paper off to moderate tension (10% to 35%) across the hand, wrist, and forearm to the medial epicondyle (Fig. A–6B).

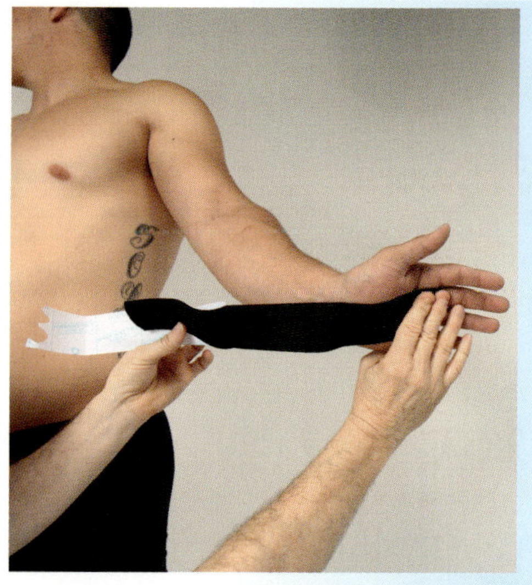

**Fig. A–6 B**

**STEP 3:** Anchor the base of the strip over the medial epicondyle with no tension. Activate the adhesive.

**STEP 4:** Apply the middle portion of the second "I" strip with moderate tension (25% to 35%) on the palmar aspect of the wrist (Fig. A–6C).

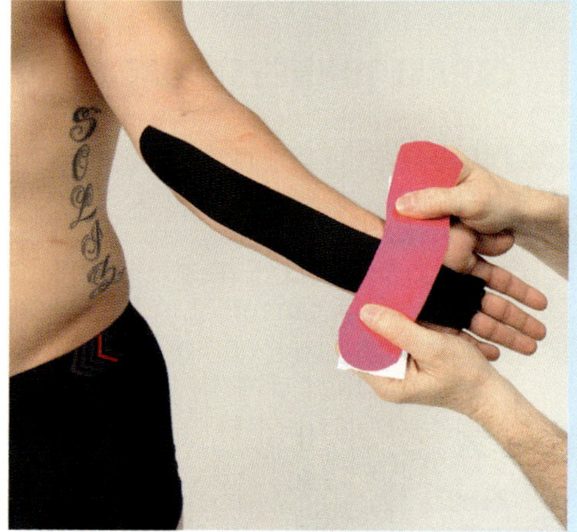

**Fig. A–6 C**

**STEP 5:** Apply the strip with 25% to 35% tension around the wrist. Release the tension in the strip at the ulnar and radial styloid process.

**STEP 6:** Anchor the strip ends on the dorsal wrist and hand with no tension. Avoid overlapping of the strip ends. Activate the adhesive (Fig. A–6D).

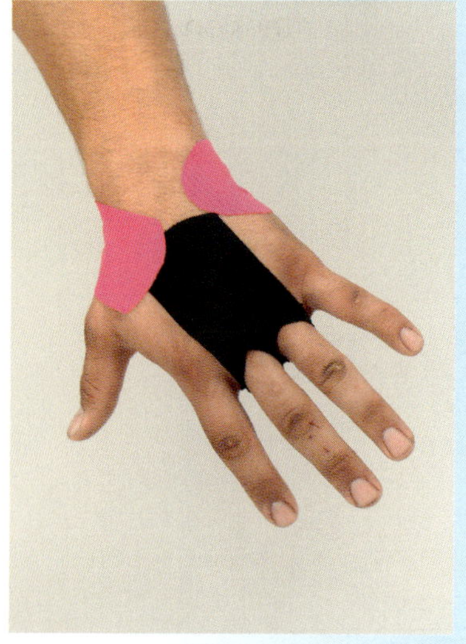

**Fig. A–6 D**

# ROTATOR CUFF IMPINGEMENT INHIBITION

➠ **Purpose:** The inhibition technique is used in the treatment of rotator cuff impingement to inhibit the supraspinatus and deltoid and provide a reduction in edema and pain.
➠ **Materials:**
  • 2 inch or 3 inch Kinesio tape and taping scissors
➠ **Position of the patient:** Standing or sitting with the involved arm placed at the side of the body.
➠ **Preparation:** Clean and dry the skin of the patient. Shaving may be necessary for effective application. Apply the tape directly to the skin. Two "Y" strips of tape are needed for the technique.
➠ **Application:**

**STEP 1:** Anchor the base of the first "Y" strip inferior to the greater tuberosity of the humerus with no tension. Activate the adhesive of the strip (Fig. A–7A). Have the patient actively position the shoulder into adduction with lateral neck flexion to the opposite side.

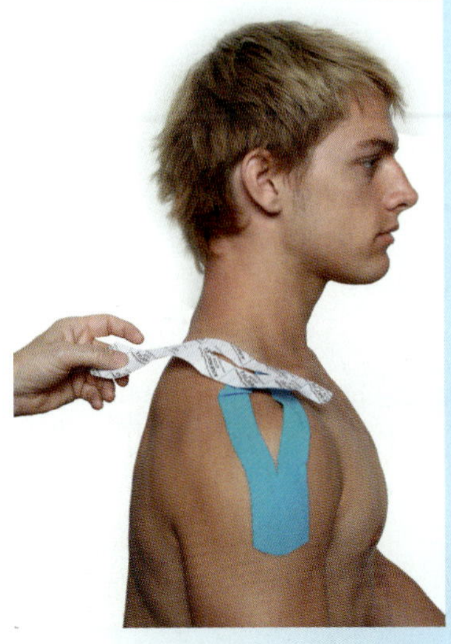

Fig. A–7 A

**STEP 2:** Apply the superior tail of the strip with light tension (15% to 25%) superior to the spinous process of the scapula, between the upper and middle trapezius, and anchor at the supraspinous fossa on the superior medial border of the scapula. Anchor the distal end with no tension. Activate the adhesive of the strip.

**STEP 3:** Apply the inferior tail of the strip with light tension (15% to 25%) along the supraspinatus. Anchor the distal end of the strip with no tension. Activate the adhesive (Fig. A–7B).

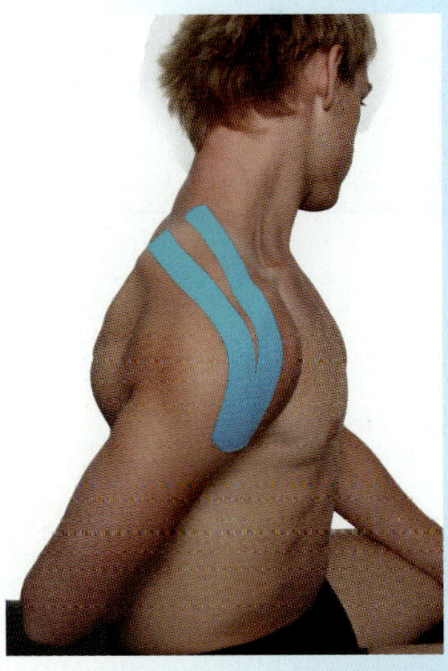

Fig. A–7 B

*Steps Cont.*

**STEP 4:** Anchor the base of the second "Y" strip to the deltoid tuberosity with no tension. Activate the adhesive of the strip (Fig. A–7C). Instruct the patient to actively horizontally abduct the shoulder and move the neck into lateral flexion in the opposite direction.

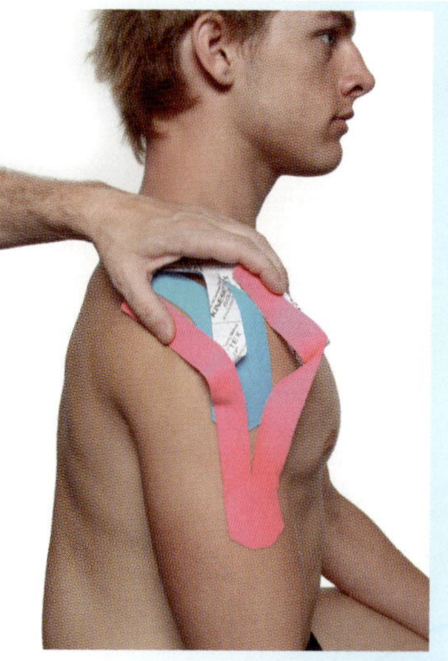

**Fig. A–7 C**

**STEP 5:** Apply the anterior tail of the strip with light tension (15% to 25%) along the anterior deltoid and anchor at the clavicle. Activate the adhesive.

**STEP 6:** Next, instruct the patient to actively adduct the involved shoulder and move the neck into lateral flexion in the opposite direction. Apply the posterior tail with light tension (15% to 25%) along the posterior deltoid and anchor at the lateral edge of the spine of the scapula. Activate the adhesive (Fig. A–7D).

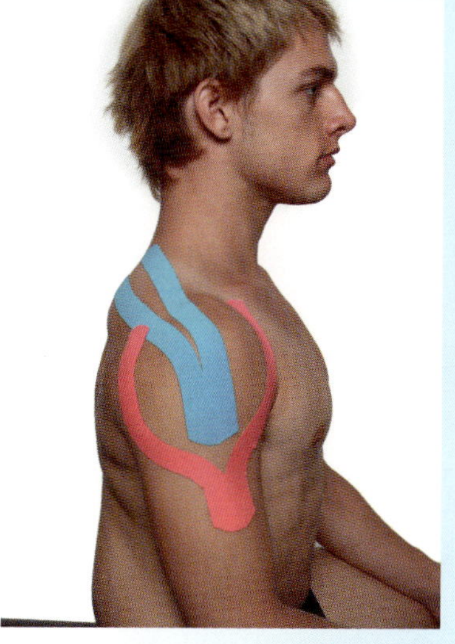

**Fig. A–7 D**

## WEB REFERENCES

### Kinesio

https://kinesiotaping.com
- This website allows access to information on Kinesio Taping products, application methods, and educational materials and resources.

http://www.shopkinesio.com
- This website provides you information about ordering Kinesio tape and technique manuals and DVDs.

## REFERENCES

1. Kase, K, Wallis, J, and Kase, T: Clinical Therapeutic Applications of the Kinesio Taping Method, ed 2. Kinesio Taping Association, Albuquerque, NM, 2003.
2. Parreira, Pdo C, Costa, Lda C, Hespanhol, LC Jr, Lopes, AD, and Costa, LO: Current evidence does not support the use of Kinesio Taping in clinical practice: A systematic review. J Physiother 60:31–39, 2014.
3. Montalvo, AM, Cara, EL, and Myer, GD: Effect of kinesiology taping on pain in individuals with musculoskeletal

injuries: Systematic review and meta-analysis. Phys Sportsmed 42:48–57, 2014.

4. Lim, EC, and Tay, MG: Kinesio taping in musculoskeletal pain and disability that lasts for more than 4 weeks: Is it time to peel off the tape and throw it out with the sweat? A systematic review with meta-analysis focused on pain and also methods of tape application. Br J Sports Med 49:1558–1566, 2015.

5. Nelson, NL: Kinesio taping for chronic low back pain: A systematic review. J Bodyw Mov Ther 20:672–681, 2016.

6. Logan, CA, Bhashyam, AR, Tisosky, AJ, Haber, DB, Jorgensen, A, Roy, A, and Provencher, MT: Systematic review of the effect of taping techniques on patellofemoral pain syndrome. Sports Health 9:456–461, 2017.

7. Csapo, R, and Alegre, LM: Effects of Kinesio taping on skeletal muscle strength—A meta-analysis of current evidence. J Sci Med Sport 18:450–456, 2015.

8. Reneker, JC, Latham, L, McGlawn, R, and Reneker, MR: Effectiveness of kinesiology tape on sports performance abilities in athletes: A systematic review. Phys Ther Sport 31:83–98, 2018.

9. Vuurberg, G, Hoorntje, A, Wink, LM, van der Doelen, BFW, van den Bekerom, MP, Dekker, R, van Dijk, CN, and et al: Diagnosis, treatment and prevention of ankle sprains: Update of an evidence-based clinical guideline. Br J Sports Med 52:956. doi: 10.1136/bjsports-2017-098106, 2018.

# Glossary

## A

**Achilles tendinitis:** Inflammation of the Achilles tendon with possible involvement of the tendon sheath. Pain can be elicited on the posterior heel with passive dorsiflexion.

**Acromioclavicular joint (AC):** Gliding joint between the distal clavicle and the acromion process.

**Adduct:** Movement of a body part toward the midline of the body.

**Amenorrhea:** Absence of menstruation.

**Annular ligament:** Encircles the radial head and neck and stabilizes the radial head with the radioulnar joint.

**Anterior:** Front surface of a body part.

**Anterior cruciate ligament (ACL):** One of two cruciate ligaments in the knee. Attaches from the anterior aspect of the tibia to the medial surface of the lateral femoral condyle and prevents the tibia from moving anteriorly on the femur, internal and external rotation of the tibia on the femur, and hyperextension of the tibia.

**Anterior dislocation/subluxation:** Complete or partial separation of humerus from glenoid fossa toward the front of the body.

**Anterior instability:** Ligamentous laxity and muscular weakness of the glenohumeral joint allowing humeral head to translate anteriorly.

**Anterior talofibular ligament:** Attaches from the lateral talus to the fibular malleolus and resists anterior movement of the talus. The most commonly injured ligament of the ankle.

**Anterior tibialis tendinitis:** Inflammation of the anterior tibialis tendon. Pain can be elicited in the lace area with passive plantar flexion.

**Anterior tibiofibular ligament:** Attaches from the distal anterior fibula to the tibia to join the bones.

**Application area:** Space in a health care facility dedicated for the application of taping, wrapping, bracing, and padding techniques.

**Avulsion fracture:** Tearing away of a piece of bone from a larger bone by force.

**Axilla:** Armpit.

## B

**Bankart lesion:** Avulsion injury causing permanent damage to the anterior rim of the glenoid labrum, often associated with an anterior dislocation and/or instability of the glenohumeral joint.

**Bimalleolar fracture:** Fracture of the medial and lateral malleoli.

**Bloodborne pathogens:** Disease-producing micro-organisms transmitted through blood and bodily fluids.

**Boxer's fracture:** Fracture of the fifth metacarpal.

**Bunion (hallux valgus):** Enlargement of the metatarsophalangeal joint of the great toe as a result of inflammation and thickening of the bursa, with the toe often becoming angled toward the second toe.

**Bunionette:** Enlargement of the metatarsophalangeal joint of the fifth toe as a result of inflammation and thickening of the bursa, with the toe often becoming angled toward the fourth toe.

**Burner:** Brachial plexus trauma resulting in a burning and/or tingling sensation often associated with numbness.

**Bursitis:** Inflammation of a bursa.

## C

**Calcaneofibular ligament:** Attaches from the lateral malleolus to the calcaneus and resists talar inversion.

**Carpal tunnel syndrome:** Compression of the median nerve in the carpal tunnel resulting in pain and tingling in the nerve distribution of the hand.

**Charley horse (thigh contusion):** Contusion to the anterior aspect of the thigh affecting the quadriceps.

**Chondral fracture:** Fracture of articular cartilage.

**Chondromalacia patella:** Softening of the articular cartilage possibly caused by compression and shear forces.

**Closed-cell foam:** Material that does not allow transfer of air from cell to cell, regains its original shape quickly, and provides minimal protection at low impact levels.

**Cock-up position:** Relating to a position of slight wrist extension.

**Contusion:** Trauma to soft tissue from a compressive force; a bruise.

**Cooper's ligament:** Supportive tissues of the breast at the thoracic wall.

## D

**Deep infrapatellar bursa:** Bursa of the knee located between the tibial tubercle and patellar tendon.

**Deltoid ligament:** Attaches from the medial malleolus to the medial talus, calcaneus, and navicular bone and resists eversion and rotation. A collective term for four medial ligaments.

**de Quervain's tenosynovitis:** Tenosynovitis of the abductor pollicis longus and extensor pollicis brevis.

**Disinfectant:** Agents applied on equipment and surfaces to destroy bacteria.

**Dislocation:** Separation or displacement of joint or articulating surfaces.

**Distal:** Away from the center of the body.

**Distal interphalangeal joint (DIP):** Synovial joint between the head of the middle phalanx and the base of the distal phalanx.

**Distal-to-proximal:** Taping and wrapping technique sequence that begins away from the center of the body and proceeds toward the center.

**Dorsal:** The back or posterior surface of a body part.

**Dorsiflexion:** Movement of a body part to the dorsal or posterior surface.

## E

**Erb's point:** An area 2–3 cm superior to the clavicle, level and in front of the transverse process of C6 vertebra.

**Eversion:** Movement of the foot outward.

**Eversion sprain:** Trauma to the ankle resulting in an opening between the medial malleolus and talus.

**Exertional compartment syndrome:** Pain and swelling within the lower leg compartments caused by vigorous exercise and relieved by rest.

**Exostosis:** Bony growth arising from the surface of a bone.

**Extension:** Positioning of the distal portion of a joint in line with the proximal portion along an axis.

**External rotation:** Turning outward of a body part on an axis.

## F

**Flexion:** Bending of a joint in which the distal and proximal parts come together.

**Foreseeable:** To see or anticipate.

**Functional position:** Relating to a position that allows an athlete/patient to perform in athletic or work activities.

## G

**Gamekeeper's thumb:** Sprain of the ulnar collateral ligament at the first metacarpophalangeal joint from forceful abduction and hyperextension of the proximal phalanx.

**Ganglion cyst:** Cystic tumor mass.

**Genu valgum:** Abnormal abduction of the lower leg in line with the thigh, knock-knee.

**Genu varus:** Abnormal adduction of the lower leg in line with the thigh, bowleg.

**Glenohumeral joint (GH):** Synovial joint between the head of the humerus and the glenoid cavity of the scapula.

**Greater trochanteric bursitis:** Inflammation of the greater trochanteric bursa causing pain over the greater trochanter with ambulation.

**Ground fault interrupter (GFI):** A device that interrupts the flow of electricity in an electrical circuit during a power surge of 5 milliamps (mA) or more.

## H

**Heterotopic ossification:** Formation of bone in an atypical location.

**Hill-Sachs lesion:** Small defect in the cartilage of the humeral head on the posterolateral aspect, often associated with an anterior glenohumeral joint dislocation.

**Hip pointer (iliac crest contusion):** Contusion of the iliac crest and surrounding tissue.

**Hyperextension:** Extension of a body part beyond its normal limit of extension.

**Hyperflexion:** Flexion of a body part beyond its normal limit of flexion.

**Hypostatic pneumonia:** Pneumonia often seen in bedridden patients who remain in one position for extended periods of time, causing alveolar collapse and supporting bacterial growth.

## I

**Iliotibial band syndrome:** Inflammation of the iliotibial band producing pain over the lateral femoral condyle and possibly the tibial insertion.

**Inferior:** Below or lower.

**Inferior dislocation/subluxation:** Complete or partial separation of humerus from the glenoid fossa in a downward direction.

**Inferior instability:** Ligamentous laxity and muscular weakness of the glenohumeral joint allowing the humeral head to translate inferiorly.

**Infrapatellar fat pad:** Fat pad of the knee located on the anterior aspect between the synovial membrane and patellar tendon.

**Interdigital neuroma:** Impingement of the interdigital nerves commonly between the third and fourth metatarsals causing pain in the web space between the toes.

**Internal rotation:** Turning inward of a body part on an axis.

**Interphalangeal joint (IP):** Synovial joint between two phalanges.

**Inversion:** Movement of the foot inward.

**Inversion sprain:** Trauma to the ankle resulting in an opening between the lateral malleolus and talus. The most common type of ankle sprain.

**Ipsilateral:** Pertaining to the same side of the body.

## L

**Lateral:** Relating to the side, away from the midline of the body.

**Lateral collateral ligament (LCL):** One of two collateral ligaments in the knee. Attaches from the lateral epicondyle of the femur to the head of the fibula and prevents the tibia from moving inward (varus stress) on the femur and external rotation of the tibia on the femur.

**Lateral epicondylitis (tennis elbow):** Inflammation of the lateral humeral epicondyle causing pain in the area of the lateral epicondyle with resistive wrist extension.

**Lateral (fibular) malleolus:** Distal end of the fibula.

**Lateral meniscus:** O-shaped fibrocartilage attached to the lateral aspect of the tibial plateau.

**Longitudinal:** Lengthwise to the body or body part.

**Longitudinal arch:** Arch of the foot in the anteroposterior direction, from the calcaneus to the metatarsal heads.

**Lumbar lordosis:** Abnormal convex curve of the lumbar spine.

## M

**Maceration:** Softening of the skin by moisture.

**Malleable:** Having the capacity to be molded, formed, or shaped by pressure.

**Mallet finger:** Rupture of the extensor digitorum tendon at the distal phalanx caused by forceful flexion of the distal phalanx.

**Medial:** Relating to the center or midline of the body.

**Medial collateral ligament (MCL):** Attaches from the medial epicondyle of the femur to the medial tibia and prevents the tibia from moving outward (valgus stress) on the femur and rotational movement of the tibia on the femur.

**Medial epicondylitis (golfer's elbow):** Inflammation of the medial humeral epicondyle causing pain distal and lateral to the medial epicondyle with resistive wrist flexion and pronation.

**Medial (tibial) malleolus:** Distal end of the tibia.

**Medial meniscus:** C-shaped fibrocartilage attached to the medial aspect of the tibial plateau. The medial meniscus is less mobile than the lateral.

**Medial tibial stress syndrome (MTSS):** Inflammation and pain in the distal third of the posteromedial tibia caused by overload and structural and muscular abnormalities.

**Metacarpophalangeal joint (MCP):** Synovial joint between the head of the metacarpal and the base of the proximal phalange.

**Metatarsal arch:** Arch of the forefoot in the medial to lateral direction, from the first to the fifth metatarsal heads.

**Metatarsalgia:** Pain around the metatarsal heads.

**Metatarsophalangeal joint (MTP):** Synovial joint between the head of the metatarsal and the base of the proximal phalange.

**Multidirectional forces:** Injurious forces that occur in more than one plane.

**Multidirectional instability:** Ligamentous laxity and muscular weakness in more than one plane.

**Myositis ossificans:** Inflammation of muscle tissue with the formation of bone.

## N

**Neutral:** Relating to an indifferent position; a relaxed anatomical position.

**Nonpliable:** Not easily bent or shaped; inflexible.

## O

**Olecranon:** The proximal end of the ulna that extends posteriorly at the elbow.

**Olecranon bursa:** Bursa of the elbow located between the olecranon and the skin.

**Oligomenorrhea:** Limited blood flow or infrequent menstruation.

**Open-cell foam:** Material that allows transfer of air from cell to cell, quickly deformed with stress, and provides low levels of shock absorption.

**Osgood-Schlatter disease (OSD):** Inflammation and degenerative changes of the tibial tubercle at the insertion of the patellar tendon.

**Osteitis pubis:** Chronic inflammation of the symphysis pubis.

**Osteochondral fracture:** Fracture of bone and articular cartilage.

**Overuse:** Cause of injuries and conditions from excessive, repetitive movement; stress; impact; or incorrect anatomical position.

## P

**Palmar:** Relating to the palm of the hand.

**Patella alta:** High-riding patella.

**Patellar tendinitis (jumper's knee):** Inflammation of the patellar tendon typically at the inferior pole of the patella or its distal insertion on the tibial tubercle.

**Patellofemoral pain (PFP):** Abnormal tracking of the patella in the femoral groove resulting in anterior knee pain.

**Periosteum:** Outer membrane of blood vessels and connective tissue cells covering bones.

**Peroneal retinaculum:** Fibrous band located on the posterior aspect of the lateral malleolus holding the peroneal tendon in its groove.

**Peroneal tendinitis:** Inflammation of the peroneal tendon. Pain can be elicited over the posterior lateral malleolus with weight-bearing movements onto the ball of the foot.

**Pes anserinus bursa:** Bursa of the knee located beneath the pes anserinus tendons (sartorius, gracilis, and semitendinosus).

**Pes anserinus tendinitis:** Inflammation of the sartorius, gracilis, and semitendinosus tendons at the distal insertion at the proximal medial tibia.

**Pes cavus:** Abnormally high longitudinal arch.

**Pes planus:** Flatfoot, absence of arch.

**Plantar:** Relating to the bottom or sole of the foot.

**Plantar fasciitis:** Pain and inflammation of the plantar fascia, commonly present on the medial heel.

**Plantar flexion:** Movement of the foot in a downward or depressed motion.

**Plica:** A fold or thickening of the synovial membrane extending into the joint cavity.

**Posterior:** Back surface of a body part.

**Posterior cruciate ligament (PCL):** Attaches from the posterior aspect of the tibia to the lateral anterior medial condyle of the femur and prevents the tibia from moving posteriorly on the femur, internal rotation of the tibia on the femur, and hyperextension of the tibia.

**Posterior dislocation/subluxation:** Complete or partial separation of humerus from glenoid fossa toward the back of the body.

**Posterior instability:** Ligamentous laxity and muscular weakness allowing the humeral head to translate posteriorly.

**Posterior talofibular ligament:** Attaches from the posterior talus and posterolateral calcaneus to the lateral malleolus and resists dorsiflexion and inversion.

**Posterior tibialis tendinitis:** Inflammation of the posterior tibial tendon. Pain can be elicited over the posterior medial malleolus with active resistive plantar flexion and inversion.

**Posterior tibiofibular ligament:** Attaches from the distal posterior fibula to the tibia to join the bones.

**Prepatellar bursa:** Bursa of the knee located between the anterior surface of the patella and the skin.

**Pronate:** Turning the palm of the hand downward with inward rotation of the forearm.

**Prophylactic:** Act of guarding or protecting from injury.

**Proximal:** Nearest the center of the body.

**Proximal interphalangeal joint (PIP):** Synovial joint between the head of the proximal phalanx and the base of the middle phalanx.

**Proximal-to-distal:** Taping and wrapping technique sequence that begins from the center of the body and proceeds away from the center.

**Pulmonary contusion:** Contusion of the heart producing chest pain, shortness of breath, and rapid breathing.

## Q

**Q angle:** Angle formed between the line of force or pull of the quadriceps and the patellar tendon used to determine patellar tracking.

## R

**Radial collateral ligament:** Attaches from the lateral epicondyle of the humerus to the annular ligament and prevents the ulna and radius from moving inward (varus stress) on the humerus.

**Radiocarpal joint:** Joint formed between the distal radius and scaphoid, lunate, and triquetrum.

**Radioulnar joint:** Joint formed between the distal ends of the radius and ulna.

**Retrocalcaneal bursitis:** Inflammation of the retrocalcaneal bursa between the Achilles tendon and calcaneus.

**Reverse Hill-Sachs lesion:** Small defect in the cartilage of the anterior humeral head often associated with a posterior glenohumeral joint dislocation.

**Rotary forces:** Injurious twisting forces.

**Rotation:** Turning of a body part on an axis.

**Rotator cuff:** Term used to describe the supraspinatus, infraspinatus, teres minor, and subscapularis muscle group of the shoulder.

## S

**Scoliosis:** A lateral curve of the spine.

**Semimembranosus bursa (Baker's cyst):** Bursa of the knee located in the popliteal fossa beneath the semimembranous tendon.

**Sesamoiditis:** Inflammation of the sesamoid bones under the first metatarsal head.

**Shoulder pointer:** Contusion of the distal clavicle and surrounding soft tissue.

**Sinding-Larsen Johansson disease (SLJ):** Inflammation and pain at the inferior pole of the patella at the origin of the patellar tendon.

**Sternoclavicular joint (SC):** Joint formed between the manubrium of the sternum and the proximal clavicle.

**Stinger:** (See Burner)

**Stress fracture:** A fracture of insidious nature.

**Subluxation:** Partial dislocation.

**Subtalar joint:** Joint formed between the talus and calcaneus at which inversion, eversion, pronation, and supination occur.

**Superior:** Above or higher.

**Superior labrum anteroposterior (SLAP) lesion:** Defect to the superior glenoid labrum of the shoulder that begins posteriorly and extends anteriorly and damages the attachment of the long head of the biceps tendon.

**Supinate:** Turning the palm of the hand upward with outward rotation of the forearm.

**Syndesmosis sprain:** Trauma to the ankle resulting in an opening of the distal tibiofibular joint.

## T

**Tackler's exostosis:** Bony growth arising from the anterolateral aspect of the humerus commonly seen in football linemen.

**Tactile:** Referring to the sense of touch.

**Talocrural joint:** Joint formed between the distal tibia and talus, medial malleolus and talus, and lateral malleolus and trochlea at which plantar flexion and dorsiflexion occur.

**Taping area:** (See Application area)

**Thenar web space:** The area of the hand between the thumb and first finger.

**Transverse arch:** Arch of the midfoot in the medial to lateral direction, from the medial cuneiform to the cuboid bones.

**Triangular fibrocartilage complex (TFCC):** Complex located between the distal ulnar head and the lunate and triquetrum, including the triangular fibrocartilage.

**Turf burn:** Abrasion to the posterior elbow and/or ulnar side of the forearm from contact with artificial grass, wood, or rubber playing surfaces.

## U

**Ulnar collateral ligament (UCL) elbow:** Composed of three bands, the UCL prevents valgus stress or medial opening of the elbow. Attaches from the medial epicondyle of the humerus to the coronoid process of the ulna and prevents the ulna and radius from moving outward (valgus stress) on the humerus.

**Ulnar collateral ligament (UCL) thumb:** Attaches from the dorsal side of the first metacarpal to the palmar aspect of the proximal first phalanx and prevents the phalanx from moving inward (varus stress) and outward (valgus stress) on the first metacarpal.

**Ulnar styloid process:** Small bony projection on the medial and posterior aspect of the ulnar head.

**Unidirectional forces:** An injurious force that occurs in one plane.

## V

**Valgus:** Distal segment of a joint bent outward, resulting in an opening on the medial aspect.

**Varus:** Distal segment of a joint bent inward, resulting in an opening on the lateral aspect.

## W

**Wryneck:** Pain and stiffness associated with spasm of the cervical neck musculature.

# INDEX

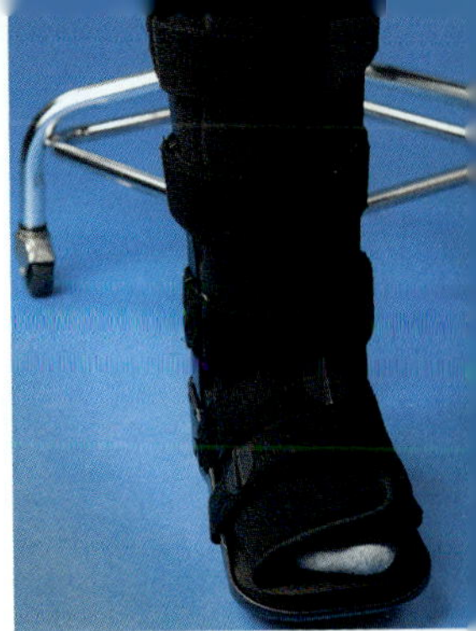

*Note:* Page numbers followed by "f" denote figures.

## A

Abdomen, 397f; *See also* Thorax, abdomen, and spine muscles of
Abrasions, elbow and forearm, 280
AC joint. *See* Acromioclavicular (AC) joint
Achilles tendinitis, 138
Achilles tendon, rupture of, 138, 138f
Achilles tendon strip technique, for ankle padding, 132
Achilles tendon taping technique, 139–143, 140f–143f
ACL. *See* Anterior cruciate ligament (ACL)
Acromioclavicular (AC) joint
  anatomy, 242, 242f
  padding techniques for, 269–273
  sprain, 242
  wrapping techniques for, 252–259
Adductor strain wrap technique, 219–222, 220f–222f
Air/gel bladder, in ankle bracing, 126–127, 127f
Allergic reactions, to tape, 12
Amenorrhea, stress fractures and, 139
Ankle, 95–135
  blisters of, 96
  bracing techniques for, 122–131
    air/gel bladder, 126–127, 127f
    evidence summary on, 130
    lace-up, 122–124, 123f–124f
    semirigid, 124–126, 125f–126f
    walking boot, 131
    wrap, 128–129, 128f–129f
  evidence-based practice on, 133–134
  fractures of, 95–96, 97f
  padding techniques for, 131–133
    Achilles tendon strips, 132
    donut pads, 132
    horseshoe pad, 131–132, 131f–132f
  sprains of, 95, 96f
  taping techniques for, 97–117
    closed basketweave, 97–108, 98f–108f
      *See also* Closed basketweave technique for ankle taping
    elastic, 109–110, 109f–110f
    evidence summary on, 130
    posterior splint, 116–117, 116f–117f
    Spartan Slipper, 111–112, 111f–112f
    spatting, 115
    subtalar sling, 113–115, 113f–114f
  wrapping techniques for, 117–121
    cloth wrap, 120–121, 120f–121f
    compression wrap as, 72–74, 72f–73f
    foot and ankle compression sleeve, 118–119, 119f
    foot and ankle compression wrap, 117–118, 118f
    soft cast, 119–120, 119f–120f
Ankle braces
  air/gel bladder, 126–127, 127f
    for lower leg, 152
  lace-up, 122–124, 123f–124f
    for lower leg, 152
  semirigid, 124–126, 125f–126f
    for lower leg, 152
Annular ligament, sprain of, 277
Anterior cruciate ligament (ACL)
  disruption of, 159–160, 161f
  sprain of, 159–160, 161f
Anterior talofibular ligament, in ankle sprains, 95
Anterior tibialis tendinitis, 138
Anterior tibiofibular ligament, in ankle sprains, 95
Application area, 34–41
  benches in, 35–36, 35f
  ceiling of, 38
  definition of, 34
  design of, 34–35
  electrical outlets in, 38–39, 39f
  evidence-based practice on, 40
  floors of, 37–38
  lighting for, 39
  plumbing for, 39
  seating in, 37
  storage in, 36–37
    for braces, 37
    for pads, 37
    for tape, 36–37, 36f
    for wraps, 37
  tables in, 35–36, 35f
  ventilation for, 39
  walls of, 38
Arch taping technique
  circular, 48–49, 48f–49f
  evidence summary on, 59
  loop, 52–53, 52f–53f
  weave, 53–55, 54f–55f
    anchor variation to, 56, 56f
  "X," 49–51, 50f–51f
    anchor variation to, 56, 56f
Arches of foot, 47f
  strains affecting, 46, 47f
  taping techniques for, 48–61
Arm, upper. *See* Shoulder and upper arm
ASTM International, 428
Athletic cups, 418, 420f
Athletic trainers (ATs), 3

## B

Avulsion fracture
  with eversion sprain of ankle, 95
  lateral malleolus, 95, 97f
  medial malleolus, 95–96, 97f

Baker's cyst, 162
Bankart lesion, 243
Baseball
  mandatory equipment for, 431
  standard equipment for, 431–432, 431f–432f
Baseball helmets
  for batter, 431, 431f
    standards and testing of, 429
  for catcher, 431–432, 432f
    with face guard, standards and testing of, 429
Benches, in application area, 35–36, 35f
Bimalleolar fracture, 95–96, 97f
Blisters
  ankle, 96
  foot, 47
    donut pads for, 84–85
  hand, fingers, and thumb, 357
  from tape, 12
  toes, 47
    donut pads for, 84–85
Bloodborne pathogens, OSHA standards for, in application area, 36
Boot
  cast, 81, 81f
  walking, 80–81, 80f–81f
Boxer's fracture, 357
Boxer's wrap technique, 377–379, 377f–379f
Brace migration, 20
Brace(s), 18–21
  ankle. *See* Ankle braces
  application of. *See also* Bracing
    pointers for, 30
    recommendations for, 20–21
  body area for, 20
  care of, 21
  custom-made, 18, 19f
  finger
    custom-made, 384–385, 384f–385f
    off-the-shelf, 382–384, 383f–384f
  fit of, 18, 19f
  functional, 19f, 20
  hand
    custom-made, 381–382, 381f–382f
    off-the-shelf, 380–381, 380f–381f
  lace-up, for ankle, 122–124, 123f–124f